PRINCIPLES AND APPLICATIONS IN ENGINEERING SERIES

Biomedical Imaging

PRINCIPLES AND APPLICATIONS IN ENGINEERING SERIES

Biomedical Imaging

Edited by

KAREN M. MUDRY
ROBERT PLONSEY
JOSEPH D. BRONZINO

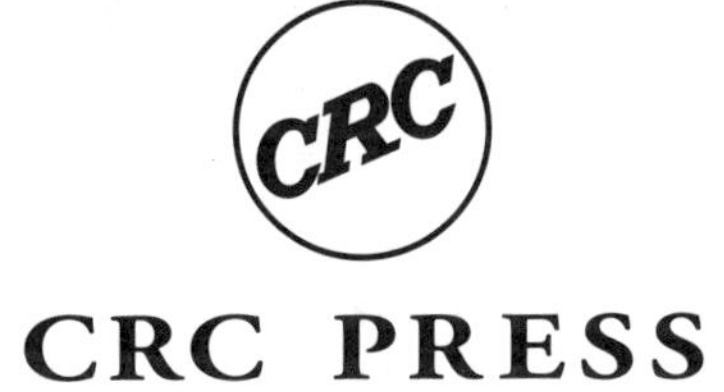

CRC PRESS

Boca Raton London New York Washington, D.C.

This material was originally published in Vol. I of *The Biomedical Engineering Handbook, Second Edition*, Joseph D. Bronzino, Ed., CRC Press, Boca Raton, FL, 2000.

Library of Congress Cataloging-in-Publication Data

Biomedical imaging / edited by Karen M. Mudry, Robert Plonsey, Joseph Bronzino.
p. cm. — (Principles and applications in engineering ; 10)
Includes bibliographical references and index.
ISBN 0-8493-1810-6 (alk. paper)
1. Imaging systems in medicine—Handbooks, manuals, etc. 2. Diagnostic imaging—Handbooks, manuals, etc. 3. Biomedical engineering—Handbooks, manuals, etc. I. Mudry, Karen M. II. Plonsey, Robert. III. Bronzino, Joseph D., 1937- IV. Series.

R857.O6B565 2003
616.07'54—dc21

2003040912

International Standard Book Number 0-8493-1810-6
Library of Congress Card Number 2003040912
Printed in the United States of America 1 2 3 4 5 6 7 8 9 0
Printed on acid-free paper

Preface

The field of medical imaging has been revolutionized by advances in computing technologies and systems resulting in new and expanded image systems finding their way into the medical environment. These systems now range from those devoted to planar imaging using x-rays to technologies that are just emerging, such as virtual reality.

Consider the following:

- Some of the systems, such as ultrasound, are relatively inexpensive, while others, such as positron emission tomography (PET) facilities, cost millions of dollars for the hardware and the employment of Ph.D.-level personnel to operate them.
- Systems that make use of x-rays have been designed to image anatomic structures, while others that make use of radioisotopes provide functional information.
- The fields of view that can be imaged range from the whole body obtained with nuclear medicine bone scans to images of cellular components using magnetic resonance (MR) microscopy.
- The designs of transducers for the imaging devices to the postprocessing of the data to allow easier interpretation of the images by medical personnel are all aspects of the medical imaging devices field.

Because of the importance of this field, *Biomedical Imaging* has been developed taking the most relevant sections to this important topic from the second edition of *The Biomedical Engineering Handbook* published by CRC Press in 2000.

The handbook begins with a section on physiologic systems, edited by Robert Plonsey, that provides an excellent overview of human systems. In this way biomedical engineers engaged in medical imaging can better understand the utilization of various imaging modalities to provide information regarding structure and physiologic function. The physiologic systems covered include cardiovascular, nervous, vision, auditory, respiratory, endocrine, and gastrointestinal.

The primary editor of *Biomedical Imaging*, Dr. Karen Mudry, then provides an overview of the main medical imaging devices as well as some of the emerging systems. The topics include x-ray, computed tomographic (CT) systems, magnetic resonance imaging, SPECT systems, ultrasound, and virtual reality, among others.

Advisory Board

Contributors

D. C. Barber
University of Sheffield
Sheffield, United Kingdom

Berj L. Bardakjian
University of Toronto
Toronto, Canada

Joseph D. Bronzino
Trinity College/The Biomedical Engineering Alliance and Consortium (BEACON)
Hartford, Connecticut

Thomas F. Budinger
University of California
Berkeley, California

Ewart R. Carson
City University
London, United Kingdom

Wei Chen
Center for Magnetic Resonance Research and the University of Minnesota Medical School
Minneapolis, Minnesota

David A. Chesler
Massachusetts General Hospital and Harvard University Medical School
Boston, Massachusetts

Ben M. Clopton
University of Washington
Seattle, Washington

Steven Conolly
Stanford University
Stanford, California

Derek G. Cramp
City University
London, United Kingdom

Barbara Y. Croft
National Institutes of Health
Kensington, Maryland

Ian A. Cunningham
Victoria Hospital, the John P. Robarts Research Institute, and the University of Western Ontario
London, Canada

K. Whittaker Ferrara
Riverside Research Institute
New York, New York

Richard L. Goldberg
University of North Carolina
Chapel Hill, North Carolina

Walter Greenleaf
Greenleaf Medical
Palo Alto, California

Xiaoping Hu
Center for Magnetic Resonance Research and the University of Minnesota Medical School
Minneapolis, Minnesota

Arthur T. Johnson
University of Maryland
College Park, Maryland

G. Allan Johnson
Duke University Medical Center
Durham, North Carolina

Philip F. Judy
Brigham and Women's Hospital and Harvard Medical School
Boston, Massachusetts

Kenneth K. Kwong
Massachusetts General Hospital and Harvard University Medical School
Boston, Massachusetts

Christopher G. Lausted
University of Maryland
College Park, Maryland

Albert Macovski
Stanford University
Stanford, California

Evangelia Micheli-Tzanakou
Rutgers University
Piscataway, New Jersey

Jack G. Mottley
University of Rochester
Rochester, New York

Karen M. Mudry
Formerly of The Whitaker Foundation
Washington, D.C.

Maqbool Patel
Center for Magnetic Resonance Research and the University of Minnesota Medical School
Minneapolis, Minnesota

John Pauly
Stanford University
Stanford, California

Tom Piantanida
Greenleaf Medical
Palo Alto, California

Robert Plonsey
Duke University
Durham, North Carolina

John Schenck
General Electric Corporate Research and Development Center
Schenectady, New York

Daniel J. Schneck
Virginia Polytechnic Institute and State University
Blacksburg, Virginia

Robert E. Shroy, Jr.
Picker International
Highland Heights, Ohio

Stephen W. Smith
Duke University
Durham, North Carolina

Francis A. Spelman
University of Washington
Seattle, Washington

George Stetten
Duke University
Durham, North Carolina

Benjamin M.W. Tsui
University of North Carolina
Chapel Hill, North Carolina

Kamil Ugurbil
Center for Magnetic Resonance Research and the University of Minnesota Medical School
Minneapolis, Minnesota

Henry F. VanBrocklin
University of California
Berkeley, California

Michael S. Van Lysel
University of Wisconsin
Madison, Wisconsin

Martin J. Yaffe
University of Toronto
Toronto, Canada

Xiaohong Zhou
Duke University Medical Center
Durham, North Carolina

Contents

SECTION I Physiologic Systems

SECTION II Imaging

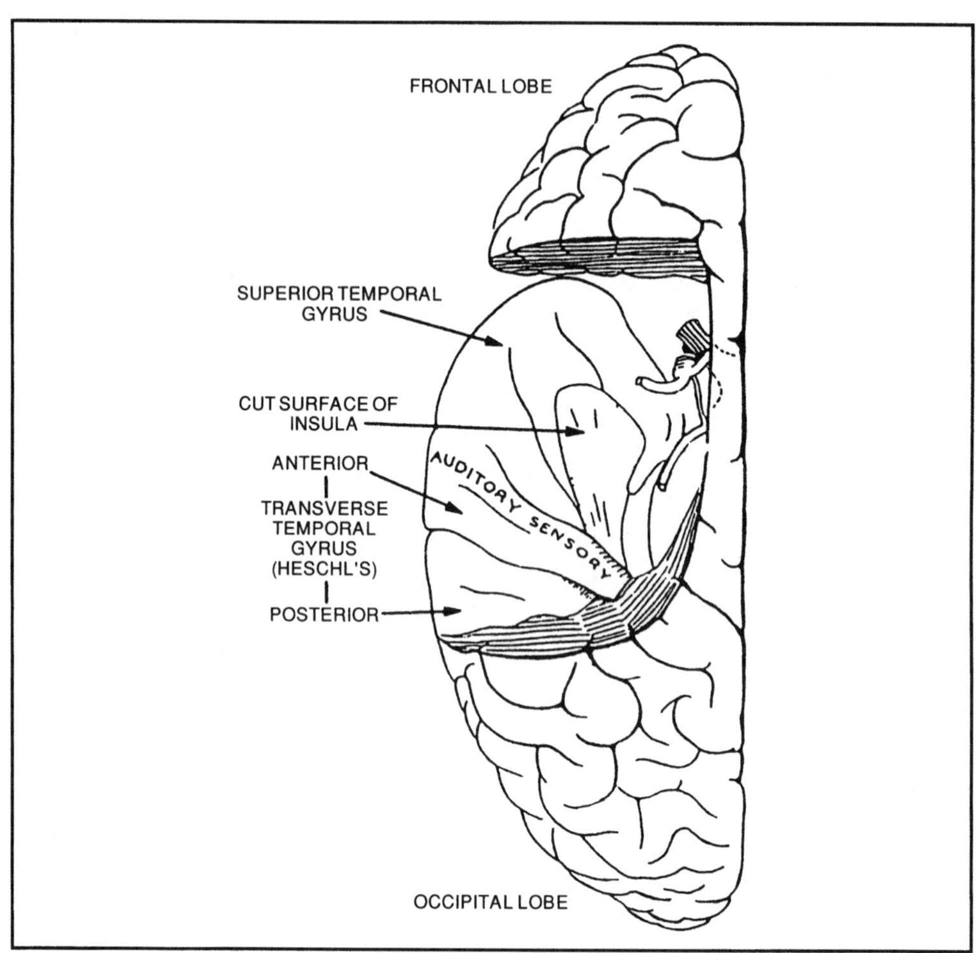

A view of the human cerebral cortex showing the underlying auditory cortex.

I

Physiologic Systems

Robert Plonsey
Duke University

THE CONTENTS OF THIS book are devoted to the subject of *biomedical imaging.* We understand biomedical engineering to involve the application of engineering science and technology to problems arising in medicine and biology. In principle, the intersection of each engineering discipline (i.e., electrical, mechanical, chemical, etc.) with each discipline in medicine (i.e., cardiology, pathology, neurology, etc.) or biology (i.e., biochemistry, pharmacology, molecular biology, cell biology, etc.) is a potential area of biomedical engineering application. As such, the discipline of biomedical engineering is potentially very extensive. However, at least to date, only a few of the aforementioned "intersections" contain active areas of research and/or development. The most significant of these are described in this book.

While the application of engineering expertise to the life sciences requires an obvious knowledge of contemporary technical theory and its applications, it also demands an adequate knowledge and understanding of relevant medicine and biology. It has been argued that the most challenging part of finding engineering solutions to problems lies in the formulation of the solution in engineering terms. In biomedical engineering, this usually demands a full understanding of the life science substrates as well as the quantitative methodologies.

This section is devoted to an overview of the major physiologic systems of current interest to biomedical engineers, on which their work is based. The overview may contain useful definitions, tables of basic physiologic data, and an introduction to the literature. Obviously these chapters must be extremely brief. However, our goal is an introduction that may enable the reader to clarify some item of interest or to indicate a way to pursue further information. Possibly the reader will find the greatest value in the references to more extensive literature.

This section contains seven chapters, and these describe each of the major organ systems of the human body. Thus we have chapters describing the cardiovascular, endocrine, nervous, visual, auditory, gastrointestinal, and respiratory systems. While each author is writing at an introductory and tutorial level, the audience is assumed to have some technical expertise, and consequently mathematical descriptions are not avoided. All authors are recognized as experts on the system which they describe, but all are also biomedical engineers.

The authors in this section noted that they would have liked more space but recognized that the main focus of this book is on "engineering." The hope is that readers will find this introductory section helpful to their understanding of later chapters of this book and, as noted above, that this section will at least provide a starting point for further investigation into the life sciences.

1

An Outline of Cardiovascular Structure and Function

Daniel J. Schneck
Virginia Polytechnic Institute and State University

Because not every cell in the human body is near enough to the environment to easily exchange with it mass (including nutrients, oxygen, carbon dioxide, and the waste products of metabolism), energy (including heat), and momentum, the physiologic system is endowed with a major highway network—organized to make available thousands of miles of access tubing for the transport to and from a different neighborhood (on the order of 10 μm or less) of any given cell whatever it needs to sustain life. This highway network, called the *cardiovascular system,* includes a pumping station, the heart; a working fluid, blood; a complex branching configuration of distributing and collecting pipes and channels, blood vessels; and a sophisticated means for both intrinsic (inherent) and extrinsic (autonomic and endocrine) control.

1.1 The Working Fluid: Blood

Accounting for about 8 ± 1% of total body weight, averaging 5200 ml, blood is a complex, heterogeneous suspension of formed elements—the *blood cells,* or *hematocytes*—suspended in a continuous, straw-colored fluid called *plasma.* Nominally, the composite fluid has a mass density of 1.057 ± 0.007 g/cm^3, and it is three to six times as viscous as water. The hematocytes (Table 1.1) include three basic types of cells: red blood cells (erythrocytes, totaling nearly 95% of the formed elements), white blood cells (leukocytes, averaging <0.15% of all hematocytes), and platelets (thrombocytes, on the order of 5% of all blood cells). Hematocytes are all derived in the active ("red") bone marrow (about 1500 g) of adults from undifferentiated stem cells called *hemocytoblasts,* and all reach ultimate maturity via a process called *hematocytopoiesis.*

The primary function of erythrocytes is to aid in the transport of blood gases—about 30 to 34% (by weight) of each cell consisting of the oxygen- and carbon dioxide–carrying protein hemoglobin (64,000 $\leq$ MW $\leq$68,000) and a small portion of the cell containing the enzyme carbonic anhydrase, which catalyzes the reversible formation of carbonic acid from carbon dioxide and water. The primary function of leukocytes is to endow the human body with the ability to identify and dispose of foreign substances (such as infectious organisms) that do not belong there—agranulocytes (lymphocytes and monocytes)

0-8493-1810-6/03/$0.00+$1.50

TABLE 1.1 Hematocytes

Cell Type	Number Cells per mm^3 Blood*	Corpuscular Diameter (μm)*	Corpuscular Surface Area (μm^2)*	Corpuscular Volume (μm^3)*	Mass Density (g/cm^3)*	Percent Water*	Percent Protein *	Percent Extractives*†
Erythrocytes (red blood cells)	4.2–5.4 × 10^6 ♀ 4.6–6.2 × 10^6 ♂ (5 × 10^6)	6–9 (7.5) Thickness 1.84–2.84 "Neck" 0.81–1.44	120–163 (140)	80–100 (90)	1.089–1.100 (1.098)	64–68 (66)	29–35 (32)	1.6–2.8 (2)
Leukocytes (white blood cells)	4000–11000 (7500)	6–10	300–625	160–450	1.055–1.085	52–60 (56)	30–36 (33)	4–18 (11)
Granulocytes								
Neutrophils: 55–70% WBC (65%)	2–6 × 10^3 (4875)	8–8.6 (8.3)	422–511 (467)	268–333 (300)	1.075–1.085 (1.080)	—	—	—
Eosinophils: 1–4% WBC (3%)	45–480 (225)	8–9 (8.5)	422–560 (491)	268–382 (321)	1.075–1.085 (1.080)	—	—	—
Basophils: 0–1.5% WBC (1%)	0–113 (75)	7.7–8.5 (8.1)	391–500 (445)	239–321 (278)	1.075–1.085 (1.080)	—	—	—
Agranulocytes								
Lymphocytes: 20–35% WBC (25%)	1000–4800 (1875)	6.75–7.34 (7.06)	300–372 (336)	161–207 (184)	1.055–1.070 (1.063)	—	—	—
Monocytes: 3–8% WBC (6%)	100–800 (450)	9–9.5 (9.25)	534–624 (579)	382–449 (414)	1.055–1.070 (1.063)	—	—	—
Thrombocytes (platelets) (2.675 × 10^5)	(1.4 ♂), 2.14 (♀)–5 × 10^5	2–4 (3) Thickness 0.9–1.3	16–35 (25)	5–10 (7.5)	1.04–1.06 (1.05)	60–68 (64)	32–40 (36)	Neg.

*Normal physiologic range, with "typical" value in parentheses.

†Extractives include mostly minerals (ash), carbohydrates, and fats (lipids).

essentially doing the "identifying" and granulocytes (neutrophils, basophils, and eosinophils) essentially doing the "disposing." The primary function of platelets is to participate in the blood clotting process.

Removal of all hematocytes from blood centrifugation or other separating techniques leaves behind the aqueous (91% water by weight, 94.8% water by volume), saline (0.15 *N*) suspending medium called *plasma*—which has an average mass density of 1.035 ± 0.005 g/cm^3 and a viscosity 1½ to 2 times that of water. Some 6.5 to 8% by weight of plasma consists of the plasma proteins, of which there are three major types—albumin, the globulins, and fibrinogen—and several of lesser prominence (Table 1.2).

TABLE 1.2 Plasma

Constituent	Concentration Range (mg/dl plasma)	Typical Plasma Value (mg/dl)	Molecular Weight Range	Typical Value	Typical size (nm)
Total protein, 7% by weight	6400–8300	7245	21,000–1,200,000	—	—
Albumin (56% TP)	2800–5600	4057	66,500–69,000	69,000	15 × 4
α_1-*Globulin* (5.5% TP)	300–600	400	21,000–435,000	60,000	5–12
α_2-*Globulin* (7.5% TP)	400–900	542	100,000–725,000	200,000	50–500
β-*Globulin* (13% TP)	500–1230	942	90,000–1,200,000	100,000	18–50
γ-*Globulin* (12% TP)	500–1800	869	150,000–196,000	150,000	23 × 4
Fibrinogen (4% TP)	150–470	290	330,000–450,000	390,000	(50–60) × (3–8)
Other (2% TP)	70–210	145	70,000–1,000,000	200,000	(15–25) × (2–6)
Inorganic ash, 0.95% by weight	930–1140	983	20–100	—	— (Radius)
Sodium	300–340	325	—	22.98977	0.102 (Na^+)
Potassium	13–21	17	—	39.09800	0.138 (K^+)
Calcium	8.4–11.0	10	—	40.08000	0.099 (Ca^{2+})
Magnesium	1.5–3.0	2	—	24,30500	0.072 (Mg^{2+})
Chloride	336–390	369	—	35.45300	0.181 (Cl^-)
Bicarbonate	110–240	175	—	61.01710	0.163 (HCO_3^-)
Phosphate	2.7–4.5	3.6	—	95.97926	0.210 (HPO_4^{2-})
Sulfate	0.5–1.5	1.0	—	96.05760	0.230 (SO_4^{2-})
Other	0–100	80.4	20–100	—	0.1–0.3
Lipids (fats), 0.80% by weight	541–1000	828	44,000–3,200,000	= Lipoproteins	Up to 200 or more
Cholesterol (34% TL)	12–105 "free" 72–259 esterified, 84–364 "total"	59 224 283	386.67	Contained mostly in intermediate to LDL β-lipoproteins; higher in women	
Phospholipid (35% TL)	150–331	292	690–1010	Contained mainly in HDL to VHDL α_1-lipoproteins	
Triglyceride (26% TL)	65–240	215	400–1370	Contained mainly in VLDL α_2-lipoproteins and chylomicrons	
Other (5% TL)	0–80	38	280–1500	Fat-soluble vitamins, prostaglandins, fatty acids	
Extractives, 0.25% by weight	200–500	259	—	—	—
Glucose	60–120, fasting	90	—	180.1572	0.86 D
Urea	20–30	25	—	60.0554	0.36 D
Carbohydrate	60–105	83	180.16–342.3	—	0.74–0.108 D
Other	11–111	61	—	—	—

The primary functions of albumin are to help maintain the osmotic (oncotic) transmural pressure differential that ensures proper mass exchange between blood and interstitial fluid at the capillary level and to serve as a transport carrier molecule for several hormones and other small biochemical constituents (such as some metal ions). The primary function of the globulin class of proteins is to act as transport carrier molecules (mostly of the α and β class) for large biochemical substances, such as fats (lipoproteins) and certain carbohydrates (muco- and glycoproteins) and heavy metals (mineraloproteins), and to work together with leukocytes in the body's immune system. The latter function is primarily the responsibility of the γ class of immunoglobulins, which have antibody activity. The primary function of fibrinogen is to work with thrombocytes in the formation of a blood clot—a process also aided by one of the most abundant of the lesser proteins, prothrombin (MW $\simeq$ 62,000).

Of the remaining 2% or so (by weight) of plasma, just under half (0.95%, or 983 mg/dl plasma) consists of minerals (inorganic ash), trace elements, and electrolytes, mostly the cations sodium, potassium, calcium, and magnesium and the anions chlorine, bicarbonate, phosphate, and sulfate—the latter three helping as buffers to maintain the fluid at a slightly alkaline pH between 7.35 and 7.45 (average 7.4). What is left, about 1087 mg of material per deciliter of plasma, includes (1) mainly (0.8% by weight) three major types of fat, i.e., cholesterol (in a free and esterified form), phospholipid (a major ingredient of cell membranes), and triglyceride, with lesser amounts of the fat-soluble vitamins (A, D, E, and K), free fatty acids, and other lipids, and (2) "extractives" (0.25% by weight), of which about two-thirds includes glucose and other forms of carbohydrate, the remainder consisting of the water-soluble vitamins (B-complex and C), certain enzymes, nonnitrogenous and nitrogenous waste products of metabolism (including urea, creatine, and creatinine), and many smaller amounts of other biochemical constituents—the list seeming virtually endless.

Removal from blood of all hematocytes and the protein fibrinogen (by allowing the fluid to completely clot before centrifuging) leaves behind a clear fluid called *serum,* which has a density of about 1.018 $\pm$ 0.003 g/cm^3 and a viscosity up to 1½ times that of water. A glimpse of Tables 1.1 and 1.2, together with the very brief summary presented above, nevertheless gives the reader an immediate appreciation for why blood is often referred to as the "river of life." This river is made to flow through the vascular piping network by two central pumping stations arranged in series: the left and right sides of the human heart.

1.2 The Pumping Station: The Heart

Barely the size of the clenched fist of the individual in whom it resides—an inverted, conically shaped, hollow muscular organ measuring 12 to 13 cm from base (top) to apex (bottom) and 7 to 8 cm at its widest point and weighing just under 0.75 lb (about 0.474% of the individual's body weight, or some 325 g)—the human heart occupies a small region between the third and sixth ribs in the central portion of the thoracic cavity of the body. It rests on the diaphragm, between the lower part of the two lungs, its base-to-apex axis leaning mostly toward the left side of the body and slightly forward. The heart is divided by a tough muscular wall—the interatrial-interventricular septum—into a somewhat crescent-shaped right side and cylindrically shaped left side (Fig. 1.1), each being one self-contained pumping station, but the two being connected in series. The left side of the heart drives oxygen-rich blood through the aortic semilunar outlet valve into the *systemic circulation,* which carries the fluid to within a differential neighborhood of each cell in the body—from which it returns to the right side of the heart low in oxygen and rich in carbon dioxide. The right side of the heart then drives this oxygen-poor blood through the pulmonary semilunar (pulmonic) outlet valve into the *pulmonary circulation,* which carries the fluid to the lungs—where its oxygen supply is replenished and its carbon dioxide content is purged before it returns to the left side of the heart to begin the cycle all over again. Because of the anatomic proximity of the heart to the lungs, the right side of the heart does not have to work very hard to drive blood through the pulmonary circulation, so it functions as a low-pressure ($P \leq 40$ mmHg gauge) pump compared with the left side of the heart, which does most of its work at a high pressure (up to 140 mmHg gauge or more) to drive blood through the entire systemic circulation to the furthest extremes of the organism.

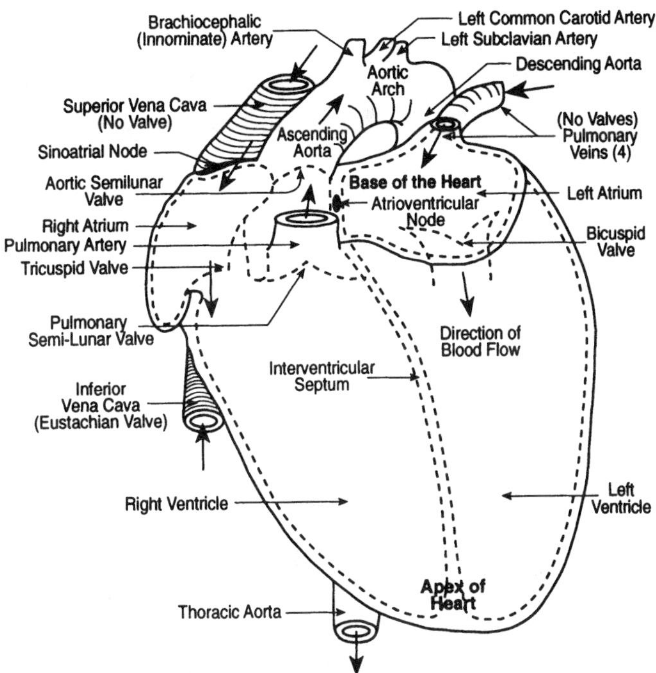

FIGURE 1.1 Anterior view of the human heart showing the four chambers, the inlet and outlet valves, the inlet and outlet major blood vessels, the wall separating the right side from the left side, and the two cardiac pacing centers—the sinoatrial node and the atrioventricular node. Boldface arrows show the direction of flow through the heart chambers, the valves, and the major vessels.

Each cardiac (heart) pump is further divided into two chambers: a small upper receiving chamber, or atrium (auricle), separated by a one-way valve from a lower discharging chamber, or ventricle, which is about twice the size of its corresponding atrium. In order of size, the somewhat spherically shaped left atrium is the smallest chamber—holding about 45 ml of blood (at rest), operating at pressures on the order of 0 to 25 mmHg gauge, and having a wall thickness of about 3 mm. The pouch-shaped right atrium is next (63 ml of blood, 0 to 10 mmHg gauge of pressure, 2-mm wall thickness), followed by the conical/cylindrically shaped left ventricle (100 ml of blood, up to 140 mmHg gauge of pressure, variable wall thickness up to 12 mm) and the crescent-shaped right ventricle (about 130 ml of blood, up to 40 mmHg gauge of pressure, and a wall thickness on the order of one-third that of the left ventricle, up to about 4 mm). All together, then, the heart chambers collectively have a capacity of some 325 to 350 ml, or about 6.5% of the total blood volume in a "typical" individual—but these values are nominal, since the organ alternately fills and expands, contracts, and then empties as it generates a *cardiac output.*

During the 480-ms or so filling phase—diastole—of the average 750-ms cardiac cycle, the inlet valves of the two ventricles (3.8-cm-diameter tricuspid valve from right atrium to right ventricle; 3.1-cm-diameter bicuspid or mitral valve from left atrium to left ventricle) are open, and the outlet valves (2.4-cm-diameter pulmonary valve and 2.25-cm-diameter aortic semilunar valve, respectively) are closed—the heart ultimately expanding to its end diastolic volume (EDV), which is on the order of 140 ml of blood for the left ventricle. During the 270-ms emptying phase—systole—electrically induced vigorous contraction of cardiac muscle drives the intraventricular pressure up, forcing the one-way inlet valves closed and the unidirectional outlet valves open as the heart contracts to its end systolic volume (ESV), which is typically on the order of 70 ml of blood for the left ventricle. Thus the ventricles normally empty about half their contained volume with each heart beat, the remainder being termed the *cardiac reserve volume.* More generally, the difference between the *actual* EDV and the *actual* ESV, called the *stroke volume* (SV), is the volume of blood expelled from the heart during each systolic interval, and the ratio of SV to EDV is called the *cardiac ejection fraction*, or *ejection ratio* (0.5 to 0.75 is normal, 0.4 to 0.5 signifies mild cardiac damage, 0.25 to 0.40 implies moderate heart damage, and <0.25 warns of severe damage to the heart's pumping ability). If the stroke volume is multiplied by the number of systolic intervals per minute, or heart rate (HR), one obtains the total cardiac output (CO):

$$\mathrm{CO} = \mathrm{HR} \times \left(\mathrm{EDV} - \mathrm{ESV}\right) \tag{1.1}$$

Dawson [1991] has suggested that the cardiac output (in milliliters per minute) is proportional to the weight W (in kilograms) of an individual according to the equation

$$\mathrm{CO} - 224W^{3/4} \tag{1.2}$$

and that "normal" heart rate obeys very closely the relation

$$\mathrm{HR} = 229W^{-1/4} \tag{1.3}$$

For a "typical" 68.7-kg individual (blood volume = 5200 ml), Eqs. (1.1), (1.2), and (1.3) yield CO = 5345 ml/min, HR = 80 beats/min (cardiac cycle period = 754 ms) and SV = CO/HR = $224W^{3/4}/229W^{-1/4}$ = $0.978W$ = 67.2 ml/beat, which are very reasonable values. Furthermore, assuming this individual lives about 75 years, his or her heart will have cycled over 3.1536 billion times, pumping a total of 0.2107 billion liters of blood (55.665 million gallons, or 8134 quarts per day)—all of it emptying into the circulatory pathways that constitute the vascular system.

1.3 The Piping Network: Blood Vessels

The vascular system is divided by a microscopic capillary network into an upstream, high-pressure, efferent arterial side (Table 1.3)—consisting of relatively thick-walled, viscoelastic tubes that carry blood away from the heart—and a downstream, low-pressure, afferent venous side (Table 1.4)—consisting of correspondingly thinner (but having a larger caliber) elastic conduits that return blood to the heart. Except for their differences in thickness, the walls of the largest arteries and veins consist of the same three distinct, well-defined, and well-developed layers. From innermost to outermost, these layers are (1) the thinnest *tunica intima*, a continuous lining (the vascular endothelium) consisting of a single layer of simple squamous (thin, sheetlike) endothelial cells "glued" together by a polysaccharide (sugar) intercellular matrix, surrounded by a thin layer of subendothelial connective tissue interlaced with a number of circularly arranged elastic fibers to form the subendothelium, and separated from the next adjacent wall layer by a thick elastic band called the *internal elastic lamina*; (2) the thickest *tunica media*, composed of numerous circularly arranged elastic fibers, especially prevalent in the largest blood vessels on the arterial side (allowing them to expand during systole and to recoil passively during diastole), a significant amount of smooth muscle cells arranged in spiraling layers around the vessel wall, especially prevalent in medium-sized arteries and arterioles (allowing them to function as control points for blood distribution), and some interlacing collagenous connective tissue, elastic fibers, and intercellular mucopolysaccharide substance (extractives), all separated from the next adjacent wall layer by another thick elastic band called the *external elastic lamina*; and (3) the medium-sized *tunica adventitia*, an outer vascular sheath consisting entirely of connective tissue.

The largest blood vessels, such as the aorta, the pulmonary artery, the pulmonary veins, and others, have such thick walls that they require a separate network of tiny blood vessels—the vasa vasorum—just to service the vascular tissue itself. As one moves toward the capillaries from the arterial side (see Table 1.3), the vascular wall keeps thinning, as if it were shedding 15-μm-thick, onion-peel-like concentric layers, and while the percentage of water in the vessel wall stays relatively constant at 70% (by weight),

TABLE 1.3 Arterial System*

Blood Vessel Type	(Systemic) Typical Number	Internal Diameter Range	Length Range†	Wall Thickness	Systemic Volume	(Pulmonary) Typical Number	Pulmonary Volume
Aorta	1	1.0–3.0 cm	30–65 cm	2–3 mm	156 ml	—	—
Pulmonary artery	—	2.5–3.1 cm	6–9 cm	2–3 cm	—	1	52 ml
Wall morphology: Complete tunica adventitia, external elastic lamina, tunica media, internal elastic lamina, tunica intima, subendothelium, endothelium, and vasa vasorum vascular supply							
Main branches	32	5 mm–2.25 cm	3.3–6 cm	≈2 mm	83.2 ml	6	41.6 ml
(Along with the aorta and pulmonary artery, the largest, most well-developed of all blood vessels)							
Large arteries	288	4.0–5.0 mm	1.4–2.8 cm	≈1 mm	104 ml	64	23.5 ml
(A well-developed tunica adventitia and vasa vasorum, although wall layers are gradually thinning)							
Medium arteries	1152	2.5–4.0 mm	1.0–2.2 cm	≈0.75 mm	117 ml	144	7.3 ml
Small arteries	3456	1.0–2.5 mm	0.6–1.7 cm	≈0.50 mm	104 ml	432	5.7 ml
Tributaries	20,736	0.5–1.0 mm	0.3–1.3 cm	≈0.25 mm	91 ml	5184	7.3 ml
(Well-developed tunica media and external elastic lamina, but tunica adventitia virtually nonexistent)							
Small rami	82,944	250–500 μm	0.2–0.8 cm	≈125 μm	57.2 ml	11,664	2.3 ml
Terminal branches	497,664	100–250 μm	1.0–6.0 mm	≈60 μm	52 ml	139,968	3.0 ml
(A well-developed endothelium, subendothelium, and internal elastic lamina, plus about two to three 15-μm-thick concentric layers forming just a very thin tunica media; no external elastic lamina)							
Arterioles	18,579,456	25–100 μm	0.2–3.8 mm	≈20–30 μm	52 ml	4,094,064	2.3 ml
Wall morphology: More than one smooth muscle layer (with nerve association in the outermost muscle layer), a well-developed internal elastic lamina; gradually thinning in 25- to 50-μm vessels to a single layer of smooth muscle tissue, connective tissue, and scant supporting tissue.							
Metarterioles	238,878,720	10–25 μm	0.1–1.8 mm	≈5–15 μm	41.6 ml	157,306,536	4.0 ml
(Well-developed subendothelium; discontinuous contractile muscle elements; one layer of connective tissue)							
Capillaries	16,124,431,360	3.5–10 μm	0.5–1.1 mm	≈0.5–1 μm	260 ml	3,218,406,696	104 ml
(Simple endothelial tubes devoid of smooth muscle tissue; one-cell-layer-thick walls)							

*Vales are approximate for a 68.7-kg individual having a total blood volume of 5200 ml.

†Average uninterrupted distance between branch origins (except aorta and pulmonary artery, which are total length).

TABLE 1.4 Venous System

Blood Vessel Type	(Systemic) Typical Number	Internal Diameter Range	Length Range	Wall Thickness	Systemic Volume	(Pulmonary) Typical Number	Pulmonary Volume
Postcapillary venules	4,408,161,734	8–30 μm	0.1–0.6 mm	1.0–5.0 μm	166.7 ml	306,110,016	10.4 ml
(Wall consists of thin endothelium exhibiting occasional pericytes (pericapillary connective tissue cells) which increase in number as the vessel lumen gradually increases)							
Collecting venules	160,444,500	30–50 μm	0.1–0.8 mm	5.0–10 μm	161.3 ml	8,503,056	1.2 ml
(One complete layer of pericytes, one complete layer of veil cells (veil-like cells forming a thin membrane), occasional primitive smooth muscle tissue fibers that increase in number with vessel size)							
Muscular venules	32,088,900	50–100 μm	0.2–1.0 mm	10–25 μm	141.8 ml	3,779,136	3.7 ml
(Relatively thick wall of smooth muscle tissue)							
Small collecting veins	10,241,508	100–200 μm	0.5–3.2 mm	≃30 μm	329.6 ml	419,904	6.7 ml
(Prominent tunica media of continuous layers of smooth muscle cells)							
Terminal branches	496,900	200–600 μm	1.0–6.0 mm	30–150 μm	206.6 ml	34,992	5.2 ml
(A well-developed endothelium, subendothelium, and internal elastic lamina; well-developed tunica media but fewer elastic fibers than corresponding arteries and much thinner walls)							
Small veins	19,968	600 μm–1.1 mm	2.0–9.0 mm	≃0.25 mm	63.5 ml	17,280	44.9 ml
Medium veins	512	1–5 mm	1–2 cm	≃0.50 mm	67.0 ml	144	22.0 ml
Large veins	256	5–9 mm	1.4–3.7 cm	≃0.75 mm	476.1 ml	48	29.5 ml
(Well-developed wall layers comparable to large arteries but about 25% thinner)							
Main branches	224	9.0 mm–2.0 cm	2.0–10 cm	≃1.00 mm	1538.1 ml	16	39.4 ml
(Along with the vena cava and pulmonary veins, the largest, most well-developed of all blood vessels)							
Vena cava	1	2.0–3.5 cm	20–50 cm	≃1.50 mm	125.3 ml	—	—
Pulmonary veins	—	1.7–2.5 cm	5–8 cm	≃1.50 mm	—	4	52 ml
Wall morphology: Essentially the same as comparable major arteries but a much thinner tunica intima, a much thinner tunica media, and a somewhat thicker tunica adventitia; contains a vasa vasorum							

Total systemic blood volume: 4394 ml—84.5% of total blood volume; 19.5% in arteries (~3:2 large:small), 5.9% in capillaries, 74.6% in veins (~3:1 large:small); 63% of volume is in vessels greater than 1 mm internal diameter

Total pulmonary blood volume: 468 ml—9.0% of total blood volume; 31.8% in arteries, 22.2% in capillaries, 46% in veins; 58.3% of volume is in vessels greater than 1 mm internal diameter; remainder of blood in heart, about 338 ml (6.5% of total blood volume)

the ratio of elastin to collagen decreases (actually reverses)—from 3:2 in large arteries (9% elastin, 6% collagen, by weight) to 1:2 in small tributaries (5% elastin, 10% collagen)—and the amount of smooth muscle tissue increases from 7.5% by weight of large arteries (the remaining 7.5% consisting of various extractives) to 15% in small tributaries. By the time one reaches the capillaries, one encounters single-cell-thick endothelial tubes—devoid of any smooth muscle tissue, elastin, or collagen—downstream of which the vascular wall gradually "reassembles itself," layer-by-layer, as it directs blood back to the heart through the venous system (Table 1.4).

Blood vessel structure is directly related to function. The thick-walled large arteries and main *distributing branches* are designed to withstand the pulsating 80 to 130 mmHg blood pressures that they must endure. The smaller elastic *conducting vessels* need only operate under steadier blood pressures in the range 70 to 90 mmHg, but they must be thin enough to penetrate and course through organs without unduly disturbing the anatomic integrity of the mass involved. Controlling arterioles operate at blood pressures between 45 and 70 mmHg but are heavily endowed with smooth muscle tissue (hence their being referred to as *muscular vessels*) so that they may be actively shut down when flow to the capillary bed they service is to be restricted (for whatever reason), and the smallest capillary *resistance vessels* (which operate at blood pressures on the order of 10 to 45 mmHg) are designed to optimize conditions for transport to occur between blood and the surrounding interstitial fluid. Traveling back up the venous side, one encounters relatively steady blood pressures continuously decreasing from around 30 mmHg all the way down to near zero, so these vessels can be thin-walled without disease consequence. However, the low blood pressure, slower, steady (time-dependent) flow, thin walls, and larger caliber that characterize the venous system cause blood to tend to "pool" in veins, allowing them to act somewhat like reservoirs. It is not surprising, then, that at any given instant, one normally finds about two-thirds of the total human blood volume residing in the venous system, the remaining one-third being divided among the heart (6.5%), the microcirculation (7% in systemic and pulmonary capillaries), and the arterial system (19.5 to 20%).

In a global sense, then, one can think of the human cardiovascular system—using an electrical analogy—as a voltage source (the heart), two capacitors (a large venous system and a smaller arterial system), and a resistor (the microcirculation taken as a whole). Blood flow and the dynamics of the system represent electrical inductance (inertia), and useful engineering approximations can be derived from such a simple model. The cardiovascular system is designed to bring blood to within a capillary size of each and every one of the more than 10^{14} cells of the body—but *which* cells receive blood at any given time, *how much* blood they get, the *composition* of the fluid coursing by them, and related physiologic considerations are all matters that are not left to chance.

1.4 Cardiovascular Control

Blood flows through organs and tissues either to nourish and sanitize them or to be itself processed in some sense—e.g., to be oxygenated (pulmonary circulation), stocked with nutrients (splanchnic circulation), dialyzed (renal circulation), cooled (cutaneous circulation), filtered of dilapidated red blood cells (splenic circulation), and so on. Thus any given vascular network normally receives blood according to the metabolic needs of the region it perfuses and/or the function of that region as a blood treatment plant and/or thermoregulatory pathway. However, it is not feasible to expect that our physiologic transport system can be "all things to all cells all of the time"—especially when resources are scarce and/or time is a factor. Thus the distribution of blood is further prioritized according to three basic criteria: (1) how essential the perfused region is to the maintenance of life itself (e.g., we can survive without an arm, a leg, a stomach, or even a large portion of our small intestine but not without a brain, a heart, and at least one functioning kidney and lung, (2) how essential the perfused region is in allowing the organism to respond to a life-threatening situation (e.g., digesting a meal is among the least of the body's concerns in a "fight or flight" circumstance), and (3) how well the perfused region can function and survive on a decreased supply of blood (e.g., some tissues—like striated skeletal and smooth muscle—have significant anaerobic capability; others—like several forms of connective tissue—can function quite effectively at a significantly decreased metabolic rate when necessary; some organs—like the liver—are larger than they really need to be; and some anatomic structures—like the eyes, ears, and limbs—have duplicates, giving them a built-in redundancy).

Within this generalized prioritization scheme, control of cardiovascular function is accomplished by mechanisms that are based either on the inherent physicochemical attributes of the tissues and organs themselves—so-called intrinsic control—or on responses that can be attributed to the effects on cardiovascular tissues of other organ systems in the body (most notably the autonomic nervous system and the endocrine system)—so-called extrinsic control. For example, the accumulation of wastes and depletion of oxygen and nutrients that accompany the increased rate of metabolism in an active tissue both lead to an *intrinsic* relaxation of local precapillary sphincters (rings of muscle)—with a consequent widening of corresponding capillary entrances—which reduces the local resistance to flow and thereby allows more blood to perfuse the active region. On the other hand, the *extrinsic* innervation by the autonomic nervous system of smooth muscle tissues in the walls of arterioles allows the central nervous system to completely shut down the flow to entire vascular beds (such as the cutaneous circulation) when this becomes necessary (such as during exposure to extremely cold environments).

In addition to prioritizing and controlling the *distribution* of blood, physiologic regulation of cardiovascular function is directed mainly at four other variables: cardiac output, blood pressure, blood volume, and blood composition. From Eq. (1.1) we see that cardiac output can be increased by increasing the heart rate (a chronotropic effect), increasing the EDV (allowing the heart to fill longer by delaying the onset of systole), decreasing the ESV (an inotropic effect), or doing all three things at once. Indeed, under the extrinsic influence of the sympathetic nervous system and the adrenal glands, heart rate can triple—to some 240 beats/min if necessary—EDV can increase by as much as 50%—to around 200 ml or more of blood—and ESV can decrease a comparable amount (the cardiac reserve)—to about 30 to 35 ml or less. The combined result of all three effects can lead to over a sevenfold increase in cardiac output—from the normal 5 to 5.5 liters/min to as much as 40 to 41 liters/min or more for very brief periods of strenuous exertion.

The control of blood pressure is accomplished mainly by adjusting at the arteriolar level the downstream resistance to flow—an increased resistance leading to a rise in arterial backpressure, and vice versa. This effect is conveniently quantified by a fluid-dynamic analogue to Ohm's famous $E = IR$ law in electromagnetic theory, voltage drop E being equated to fluid pressure drop ΔP, electric current I corresponding to flow—cardiac output (CO)—and electric resistance R being associated with an analogous vascular "peripheral resistance" (PR). Thus one may write

$$\Delta P = (\mathrm{CO})(\mathrm{PR}) \tag{1.4}$$

Normally, the total systemic peripheral resistance is 15 to 20 mmHg/liter/min of flow but can increase significantly under the influence of the vasomotor center located in the medulla of the brain, which controls arteriolar muscle tone.

The control of blood volume is accomplished mainly through the excretory function of the kidney. For example, antidiuretic hormone (ADH) secreted by the pituitary gland acts to prevent renal fluid loss (excretion via urination) and thus increases plasma volume, whereas perceived extracellular fluid overloads such as those that result from the peripheral vasoconstriction response to cold stress lead to a sympathetic/adrenergic receptor-induced renal diuresis (urination) that tends to decrease plasma volume—if not checked, to sometimes dangerously low dehydration levels. Blood composition, too, is maintained primarily through the activity of endocrine hormones and enzymes that enhance or repress specific biochemical pathways. Since these pathways are too numerous to itemize here, suffice it to say that in the body's quest for homeostasis and stability, virtually nothing is left to chance, and every biochemical end can be arrived at through a number of alternative means. In a broader sense, as the organism strives to maintain life, it coordinates a wide variety of different functions, and central to its ability to do just that is the role played by the cardiovascular system in transporting mass, energy, and momentum.

Defining Terms

Atrioventricular (AV) node: A highly specialized cluster of neuromuscular cells at the lower portion of the right atrium leading to the interventricular septum; the AV node delays sinoatrial (SA) node–generated electrical impulses momentarily (allowing the atria to contract first) and then conducts the depolarization wave to the bundle of His and its bundle branches.

Autonomic nervous system: The functional division of the nervous system that innervates most glands, the heart, and smooth muscle tissue in order to maintain the internal environment of the body.

Cardiac muscle: Involuntary muscle possessing much of the anatomic attributes of skeletal voluntary muscle and some of the physiologic attributes of involuntary smooth muscle tissue; SA node–induced contraction of its interconnected network of fibers allows the heart to expel blood during systole.

Chronotropic: Affecting the periodicity of a recurring action, such as the slowing (bradycardia) or speeding up (tachycardia) of the heartbeat that results from extrinsic control of the SA node.

Endocrine system: The system of ductless glands and organs secreting substances directly into the blood to produce a specific response from another "target" organ or body part.

Endothelium: Flat cells that line the innermost surfaces of blood and lymphatic vessels and the heart.

Homeostasis: A tendency to uniformity or stability in an organism by maintaining within narrow limits certain variables that are critical to life.

Inotropic: Affecting the contractility of muscular tissue, such as the increase in cardiac *power* that results from extrinsic control of the myocardial musculature.

Precapillary sphincters: Rings of smooth muscle surrounding the entrance to capillaries where they branch off from upstream metarterioles. Contraction and relaxation of these sphincters close and open the access to downstream blood vessels, thus controlling the irrigation of different capillary networks.

Sinoatrial (SA) node: Neuromuscular tissue in the right atrium near where the superior vena cava joins the posterior right atrium (the sinus venarum); the SA node generates electrical impulses that initiate the heartbeat, hence its nickname the cardiac "pacemaker."

Stem cell: A generalized parent cell spawning descendants that become individually specialized.

Acknowledgments

The author gratefully acknowledges the assistance of Professor Robert Hochmuth in the preparation of Table 1.1 and the Radford Community Hospital for its support of the Biomedical Engineering Program at Virginia Tech.

References

Bhagavan NV. 1992. Medical Biochemistry. Boston, Jones and Bartlett.

Beall HPT, Needham D, Hochmuth RM. 1993. Volume and osmotic properties of human neutrophils. Blood 81(10):2774–2780.

Caro CG, Pedley TJ, Schroter RC, Seed WA. 1978. The Mechanics of the Circulation. New York, Oxford University Press.

Chandran KB. 1992. Cardiovascular Biomechanics. New York, New York University Press.

Frausto da Silva JJR, Williams RJP. 1993. The Biological Chemistry of the Elements. New York, Oxford University Press/Clarendon.

Dawson TH. 1991. Engineering Design of the Cardiovascular System of Mammals. Englewood Cliffs, NJ, Prentice-Hall.

Duck FA. 1990. Physical Properties of Tissue. San Diego, Academic Press.

Kaley G, Altura BM (Eds). Microcirculation, vol I (1977), vol II (1978), vol III (1980). Baltimore, University Park Press.

Kessel RG, Kardon RH. 1979. Tissue and Organs—A Text-Atlas of Scanning Electron Microscopy. San Francisco, WH Freeman.

Lentner C (Ed). Geigy Scientific Tables, vol 3: Physical Chemistry, Composition of Blood, Hematology and Somatometric Data, 8th ed. 1984. New Jersey, Ciba-Geigy.

———Vol 5: Heart and Circulation, 8th ed. 1990. New Jersey, Ciba-Geigy.

Schneck DJ. 1990. Engineering Principles of Physiologic Function. New York, New York University Press.

Tortora GJ, Grabowski SR. 1993. Principles of Anatomy and Physiology, 7th ed. New York, HarperCollins.

2

Endocrine System

Derek G. Cramp
City University, London

Ewart R. Carson
City University, London

The body, if it is to achieve optimal performance, must possess mechanisms for sensing and responding appropriately to numerous biologic cues and signals in order to control and maintain its internal environment. This complex role is effected by the integrative action of the endocrine and neural systems. The endocrine contribution is achieved through a highly sophisticated set of communication and control systems involving signal generation, propagation, recognition, transduction, and response. The signal entities are chemical messengers or hormones that are distributed through the body by the blood circulatory system to their respective target organs to modify their activity in some fashion.

Endocrinology has a comparatively long history, but real advances in the understanding of endocrine physiology and mechanisms of regulation and control began only in the late 1960s with the introduction of sensitive and relatively specific analytical methods; these enabled low concentrations of circulating hormones to be measured reliably, simply, and at relatively low cost. The breakthrough came with the development and widespread adoption of competitive protein binding and radioimmunoassays that superseded existing cumbersome bioassay methods. Since then, knowledge of the physiology of individual endocrine glands and of the neural control of the pituitary gland and the overall feedback control of the endocrine system has progressed and is growing rapidly. Much of this has been accomplished by applying to endocrinological research the methods developed in cellular and molecular biology and recombinant DNA technology. At the same time, theoretical and quantitative approaches using mathematical modeling complemented experimental studies have been of value in gaining a greater understanding of endocrine dynamics.

2.1 Endocrine System: Hormones, Signals, and Communication between Cells and Tissues

Hormones are synthesized and secreted by specialized endocrine glands to act locally or at a distance, having been carried in the bloodstream (classic endocrine activity) or secreted into the gut lumen (lumocrine activity) to act on target cells that are distributed elsewhere in the body. Hormones are chemically diverse, physiologically potent molecules that are the primary vehicle for intercellular communication with the

0-8493-1810-6/03/$0.00+$1.50

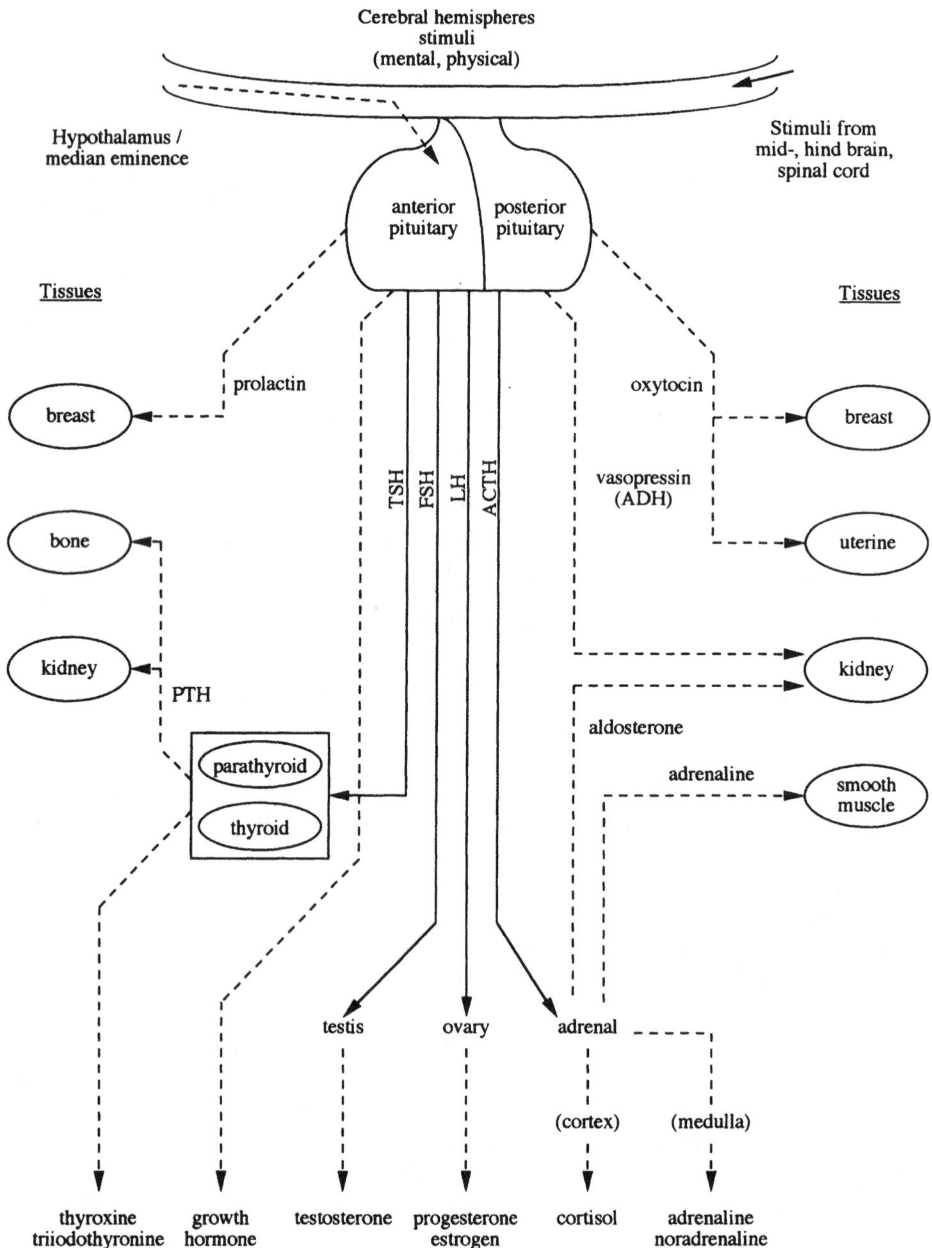

FIGURE 2.1 Representation of the forward pathways of pituitary and target gland hormone release and action: —— tropic hormones; - - - tissue-affecting hormones.

capacity to override the intrinsic mechanisms of normal cellular control. They can be classified broadly into three groups according to their physicochemical characteristics: (1) steroid hormones produced by chemical modification of cholesterol, (2) peptide and protein hormones, and (3) those derived from the aromatic amino acid tyrosine. The peptide and protein hormones are essentially hydrophilic and are therefore able to circulate in the blood in the free state; however, the more hydrophobic lipid-derived molecules have to be carried in the circulation bound to specific transport proteins. Figure 2.1 and Table 2.1 show, in schematic and descriptive form, respectively, details of the major endocrine glands of the body and the endocrine pathways.

TABLE 2.1 Main Endocrine Glands and the Hormones They Produce and Release

Gland	Hormone	Chemical Characteristics
Hypothalamus/median eminence	Thyrotropin-releasing hormone (TRH)	Peptides
	Somatostatin	
	Gonadotropin-releasing hormone	Amine
	Growth hormone-releasing hormone	
	Corticotropin-releasing hormone	
	Prolactin inhibitor factor	
Anterior pituitary	Thyrotropin (TSH)	Glycoproteins
	Luteinizing hormone	
	Follicle-stimulating hormone (FSH)	Proteins
	Growth hormone	
	Prolactin	
	Adrenocorticotropin (ACTH)	
Posterior pituitary	Vasopressin (antidiuretic hormone, ADH)	
	Oxytocin	Peptides
Thyroid	Triidothyronine (T3)	Tyrosine derivatives
	Thyroxine (T4)	
Parathyroid	Parathyroid hormone (PTH)	Peptide
Adrenal cortex	Cortisol	Steroids
	Aldosterone	
Adrenal medulla	Epinephrine	Catecolamines
	Norepinephrine	
Pancreas	Insulin	Proteins
	Glucagon	
	Somatostatin	
Gonads: Testes	Testosterone	Steroids
Ovaries	Estrogen	
	Progesterone	

The endocrine and nervous system are physically and functionally linked by a specific region of the brain called the *hypothalamus*, which lies immediately above the pituitary gland, to which it is connected by an extension called the *pituitary stalk.* The integrating function of the hypothalamus is mediated by cells that possess the properties of both nerve and processes that carry electrical impulses and on stimulation can release their signal molecules into the blood. Each of the hypothalamic neurosecretory cells can be stimulated by other nerve cells in higher regions of the brain to secrete specific peptide hormones or release factors into the adenohypophyseal portal vasculature. These hormones can then specifically stimulate or suppress the secretion of a second hormone from the anterior pituitary.

The pituitary hormones in the circulation interact with their target tissues, which, if endocrine glands, are stimulated to secrete further (third) hormones that feed back to inhibit the release of the pituitary hormones. It will be seen from Fig. 2.1 and Table 2.1 that the main targets of the pituitary are the adrenal cortex, the thyroid, and the gonads. These axes provide good examples of the control of pituitary hormone release by negative-feedback inhibition; e.g., adrenocorticotropin (ACTH), luteinizing hormone (LH), and follicle-stimulating hormone (FSH) are selectively inhibited by different steroid hormones, as is thyrotropin (TSH) release by the thyroid hormones.

In the case of growth hormone (GH) and prolactin, the target tissue is not an endocrine gland and thus does not produce a hormone; then the feedback control is mediated by inhibitors. Prolactin is under dopamine inhibitory control, whereas hypothalamic releasing and inhibitory factors control GH release. The two posterior pituitary (neurohypophyseal) hormones, oxytocin and vasopressin, are synthesized in the supraoptic and paraventricular nuclei and are stored in granules at the end of the nerve fibers in the posterior pituitary. Oxytocin is subsequently secreted in response to peripheral stimuli from the cervical stretch receptors or the suckling receptors of the breast. In a like manner, antidiuretic hormone (ADH, vasopressin) release is stimulated by the altered activity of hypothalamic osmoreceptors responding to changes in plasma solute concentrations.

It will be noted that the whole system is composed of several endocrine axes with the hypothalamus, pituitary, and other endocrine glands together forming a complex hierarchical regulatory system. There is no doubt that the anterior pituitary occupies a central position in the control of hormone secretion and, because of its important role, was often called the "conductor of the endocrine orchestra." However, the release of pituitary hormones is mediated by complex feedback control, so the pituitary should be regarded as having a permissive role rather than having the overall control of the endocrine system.

2.2 Hormone Action at the Cell Level: Signal Recognition, Signal Transduction, and Effecting a Physiological Response

The ability of target glands or tissues to respond to hormonal signals depends on the ability of the cells to recognize the signal. This function is mediated by specialized proteins or glycoproteins in or on the cell plasma membrane that are specific for a particular hormone, able to recognize it, bind it with high affinity, and react when very low concentrations are present. Recognition of the hormonal signal and activation of the cell surface receptors initiates a flow of information to the cell interior which triggers a chain of intracellular events in a pre-programmed fashion that produces a characteristic response. It is useful to classify the site of such action of hormones into two groups: those which act at the cell surface without, generally, traversing the cell membrane and those which actually enter the cell before effecting a response. In the study of this multi-step sequence, two important events can be readily studied, namely, the binding of the hormone to its receptor and activation of cytoplasmic effects. However, it is some of the steps between these events, such as receptor activation and signal generation, that are still relatively poorly defined. One method employed in an attempt to elucidate the intermediate steps has been to use ineffective mutant receptors, which when assayed are either defective in their hormone binding capabilities or in effector activation and thus unable to transduce a meaningful signal to the cell. But the difficulty with these studies has been to distinguish receptor-activation and signal-generation defects from hormone binding and effector activation defects.

Hormones Acting at the Cell Surface

Most peptide and protein hormones are hydrophilic and thus unable to traverse the lipid-containing cell membrane and must therefore act through activation of receptor proteins on the cell surface. When these receptors are activated by the binding of an extracellular signal ligand, the ligand-receptor complex initiates a series of protein interactions within or adjacent to the inner surface of the plasma membrane, which in turn brings about changes in intracellular activity. This can happen in one of two ways. The first involves the so-called second messenger, by altering the activity of a plasma membrane-bound enzyme, which in turn increases (or sometimes decreases) the concentration of an intracellular mediator. The second involves activation of other types of cell surface receptors, which leads to changes in the plasma membrane electrical potential and the membrane permeability, resulting in altered transmembrane transport of ions or metabolites. If the hormone is thought of as the "first messenger," cyclic adenosine monophosphate (cAMP) can be regarded as the "second messenger," capable of triggering a cascade of intracellular biochemical events that can lead either to a rapid secondary response such as altered ion transport, enhanced metabolic pathway flux, steroidogenesis or to a slower response such as DNA, RNA, and protein synthesis resulting in cell growth or cell division.

The peptide and protein hormones circulate at very low concentrations relative to other proteins in the blood plasma. These low concentrations are reflected in the very high affinity and specificity of the receptor sites, which permits recognition of the relevant hormones amid the profusion of protein molecules in the circulation. Adaptation to a high concentration of a signal ligand in a time-dependent reversible manner enables cells to respond to changes in the concentration of a ligand instead of to its absolute concentration. The number of receptors in a cell is not constant; synthesis of receptors may be induced or repressed by other hormones or even by their own hormones. Adaptation can occur in several ways. Ligand binding can inactivate a cell surface receptor either by inducing its internalization and degradation or by causing the receptor to adopt an inactive conformation. Alternatively, it may result from the changes in one of the non-receptor proteins involved in signal transduction following receptor activation. Downregulation is the name given to the process whereby a cell decreases the number of receptors in response to intense or frequent stimulation and can occur by degradation or more temporarily by phosphorylation and sequestration. Upregulation is the process of increasing receptor expression either by other hormones or in response to altered stimulation.

The cell surface receptors for peptide hormones are linked functionally to a cell membrane-bound enzyme that acts as the catalytic unit. This receptor complex consists of three components: (1) the receptor itself which recognizes the hormone, (2) a regulatory protein called a G-protein that binds guanine nucleotides and is located on the cytosolic face of the membrane, and (3) adenylate cyclase which catalyzes the conversion of ATP to cAMP. As the hormone binds at the receptor site, it is coupled through a regulatory protein, which acts as a transducer, to the enzyme adenyl cyclase, which catalyzes the formation of cAMP from adenosine triphosphate (ATP). The G-protein consists of three subunits, which in the unstimulated state form a heterotrimer to which a molecule of GDP is bound. Binding of the hormone to the receptor causes the subunit to exchange its GDP for a molecule of GTP (guanine triphosphate) which then dissociates from the subunits. This in turn decreases the affinity of the receptor for the hormone and leads to its dissociation. The GTP subunit not only activates adenylate cyclase, but also has intrinsic GTPase activity and slowly converts GTP back to GDP, thus allowing the subunits to reassociate and so regain their initial resting state. There are hormones, such as somatostatin, that possess the ability to inhibit AMP formation but still have similarly structured receptor complexes. The G-protein of inhibitory complexes consists of an inhibitory subunit complexed with a subunit thought to be identical to the subunits of the stimulatory G-protein. However, it appears that a single adenylate cyclase molecule can be simultaneously regulated by more than one G-protein enabling the system to integrate opposing inputs.

The adenylate cyclase reaction is rapid, and the increased concentration of intracellular cAMP is short-lived, since it is rapidly hydrolyzed and destroyed by the enzyme cAMP phosphodiesterase which terminates the hormonal response. The continual and rapid removal of cAMP and free calcium ions from the cytosol makes for both the rapid increase and decrease of these intracellular mediators when the cells respond to signals. Rising cAMP concentrations affect cells by stimulating cAMP-dependent protein kinases to phosphorylate specific target proteins. Phosphorylation of proteins leads to conformational changes that enhance their catalytic activity, thus providing a signal amplification pathway from hormone to effector. These effects are reversible because phosphorylated proteins are rapidly dephosphorylated by protein phosphatases when the concentration of cAMP falls. A similar system involving cyclic GMP, although less common and less well studied, plays an analogous role to that of cAMP. The action of thyrotropin-releasing hormone (TRH), parathyroid hormone (PTH), and epinephrine is catalyzed by adenyl cyclase, and this can be regarded as the classic reaction.

However, there are variant mechanisms. In the phosphatidylinositol-diacylglycerol (DAG)/inositol triphosphate (IP3) system, some surface receptors are coupled through another G-protein to the enzyme phospholipase C which cleaves the membrane phospholipid to form DAG and IP3 or phospholipase D which cleaves phosphatidyl choline to DAG via phosphatidic acid. DAG causes the calcium, phospholipid-dependent protein kinase C to translocate to the cell membrane from the cytosolic cell compartment becoming 20 times more active in the process. IP3 mobilizes calcium from storage sites associated with the plasma and intracellular membranes thereby contributing to the activation of protein kinase C as well as other calcium-dependent processes. DAG is cleared from the cell either by conversion to phosphatidic acid which may be recycled to phospholipid or it may be broken down to fatty acids and glycerol. The DAG derived from phosphatidylinositol usually contains arachidonic acid esterified to the middle carbon of glycerol. Arachidonic acid is the precursor of the prostaglandins and leukotrienes which are biologically active eicosanoids.

Thyrotropin and vasopressin modulate an activity of phospholipase C that catalyzes the conversion of phosphatidylinositol to diacylglycerol and inositol, l,4,5-triphosphate, which act as the second messengers. They mobilize bound intracellular calcium and activate a protein kinase, which in turn alters the activity of other calcium-dependent enzymes within the cell.

Increased concentrations of free calcium ions affect cellular events by binding to and altering the molecular conformation of calmodulin; the resulting calcium ion-calmodulin complex can activate many different target proteins, including calcium ion-dependent protein kinases. Each cell type has a characteristic set of target proteins that are so regulated by cAMP-dependent kinases and/or calmodulin that it will respond in a specific way to an alteration in cAMP or calcium ion concentrations. In this way, cAMP or calcium ions act as second messengers in such a way as to allow the extracellular signal not only to be greatly amplified but, just as importantly, also to be made specific for each cell type.

The action of the important hormone insulin that regulates glucose metabolism depends on the activation of the enzyme tyrosine kinase catalyzing the phosphorylation of tyrosyl residues of proteins. This effects changes in the activity of calcium-sensitive enzymes, leading to enhanced movement of glucose and fatty acids across the cell membrane and modulating their intracellular metabolism. The binding of insulin to its receptor site has been studied extensively; the receptor complex has been isolated and characterized. It was such work that highlighted the interesting aspect of feedback control at the cell level, downregulation: the ability of peptide hormones to regulate the concentration of cell surface receptors. After activation, the receptor population becomes desensitized, or "downregulated," leading to a decreased availability of receptors and thus a modulation of transmembrane events.

Hormones Acting within the Cell

Steroid hormones are small hydrophobic molecules derived from cholesterol that are solubilized by binding reversibly to specify carrier proteins in the blood plasma. Once released from their carrier proteins, they readily pass through the plasma membrane of the target cell and bind, again reversibly, to steroid hormone receptor proteins in the cytosol. This is a relatively slow process when compared to protein hormones. The latter second messenger–mediated phosphorylation-dephosphorylation reactions modify enzymatic processes rapidly with the physiologic consequences becoming apparent in seconds or minutes and are as rapidly reversed. Nuclear-mediated responses, on the other hand, lead to transcription/translation-dependent changes that are slow in onset and tend to persist since reversal is dependent on degradation of the induced proteins. The protein component of the steroid hormone-receptor complex has an affinity for DNA in the cell nucleus, where it binds to nuclear chromatin and initiates the transcription of a small number of genes. These gene products may, in turn, activate other genes and produce a secondary response, thereby amplifying the initial effect of the hormone. Each steroid hormone is recognized by a separate receptor protein, but this same receptor protein has the capacity to regulate several different genes in different target cells. This, of course, suggests that the nuclear chromatin of each cell type is organized so that only the appropriate genes are made available for regulation by the hormone-receptor complex. The thyroid hormone triiodothyronine (T3) also acts, though by a different mechanism than the steroids, at the cell nucleus level to initiate genomic transcription. The hormonal activities of GH and prolactin influence cellular gene transcription and translation of messenger RNA by complex mechanisms.

2.3 Endocrine System: Some Other Aspects of Regulation and Control

From the foregoing sections it is clear that the endocrine system exhibits complex molecular and metabolic dynamics which involve many levels of control and regulation. Hormones are chemical signals released from a hierarchy of endocrine glands and propagated through the circulation to a hierarchy of cell types. The integration of this system depends on a series of what systems engineers call "feedback

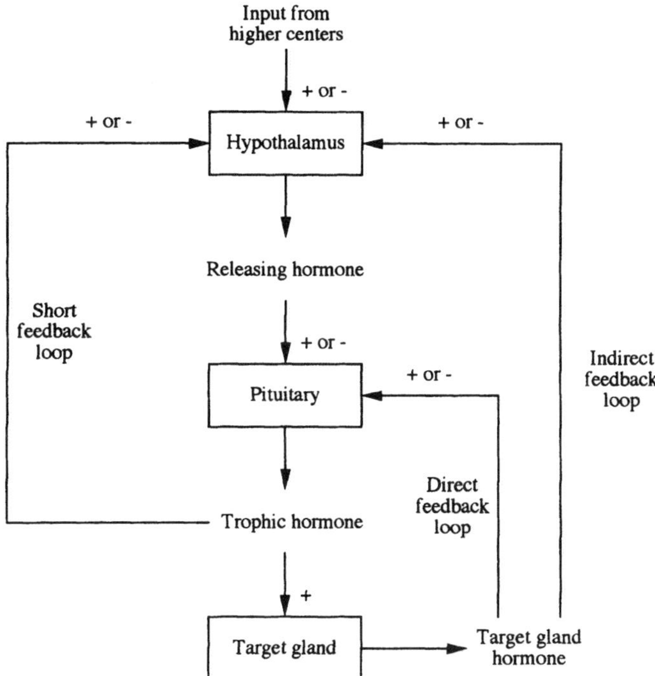

FIGURE 2.2 Illustration of the complexity of hormonal feedback control (+ indicates a positive or augmenting effect; – indicates a negative or inhibiting effect).

loops"; feedback is a reflection of mutual dependence of the system variables: variable x affects variable y, and y affects x. Further, it is essentially a closed-loop system in which the feedback of information from the system output to the input has the capacity to maintain homeostasis. A diagrammatic representation of the ways in which hormone action is controlled is shown in Fig. 2.2. One example of this control structure arises in the context of the thyroid hormones. In this case, TRH, secreted by the hypothalamus, triggers the anterior pituitary into the production of TSH. The target gland is the thyroid, which produces T3 and thyroxine (T4). The complexity of control includes both direct and indirect feedback of T3 and T4, as outlined in Fig. 2.2, together with TSH feedback on to the hypothalamus.

Negative Feedback

If an increase in y causes a change in x which in turn tends to decrease y, feedback is said to be *negative;* in other words, the signal output induces a response that feeds back to the signal generator to decrease its output. This is the most common form of control in physiologic systems, and examples are many. For instance, as mentioned earlier, the anterior pituitary releases trophic or stimulating hormones that act on peripheral endocrine glands such as the adrenals or thyroid or on gonads to produce hormones that act back on the pituitary to decrease the secretion of the trophic hormones. These are examples of what is called *long-loop feedback* (see Fig. 2.2). (**Note:** The adjectives *long* and *short* reflect the spatial distance or proximity of effector and target sites.) The trophic hormones of the pituitary are also regulated by feedback action at the level of their releasing factors. *Ultrashort-loop feedback* is also described. There are numerous examples of *short-loop feedback* as well, the best being the reciprocal relation between insulin and blood glucose concentrations, as depicted in Fig. 2.3. In this case, elevated glucose concentration (and positive rate of change, implying not only proportional but also derivative control) has a positive effect on the pancreas, which secretes insulin in response. This has an inhibiting effect on glucose metabolism, resulting in a reduction of blood glucose toward a normal concentration; in other words, classic negative-feedback control.

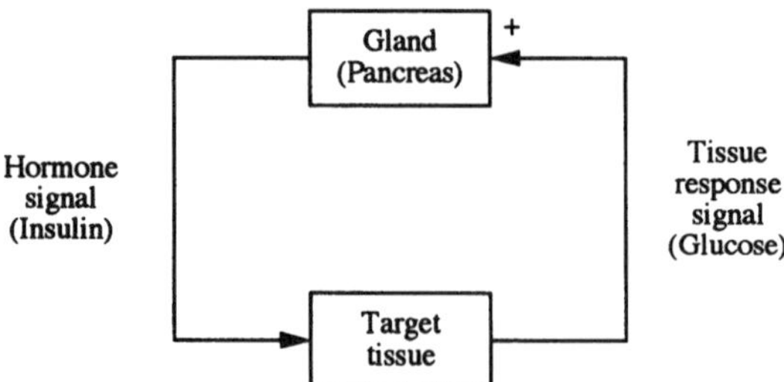

FIGURE 2.3 The interaction of insulin as an illustration of negative feedback within a hormonal control system.

Positive Feedback

If increase in y causes a change in x which tends to increase y, feedback is said to be *positive*; in other words, a further signal output is evoked by the response it induces or provokes. This is intrinsically an unstable system, but there are physiologic situations where such control is valuable. In the positive feedback situation, the signal output will continue until no further response is required. Suckling provides an example; stimulation of nipple receptors by the suckling child provokes an increased oxytocin release from the posterior pituitary with a corresponding increase in milk flow. Removal of the stimulus causes cessation of oxytocin release.

Rhythmic Endocrine Control

Many hormone functions exhibit rhythmically in the form of pulsatile release of hormones. The most common is the approximately 24-h cycle (circadian or diurnal rhythm). For instance, blood sampling at frequent intervals has shown that ACTH is secreted episodically, each secretory burst being followed 5 to 10 min later by cortisol secretion. These episodes are most frequent in the early morning, with plasma cortisol concentrations highest around 7 to 8 AM and lowest around midnight. ACTH and cortisol secretion vary inversely, and the parallel circadian rhythm is probably due to a cyclic change in the sensitivity of the hypothalamic feedback center to circulating cortisol. Longer cycles are also known, e.g., the infradian menstrual cycle.

It is clear that such inherent rhythms are important in endocrine communication and control, suggesting that its physiologic organization is based not only on the structural components of the system but also on the dynamics of their interactions. The rhythmic, pulsatile nature of release of many hormones is a means whereby time-varying signals can be encoded, thus allowing large quantities of information to be transmitted and exchanged rapidly in a way that small, continuous changes in threshold levels would not allow.

References

Inevitably, our brief exposition has been able to touch upon an enormous subject only by describing some of the salient features of this fascinating domain, but it is hoped that it may nevertheless stimulate a further interest. However, not surprisingly the endocrinology literature is massive and it is suggested that anyone wishing to read further turn initially to one of the many excellent textbooks and go on from there. Those we have found useful include:

Goodman HM. 1994. *Basic Medical Endocrinology,* New York, Raven Press. 2nd ed.

Greenspan FS, Strewler GJ (Eds.). 1997. *Basic and Clinical Endocrinology,* Norwalk, CT, Appleton & Lange. 5th ed.

O'Malley BW, Birnbaumer L, Hunter T (Eds.). 1998. *Hormones and Signaling.* (Vol. 1). New York, Academic Press.

Wilson JD, Foster DW, Kronenberg HM (Eds.). 1998. *Williams Textbook of Endocrinology,* Philadelphia, WB Saunders. 9th ed.

3

Nervous System

Evangelia Micheli-Tzanakou
Rutgers University

The nervous system, unlike other organ systems, is concerned primarily with signals, information encoding and processing, and control rather than manipulation of energy. It acts like a communication device whose components use substances and energy in processing signals and in reorganizing them, choosing, and commanding, as well as in developing and learning. A central question that is often asked is how nervous systems work and what are the principles of their operation. In an attempt to answer this question, we will, at the same time, ignore other fundamental questions, such as those relating to anatomic or neurochemical and molecular aspects. We will concentrate rather on relations and transactions between neurons and their assemblages in the nervous system. We will deal with neural signals (encoding and decoding), the evaluation and weighting of incoming signals, and the formulation of outputs. A major part of this chapter is devoted to higher aspects of the nervous system, such as memory and learning, rather than individual systems, such as vision and audition, which are treated extensively elsewhere in this book.

3.1 Definitions

Nervous systems can be defined as organized assemblies of nerve cells as well as nonnervous cells. Nerve cells, or *neurons*, are specialized in the generation, integration, and conduction of incoming signals from the outside world or from other neurons and deliver them to other excitable cells or to *effectors* such as muscle cells. Nervous systems are easily recognized in higher animals but not in the lower species, since the defining criteria are difficult to apply.

A central nervous system (CNS) can be distinguished easily from a peripheral nervous system (PNS), since it contains most of the motor and nucleated parts of neurons that innervate muscles and other effectors. The PNS contains all the sensory nerve cell bodies, with some exceptions, plus local *plexuses*, local *ganglia*, and peripheral axons that make up the *nerves*. Most sensory axons go all the way into the CNS, while the remaining sensory axons relay in peripheral plexuses. Motor axons originating in the CNS innervate effector cells.

The nervous system has two major roles: (1) to regulate, acting homeostatically in restoring some conditions of the organism after some external stimulus, and (2) to act to alter a preexisting condition by replacing it or modifying it. In both cases — regulation or initiation of a process — learning can be superimposed. In most species, learning is a more or less adaptive mechanism, combining and timing species-characteristic acts with a large degree of evolution toward perfection.

0-8493-1810-6/03/$0.00+$1.50

The nervous system is a complex structure for which realistic assumptions have led to irrelevant oversimplifications. One can break the nervous system down into four components: sensory transducers, neurons, axons, and muscle fibers. Each of these components gathers, processes, and transmits information impinging on it from the outside world, usually in the form of complex stimuli. The processing is carried out by exitable tissues — neurons, axons, sensory receptors, and muscle fibers. Neurons are the basic elements of the nervous system. If put in small assemblies or clusters, they form neuronal assemblies or neuronal networks communicating with each other either chemically via *synaptic junctions* or electrically via *tight* junctions. The main characteristics of a cell are the *cell body,* or *soma,* which contains the *nucleus,* and a number of processes originating from the cell body, called the *dendrites,* which reach out to surroundings to make contacts with other cells. These contacts serve as the incoming information to the cell, while the outgoing information follows a conduction path, the axon. The incoming information is integrated in the cell body and generates its action potential at the *axon hillock.* There are two types of outputs that can be generated and therefore two types of neurons: those which generate *graded* potentials that attenuate with distance and those which generate *action* potentials. The latter travel through the axon, a thin, long process that passively passes the action potential or rather a train of action potentials without any attenuation (*all-or-none effect*). A number of action potentials is often called a *spike train.* A threshold built into the hillock, depending on its level, allows or stops the generation of the spike train. Axons usually terminate on other neurons by means of *synaptic terminals* or *boutons* and have properties similar to those of an electric cable with varying diameters and speeds of signal transmission. Axons can be of two types: *myelinated* or *unmyelinated.* In the former case, the axon is surrounded by a thick fatty material, the myelin sheath, which is interrupted at regular intervals by gaps called the *nodes of Ranvier.* These nodes provide for the *saltatory* conduction of the signal along the axon. The axon makes functional connections with other neurons at synapses on the cell body, or the dendrites, or the axons. There exist two kinds of synapses: *excitatory* and *inhibitory,* and as the names imply, they either increase the *firing* frequency of the postsynaptic neurons or decrease it, respectively.

Sensory receptors are specialized cells that, in response to an incoming stimulus, generate a corresponding electrical signal, a graded receptor potential. Although the mechanisms by which the sensory receptors generate receptor potentials are not known exactly, the most plausible scenario is that an external stimulus alters the membrane permeabilities. The receptor potential, then, is the change in intracellular potential relative to the *resting* potential.

It is important to notice here that the term *receptor* is used in physiology to refer not only to sensory receptors but also, in a different sense, to proteins that bind neurotransmitters, hormones, and other substances with great affinity and specificity as a first step in starting up physiologic responses. This receptor is often associated with nonneural cells that surround it and form a *sense organ.* The forms of energy converted by the receptors include mechanical, thermal, electromagnetic, and chemical energy. The particular form of energy to which a receptor is most sensitive is called its *adequate stimulus.* The problem of how receptors convert energy into action potentials in the sensory nerves has been the subject of intensive study. In the complex sense organs, such as those concerned with hearing and vision, there exist separate receptor cells and synaptic junctions between receptors and afferent nerves. In other cases, such as the cutaneous sense organs, the receptors are specialized. Where a stimulus of constant strength is applied to a receptor repeatedly, the frequency of the action potentials in its sensory nerve declines over a period of time. This phenomenon is known as *adaptation.* If the adaptation is very rapid, then the receptors are called *phasic*; otherwise, they are called *tonic.*

Another important issue is the *coding* of sensory information. Action potentials are similar in all nerves, although there are variations in their speed of conduction and other characteristics. However, if the action potentials were the same in most cells, then what makes the visual cells sensitive to light and not to sound and the touch receptors sensitive to touch and not to smell? And how can we tell if these sensations are strong or not? These sensations depend on what is called the *doctrine of specific nerve energies,* which has been questioned over time by several researchers. No matter where a particular sensory pathway is stimulated along its course to the brain, the sensation produced is referred to the location of the receptor. This is the *law of projections.* An example of this law is the "phantom limb," in which an amputee complains about an itching sensation in the amputated limb.

3.2 Functions of the Nervous System

The basic unit of integrated activity is the *reflex arc.* This arc consists of a sense organ, afferent neuron, one or more synapses in a central integrating station (or sympathetic ganglion), an efferent neuron, and an effector. The simplest reflex arc is the *monosynaptic* one, which has only one synapse between the afferent and efferent neurons. With more than one synapse, the reflex arc is called *polysynaptic.* In each of these cases, activity is modified by both spatial and temporal facilitation, occlusion, and other effects.

In mammals, the concentration between afferent and efferent somatic neurons is found either in the brain or in the spinal cord. The Bell-Magendie law dictates that in the spinal cord the dorsal roots are sensory, while the ventral roots are motor. The action potential message that is carried by an axon is eventually fed to a muscle, to a secretory cell, or to the dendrite of another neuron. If an axon is carrying a graded potential, its output is too weak to stimulate a muscle, but it can terminate on a secretory cell or dendrite. The latter can have as many as 10,000 inputs. If the endpoint is a motor neuron, which has been found experimentally in the case of fibers from the primary endings, then there is a lag between the time when the stimulus was applied and when the response is obtained from the muscle. This time interval is called the *reaction time* and in humans is approximately 20 ms for a stretch reflex. The distance from the spinal cord can be measured, and since the conduction velocities of both the efferent and afferent fibers are known, another important quality can be calculated: the *central delay.* This delay is the portion of the reaction time that was spent for conduction to and from the spinal cord. It has been found that muscle spindles also make connections that cause muscle contraction via polysynaptic pathways, while the afferents from secondary endings make connections that excite extensor muscles. When a motor neuron sends a burst of action potentials to its skeletal muscle, the amount of contraction depends largely on the discharge frequency but also on many other factors, such as the history of the load on the muscle and the load itself. The *stretch error* can be calculated from the desired motion minus the actual stretch. If this error is then fed back to the motor neuron, its discharge frequency is modified appropriately. This corresponds to one of the three feedback loops that are available locally. Another loop corrects for overstretching beyond the point that the muscle or tendon may tear. Since a muscle can only contract, it must be paired with another muscle (*antagonist*) in order to effect the return motion. Generally speaking, a flexor muscle is paired with an extensor muscle that cannot be activated simultaneously. This means that the motor neurons that affect each one of these are not activated at the same time. Instead, when one set of motor neurons is activated, the other is inhibited, and vice versa. When movement involves two or more muscles that normally cooperate by contracting simultaneously, the excitation of one causes facilitation of the other *synergistic* members via cross-connections. All these networks form feedback loops. An engineer's interpretation of how these loops work would be to assume dynamic conditions, as is the case in all parts of the nervous system. This has little value in dealing with stationary conditions, but it provides for an ability to adjust to changing conditions.

The nervous system, as mentioned earlier, is a control system of processes that adjust both internal and external operations. As humans, we have experiences that change our perceptions of events in our environment. The same is true for higher animals, which, besides having an internal environment the status of which is of major importance, also share an external environment of utmost richness and variety. Objects and conditions that have direct contact with the surface of an animal directly affect the future of the animal. Information about changes at some point provides a prediction of possible future status. The amount of information required to represent changing conditions increases as the required temporal resolution of detail increases. This creates a vast amount of data to be processed by any finite system. Considering that the information reaching sensory receptors is too extensive and redundant, as well as modified by external interference (noise), the nervous system has a tremendously difficult task to accomplish. Enhanced responsiveness to a particular stimulus can be produced by structures that either increase the energy converging on a receptor or increase the effectiveness of coupling of a specific type of stimulus with its receptor. Different species have sensory systems that respond to stimuli that are important to them for survival. Often one nervous system responds to conditions that are not sensed by another nervous system. The transduction, processing, and transmission of signals in any nervous system produce a survival mechanism for an organism but only after these signals have been further modified by effector organs. Although the nerve impulses that drive a muscle, as explained earlier, are discrete events, a muscle twitch takes much longer to happen, a fact that allows for their responses to overlap and produce a much smoother output. Neural control of motor activity of skeletal muscle is accomplished entirely by the modification of muscle excitation, which involves changes in velocity, length, stiffness, and heat production. The importance of accurate timing of inputs and the maintenance of this timing across several synapses is obvious in sensory pathways of the nervous system. Cells are located next to other cells that have overlapping or adjacent receptor or motor fields. The dendrites provide important and complicated sites of interactions as well as channels of variable effectiveness for excitatory inputs, depending on their position relative to the cell body. Among the best examples are the cells of the medial superior olive in the auditory pathway. These cells have two major dendritic trees extending from opposite poles of the cell body. One receives synaptic inhibitory input from the ipsilateral cochlear nucleus, the other from the contralateral nucleus that normally is an excitatory input. These cells deal with the determination of the azimuth of a sound. When a sound is present on the contralateral side, most cells are excited, while ipsilateral sounds cause inhibition. It has been shown that the cells can go from complete excitation to full inhibition with a difference of only a few hundred milliseconds in arrival time of the two inputs.

The question then arises: How does the nervous system put together the signals available to it so that a determination of output can take place? To arrive at an understanding of how the nervous system intergrates incoming information at a given moment of time, we must understand that the processes that take place depend both on cellular forms and a topologic architecture and on the physiologic properties that relate input to output. That is, we have to know the *transfer* functions or *coupling* functions. Integration depends on the weighting of inputs. One of the important factors determining weighting is the area of synaptic contact. The extensive dendrites are the primary integrating structures. Electronic spread is the means of mixing, smoothing, attenuating, delaying, and summing postsynaptic potentials. The spatial distribution of input is often not random but systematically restricted. Also, the wide variety of characteristic geometries of synapses is no doubt important not only for the weighting of different combinations of inputs. When repeated stimuli are presented at various intervals at different junctions, increasing synaptic potentials are generated if the intervals between them are not too short or too long. This increase is due to a phenomenon called *facilitation.* If the response lasts longer than the interval between impulses, such that the second response rises from the residue of the first, then it is temporal summation. If, in addition, the response increment due to the second stimulus is larger than the preceding one, then it is facilitation. Facilitation is an important function of the nervous system and is found in quite different forms and durations ranging from a few milliseconds to tenths of seconds. Facilitation may grade from forms of sensitization to learning, especially at long intervals. A special case is the so-called *posttetanic potentiation* that is the result of high-frequency stimulation for long periods of time (about 10 s). This is an interesting case, since no effects can be seen during stimulation, but afterwards, any test stimulus at various intervals creates a marked increase in response up to many times more than the "tetanic" stimulus. *Antifacilitation* is the phenomenon where a decrease of response from the neuron is observed at certain junctions due to successive impulses. Its mechanism is less understood than facilitation. Both facilitation and antifacilitation may be observed on the same neuron but in different functions of it.

3.3 Representation of Information in the Nervous System

Whenever information is transferred between different parts of the nervous system, some communication paths have to be established, and some parameters of impulse firing relevant to communication must be set up. Since what is communicated is nothing more than impulses — spike trains — the only basic variables in a train of events are the number and intervals between spikes. With respect to this, the nervous system acts like a pulse-coded analog device, since the intervals are continuously graded. There exists a distribution of interval lengths between individual spikes, which in any sample can be expressed by the shape of the interval histogram. If one examines different examples, their distributions differ markedly. Some histograms look like Poisson distributions; some others exhibit Gaussian or bimodal shapes. The coefficient of variation — expressed as the standard deviation over the mean — in some cases is constant, while in others it varies. Some other properties depend on the sequence of longer and shorter intervals than the mean. Some neurons show no linear dependence; some others show positive or negative correlations of successive intervals. If a stimulus is delivered and a discharge from the neuron is observed, a *poststimulus time histogram* can be used, employing the onset of the stimulus as a reference point and averaging many responses in order to reveal certain consistent features of temporal patterns. Coding of information can then be based on the average frequency, which can represent relevant gradations of the input. Mean frequency is the code in most cases, although no definition of it has been given with respect to measured quantities, such as averaging time, weighting functions, and forgetting functions. Characteristic transfer functions have been found, which suggests that there are several distinct coding principles in addition to the mean frequency. Each theoretically possible code becomes a candidate code as long as there exists some evidence that is readable by the system under investigation. Therefore, one has to first test for the availability of the code by imposing a stimulus that is considered "normal." After a response has been observed, the code is considered to be available. If the input is then changed to different levels of one parameter and changes are observed at the postsynaptic level, the code is called *readable.* However, only if both are formed in the same preparation and no other parameter is available and readable can the code be said to be the *actual* code employed. Some such parameters follow:

1. Time of firing
2. Temporal pattern
3. Number of spikes in the train
4. Variance of interspike intervals
5. Spike delays or latencies
6. Constellation code

The last is a very important parameter, especially when used in conjunction with the concept of *receptive fields* of units in the different sensory pathways. The unit receptors do not need to have highly specialized abilities to permit encoding of a large number of distinct stimuli. Receptive fields are topographic and overlap extensively. Any given stimulus will excite a certain constellation of receptors and is therefore encoded in the particular set that is activated. A large degree of uncertainty prevails and requires the brain to operate probabilistically. In the nervous system there exists a large amount of *redundancy,* although neurons might have different thresholds. It is questionable, however, if these units are entirely equivalent, although they share parts of their receptive fields. The nonoverlapping parts might be of importance and critical to sensory function. On the other hand, redundancy does not necessarily mean unspecified or random connectivity. Rather, it allows for greater sensitivity and resolution, improvement of signal-to-noise ratio, while at the same time it provides stability of performance.

Integration of large numbers of converging inputs to give a single output can be considered as an averaging or probabilistic operation. The "decisions" made by a unit depend on its inputs, or some intrinsic states, and reaching a certain threshold. This way every unit in the nervous system can make a decision when it changes from one state to a different one. A theoretical possibility also exists that a mass of randomly connected neurons may constitute a trigger unit and that activity with a sharp threshold can spread through such a mass redundancy. Each part of the nervous system, and in particular the receiving side, can be thought of as a filter. Higher-order neurons do not merely pass their information on, but instead they use convergence from different channels, as well as divergence of the same channels and other processes, in order to modify incoming signals. Depending on the structure and coupling functions of the network, what gets through is determined. Similar networks exist at the output side.

They also act as filters, but since they formulate decisions and commands with precise *spatiotemporal* properties, they can be thought of as *pattern generators.*

3.4 Lateral Inhibition

This discussion would be incomplete without a description of a very important phenomenon in the nervous system. This phenomenon, called *lateral inhibition,* is used by the nervous system to improve spatial resolution and contrast. The effectiveness of this type of inhibition decreases with distance. In the retina, for example, lateral inhibition is used extensively in order to improve contrast. As the stimulus approaches a certain unit, it first excites neighbors of the recorded cell. Since these neighbors inhibit that unit, it responds by a decrease in firing frequency. If the stimulus is exactly over the recorded unit, this unit is excited and fires above its normal rate, and as the stimulus moves out again, the neighbors are excited, while the unit under consideration fires less. If we now examine the output of all the units as a whole, and while half the considered array is stimulated and the other half is not, we will notice that at the point of discontinuity of the stimulus going from stimulation to nonstimulation, the firing frequencies of the two halves have been differentiated to the extreme at the stimulus edge, which has been enhanced. The neuronal circuits responsible for lateral shifts are relatively simple. Lateral inhibition can be considered to give the negative of the second spatial derivative of the input stimulus. A second layer of neurons could be constructed to perform this spatial differentiation on the input signal to detect the edge only. It is probably lateral inhibition that explains the psychophysical illusion known as *Mach bands.* It is probably the same principle that operates widely in the nervous system to enhance the sensitivity to contrast in the visual system in particular and in all other modalities in general. Through the years, different models have been developed to describe lateral inhibition mathematically, and various methods of analysis have been employed. Such methods include:

Functional notations
Graphic solutions
Tabular solution
Taylor's series expansions
Artificial neural network modeling

These models include both one-dimensional examination of the phenomenon and two-dimensional treatment, where a two-dimensional array is used as a stimulus. This two-dimensional treatment is justified because most of the sensory receptors of the body form two-dimensional maps (receptive fields). In principle, if a one-dimensional lateral inhibition system is linear, one can extend the analysis to two dimensions by means of superposition. The two-dimensional array can be thought of as a function $f(x, y)$, and the lateral inhibition network itself is embodied in a separate $N \times N$ array, the central square of which has a positive value and can be thought of as a direct input from an incoming axon. The surrounding squares have negative values that are higher than the corner values, which are also negative. The method consists of multiplying the input signal values $f(x, y)$ and their contiguous values by the lateral inhibitory network's weighting factors to get a corresponding $g(x, y)$. Figure 3.1 presents an example of such a process. The technique illustrated here is used in the contrast enhancement of photographs. The objective is the same as that of the nervous system: to improve image sharpness without introducing too much distortion. This technique requires storage of each picture element and lateral "inhibitory" interactions between adjacent elements. Since a picture may contain millions of elements, high-speed computers with large-scale memories are required.

At a higher level, similar algorithms can be used to evaluate decision-making mechanisms. In this case, many inputs from different sensory systems are competing for attention. The brain evaluates each one of the inputs as a function of the remaining ones. One can picture a decision-making mechanism resembling a "locator" of stimulus peaks. The final output depends on what weights are used at the inputs of a push-pull mechanism. Thus a decision can be made depending on the weights as an individual's

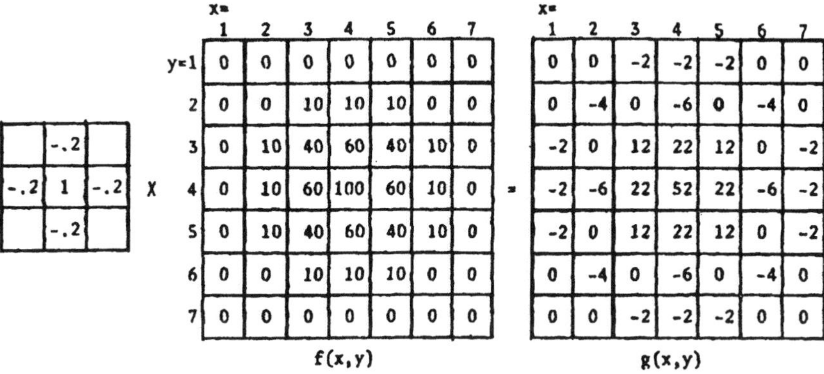

FIGURE 3.1 An example of two-dimensional lateral inhibition. On the left, the 3 × 3 array corresponds to the values of the synaptic junctions weighting coefficients. For simplicity, the corner weights are assumed to be zero. $g(x, y)$ represents the output matrix after lateral inhibition has been applied to the input matrix.

brain is applying to the incoming information about a situation under consideration. The most important information is heavily weighted, while the rest is either totally masked or weighted very lightly.

3.5 Higher Functions of the Nervous System

Pattern Recognition

One way of understanding human perception is to study the mechanism of information processing in the brain. The recognition of patterns of sensory input is one of the functions of the brain, a task accomplished by neuronal circuits, the *feature extractors.* Although such neuronal information is more likely to be processed globally by a large number of neurons, in animals, single-unit recording is one of the most powerful tools in the hands of the physiologist. Most often, the concept of the *receptive field* is used as a method of understanding sensory information processing. In the case of the visual system, one could call the receptive field a well-defined region of the visual field which, when stimulated, will change the firing rate of a neuron in the visual pathway. The response of that neuron will usually depend on the distribution of light in the receptive field. Therefore, the information collected by the brain from the outside world is transformed into spatial as well as temporal patterns of neuronal activity.

The question often asked is how do we perceive and recognize faces, objects, and scenes. Even in those cases where only noisy representations exist, we are still able to make some inference as to what the pattern represents. Unfortunately, in humans, single-unit recording, as mentioned above, is impossible. As a result, one has to use other kinds of measurements, such as *evoked potentials* (EPs). Although physiologic in nature, EPs are still far from giving us information at the neuronal level. Yet EPs have been used extensively as a way of probing human (and animal) brains because of their noninvasive character. EPs can be considered to be the result of integrations of the neuronal activity of many neurons some place in the brain. This gross potential can then be used as a measure of the response of the brain to sensory input.

The question then becomes: Can we somehow use this response to influence the brain in producing patterns of activity that we want? None of the efforts of the past closed this loop. How do we explain then the phenomenon of selective attention by which we selectively direct our attention to something of interest and discard the rest? And what happens with the evolution of certain species that change appearance according to their everyday needs? All these questions tend to lead to the fact that somewhere in the brain there is a loop where previous knowledge or experience is used as a feedback to the brain itself. This feedback then modifies the ability of the brain to respond in a different way to the same stimulus the next time it is presented. In a way, then, the brain creates mental "images" independent of the stimulus which tend to modify the representation of the stimulus in the brain.

This section describes some efforts in which different methods have been used in trying to address the difficult task of feedback loops in the brain. However, no attempt will be made to explain or even postulate where these feedback loops might be located. If one considers the brain as a huge set of neural nets, then one question has been debated for many years: What is the role of the individual neuron in the net, and what is the role of each network in the holistic process of the brain? More specifically, does the neuron act as an analyzer or a detector of specific features, or does it merely reflect the characteristic response of a population of cells of which it happens to be a member? What invariant relationships exist between sensory input and the response of a single neuron, and how much can be "read" about the stimulus parameters from the record of a single EP? In turn, then, how much feedback can one use from a single EP in order to influence the stimulus, and how successful can that influence be? Many physiologists express doubts that simultaneous observations of large numbers of individual neuronal activities can be readily interpreted. The main question we are asking is: Can a feedback process influence and modulate the stimuli patterns so that they appear optimal? If this is proved to be true, it would mean that we can reverse the pattern-recognition process, and instead of recognizing a pattern, we would be able to create a pattern from a vast variety of possible patterns. It would be like creating a link between our brain and a computer; equivalent to a brain-computer system network. Figure 3.2 is a schematic representation of such a process involved in what we call the *feedback loop* of the system. The pattern-recognition device (PRD) is connected to an ALOPEX system (a computer algorithm and an image processor in this case) and faces a display monitor where different-intensity patterns can be shown. Thin arrows representing response information and heavy arrows representing detailed pattern information are generated by the computer and relayed by the ALOPEX system to the monitor. ALOPEX is a set of algorithms described in detail elsewhere in this book. If this kind of arrangement is used for the determination of visual receptive fields of neurons, then the PRD is nothing more than the brain of an experimental animal. This way the neuron under investigation does its own selection of the best stimulus or trigger feature and reverses the role of the neuron from being a feature extractor to becoming a feature generator, as mentioned earlier. The idea is to find the response of the neuron to a stimulus and use this response as a positive feedback in the directed evaluation of the initially random pattern. Thus the cell involved filters out the key trigger features from the stimulus and reinforces them with the feedback.

As a generalization of this process, one might consider that a neuron N receives a visual input from a pattern P which is transmitted in a modified form P' to an analyzer neuron AN (or even a complex of

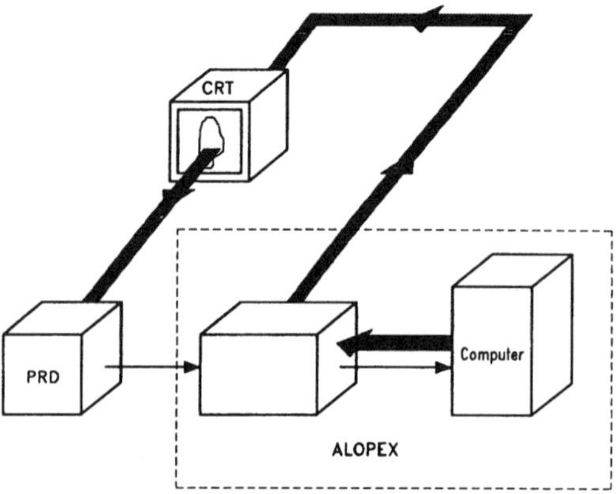

FIGURE 3.2 An ALOPEX system. The stimulus is presented on the CRT. The observer or any pattern-recognition device (PRD) faces the CRT; the subject's response is sent to the ALOPEX interface unit, where it is recorded and integrated, and the final response is sent to the computer. The computer calculates the values of the new pattern to be presented on the CRT according to the ALOPEX algorithm, and the process continues until the desired pattern appears on the CRT. At this point, the response is considered to be optimal and the process stops.

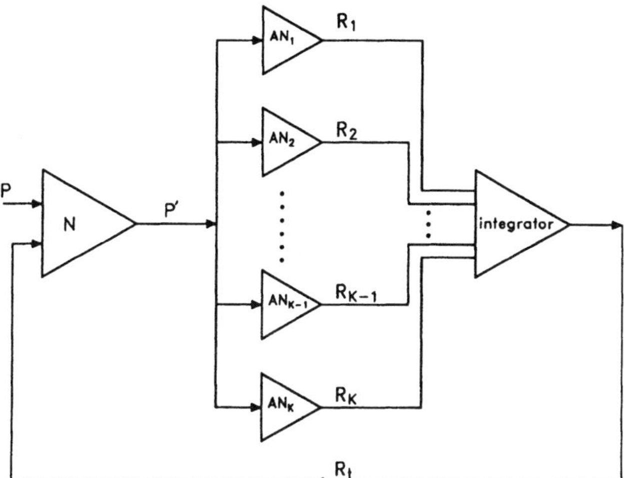

FIGURE 3.3 Diagrammatic representation of the ALOPEX "inverse" pattern-recognition scheme. Each neuron represents a feature analyzer that responds to the stimulus with a scalar quantity R called the *response.* R is then fed back to the system, and the pattern is modified accordingly. This process continues until there is a close correlation between the desired output and the original pattern.

neurons), as shown in Fig. 3.3. The analyzer responds with a scalar variable R that is then fed back to the system, and the pattern is modified accordingly. The process continues in small steps until there is an almost perfect correlation between the original pattern (template) and the one that neuron N indirectly created. This integrator sends the response back to the original modifier. The integrator need not be a linear summator. It could take any nonlinear form, a fact that is a more realistic representation of the visual cortex. One can envision the input patterns as templates preexisting in the memory of the system, a situation that might come about with visual experience. For a "naive" system, any initial pattern will do. As experience is gained, the patterns become less random. If one starts with a pattern that has some resemblance to one of the preexisting patterns, evolution will take its course. In nature, there might exist a mechanism similar to that of ALOPEX. By filtering the characteristics most important for the survival of the species, changes would be triggered. Perception, therefore, could be considered to be an interaction between sensory inputs and past experience in the form of templates stored in the memory of the perceiver and specific to the perceiver's needs. These templates are modifiable with time and adjusted accordingly to the input stimuli. With this approach, the neural nets and ensembles of nets under observation generate patterns that describe their thinking and memory properties. The normal flow of information is reversed and controls the afferent systems.

The perception processes as well as feature extraction or suppression of images or objects can be ascribed to specific neural mechanisms due to some sensory input or even due to some "wishful thinking" of the PRD. If it is true that the association cortex is affecting the sensitivity of the sensory cortex, then an ALOPEX mechanism is what one needs to close the loop for memory and learning.

Memory and Learning

If we try to define what memory is, we will face the fact that memory is not a single mental faculty but is rather composed of multiple abilities mediated by separate and distinct brain systems. Memory for a recent event can be expressed *explicitly* as a conscious recollection or *implicitly* as a facilitation of test performance without conscious recollection. The major distinction between these two memories is that explicit or *declarative* memory depends on limbic and diencephalic structures and provides the basis for recollection of events, while implicit or *nondeclarative* memory supports skills and habit learning, single conditioning, and the well-researched phenomenon of *priming.*

Declarative memory refers to memory of recent events and is usually assessed by tests of recall or recognition for specific single items. When the list of items becomes longer, a subject not only learns about each item on the list but also makes associations about what all these items have in common; i.e., the subject learns about the category that the items belong to. Learning leads to changes that increase or decrease the effectiveness of impulses arriving at the junctions between neurons, and the cumulative effect of these changes constitutes memory. Very often a particular pattern of neural activity leads to a result that occurs some time after the activity has ended. Learning then requires some means of relating the activity that is to be changed to the evaluation that can be made only by the delayed consequence. This phenomenon in physics is called *hysteresis* and refers to any modifications of future actions due to past actions. *Learning* then could be defined as change in any neuronal response resulting from previous experiences due to an external stimulus. Memory, in turn, would be the maintenance of these changes over time. The collection of neural changes representing memory is commonly known as the *engram*, and a major part of recent work has been to identify and locate engrams in the brain, since specific parts of the nervous system are capable of specific types of learning. The view of memory that has recently emerged is that information storage is tied to specific processing areas that are engaged during learning. The brain is organized so that separate regions of neocortex simultaneously carry out computations on specific features or characteristics of the external stimulus, no matter how complex that stimulus might be. If the brain learns specific properties or features of the stimulus, then we talk about the *nonassociative memory.* Associated with this type of learning is the phenomenon of *habituation*, in which if the same stimulus is presented repeatedly, the neurons respond less and less, while the introduction of a new stimulus increases the sensitization of the neuron. If the learning includes two related stimuli, then we talk about associative learning. This type of learning includes two types: *classic conditioning* and *operant conditioning.* The first deals with relationships among stimuli, while the latter deals with the relationship of the stimulus to the animal's own behavior. In humans, there exist two types of memory: *short-term* and *long-term memories.* The best way to study any physiologic process in humans, and especially memory, is to study its pathology. The study of amnesia has provided strong evidence distinguishing between these types of memory. Amnesic patients can keep a short list of numbers in mind for several minutes if they pay attention to the task. The difficulty comes when the list becomes longer, especially if the amount to be learned exceeds the brain capacity of what can be held in immediate memory. It could be that this happens because more systems have to be involved and that temporary information storage may occur within each brain area where stable changes in synaptic efficacy can eventually develop. *Plasticity* within existing pathways can account for most of the observations, and short-term memory occurs too quickly for it to require any major modifications of neuronal pathways. The capacity of long-term memory requires the integrity of the medial temporal and diencephalic regions in conjunction with neurons for storage of information. Within the domain of long-term memory, amnesic patients demonstrate intact learning and retention of certain motor, perceptual, and cognitive skills and intact priming effects. These patients do not exhibit any learning deficits but have no conscious awareness of prior study sessions or recognition of previously presented stimuli.

Priming effects can be tested by presenting words and then providing either the first few letters of the word or the last part of the word for recognition by the patient. Normal subjects, as expected, perform better than amnesic subjects. However, if these patients are instructed to "read" the incomplete word instead of memorizing it, then they perform as well as the normal individuals. Also, these amnesic patients perform well if words are cued by category names. Thus priming effects seem to be independent of the processes of recall and recognition memory, which is also observed in normal subjects. All this evidence supports the notion that the brain has organized its memory functions around fundamentally different information storage systems. In perceiving a word, a preexisting array of neurons is activated that have concurrent activities that produce perception, and priming is one of these functions.

Memory is not fixed immediately after learning but continues to grow toward stabilization over a period of time. This stabilization is called *consolidation of memory.* Memory consolidation is a *dynamic* feature of long-term memory, especially the declarative memory, but it is neither an automatic process with fixed lifetime nor is it determined at the time of learning. It is rather a process of reorganization of stored information. As time passes, some not yet consolidated memories fade out by remodeling the neural circuitry that is responsible for the original representation or by establishing new representations, since the original one can be forgotten.

The problems of learning and memory are studied continuously and with increased interest these days, especially because artificial systems such as neural networks can be used to mimic functions of the nervous system.

References

Cowan WM, Cuenod M (Eds). 1975. Use of Axonal Transport for Studies of Neuronal Connectivity. New York, Elsevier.

Deutsch S, Micheli-Tzanakou E. 1987. Neuroelectric Systems. New York, New York University Press.

Ganong WF. 1989. Review of Medical Physiology, 14th ed. Norwalk, CT, Appleton & Lange.

Hartzell HC. 1981. Mechanisms of slow postsynaptic potentials. Nature 291:593.

McMahon TA. 1984. Muscles, Reflexes and Locomotion. Princeton, NJ, Princeton University Press.

Partridge LD, Partridge DL. 1993. The Nervous System: Its Function and Interaction with the World. Cambridge, MA, MIT Press.

Shepherd GM. 1978. Microcircuits in the nervous system. Sci Am 238(2):92–103.

4

Vision System

George Stetten
Duke University

David Marr, an early pioneer in computer vision, defined *vision* as extracting "from images of the external world, a description that is useful for the viewer and not cluttered with irrelevant information" [Marr, 1982]. Advances in computers and video technology in the past decades have created the expectation that artificial vision should be realizable. The nontriviality of the task is evidenced by the continuing proliferation of new and different approaches to computer vision without any observable application in our everyday lives. Actually, computer vision is already offering practical solutions in industrial assembly and inspection, as well as for military and medical applications, so it seems we are beginning to master some of the fundamentals. However, we have a long way to go to match the vision capabilities of a 4-year-old child. In this chapter we will explore what is known about how nature has succeeded at this formidable task — that of interpreting the visual world.

4.1 Fundamentals of Vision Research

Research into biologic vision systems has followed several distinct approaches. The oldest is psychophysics, in which human and animal subjects are presented with visual stimuli and their responses recorded. Important early insights also were garnered by correlating clinical observations of visual defects with known neuroanatomic injury. In the past 50 years, a more detailed approach to understanding the mechanisms of vision has been undertaken by inserting small electrodes deep within the living brain to monitor the electrical activity of individual neurons and by using dyes and biochemical markers to track the anatomic course of nerve tracts. This research has led to a detailed and coherent, if not complete, theory of a visual system capable of explaining the discrimination of form, color, motion, and depth. This theory has been confirmed by noninvasive radiologic techniques that have been used recently to study the physiologic responses of the visual system, including positron emission tomography [Zeki et al., 1991] and functional magnetic resonance imaging [Belliveau et al., 1992; Cohen and Bookheimer, 1994], although these noninvasive techniques provide far less spatial resolution and thus can only show general regions of activity in the brain.

4.2 A Modular View of the Vision System

The Eyes

Movement of the eyes is essential to vision, not only allowing rapid location and tracking of objects but also preventing stationary images on the retina, which are essentially invisible. Continual movement of the image on the retina is essential to the visual system.

0-8493-1810-6/03/$0.00+$1.50

The eyeball is spherical and therefore free to turn in both the horizontal and vertical directions. Each eye is rotated by three pairs of mutually opposing muscles, innervated by the oculomotor nuclei in the brainstem. The eyes are coordinated as a pair in two useful ways: turning together to find and follow objects and turning inward to allow adjustment for parallax as objects become closer. The latter is called *convergence.*

The optical portion of the eye, which puts an image on the retina, is closely analogous to a photographic or television camera. Light enters the eye, passing through a series of transparent layers — the cornea, the aqueous humor, the lens, and the vitreous body — to eventually project on the retina.

The *cornea,* the protective outer layer of the eye, is heavily innervated with sensory neurons, triggering the blink reflex and tear duck secretion in response to irritation. The cornea is also an essential optical element, supplying two-thirds of the total refraction in the eye. Behind the cornea is a clear fluid, the *aqueous humor,* in which the central aperture of the iris, the pupil, is free to constrict or dilate. The two actions are accomplished by opposing sets of muscles.

The *lens,* a flexible transparent object behind the iris, provides the remainder of refraction necessary to focus an image on the retina. The ciliary muscles surrounding the lens can increase the lens' curvature, thereby decreasing its focal length and bringing nearer objects into focus. This is called *accommodation.* When the ciliary muscles are at rest, distant objects are in focus. There are no contradictory muscles to flatten the lens. This depends simply on the elasticity of the lens, which decreases with age. Behind the lens is the *vitreous humor,* consisting of a semigelatinous material filling the volume between the lens and the retina.

The Retina

The retina coats the back of the eye and is therefore spherical, not flat, making optical magnification constant at 3.5° of scan angle per millimeter. The retina is the neuronal front end of the visual system, the image sensor. In addition, it accomplishes the first steps in edge detection and color analysis before sending the processed information along the optic nerve to the brain. The retina contains five major classes of cells, roughly organized into layers. The dendrites of these cells each occupy no more than 1 to 2 mm^2 in the retina, limiting the extent of spatial integration from one layer of the retina to the next.

First come the *receptors,* which number approximately 125 million in each eye and contain the light-sensitive pigments responsible for converting photons into chemical energy. Receptor cells are of two general varieties: *rods* and *cones.* The cones are responsible for the perception of color, and they function only in bright light. When the light is dim, only rods are sensitive enough to respond. Exposure to a single photon may result in a measurable increase in the membrane potential of a rod. This sensitivity is the result of a chemical cascade, similar in operation to the photo multiplier tube, in which a single photon generates a cascade of electrons. All rods use the same pigment, whereas three different pigments are found in three separate kinds of cones.

Examination of the retina with an otoscope reveals its gross topography. The yellow circular area occupying the central 5° of the retina is called the *macula lutea,* within which a small circular pit called the *fovea* may be seen. Detailed vision occurs only in the fovea, where a dense concentration of cones provides visual activity to the central 1° of the visual field.

On the inner layer of the retina one finds a layer of *ganglion cells,* whose axons make up the optic nerve, the output of the retina. They number approximately 1 million, or less than 1% of the number of receptor cells. Clearly, some data compression has occurred in the space between the receptors and the ganglion cells. Traversing this space are the *bipolar cells,* which run from the receptors through the retina to the ganglion cells. Bipolar cells exhibit the first level of information processing in the visual system; namely, their response to light on the retina demonstrates "center/surround" receptive fields. By this I mean that a small dot on the retina elicits a response, while the area surrounding the spot elicits the opposite response. If both the center and the surround are illuminated, the net result is no response.

Thus bipolar cells respond only at the border between dark and light areas. Bipolar cells come in two varieties, on-center and off-center, with the center brighter or darker, respectively, than the surround.

The center response of bipolar cells results from direct contact with the receptors. The surround response is supplied by the *horizontal cells,* which run parallel to the surface of the retina between the receptor layer and the bipolar layer, allowing the surrounding area to oppose the influence of the center. The *amacrine cells,* a final cell type, also run parallel to the surface but in a different layer, between the bipolar cells and the ganglion cells, and are possibly involved in the detection of motion.

Ganglion cells, since they are triggered by bipolar cells, also have center/surround receptive fields and come in two types, on-center and off-center. On-center ganglion cells have a receptive field in which illumination of the center increases the firing rate and a surround where it decreases the rate. Off-center ganglion cells display the opposite behavior. Both types of ganglion cells produce little or no change in firing rate when the entire receptive field is illuminated, because the center and surround cancel each other. As in many other areas of the nervous system, the fibers of the optic nerve use frequency encoding to represent a scalar quantity.

Multiple ganglion cells may receive output from the same receptor, since many receptive fields overlap. However, this does not limit overall spatial resolution, which is maximum in the fovea, where two points separated by 0.5 min of arc may be discriminated. This separation corresponds to a distance on the retina of 2.5 μm, which is approximately the center-to-center spacing between cones. Spatial resolution falls off as one moves away from the fovea into the peripheral vision, where resolution is as low as 1° of arc.

Several aspects of this natural design deserve consideration. Why do we have center/surround receptive fields? The ganglion cells, whose axons make up the optic nerve, do not fire unless there is meaningful information, i.e., a border, falling within the receptive field. It is the edge of a shape we see rather than its interior. This represents a form of data compression. Center/surround receptive fields also allow for relative rather than absolute measurements of color and brightness. This is essential for analyzing the image independent of lighting conditions. Why do we have both on-center and off-center cells? Evidently, both light and dark are considered information. The same shape is detected whether it is lighter or darker than the background.

Optic Chiasm

The two optic nerves, from the left and right eyes, join at the optic chiasm, forming a *hemidecussation,* meaning that half the axons cross while the rest proceed uncrossed. The resulting two bundles of axons leaving the chiasm are called the *optic tracts.* The left optic tract contains only axons from the left half of each retina. Since the images are reversed by the lens, this represents light from the right side of the visual field. The division between the right and left optic tracts splits the retina down the middle, bisecting the fovea. The segregation of sensory information into the contralateral hemispheres corresponds to the general organization of sensory and motor centers in the brain.

Each optic tract has two major destinations on its side of the brain: (1) the superior colliculus and (2) the lateral geniculate nucleus (LGN). Although topographic mapping from the retina is scrambled within the optic tract, it is reestablished in both major destinations so that right, left, up, and down in the image correspond to specific directions within those anatomic structures.

Superior Colliculus

The *superior colliculus* is a small pair of bumps on the dorsal surface of the midbrain. Another pair, the *inferior colliculus,* is found just below it. Stimulation of the superior colliculus results in contralateral eye movement. Anatomically, output tracts from the superior colliculus run to areas that control eye and neck movement. Both the inferior and superior colliculi are apparently involved in locating sound. In the bat, the inferior colliculus is enormous, crucial to that animal's remarkable echolocation abilities.

The superior colliculus processes information from the inferior colliculus, as well as from the retina, allowing the eyes to quickly find and follow targets based on visual and auditory cues.

Different types of eye movements have been classified. The *saccade* (French, for "jolt") is a quick motion of the eyes over a significant distance. The saccade is how the eyes explore an image, jumping from landmark to landmark, rarely stopping in featureless areas. *Nystagmus* is the smooth pursuit of a moving image, usually with periodic backward saccades to lock onto subsequent points as the image moves by. *Microsaccades* are small movements, several times per second, over 1 to 2 min of arc in a seemingly random direction. Microsaccades are necessary for sight; their stabilization leads to effective blindness.

LGN

The thalamus is often called "the gateway to the cortex" because it processes much of the sensory information reaching the brain. Within the thalamus, we find the *lateral geniculate nucleus* (LGN), a peanut-sized structure that contains a single synaptic stage in the major pathway of visual information to higher centers. The LGN also receives information back from the cortex, so-called reentrant connections, as well as from the nuclei in the brainstem that control attention and arousal.

The cells in the LGN are organized into three pairs of layers. Each pair contains two layers, one from each eye. The upper two pairs consist of parvocellular cells (*P cells*) that respond with preference to different colors. The remaining lower pair consists of magnocellular cells (*M cells*) with no color preference (Fig. 4.1). The topographic mapping is identical for all six layers; i.e., passing through the layers at a given point yields synapses responding to a single area of the retina. Axons from the LGN proceed to the primary visual cortex in broad bands, the *optic radiations*, preserving this topographic mapping and displaying the same center/surround response as the ganglion cells.

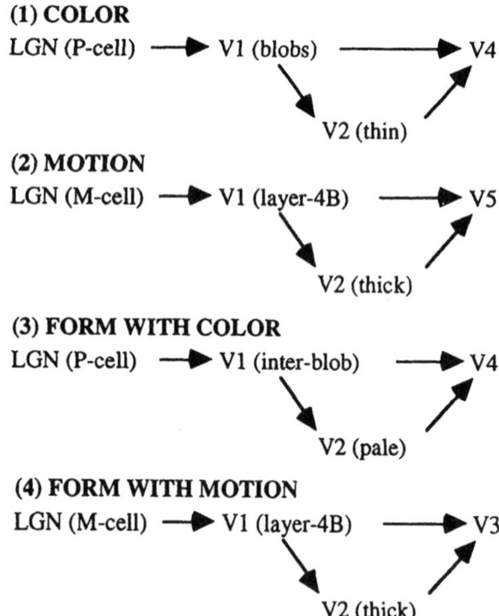

FIGURE 4.1 Visual pathways to cortical areas showing the separation of information by type. The lateral geniculate nucleus (LGN) and areas V1 and V2 act as gateways to more specialized higher areas.

Area V1

The LGN contains approximately 1.5 million cells. By comparison, the *primary visual cortex*, or *striate cortex*, which receives the visual information from the LGN, contains 200 million cells. It consists of a thin (2-mm) layer of gray matter (neuronal cell bodies) over a thicker collection of white matter (myelinated axons) and occupies a few square inches of the occipital lobes. The primary visual cortex has been called *area 17* from the days when the cortical areas were first differentiated by their cytoarchitectonics (the microscopic architecture of their layered neurons). In modern terminology, the primary visual cortex is often called *visual area 1*, or simply *V1*.

Destroying any small piece of V1 eliminates a small area in the visual field, resulting in *scotoma*, a local blind spot. Clinical evidence has long been available that a scotoma may result from injury, stroke, or tumor in a local part of V1. Between neighboring cells in V1's gray matter, horizontal connections are at most 2 to 5 mm in length. Thus, at any given time, the image from the retina is analyzed piecemeal in V1. Topographic mapping from the retina is preserved in great detail. Such mapping is seen elsewhere in the brain, such as in the somatosensory cortex [Mountcastle, 1957]. Like all cortical surfaces, V1 is a highly convoluted sheet, with much of its area hidden within its folds. If unfolded, V1 would be roughly pear shaped, with the top of the pear processing information from the fovea and the bottom of the pear processing the peripheral vision. Circling the pear at a given latitude would correspond roughly to circling the fovea at a fixed radius.

The primary visual cortex contains six layers, numbered 1 through 6. Distinct functional and anatomic types of cells are found in each layer. Layer 4 contains neurons that receive information from the LGN. Beyond the initial synapses, cells demonstrate progressively more complex responses. The outputs of V1 project to an area known as *visual area 2 (V2)*, which surrounds V1, and to higher visual areas in the occipital, temporal, and parietal lobes as well as to the superior colliculus. V1 also sends reentrant projections back to the LGN. Reentrant projections are present at almost every level of the visual system [Felleman and Essen, 1991; Edelman, 1978].

Cells in V1 have been studied extensively in animals by inserting small electrodes into the living brain (with surprisingly little damage) and monitoring the individual responses of neurons to visual stimuli. Various subpopulations of cortical cells have thus been identified. Some, termed *simple cells,* respond to illuminated edges or bars at specific locations and at specific angular orientations in the visual field. The angular orientation must be correct within 10° to 20° for the particular cell to respond. All orientations are equally represented. Moving the electrode parallel to the surface yields a smooth rotation in the orientation of cell responses by about 10° for each 50 μm that the electrode is advanced. This rotation is subject to reversals in direction, as well as "fractures," or sudden jumps in orientation.

Other cells, more common than simple cells, are termed *complex cells.* Complex cells respond to a set of closely spaced parallel edges within a particular receptive field. They may respond specifically to movement perpendicular to the orientation of the edge. Some prefer one direction of movement to the other. Some complex and simple cells are *end-stopped,* meaning they fire only if the illuminated bar or edge does not extend too far. Presumably, these cells detect corners, curves, or discontinuities in borders and lines. End-stopping takes place in layers 2 and 3 of the primary visual cortex. From the LGN through the simple cells and complex cells, there appears to be a sequential processing of the image. It is probable that simple cells combine the responses of adjacent LGN cells and that complex cells combine the responses of adjacent simple cells.

A remarkable feature in the organization of V1 is binocular convergence, in which a single neuron responds to identical receptive fields in both eyes, including location, orientation, and directional sensitivity to motion. It does not occur in the LGN, where axons from the left and right eyes are still segregated into different layers. Surprisingly, binocular connections to neurons are present in V1 at birth. Some binocular neurons are equally weighted in terms of responsiveness to both eyes, while others are more sensitive to one eye than to the other. One finds columns containing the latter type of cells in which one eye dominates, called *ocular dominance columns,* in uniform bands approximately 0.5 mm wide everywhere in V1. Ocular dominance columns occur in adjacent pairs, one for each eye, and are prominent in animals with forward-facing eyes, such as cats, chimpanzees, and humans. They are nearly absent in rodents and other animals whose eyes face outward.

The topography of orientation-specific cells and of ocular dominance columns is remarkably uniform throughout V1, which is surprising because the receptive fields near the fovea are 10 to 30 times smaller than those at the periphery. This phenomenon is called magnification. The fovea maps to a greater relative distance on the surface of V1 than does the peripheral retina, by as much as 36-fold [Daniel and Whitteridge, 1961]. In fact, the majority of V1 processes only the central 10° of the visual field. Both simple and complex cells in the foveal portion can resolve bars as narrow as 2 min of arc. Toward the periphery, the resolution falls off to 1° of arc.

As an electrode is passed down through the cortex *perpendicular* to the surface, each layer demonstrates receptive fields of characteristic size, the smallest being at layer 4, the input layer. Receptive fields are larger in other layers due to lateral integration of information. Passing the electrode *parallel* to the surface of the cortex reveals another important uniformity to V1. For example, in layer 3, which sends output fibers to higher cortical centers, one must move the electrode approximately 2 mm to pass from one collection of receptive fields to another that does not overlap. An area approximately 2 mm across thus represents the smallest unit piece of V1, i.e., that which can completely process the visual information.

Indeed, it is just the right size to contain a complete set of orientations and more than enough to contain information from both eyes. It receives a few tens of thousands of fibers from the LGN, produces perhaps 50,000 output fibers, and is fairly constant in cytoarchitectonics whether at the center of vision, where it processes approximately 30 min of arc, or at the far periphery, where it processes 7° to 8° of arc.

The topographic mapping of the visual field onto the cortex suffers an abrupt discontinuity between the left and right hemispheres, and yet our perception of the visual scene suffers no obvious rift in the midline. This is due to the *corpus collousum,* an enormous tract containing at least 200 million axons, that connects the two hemispheres. The posterior portion of the corpus collousum connects the two halves of V1, linking cells that have similar orientations and whose receptive fields overlap in the vertical midline. Thus a perceptually seamless merging of left and right visual fields is achieved. Higher levels of the visual system are likewise connected across the corpus collousum. This is demonstrated, for example, by the clinical observation that cutting the corpus collousum prevents a subject from verbally describing objects in the left field of view (the right hemisphere). Speech, which normally involves the left hemisphere, cannot process visual objects from the right hemisphere without the corpus collousum.

By merging the information from both eyes, V1 is capable of analyzing the distance to an object. Many cues for depth are available to the visual system, including occlusion, parallax (detected by the convergence of the eyes), optical focusing of the lens, rotation of objects, expected size of objects, shape based on perspective, and shadow casting. Stereopsis, which uses the slight difference between images due to the parallax between the two eyes, was first enunciated in 1838 by Sir Charles Wheatstone and it is probably the most important cue [Wheatstone, 1838]. Fixating on an object causes it to fall on the two foveas. Other objects that are nearer become outwardly displaced on the two retinas, while objects that are farther away become inwardly displaced. About 2° of horizontal disparity is tolerated, with fusion by the visual system into a single object. Greater horizontal disparity results in double vision. Almost no vertical displacement (a few minutes of arc) is tolerated. Physiologic experiments have revealed a particular class of complex cells in V1 which are *disparity tuned.* They fall into three general classes. One class fires only when the object is at the fixation distance, another only when the object is nearer, and a third only when it is farther away [Poggio and Talbot, 1981]. Severing the corpus collousum leads to a loss of stereopsis in the vertical midline of the visual field.

When the inputs to the two retinas cannot be combined, one or the other image is rejected. This phenomenon is known as *retinal rivalry* and can occur in a piecewise manner or can even lead to blindness in one eye. The general term *amblyopia* refers to the partial or complete loss of eyesight not caused by abnormalities in the eye. The most common form of amblyopia is caused by *strabismus,* in which the eyes are not aimed in a parallel direction but rather are turned inward (cross-eyed) or outward (wall-eyed). This condition leads to habitual suppression of vision from one of the eyes and sometimes to blindness in that eye or to *alternation,* in which the subject maintains vision in both eyes by using only one eye at a time. Cutting selected ocular muscles in kittens causes strabismus, and the kittens respond by alternation, preserving functional vision in both eyes. However, the number of cells in the cortex displaying binocular responses is greatly reduced. In humans with long-standing alternating strabismus, surgical repair making the eyes parallel again does not bring back a sense of depth. Permanent damage has been caused by the subtle condition of the images on the two retinas not coinciding. This may be explained by the Hebb model for associative learning, in which temporal association between inputs strengthens synaptic connections [Hebb, 1961].

Further evidence that successful development of the visual system depends on proper input comes from clinical experience with children who have *cataracts* at birth. Cataracts constitute a clouding of the lens, permitting light, but not images, to reach the retina. If surgery to remove the cataracts is delayed until the child is several years old, the child remains blind even though images are restored to the retina. Kittens and monkeys whose eyelids are sewn shut during a critical period of early development stay blind even when the eyes are opened. Physiologic studies in these animals show very few cells responding in the visual cortex. Other experiments depriving more specific elements of an image, such as certain orientations or motion in a certain direction, yield a cortex without the corresponding cell type.

Color

Cones, which dominate the fovea, can detect wavelengths between 400 and 700 nm. The population of cones in the retina can be divided into three categories, each containing a different pigment. This was established by direct microscopic illumination of the retina [Wald, 1974; Marks et al., 1964]. The pigments have a bandwidth on the order of 100 nm, with significant overlap, and with peak sensitivities at 560 nm (yellow-green), 530 nm (blue-green), and 430 nm (violet). These three cases are commonly known as red, green, and blue. Compared with the auditory system, whose array of cochlear sensors can discriminate thousands of different sonic frequencies, the visual system is relatively impoverished with only three frequency parameters. Instead, the retina expends most of its resolution on spatial information. Color vision is absent in many species, including cats, dogs, and some primates, as well as in most nocturnal animals, since cones are useless in low light.

By having three types of cones at a given locality on the retina, a simplified spectrum can be sensed and represented by three independent variables, a concept known as *trichromacy.* This model was developed by Thomas Young and Hermann von Helmholtz in the 19th century before neurobiology existed and does quite well at explaining the retina [Young, 1802; Helmholtz, 1889]. The model is also the underlying basis for red-green-blue (RGB) video monitors and color television [Ennes, 1981]. Rods do not help in discriminating color, even though the pigment in rods does add a fourth independent sensitivity peak.

Psychophysical experimentation yields a complex, redundant map between spectrum and perceived color, or *hue,* including not only the standard red, orange, yellow, green, and blue but hues such as pink, purple, brown, and olive green that are not themselves in the rainbow. Some of these may be achieved by introducing two more variables: *saturation,* which allows for mixing with white light, and *intensity,* which controls the level of color. Thus three variables are still involved: hue, saturation, and intensity.

Another model for color vision was put forth in the 19th century by Ewald Hering [Hering, 1864]. This theory also adheres to the concept of trichromacy, espousing three independent variables. However, unlike the Young-Helmholtz model, these variables are signed; they can be positive, negative, or zero. The resulting three axes are *red-green, yellow-blue,* and *black-white.* The Hering model is supported by the physiologic evidence for the center/surround response, which allows for positive as well as negative information. In fact, two populations of cells, activated and suppressed along the red-green and yellow-blue axes, have been found in monkey LGN. Yellow is apparently detected by a combination of red and green cones.

The Hering model explains, for example, the perception of the color brown, which results only when orange or yellow is surrounded by a brighter color. It also accounts for the phenomenon of color constancy, in which the perceived color of an object remains unchanged under differing ambient light conditions provided background colors are available for comparison. Research into color constancy was pioneered in the laboratory of Edwin Land [Land and McCann, 1971]. As David Hubel says, "We require color borders for color, just as we require luminance borders for black and white" [Hubel, 1988, p. 178]. As one might expect, when the corpus collousum is surgically severed, color constancy is absent across the midline.

Color processing in V1 is confined to small circular areas, known as *blobs,* in which *double-opponent cells* are found. They display a center/surround behavior based on the red-green and yellow-blue axes but lack orientation selectivity. The V1 blobs were first identified by their uptake of certain enzymes, and only later was their role in color vision discovered [Livingstone and Hubel, 1984]. The blobs are especially prominent in layers 2 and 3, which receive input from the P cells of the LGN.

Higher Cortical Centers

How are the primitive elements of image processing so far discussed united into an understanding of the image? Beyond V1 are many higher cortical centers for visual processing, at least 12 in the occipital lobe and others in the temporal and parietal lobes. Areas V2 receives axons from both the blob and interblob areas of V1 and performs analytic functions such as filling in the missing segments of an edge. V2 contains three areas categorized by different kinds of stripes: *thick stripes* which process relative horizontal position and stereopsis, *thin stripes* which process color without orientations, and *pale stripes* which extend the process of end-stopped orientation cells.

Beyond V2, higher centers have been labeled V3, V4, V5, etc. Four parallel systems have been delineated [Zeki, 1992], each system responsible for a different attribute of vision, as shown in Fig. 4.1. This is obviously an oversimplification of a tremendously complex system.

Corroborative clinical evidence supports this model. For example, lesions in V4 lead to *achromatopsia,* in which a patient can only see gray and cannot even recall colors. Conversely, a form of poisoning, *carbon monoxide chromatopsia,* results when the V1 blobs and V2 thin stripes selectively survive exposure to carbon monoxide thanks to their rich vasculature, leaving the patient with a sense of color but not of shape. A lesion in V5 leads to *akinetopsia,* in which objects disappear.

As depicted in Fig. 4.1, all visual information is processed through V1 and V2, although discrete channels within these areas keep different types of information separate. A total lesion of V1 results in the perception of total blindness. However, not all channels are shown in Fig. 4.1, and such a "totally blind" patient may perform better than randomly when forced to guess between colors or between motion in different directions. The patient with this condition, called *blindsight,* will deny being able to see anything [Weiskrantz, 1990].

Area V1 preserves retinal topographic mapping and shows receptive fields, suggesting a piecewise analysis of the image, although a given area of V1 receives sequential information from disparate areas of the visual environment as the eyes move. V2 and higher visual centers show progressively larger receptive fields and less defined topographic mapping but more specialized responses. In the extreme of specialization, neurobiologists joke about the "grandmother cell," which would respond only to a particular face. No such cell has yet been found. However, cortical regions that respond to faces in general have been found in the temporal lobe. Rather than a "grandmother cell," it seems that face-selective neurons are members of ensembles for coding facts [Gross and Sergen, 1992].

Defining Terms

Binocular convergence: The response of a single neuron to the same location in the visual field of each eye.

Color constancy: The perception that the color of an object remains constant under different lighting conditions. Even though the spectrum reaching the eye from that object can be vastly different, other objects in the field of view are used to compare.

Cytoarchitectonics: The organization of neuron types into layers as seen by various staining techniques under the microscope. Electrophysiologic responses of individual cells can be correlated with their individual layer.

Magnification: The variation in amount of retinal area represented per unit area of V1 from the fovea to the peripheral vision. Even though the fovea takes up an inordinate percentage of V1 compared with the rest of the visual field, the scale of the cellular organization remains constant. Thus the image from the fovea is, in effect, magnified before processing.

Receptive field: The area in the visual field that evokes a response in a neuron. Receptive fields may respond to specific stimuli such as illuminated bars or edges with particular directions of motion, etc.

Stereopsis: The determination of distance to objects based on relative displacement on the two retinas because of parallax.

Topographic mapping: The one-to-one correspondence between location on the retina and location within a structure in the brain. Topographic mapping further implies that contiguous areas on the retina map to contiguous areas in the particular brain structure.

References

Belliveau JH, Kwong KK, et al. 1992. Magnetic resonance imaging mapping of brain function: Human visual cortex. Invest Radiol 27(suppl 2):S59.

Cohen MS, Bookheimer SY. 1994. Localization of brain function using magnetic resonance imaging. Trends Neurosci 17(7):268.

Daniel PM, Whitteridge D. 1961. The representation of the visual field on the cerebral cortex in monkeys. J Physiol 159:203.

Edelman GM. 1978. Group selection and phasic reentrant signalling: A theory of higher brain function. In GM Edelman and VB Mountcastle (eds), The Mindful Brain, pp 51–100, Cambridge, MA, MIT Press.

Ennes HE. 1981. NTSC color fundamentals. In Television Broadcasting: Equipment, Systems, and Operating Fundamentals. Indianapolis, Howard W. Sams & Co.

Felleman DJ, V Essen DC. 1991. Distributed hierarchical processing in the primate cerebral cortex. Cerebral Cortex 1(1):1.

Gross CG, Sergen J. 1992. Face recognition. Curr Opin Neurobiol 2(2):156.

Hebb DO. 1961. The Organization of Behavior. New York, Wiley.

Helmholtz H. 1889, Popular Scientific Lectures. London, Longmans.

Hering E. 1864. Outlines of a Theory of Light Sense. Cambridge, MA, Harvard University Press.

Hubel DH. 1995. Eye, Brain, and Vision. New York, Scientific American Library.

Land EH, McCann JJ. 1971. Lightness and retinex theory. J Opt Soc Am 61:1.

Livingstone MS, Hubel DH. 1984. Anatomy and physiology of a color system in the primate visual cortex. J Neurosci 4:309.

Marks WB, Dobelle WH, MacNichol EF. 1964. Visual pigments of single primate cones. Science 143:1181.

Marr D. 1982. Vision. San Francisco, WH Freeman.

Mountcastle VB. 1957. Modality and topographic properties of single neurons of cat's somatic sensory cortex. J Neurophysiol 20(3):408.

Poggio GF, Talbot WH. 1981. Mechanisms of static and dynamic stereopsis in foveal cortex of the rhesus monkey. J Physiol 315:469.

Wald G. 1974. Proceedings: Visual pigments and photoreceptors — Review and outlook. Exp Eye Res 18(3):333.

Weiskrantz L. 1990. The Ferrier Lecture: Outlooks for blindsight: Explicit methodologies for implicit processors. Proc R Soc Lond B239:247.

Wheatstone SC. 1838. Contribution to the physiology of vision. Philos Trans R Soc Lond.

Young T. 1802. The Bakerian Lecture: On the theory of lights and colours. Philos Trans R Soc Lond 92:12.

Zeki S. 1992. The visual image in mind and brain. Sci Am, Sept., p. 69.

Zeki S, Watson JD, Lueck CJ, et al. 1991. A direct demonstration of functional specialization in human visual cortex. J Neurosci 11(3):641.

Further Reading

An excellent introductory text about the visual system is *Eye, Brain, and Vision,* by Nobel laureate, David H. Hubel (1995, Scientific American Library, New York). A more recent general text with a thorough treatment of color vision, as well as the higher cortical centers, is *A Vision of the Brain,* by Semir Zeki (1993, Blackwell Scientific Publications, Oxford).

Other useful texts with greater detail about the nervous system are *From Neuron to Brain,* by Nicholls, Martin, Wallace, and Kuffler (3rd ed., 1992, Sinauer Assoc., Sunderand, MA), *The Synaptic Organization of the Brain,* by Shepherd (4th ed., 1998, Oxford University Press, New York), and *Fundamental Neuroanatomy,* by Nauta and Feirtag (1986, WH Freeman, New York).

A classic text that laid the foundation of computer vision is *Vision,* by David Marr (1982, WH Freeman, New York). Other texts dealing with the mathematics of image processing and image analysis are *Digital Image Processing,* by Pratt (1991, Wiley, New York), and *Digital Imaging Processing and Computer Vision,* by Schalkoff (1989, Wiley, New York).

5

Auditory System

Ben M. Clopton
University of Washington

Francis A. Spelman
University of Washington

The auditory system can be divided into two large subsystems, peripheral and central. The peripheral auditory system converts the condensations and rarefactions that produce sound into neural codes that are interpreted by the central auditory system as specific sound tokens that may affect behavior.

The peripheral auditory system is subdivided into the external ear, the middle ear, and the inner ear (Fig. 5.1). The external ear collects sound energy as pressure waves, which are converted to mechanical motion at the *eardrum.* This motion is transformed across the *middle ear* and transferred to the *inner ear,* where it is frequency analyzed and converted into neural codes that are carried by the eighth cranial nerve, or *auditory nerve,* to the central auditory system.

Sound information, encoded as discharges in an array of thousands of auditory nerve fibers, is processed in nuclei that make up the central auditory system. The major centers include the *cochlear nuclei* (CN), the *superior olivary complex* (SOC), the *nuclei of the lateral lemniscus* (NLL), the *inferior colliculi* (IC), the *medial geniculate body* (MGB) of the thalamus, and the *auditory cortex* (AC). The CN, SOC, and NLL are brainstem nuclei; the IC is at the midbrain level; and the MGB and AC constitute the auditory thalamocortical system.

While interesting data have been collected from groups other than mammals, this chapter will emphasize the mammalian auditory system. This chapter ignores the structure and function of the vestibular system. While a few specific references are included, most are general in order to provide a more introductory entry into topics.

5.1 Physical and Psychological Variables

Acoustics

Sound is produced by time-varying motion of the particles in air. The motions can be defined by their pressure variations or by their volume velocities. *Volume velocity* is defined as the average particle velocity produced across a cross-sectional area and is the acoustic analogue of electric current. *Pressure* is the acoustic analogue of voltage. *Acoustic intensity* is the average rate of the flow of energy through a unit

0-8493-1810-6/03/$0.00+$1.50

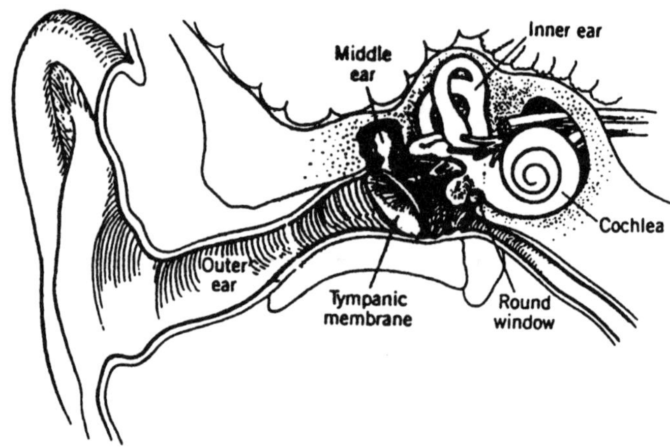

FIGURE 5.1 The peripheral auditory system showing the ear canal, tympanic membrane, middle ear and ossicles, and the inner ear consisting of the cochlea and semicircular canals of the vestibular system. Nerves communicating with the brain are also shown.

area normal to the direction of the propagation of the sound wave. It is the product of the acoustic pressure and the volume velocity and is analogous to electric power. *Acoustic impedance,* the analogue of electrical impedance, is the complex ratio of acoustic pressure and volume velocity. Sound is often described in terms of either acoustic pressure or acoustic intensity [Kinsler and Frey, 1962].

The auditory system has a wide dynamic range; i.e., it responds to several decades of change in the magnitude of sound pressure. Because of this wide dynamic range, it is useful to describe the independent variables in terms of decibels, where acoustic intensity is described by $\text{dB} = 10 \log(I/I_0)$, where I_0 is the reference intensity, or equivalently for acoustic pressure, $\text{dB} = 20 \log(P/P_0)$, where P_0 is the reference pressure.

Psychoacoustics

Physical variables, such as *frequency* and *intensity,* may have correlated psychological variables, such as *pitch* and *loudness.* Relationships between acoustic and psychological variables, the subject of the field of *psychoacoustics,* are generally not linear and may be very complex, but measurements of human detection and discrimination can be made reliably. Humans without hearing loss detect tonal frequencies from 20 Hz to 20 kHz. At 2 to 4 kHz their *dynamic range,* the span between threshold and pain, is approximately 120 dB. The minimum threshold for sound occurs between 2 and 5 kHz and is about 20 μPa. At the low end of the auditory spectrum, threshold is 80 dB higher, while at the high end, it is 70 dB higher. Intensity differences of 1 dB can be detected, while frequency differences of 2 to 3 Hz can be detected at frequencies below about 3 kHz [Fay, 1988].

5.2 The Peripheral Auditory System

The External Ear

Ambient sounds are collected by the *pinna,* the visible portion of the external ear, and guided to the middle ear by the *external auditory meatus,* or ear canal. The pinna acquires sounds selectively due to its geometry and the sound shadowing effect produced by the head. In those species whose ears can be moved voluntarily through large angles, selective scanning of the auditory environment is possible.

The ear canal serves as an acoustic waveguide that is open at one end and closed at the other. The open end at the pinna approximates a short circuit (large volume velocity and small pressure variation), while that at the closed end is terminated by the *tympanic membrane* (eardrum). The tympanic membrane has a relatively high acoustic impedance compared with the characteristic impedance of the meatus and looks like an open circuit. Thus the ear canal can resonate at those frequencies for which its length is an odd number of quarter wavelengths. The first such frequency is at about 3 kHz in the human. The meatus is antiresonant for those frequencies for which its length is an integer number of half wavelengths. For a discussion of resonance and antiresonance in an acoustic waveguide, see a text on basic acoustics, e.g., Kinsler and Frey [1962].

The acoustic properties of the external ear produce differences between the sound pressure produced at the tympanic membrane and that at the opening of the ear canal. These differences are functions of frequency, with larger differences found at frequencies between 2 and 6 kHz than those below 2 kHz. These variations have an effect on the frequency selectivity of the overall auditory system.

The Middle Ear

Anatomy

Tracing the acoustic signal, the boundaries of the middle ear include the tympanic membrane at the input and the oval window at the output. The middle ear bones, the ossicles, lie between. Pressure relief for the tympanic membrane is provided by the eustachian tube. The middle ear is an air-filled cavity.

The Ossicles

The three bones that transfer sound from the tympanic membrane to the *oval window* are called the *malleus* (hammer), *incus* (anvil), and *stapes* (stirrup). The acoustic impedance of the atmospheric source is much less than that of the aqueous medium of the load. The ratio is 3700 in an open medium, or 36 dB [Kinsler and Frey, 1962]. The ossicles comprise an impedance transformer for sound, producing a mechanical advantage that allows the acoustic signal at the tympanic membrane to be transferred with low loss to the round window of the cochlea (inner ear). The air-based sound source produces an acoustic signal of low-pressure and high-volume velocity, while the mechanical properties of the inner ear demand a signal of high-pressure and low-volume velocity.

The impedance transformation is produced in two ways: The area of the tympanic membrane is greater than that of the footplate of the stapes, and the lengths of the malleus and incus produce a lever whose length is greater on the side of the tympanic membrane than it is on the side of the oval window. In the human, the mechanical advantage is about 22:1 [Dobie and Rubel, 1989] and the impedance ratio of the transformer is 480, 27 dB, changing the mismatch from 3700:1 to about 8:1.

This simplified discussion of the function of the ossicles holds at low frequencies, those below 2 kHz. First, the tympanic membrane does not behave as a piston at higher frequencies but can support modes of vibration. Second, the mass of the ossicles becomes significant. Third, the connections between the ossicles is not lossless, nor can the stiffness of these connections be ignored. Fourth, pressure variations in the middle ear cavity can change the stiffness of the tympanic membrane. Fifth, the cavity of the middle ear produces resonances at acoustic frequencies.

Pressure Relief

The eustachian tube is a bony channel that is lined with soft tissue. It extends from the middle ear to the nasopharynx and provides a means by which pressure can be equalized across the tympanic membrane. The function is clearly observed with changes in altitude or barometric pressure. A second function of the eustachian tube is to aerate the tissues of the middle ear.

The Inner Ear

The mammalian inner ear is a spiral structure, the *cochlea* (snail), consisting of three fluid-filled chambers, or scalae, the *scala vestibuli,* the *scala media,* and the *scala tympani* (Fig. 5.2). The stapes footplate introduces mechanical displacements into the scala vestibuli through the oval window at the *base* of the

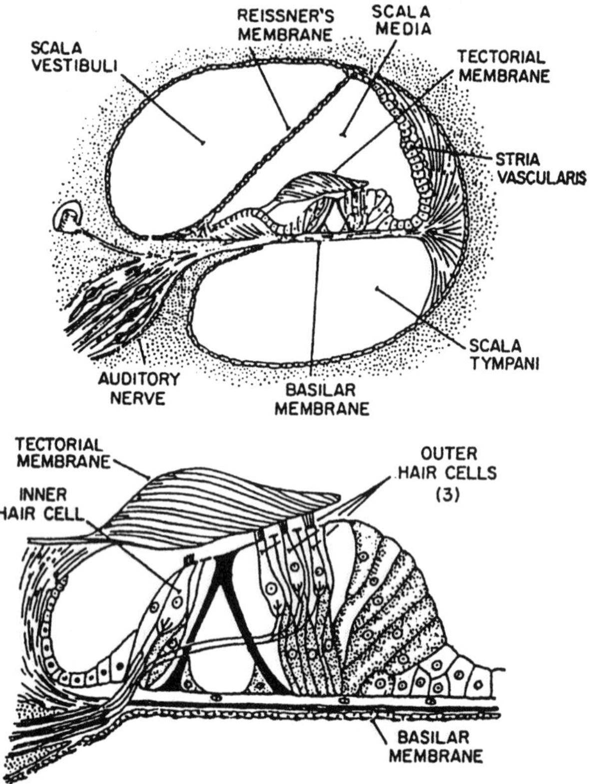

FIGURE 5.2 Cross section of one turn of the cochlea showing the scala vestibuli, scala media, and scala tympani. Reissner's membrane separates the SM and SV, while the basilar membrane and organ of Corti separate the SM and ST.

cochlea. At the other end of the spiral, the *apex* of the cochlea, the scala vestibuli and the scala tympani communicate by an opening, the *helicotrema.* Both are filled with an aqueous medium, the *perilymph.* The scala media spirals between them and is filled with *endolymph,* a medium that is high in K^+ and low in Na^+. The scala media is separated from the scala vestibuli by *Reissner's membrane,* which is impermeable to ions, and the scala media is separated from the scala tympani by the *basilar membrane* (BM) and *organ of Corti.* The organ of Corti contains the hair cells that transduce acoustic signals into neural signals, the cells that support the hair cells, and the tectorial membrane to which the outer hair cells are attached. The BM provides the primary filter function of the inner ear and is permeable so that the cell bodies of the hair cells are bathed in perilymph.

Fluid and tissue displacements travel from the footplate of the stapes along the cochlear spiral from base to apex. Pressure relief is provided for the incompressible fluids of the inner ear by the round window membrane; e.g., if a transient pressure increase at the stapes displaces its footplate inward, there will be a compensatory outward displacement of the round window membrane.

The Basilar Membrane

Physiology

The BM supports the hair cells and their supporting cells (see Fig. 5.2). Sound decomposition into its frequency components is a major code of the BM. A transient sound, such as a click, initiates a *traveling wave* of displacement in the BM, and this motion has frequency-dependent characteristics which arise from properties of the membrane and its surrounding structures [Bekesy, 1960]. The membrane's width varies as it traverses the cochlear duct: It is narrower at its basal end than at its apical end. It is stiffer at the base than at the apex, with stiffness varying by about two orders of magnitude [Dobie and Rubel, 1989]. The membrane is a distributed structure, which acts as a delay line, as suggested by the nature of the traveling wave [Lyon and Mead, 1989]. The combination of mechanical properties of the BM produces a structure that demonstrates a distance-dependent displacement when the ear is excited sinusoidally. The distance from the apex to the maximum displacement is logarithmically related to the frequency of a sinusoidal tone [LePage, 1991].

Tuning is quite sharp for sinusoidal signals. The slope of the tuning curve is much greater at the high-frequency edge than at the low-frequency edge, with slopes of more than 100 dB per octave at the high edge and about half that at the low edge [Lyon and Mead, 1989]. The filter is sharp, with a 10-dB bandwidth of 10 to 25% of the center frequency.

The auditory system includes both passive and active properties. The outer hair cells (see below) receive efferent output from the brain and actively modify the characteristics of the auditory system. The result is to produce a "cochlear amplifier," which sharpens the tuning of the BM [Lyon and Mead, 1989], as well as adding nonlinear properties to the system [Geisler, 1992; Cooper and Rhode, 1992], along with otoacoustic emissions [LePage, 1991].

The Organ of Corti

The organ of Corti is attached to the BM on the side of the aqueous fluid of the scala media. It is comprised of the supporting cells for the hair cells, the hair cells themselves, and the *tectorial membrane.* The cilia of the *inner hair cells* (IHCs) do not contact the tectorial membrane, while those of the *outer hair cells* (OHCs) do. Both IHCs and OHCs have precise patterns of stereocilia at one end which are held within the tectorial plate next to the overlying tectorial membrane. The IHCs synapse with *spiral ganglion cells,* the afferent neurons, while the OHCs synapse with efferent neurons. Both IHCs and OHCs are found along the length of the organ of Corti. The IHCs are found in a single line, numbering between about 3000 and 4000 in human. There are three lines of OHCs, numbering about 12,000 in human [Nadol, 1988].

Inner Hair Cells

The stereocilia of the IHCs are of graded, decreasing length from one side of the cell where a kinocilium is positioned early in ontogeny. If the cilia are deflected in a direction toward this position, membrane channels are further opened to allow potassium to enter and depolarize the cell [Hudspeth, 1987]. Displacement in the other direction reduces channel opening and produces a relative hyperpolarization [Hudspeth and Corey, 1977]. These changes in intracellular potential modulate transmitter release at the base of the IHCs.

The IHCs are not attached to the tectorial membrane, so their response to motion of the membrane is proportional to the velocity of displacement rather than to displacement itself, since the cilia of the hair cells are bathed in endolymph. When the membrane vibrates selectively in response to a pure tone, the stereocilia are bent atop a small number of hair cells, which depolarize in response to the mechanical event. Thus, the *tonotopic organization* of the BM is transferred to the hair cells and to the rest of the auditory system. The auditory system is organized tonotopically, i.e., in order of frequency, because the frequency ordering of the cochlea is mapped through successive levels of the system. While this organization is preserved throughout the system, it is much more complex than a huge set of finely tuned filters.

Hair cells in some species exhibit frequency tuning when isolated [Crawford and Fettiplace, 1985], but mammalian hair cells exhibit no tuning characteristics. The tuning of the mammalian auditory system depends on the mechanical characteristics of the BM as modified by the activity of the OHCs.

Outer Hair Cells

The OHCs have cilia that are attached to the tectorial membrane. Since their innervation is overwhelmingly efferent, they do not transfer information to the brain but are modulated in their mechanical action by the brain. There are several lines of evidence that lead to the conclusion that the OHCs play an active role in the processes of the inner ear. First, OHCs change their length in response to neurotransmitters

[Dobie and Rubel, 1989]. Second, observation of the Henson's cells, passive cells that are intimately connected to OHCs, shows that spontaneous vibrations are produced by the Henson's cells in mammals and likely in the OHCs as well. These vibrations exhibit spectral peaks that are appropriate in frequency to their locations on the BM [Khanna et al., 1993]. Third, action of the OHCs as amplifiers leads to spontaneous otoacoustic emissions [Kim, 1984; Lyon and Mead, 1989] and to changes in the response of the auditory system [Lyon and Mead, 1989; Geisler, 1992]. Fourth, AC excitation of the OHCs of mammals produces changes in length [Cooke, 1993].

The OHCs appear to affect the response of the auditory system in several ways. They enhance the tuning characteristics of the system to sinusoidal stimuli, decreasing thresholds and narrowing the filter's bandwidth [Dobie and Rubel, 1989]. They likely influence the damping of the BM dynamically by actively changing its stiffness.

Spiral Ganglion Cells and the Auditory Nerve

Anatomy

The auditory nerve of the human contains about 30,000 fibers consisting of myelinated proximal processes of spiral ganglion cells (SGCs). The somas of spiral ganglion cells (SGCs) lie in *Rosenthal's canal,* which spirals medial to the three scalae of the cochlea. Most (93%) are large, heavily myelinated, *type I* SGCs whose distal processes synapse on IHCs. The rest are smaller *type II* SGCs, which are more lightly myelinated. Each IHC has, on average, a number of fibers that synapse with it, 8 in the human and 18 in the cat, although some fibers contact more than one IHC. In contrast, each type II SGC contacts OHCs at a rate of about 10 to 60 cells per fiber.

The auditory nerve collects in the center of the cochlea, its *modiolus,* as SGC fibers join it. Low-frequency fibers from the apex join first, and successively higher frequency fibers come to lie concentrically on the outer layers of the nerve in a spiraling fashion before it exits the modiolus to enter the internal auditory meatus of the temporal bone. A precise tonotopic organization is retrained in the concentrically wrapped fibers.

Physiology

Discharge spike patterns from neurons can be recorded extracellularly while repeating tone bursts are presented. A *threshold level* can be identified from the resulting *rate-level function* (RLF). In the absence of sound and at lower, subthreshold levels, a *spontaneous rate* of discharge is measured. In the nerve this ranges from 50 spikes per second to fewer than 10. As intensity is raised, the *threshold level* is encountered, where the evoked discharge rate significantly exceeds the spontaneous discharge rate. The plot of threshold levels as a function of frequency is the neuron's *threshold tuning curve.* The tuning curves for axons in the auditory nerve show a minimal threshold (maximum sensitivity) at a *characteristic frequency* (CF) with a narrow frequency range of responding for slightly more intense sounds. At high intensities, a large range of frequencies elicits spike discharges. RLFs for nerve fibers are *monotonic* (i.e., spike rate increases with stimulus intensity), and although a saturation rate is usually approached at high levels, the spike rate does not decline. Mechanical tuning curves for the BM and neural threshold tuning curves are highly similar (Fig. 5.3). Mechanical frequency analysis in the cochlea and the orderly projection of fibers through the nerve lead to correspondingly orderly maps for CFs in the nerve and the nuclei of the central pathways.

Sachs and Young [1979] found that the frequency content of lower intensity vowel sounds is represented as corresponding tonotopic rate peaks in nerve activity, but for higher intensities this rate code is lost as fibers tend toward equal discharge rates. At high intensities spike synchrony to frequencies near CF continue to signal the relative spectral content of vowels, a temporal code. These results hold for *high-spontaneous-rate fibers* (over 15 spikes per second), which are numerous. Less common, *low-spontaneous-rate fibers* (less than 15 spikes per second) appear to maintain the rate code at higher intensities, suggesting different coding roles for these two fiber populations.

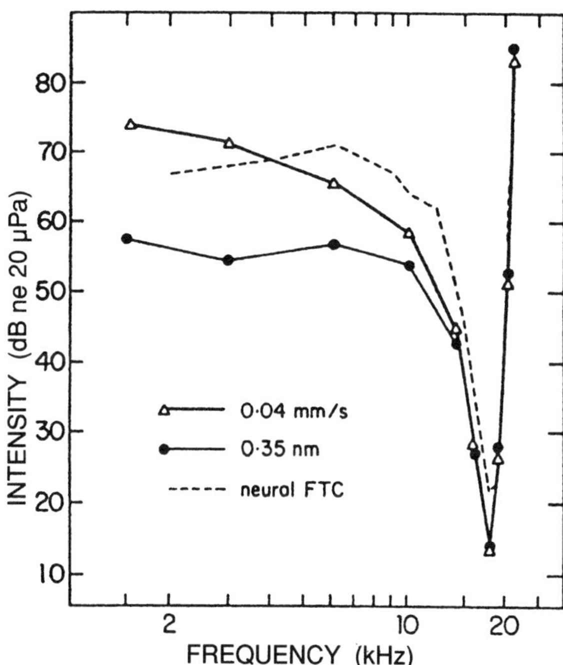

FIGURE 5.3 Mechanical and neural turning curves from the BM and auditory nerve, respectively. The two mechanical curves show the intensity and frequency combinations for tones required to obtain a criterion displacement or velocity, while the neural curve shows the combinations needed to increase neural discharge rates a small amount over spontaneous rate.

5.3 The Central Auditory System

Overview

In ascending paths, obligatory synapses occur at the CN, IC, MGB, and AC, but a large number of alternative paths exist with ascending and descending internuclear paths and the shorter intranuclear connections between neighboring neurons and subdivisions within a major nuclear group. Each of the centers listed contains subpopulations of neurons that differ in aspects of their morphologies, discharge patterns to sounds, segregation in the nucleus, biochemistry, and synaptic connectivities. The arrangement of the major ascending auditory pathways is schematically illustrated in Fig. 5.4. For references, see Altschuler et al. [1991].

Neural Bases of Processing

The Cochlear Nuclei

Anatomy of the Cochlear Nuclei. The CN can be subdivided into at least three distinct regions, the *anteroventral CN* (AVCN), the *posteroventral CN* (PVCN), and the *dorsal CN* (DCN). Each subdivision has one or more distinctive neuron types and unique intra- and internuclear connections. The axon from each type I SGC in the nerve branches to reach each of the three divisions in an orderly manner so that tonotopic organization is maintained. Neurons with common morphologic classifications are found in all three divisions, especially *granule cells,* which tend to receive connections from type II spiral ganglion cells.

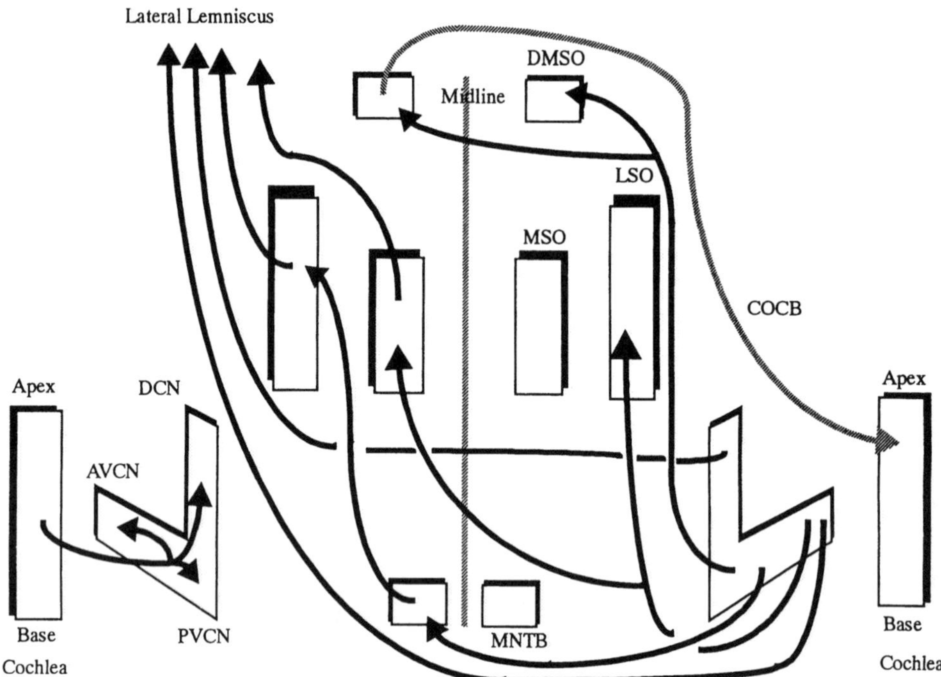

FIGURE 5.4 A schematic of major connections in the auditory brainstem discussed in the text. All structures and connections are bilaterally symmetrical, but connections have been shown on one side only for clarity. No cell types are indicated, but the subdivisions of origin are suggested in the CN. Note that the LSO and MSO receive inputs from both CN.

Morphologic classification of neurons based on the shapes of their dendritic trees and somas show that the anterior part of the AVCN contains many *spherical bushy cells,* while in its posterior part both *globular bushy cells* and spherical bushy cells are found. Spherical bushy cells receive input from one type I ganglion cell through a large synapse formation containing end bulbs of Held, while the globular cells may receive inputs from a few afferent fibers. These endings cover a large part of the soma surface and parts of the proximal dendrite, especially in spherical bushy cells, and they have rounded vesicles presynaptically, indicating excitatory input to the bushy cells, while other synaptic endings of noncochlear origins tend to have flattened vesicles associated with inhibitory inputs. *Stellate cells* are found throughout the AVCN, as well as in the lower layers of the DCN. The AVCN is tonotopically organized, and neurons having similar CFs have been observed to lie in layers or laminae [Bourk et al., 1981]. *Isofrequency laminae* also have been indicated in other auditory nuclei.

The predominant neuron in the PVCN is the *octopus cell,* a label arising from its distinctive shape with asymmetrically placed dendrites. Octopus cells receive cochlear input from type I SGCs on their somas and proximal dendrites. Their dendrites cross the incoming array of cochlear fibers, and these often branch to follow the dendrite toward the soma.

The DCN is structurally the most intricate of the CN. In many species, four or five layers are noticeable, giving it a "cortical" structure, and its local circuitry has been compared with that of the cerebellum. *Fusiform cells* are the most common morphologic type. Their somas lie in the deeper layers of the DCN, and their dendrites extend toward the surface of the nucleus and receive primarily noncochlear inputs. Cochlear fibers pass deeply in the DCN and turn toward the surface to innervate fusiform and *giant cells* that lie in the deepest layer of the DCN. The axons of fusiform and giant cells project out of the DCN to the contralateral IC.

Intracellular recording in slice preparation is beginning to identify the membrane characteristics of neuronal types in the CN. The diversity of neuronal morphologic types, their participation in local

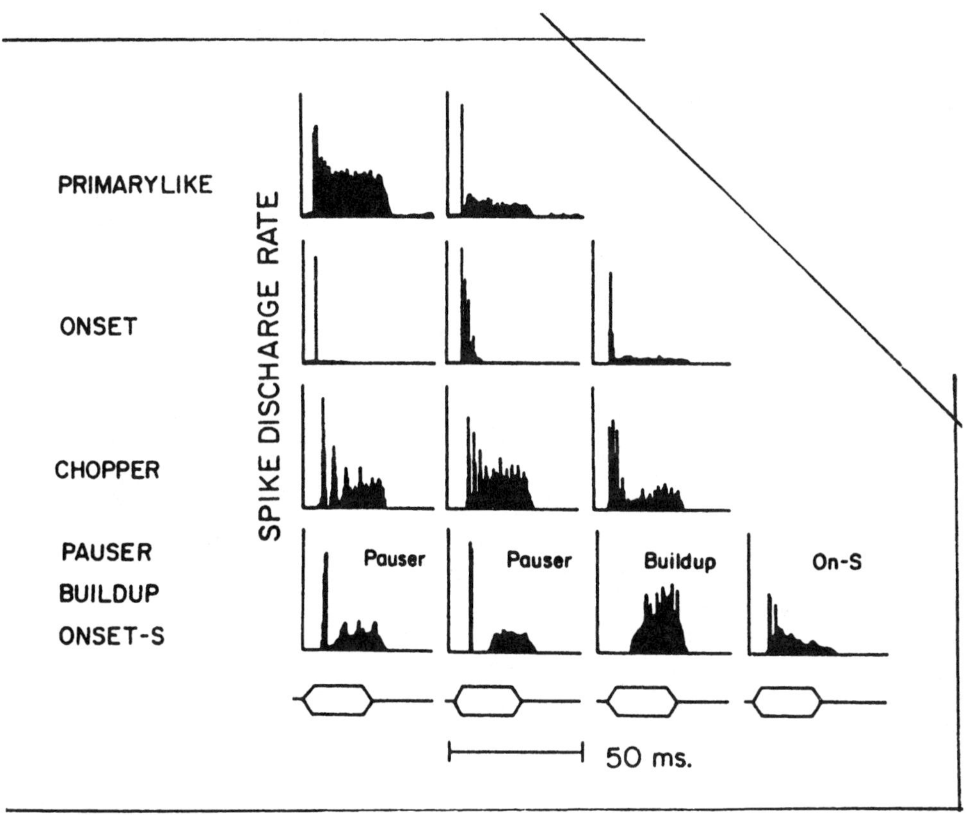

FIGURE 5.5 Peristimulus time histogram patterns obtained in the CN and nerve. Repeated presentations of a tone burst at CF are used to obtain these estimates of discharge rate during the stimulus. (Adapted from Young, 1984.)

circuits, and the emerging knowledge of their membrane biophysics are motivating detailed compartmental modeling [Arle and Kim, 1991].

Spike Discharge Patterns. Auditory nerve fibers and neurons in central nuclei may discharge only a few times during a brief tone burst, but if a histogram of spike events is synchronized to the onset of the tone burst, a *peristimulus time histogram* (PSTH) is obtained that is more representative of the neuron's response than any single one. The PSTH may be expressed in terms of spike counts, spike probability, or spike rate as a function of time, but all these retain the underlying temporal pattern of the response. PSTHs taken at the CF for a tone burst intensity roughly 40 dB above threshold have shapes that are distinctive to different nuclear subdivisions and even different morphologic types. They have been used for functionally classifying auditory neurons.

Figure 5.5 illustrates some of the major pattern types obtained from the auditory nerve and CN. Auditory nerve fibers and spherical bushy cells in AVCN have *primary-like* patterns in their PSTHs, an elevated spike rate after tone onset, falling to a slowly adapting level until the tone burst ends. Globular bushy cells may have primary-like, *pri-notch* (primary-like with a brief notch after onset), or chopper patterns. Stellate cells have non-primary-like patterns. *Onset* response patterns, one or a few brief peaks of discharge at onset with little or no discharges afterward, are observed in the PVCN from octopus cells. *Chopper, pauser,* and *buildup* patterns are observed in many cells of the DCN. For most neurons of the CN, these patterns are not necessarily stable over different stimulus intensities; a primary-like pattern may change to a pauser pattern and then to a chopper pattern as intensity is raised [Young, 1984].

Functional classification also has been based on the *response map,* a plot of a neuron's spike discharge rate as a function of tonal frequency and intensity. Fibers and neurons with primary-like PSTHs generally have response maps with only an *excitatory region* of elevated rate. The lower edges of this region approximate the threshold tuning curve. Octopus cells often have very broad tuning curves and extended response maps, as suggested by their frequency-spanning dendritic trees. More complex response maps are observed for some neurons, such as those in the DCN. Inhibitory regions alone, a frequency-intensity area of suppressed spontaneous discharge rates, or combinations of excitatory regions and inhibitory regions have been observed. Some neurons are excited only within islands of frequency-intensity combinations, demonstrating a CF but having no response to high-intensity sounds. In these cases, an RLF at CF would be *nonmonotonic;* i.e., spike rate decreases as the level is raised. Response maps in the DCN containing both excitatory and inhibitory regions have been shown to arise from a convergence of inputs from neurons with only excitatory or inhibitory regions in their maps [Young and Voigt, 1981].

Superior Olivary Complex (SOC)

The SOC contains 10 or more subdivisions in some species. It is the first site at which connections from the two ears converge and is therefore a center for binaural processing that underlies sound localization. There are large differences in the subdivisions between mammalian groups such as bats, primates, cetaceans, and burrowing rodents that utilize vastly different binaural cues. Binaural cues to the locus of sounds include *interaural level differences* (ILDs), *interaural time differences* (ITDs), and detailed spectral differences for multispectral sounds due to head and pinna filtering characteristics.

Neurons in the *medial superior olive* (MSO) and *lateral superior olive* (LSO) tend to process ITDs and ILDs, respectively. A neuron in the MSO receives projections from spherical bushy cells of the CN from both sides and thereby the precise timing and tuning cues of nerve fibers passed through the large synapses mentioned. The time accuracy of the pathways and the comparison precision of MSO neurons permit the discrimination of changes in ITD of a few tens of microseconds. MSO neurons project to the ipsilateral IC through the lateral lemniscus. Globular bushy cells of the CN project to the medial nucleus of the trapezoid body (MNTB) on the contralateral side, where they synapse on one and only one neuron in a large, excitatory synapse, the calyx of Held. MNTB neurons send inhibitory projections to neurons of the LSO on the same side, which also receives excitatory input from spherical bushy cells from the AVCN on the same side. Sounds reaching the ipsilateral side will excite discharges from an LSO neuron, while those reaching the contralateral side will inhibit its discharge. The relative balance of excitation and inhibition is a function of ILD over part of its physiological range, leading to this cue being encoded in discharge rate.

One of the subdivisions of the SOC, the *dorsomedial periolivary nucleus* (DMPO), is a source of efferent fibers that reach the contralateral cochlea in the *crossed olivocochlear bundle* (COCB). Neurons of the DMPO receive inputs from collaterals of globular bushy cell axons of the contralateral ACVN that project to the MNTB and from octopus cells on both sides. The functional role of the feedback from the DMPO to the cochlea is not well understood.

Nuclei of the Lateral Lemniscus (NLL)

The lateral lemniscus consists of ascending axons from the CN and LSO. The NLL lie within this tract, and some, such as the dorsal nucleus (DNLL), are known to process binaural information, but less is known about these nuclei as a group than others, partially due to their relative inaccessibility.

Inferior Colliculi (IC)

The IC are paired structures lying on the dorsal surface of the rostral brainstem. Each colliculus has a large *central nucleus* (ICC), a surface cortex, and paracentral nuclei. Each colliculus receives afferents from a number of lower brainstem nuclei, projects to the MGB through the *brachium,* and communicates with the other colliculus through a *commissure.* The ICC is the major division and has distinctive laminae in much of its volume. The laminae are formed from *disk-shaped cells* and afferent fibers. The disk-shaped cells, which make up about 80% of the ICC neuronal population, have flattened dendritic fields that lie in the laminar plane. The terminal endings of afferents form fibrous layers between laminae. The remaining neurons in the ICC are *stellate cells* that have dendritic trees spanning laminae. Axons from these two cell types make up much of the ascending ICC output.

Tonotropic organization is preserved in the ICC laminae, each corresponding to an *isofrequency lamina.* Both monaural and binaural information converges at the IC through direct projections from the CN and from the SOC and NLL. Crossed CN inputs and those from the ipsilateral MSO are excitatory. Inhibitory synapses in the ICC arise from the DNLL, mediated by gamma-aminobutyric acid (GABA), and from the ipsilateral LSO, mediated by glycine.

These connections provide an extensive base for identifying sound direction at this midbrain level, but due to their convergence, it is difficult to determine what binaural processing occurs at the IC as opposed to being passed from the SOC and NLL. Many neurons in the IC respond differently depending on binaural parameters. Varying ILDs for clicks or high-frequency tones often indicates that contralateral sound is excitatory. Ipsilateral sound may have no effect on responses to contralateral sound, classifying the cell as E0, or it may inhibit responses, in which case the neuron is classified as EI, or maximal excitation may occur for sound at both ears, classifying the neuron as EE. Neurons responding to lower frequencies are influenced by ITDs, specifically the phase difference between sinusoids at the ears. Spatial receptive fields for sounds are not well documented in the mammalian IC, but barn owls, who use the sounds of prey for hunting at night, have sound-based spatial maps in the homologous structure. The superior colliculus, situated just rostral to the IC, has spatial auditory receptive field maps for mammals and owl.

Auditory Thalamocortical System

Medial Geniculate Body (MGB). The MGB and AC form the auditory thalamocortical system. As with other sensory systems, extensive projections to and from the cortical region exist in this system. The MGB has three divisions, the *ventral, dorsal,* and *medial.* The ventral division is the largest and has the most precise tonotopic organization. Almost all its input is from the ipsilateral ICC through the brachium of the IC. Its large *bushy cells* have dendrites oriented so as to lie in isofrequency layers, and the axons of these neurons project to the AC, terminating in layers III and IV.

Auditory Cortex. The auditory cortex (AC) consists of areas of the cerebral cortex that respond to sounds. In mammals, the AC is bilateral and has a primary area with surrounding secondary areas. In nonprimates, the AC is on the lateral surface of the cortex, but in most primates, it lies within the lateral fissure on the superior surface of the temporal lobe. Figure 5.6 reveals the area of the temporal lobe involved with auditory function in humans. Tonotopic mapping is usually evident in these areas as isofrequency surface lines. The primary AC responds most strongly and quickly to sounds. In echolocating bats, the cortex has a large tonotopic area devoted to the frequency region of its emitted cries and cues related to its frequency modulation and returned Doppler shift [Aitkin, 1990].

The cytoarchitecture of the primary AC shows layers I (surface) through VI (next to white matter), with the largest neurons in layers V and VI. Columns with widths of 50 to 75 μm are evident from dendritic organization in layers III and IV, with fibers lying between the columns. A description of cell types is beyond this treatment.

Discharge patterns in the AC for sound stimuli are mainly of the onset type. Continuous stimuli often evoke later spikes, after the onset discharge, in unanesthetized animals. About half the neurons in the primary AC have monotonic RLFs, but the proportion of nonmonotonic RLFs in secondary areas is much higher. A number of studies have used complex sounds to study cortical responses. Neural responses to species-specific cries, speech, and other important sounds have proved to be labile and to a great extent dependent on the arousal level and behavioral set of the animal.

Cortical lesions in humans rarely produce deafness, although deficits in speech comprehension and generation may exist. Audiometric tests will generally indicate that sensitivity to tonal stimuli is retained. It has been known for some time that left-hemisphere lesions in the temporal region can disrupt comprehension (Wernicke's area) and in the region anterior to the precentral gyrus (Broca's area) can interfere with speech production. It is difficult to separate the effects of these areas because speech comprehension provides vital feedback for producing correct speech.

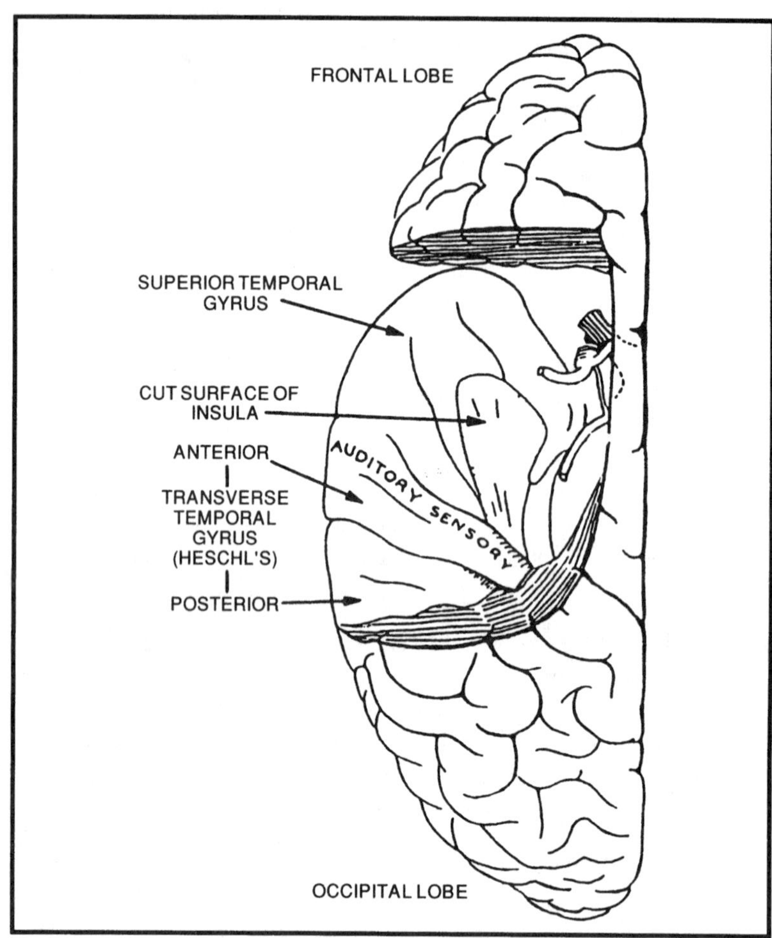

FIGURE 5.6 A view of the human cerebral cortex showing the auditory cortex on the superior surface of the left temporal lobe after removal of the overlying parietal cortex.

5.4 Pathologies

Hearing loss results from conductive and neural deficits. Conductive hearing loss due to attenuation in the outer or middle ear often can be alleviated by amplification provided by hearing aids and may be subject to surgical correction. Sensorineural loss due to the absence of IHCs results from genetic deficits, biochemical insult, exposure to intense sound, or aging (*presbycusis*). For some cases of sensorineural loss, partial hearing function can be restored with the cochlear prosthesis, electrical stimulation of remaining SGCs using small arrays of electrodes inserted into the scala tympani [Miller and Spelman, 1990]. In a few patients having no auditory nerve, direct electrical stimulation of the CN has been used experimentally to provide auditory sensation. Lesions of the nerve and central structures occur due to trauma, tumor growth, and vascular accidents. These may be subject to surgical intervention to prevent further damage and promote functional recovery.

5.5 Models of Auditory Function

Hearing mechanisms have been modeled for many years at a phenomenologic level using psychophysical data. As physiologic and anatomic observations have provided detailed parameters for peripheral and central processing, models of auditory encoding and processing have become more quantitative and physically based. Compartmental models of single neurons, especially SGCs and neurons in the CN, having accurate morphometric geometries, electrical properties, membrane biophysics, and local circuitry are seeing increasing use.

References

Aitkin L. 1990. The Auditory Cortex: Structural and Functional Bases of Auditory Perception. London, Chapman & Hall.

Altschuler RA, Bobbin RP, Clopton BM, Hoffman DW (Eds). 1991. Neurobiology of Hearing: The Central Auditory System. New York, Raven Press.

Arle JE, Kim DO. 1991. Neural modeling of intrinsic and spike-discharge properties of cochlear nucleus neurons. Biol Cybern 64:273.

Bekesy G. von. 1960. Experiments in Hearing. New York, McGraw-Hill.

Bourk TR, Mielcarz JP, Norris BE. 1981. Tonotopic organization of the anteroventral cochlear nucleus of the cat. Hear Res 4:215.

Cooke M. 1993. Modelling Auditory Processing and Organisation. Cambridge, England, Cambridge University Press.

Cooper NP, Rhode WS. 1992. Basilar membrane mechanics in the hook region of cat and guinea-pig cochleae: Sharp tuning and nonlinearity in the absence of baseline position shifts. Hear Res 63:163.

Crawford AC, Fettiplace R. 1985. The mechanical properties of ciliary bundles of turtle cochlear hair cells. J Physiol 364:359.

Dobie RA, Rubel EW. 1989. The auditory system: Acoustics, psychoacoustics, and the periphery. In HD Patton et al. (Eds), Textbook of Physiology, vol 1: Excitable Cells and Neurophysiology, 21st ed. Philadelphia, Saunders.

Fay RR. 1988. Hearing in Vertebrates: A Psychophysics Databook. Winnetka, Hill-Fay Associates.

Geisler CD. 1992. Two-tone suppression by a saturating feedback model of the cochlear partition. Hear Res 63:203.

Hudspeth AJ. 1987. Mechanoelectrical transduction by hair cells in the acousticolateralis sensory system. Annu Rev Neurosci 6:187.

Hudspeth AJ, Corey DP. 1977. Sensitivity, polarity, and conductance change in the response of vertebrate hair cells to controlled mechanical stimuli. Proc Natl Acad Sci USA 74:2407.

Khanna SM, Keilson SE, Ulfendahl M, Teich MC. 1993. Spontaneous cellular vibrations in the guinea-pig temporal-bone preparation. Br J Audiol 27:79.

Kim DO. 1984. Functional roles of the inner- and outer-hair-cell subsystems in the cochlea and brainstem. In CI Berlin (Ed), Hearing Science: Recent Advances. San Diego, College-Hill Press.

Kinsler LE, Frey AR. 1962. Fundamentals of Acoustics. New York, Wiley.

LePage EL. 1991. Helmholtz revisited: Direct mechanical data suggest a physical model for dynamic control of mapping frequency to place along the cochlear partition. In Lecture Notes in Biomechanics. New York, Springer-Verlag.

Lyon RF, Mead C. 1989. Electronic cochlea. In C Mead (Ed), Analog VLSI and Neural Systems. Reading, MA, Addison-Wesley.

Miller JM, Spelman FA (Eds). 1990. Cochlear Implants: Models of the Electrically Stimulated Ear. New York, Springer-Verlag.

Nadol JB Jr. 1988. Comparative anatomy of the cochlea and auditory nerve in mammals. Hear Res 34:253.

Sachs MB, Young ED. 1979. Encoding of steady-state vowels in the auditory nerve: Representation in terms of discharge rate. J Acoust Soc Am 66:470.

Young ED, Voigt HF. 1981. The internal organization of the dorsal cochlear nucleus. In J Syka and L Aitkin (Eds), Neuronal Mechanisms in Hearing, pp 127–133. New York, Plenum Press.

Young ED. 1984. Response characteristics of neurons of the cochlear nuclei. In CI Berlin (Ed), Hearing Science: Recent Advances. San Diego, College-Hill Press.

6

Gastrointestinal System

Berj L. Bardakjian
University of Toronto

6.1 Introduction

The primary function of the gastrointestinal system (Fig. 6.1) is to supply the body with nutrients and water. The ingested food is moved along the alimentary canal at an appropriate rate for digestion, absorption, storage, and expulsion. To fulfill the various requirements of the system, each organ has adapted one or more functions. The esophagus acts as a conduit for the passage of food into the stomach for trituration and mixing. The ingested food is then emptied into the small intestine, which plays a major role in the digestion and absorption processes. The chyme is mixed thoroughly with secretions and it is propelled distally (1) to allow further gastric emptying, (2) to allow for uniform exposure to the absorptive mucosal surface of the small intestine, and (3) to empty into the colon. The vigor of mixing and the rate of propulsion depend on the required contact time of chyme with enzymes and the mucosal surface for efficient performance of digestion and absorption. The colon absorbs water and electrolytes from the chyme, concentrating and collecting waste products that are expelled from the system at appropriate times. All of these motor functions are performed by contractions of the muscle layers in the gastrointestinal wall.

6.2 Gastrointestinal Electrical Oscillations

Gastrointestinal motility is governed by myogenic, neural, and chemical control systems (Fig. 6.2). The myogenic control system is manifest by periodic depolarizations of the smooth muscle cells, which constitute autonomous electrical oscillations called the electrical control activity (ECA) or slow waves [Daniel and Chapman, 1963]. The properties of this myogenic system and its electrical oscillations dictate to a large extent the contraction patterns in the stomach, small intestine, and colon [Szurszewski, 1987].

0-8493-1810-6/03/$0.00+$1.50

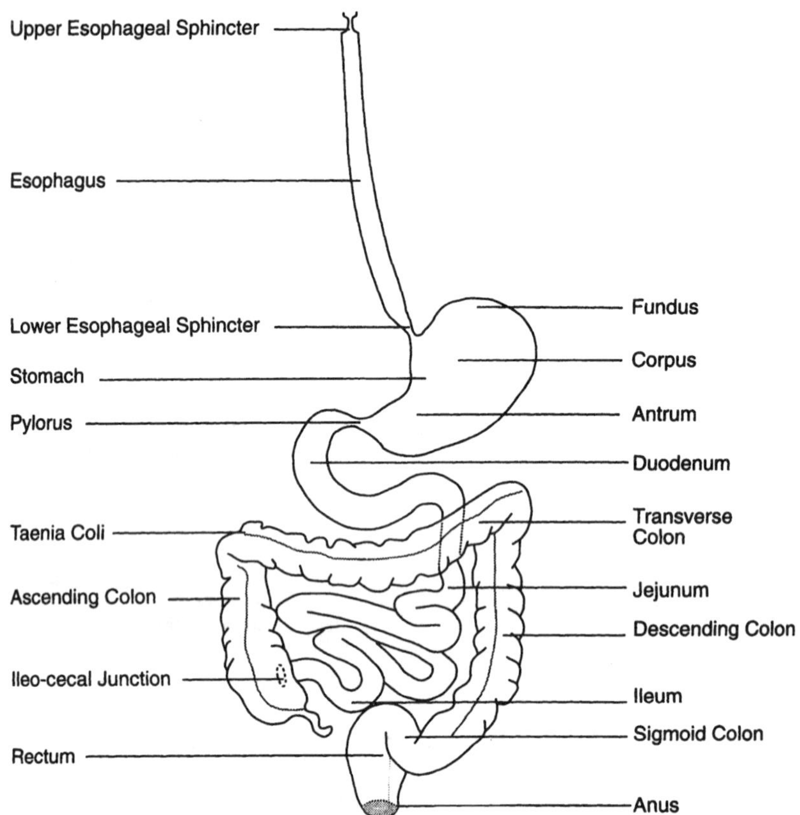

FIGURE 6.1 The gastrointestinal tract.

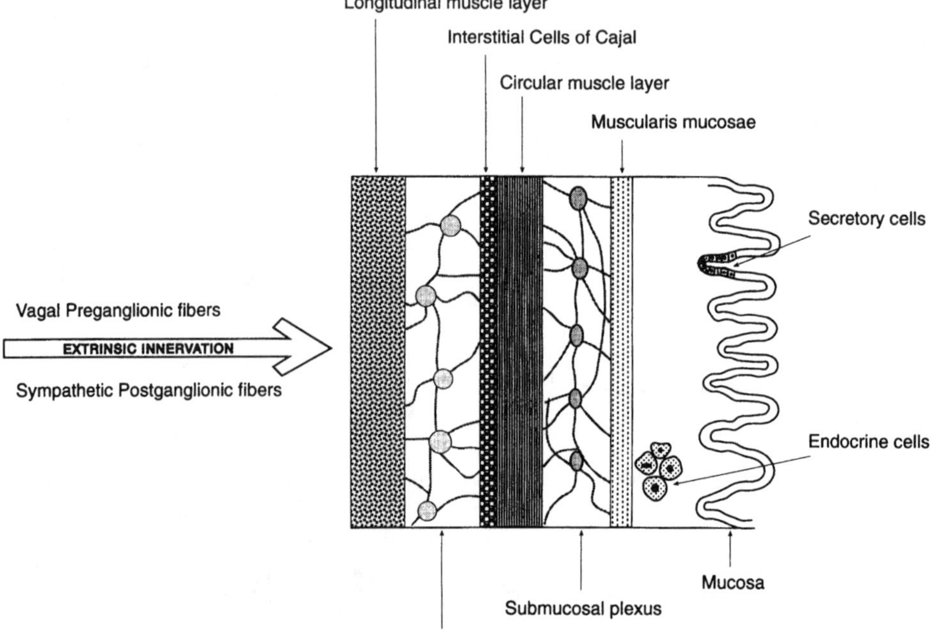

FIGURE 6.2 The layers of the gastrointestinal wall.

The ECA controls the contractile excitability of smooth muscle cells since the cells may contract only when depolarization of the membrane voltage exceeds an excitation threshold. The normal spontaneous amplitude of ECA depolarization does not exceed this excitation threshold except when neural or chemical excitation is present. The myogenic system affects the frequency, direction, and velocity of the contractions. It also affects the coordination or lack of coordination between adjacent segments of the gut wall. Hence, the electrical activities in the gut wall provide an electrical basis for gastrointestinal motility.

In the distal stomach, small intestine, and colon, there are intermittent bursts of rapid electrical oscillations, called the electrical response activity (ERA) or spike bursts. The ERA occurs during the depolarization plateaus of the ECA if a cholinergic stimulus is present, and it is associated with muscular contractions (Fig. 6.3). Thus, neural and chemical control systems determine whether contractions will occur or not, but when contractions are occurring, the myogenic control system (Fig. 6.4) determines the spatial and temporal patterns of contractions.

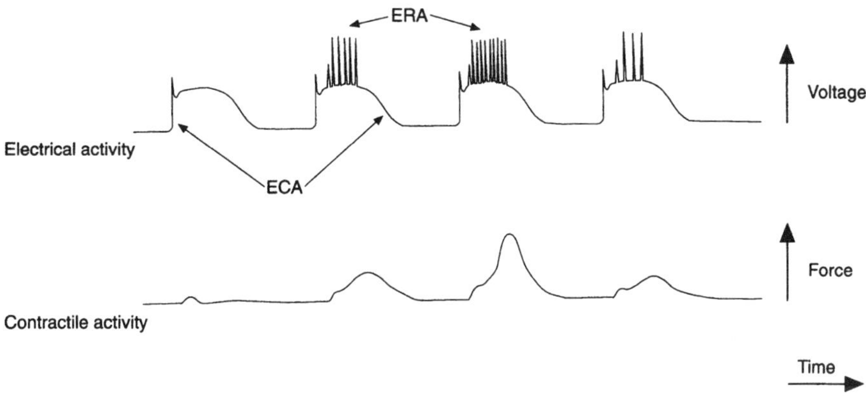

FIGURE 6.3 The relationships between ECA, ERA, and muscular contractions. The ERA occurs in the depolarized phase of the ECA. Muscular contractions are associated with the ERA, and their amplitude depends on the frequency of response potentials within an ERA burst.

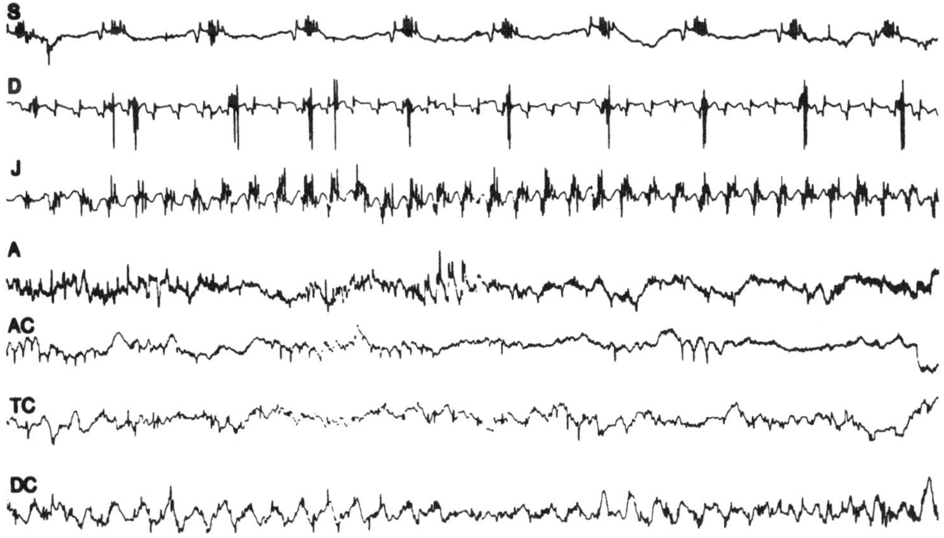

FIGURE 6.4 The gastrointestinal ECA and ERA, recorded in a conscious dog from electrode sets implanted subserosally on stomach (S), duodenum (D), jejunum (J), proximal ascending colon (A), distal ascending colon (AC), transverse colon (TC), and descending colon (DC), respectively. Each trace is of 2 min duration.

There is also a cyclical pattern of of distally propagating ERA that appears in the small intestine during the fasted state [Szurszewski, 1969], called the migrating motility complex (MMC). This pattern consists of four phases [Code and Marlett, 1975]: Phase I has little or no ERA, phase II consists of irregular ERA bursts, phase III consists of intense repetitive ERA bursts where there is an ERA burst on each ECA cycle, and phase IV consists of irregular ERA bursts but is usually much shorter than phase II and may not be always present. The initiation and propagation of the MMC is controlled by enteric cholinergic neurons in the intestinal wall (Fig. 6.2). The propagation of the MMC may be modulated by inputs from extrinsic nerves or circulating hormones [Sarna et al., 1981]. The MMC keeps the small intestine clean of residual food, debris, and desquamated cells.

6.3 A Historical Perspective

Minute Rhythms

Alvarez and Mahoney [1922] reported the presence of a rhythmic electrical activity (which they called "action currents") in the smooth muscle layers of the stomach, small intestine, and colon. Their data were acquired from cat (stomach, small intestine), dog (stomach, small intestine, colon), and rabbit (small intestine, colon). They also demonstrated the existence of frequency gradients in excised stomach and bowel. Puestow [1933] confirmed the presence of a rhythmic electrical activity (which he called "waves of altered electrical potential") and a frequency gradient in isolated canine small intestinal segments. He also demonstrated the presence of an electrical spiking activity (associated with muscular contractions) superimposed on the rhythmic electrical activity. He implied that the rhythmic electrical activity persisted at all times, whereas the electrical spike activity was of an intermittent nature. Bozler [1938, 1939, 1941] confirmed the occurrence of an electrical spiking activity associated with muscular contractions both *in vitro* in isolated longitudinal muscle strips from guinea pig (colon, small intestine) and rabbit (small intestine), and *in situ* in exposed loops of small intestine of anesthetized cat, dog, and rabbit as well as in cat stomach. He also suggested that the strength of a spontaneous muscular contraction is proportional to the frequency and duration of the spikes associated with it.

The presence of two types of electrical activity in the smooth muscle layers of the gastrointestinal tract in several species has been established [Milton and Smith, 1956; Bulbring et al., 1958; Burnstock et al., 1963; Daniel and Chapman, 1963; Bass, 1965; Gillespie, 1962; Duthie, 1974; Christensen, 1975; Daniel, 1975; Sarna, 1975a]. The autonomous electrical rhythmic activity is an omnipresent myogenic activity [Burnstock et al., 1963] whose function is to control the appearance *in time and space* of the electrical spiking activity (an intermittent activity associated with muscular contractions) when neural and chemical factors are appropriate [Daniel and Chapman, 1963]. Neural and chemical factors determine whether or not contractions will occur, but when contractions are occurring, the myogenic control system determines the *spatial and temporal* patterns of contractions.

Isolation of a distal segment of canine small intestine from a proximal segment (using surgical transection or clamping) has been reported to produce a decrease in the frequency of both the rhythmic muscular contractions [Douglas, 1949; Milton and Smith, 1956] and the electrical rhythmic activity [Milton and Smith, 1956] of the distal segment, suggesting frequency entrainment or pulling of the distal segment by the proximal one. It was demonstrated [Milton and Smith, 1956] that the repetition of the electrical spiking activity changed in the same manner as that of the electrical rhythmic activity, thus confirming a one-to-one temporal relationship between the frequency of the electrical rhythmic activity, the repetition rate of the electrical spiking activity, and the frequency of the muscular contractions (when all are present at any one site). Nelson and Becker [1968] suggested that the electrical rhythmic activity of the small intestine behaves like a system of coupled relaxation oscillators. They used two forward coupled relaxation oscillators, having different intrinsic frequencies, to demonstrate frequency entrainment of the two coupled oscillators. Uncoupling of the two oscillators caused a decrease in the frequency of the distal oscillator simulating the effect of transection of the canine small intestine.

The electrical rhythmic activity in canine stomach [Sarna et al., 1972], canine small intestine [Nelson and Becker, 1968; Diamant et al., 1970; Sarna et al., 1971], human small intestine [Robertson-Dunn and Linkens, 1974], human colon [Bardakjian and Sarna, 1980], and human rectosigmoid [Linkens et al., 1976] has been modeled by populations of coupled nonlinear oscillators. The interaction between coupled nonlinear oscillators is governed by both intrinsic oscillator properties and coupling mechanisms.

Hour Rhythms

The existence of periodic gastric activity in the fasted state in both dog [Morat, 1882] and man [Morat, 1893] has been reported. The occurrence of a periodic pattern of motor activity, comprising bursts of contractions alternating with "intervals of repose," in the gastrointestinal tracts of fasted animals was noted early in the 20th century by Boldireff [1905]. He observed that (1) the bursts recurred with a periodicity of about 1.5 to 2.5 h, (2) the amplitude of the gastric contractions during the bursts were larger than those seen postprandially, (3) the small bowel was also involved, and (4) with longer fasting periods, the bursts occurred less frequently and had a shorter duration. Periodic bursts of activity were also observed in (1) the lower esphageal sphincter [Cannon and Washburn, 1912] and (2) the pylorus [Wheelon and Thomas, 1921]. Further investigation of the fasting contractile activity in the upper small intestine was undertaken in the early 1920s with particular emphasis on the coordination between the stomach and duodenum [Wheelon and Thomas, 1922; Alvarez and Mahoney, 1923]. More recently, evidence was obtained [Itoh et al., 1978] that the cyclical activity in the lower esophageal sphincter noted by Cannon and Washburn [1912] was also coordinated with that of the stomach and small intestine.

With the use of implanted strain gauges, it was possible to observe contractile activity over long periods of time and it was demonstrated that the cyclical fasting pattern in the duodenum was altered by feeding [Jacoby et al., 1963]. The types of contractions observed during fasting and feeding were divided into four groups [Reinke et al., 1967; Carlson et al., 1972]. Three types of contractile patterns were observed in fasted animals: (1) quiescent interval, (2) a shorter interval of increasing activity, and (3) an interval of maximal activity. The fourth type was in fed animals and it consisted of randomly occurring contractions of varying amplitudes. With the use of implanted electrodes in the small intestine of fasted dogs, Szurszewski [1969] demonstrated that the cyclical appearance of electrical spiking activity at each electrode site was due to the migration of the cyclical pattern of quiescence, increasing activity and maximal electrical activity down the small intestine from the duodenum to the terminal ileum. He called this electrical pattern the *migrating myoelectric complex* (MMC). Grivel and Ruckebusch [1972] demonstrated that the mechanical correlate of this electrical pattern, which they called the *migrating motor complex*, occurs in other species such as sheep and rabbits. They also observed that the velocity of propagation of the maximal contractile activity was proportional to the length of the small intestine. Code and Marlett [1975] observed the electrical correlate of the cyclical activity in dog stomach that was reported by Morat [1882, 1893], and they demonstrated that the stomach MMC was coordinated with the duodenal MMC.

The MMC pattern has been demonstrated in other mammalian species [Ruckebusch and Fioramonti, 1975; Ruckebusch and Bueno, 1976], including humans. Bursts of distally propagating contractions has been noted in the gastrointestinal tract of man [Beck et al., 1965], and their cyclical nature was reported by Stanciu and Bennet [1975]. The MMC has been described in both normal volunteers [Vantrappen et al., 1977; Fleckenstein, 1978; Thompson et al., 1980; Kerlin and Phillips, 1982; Rees et al., 1982] and in patients [Vantrappen et al., 1977; Thompson et al., 1982; Summers et al., 1982].

Terminology

A nomenclature to describe the gastrointestinal electrical activities has been proposed to describe the minute rhythm [Sarna, 1975b] and the hour rhythm [Carlson et al., 1972; Code and Marlett, 1975].

Control cycle is one depolarization and repolarization of the transmembrane voltage. *Control wave* (*or slow wave*) is the continuing rhythmic electrical activity recorded at any one site. It was assumed to be generated by the smooth muscle cells behaving like a relaxation oscillator at that site. However, recent evidence [Hara et al., 1986; Suzuki et al., 1986; Barajas-Lopez et al., 1989; Serio et al., 1991] indicates that it is generated by a system of interstitial cells of Cajal (ICC) and smooth muscle cells at that site. *Electrical Control Activity* (ECA) is the totality of the control waves recorded at one or several sites. *Response Potentials* (or *spikes*) are the rapid oscillations of transmembrane voltage in the depolarized state of smooth muscle cells. They are associated with muscular contraction and their occurrence is assumed to be in response to a control cycle when acetylcholine is present. *Electrical Response Activity* (ERA) is the totality of the groups of response potentials at one or several sites.

Migrating Motility Complex (MMC) is the entire cycle which is composed of four phases. Initially, the electrical and mechanical patterns were referred to as the migrating myoelectric complex and the migrating motor complex, respectively. *Phase I* is the interval during which fewer than 5% of ECA have associated ERA, and no or very few contractions are present. *Phase II* is the interval when 5 to 95% of the ECA has associated ERA, and intermittent contractions are present. *Phase III* is the interval when more than 95% of ECA have associated ERA, and large cyclical contractions are present. *Phase IV* is a short and waning interval of intermittent ERA and contractions. Phases II and IV are not always present and are difficult to characterize, whereas phases I and III are always present. *MMC Cycle Time* is the interval from the end of one phase III to the end of a subsequent phase III at any one site. *Migration Time* is the time taken for the MMC to migrate from the upper duodenum to the terminal ileum.

6.4 The Stomach

Anatomical Features

The stomach is somewhat pyriform in shape with its large end directed upward at the lower esophageal sphincter and its small end bent to the right at the pylorus. It has two curvatures, the greater curvature which is four to five times as long as the lesser curvature, and it consists of three regions: the fundus, corpus (or body), and antrum. It has three smooth muscle layers. The outermost layer is the longitudinal muscle layer, the middle is the circular muscle layer, and the innermost is the oblique muscle layer. These layers thicken gradually in the distal stomach toward the pylorus, which is consistent with stomach function since trituration occurs in the distal antrum. The size of the stomach varies considerably among subjects. In an adult male, its greatest length when distended is about 25 to 30 cm and its widest diameter is about 10 to 12 cm [Pick and Howden, 1977].

The structural relationships of nerve, muscle, and interstitial cells of Cajal in the canine corpus indicated a high density of gap junctions indicating very tight coupling between cells. Nerves in the corpus are not located close to circular muscle cells but are found exterior to the muscle bundles, whereas ICCs have gap junction contact with smooth muscle cells and are closely innervated [Daniel and Sakai, 1984].

Gastric ECA

In the canine stomach, the fundus does not usually exhibit spontaneous electrical oscillations, but the corpus and antrum do exhibit such oscillations. In the intact stomach, the ECA is entrained to a frequency of about 5 cpm (about 3 cpm in humans) throughout the electrically active region with phase lags in both the longitudinal and circumferential directions [Sarna et al., 1972]. The phase lags decrease distally from corpus to antrum.

There is a marked intrinsic frequency gradient along the axis of the stomach and a slight intrinsic frequency gradient along the circumference. The intrinsic frequency of gastric ECA in isolated circular muscle of the orad and mid corpus is the highest (about 5 cpm) compared to about 3.5 cpm in the rest of the corpus, and about 0.5 cpm in the antrum. Also, there is an orad to aborad intrinsic gradient in resting membrane potential, with the terminal antrum having the most negative resting membrane potential, about 30 mV more negative than the fundal regions [Szurszewski, 1987]. The relatively depolarized state of the fundal muscle may explain its electrical inactivity since the voltage-sensitive ionic channels may be kept in a state of inactivation. Hyperpolarization of the fundus to a transmembrane voltage of –60 mV produces fundal control waves similar to those recorded from mid and orad corpus.

The ECA in canine stomach was modeled [Sarna et al., 1972] using an array of 13 bidirectionally coupled relaxation oscillators. The model featured (1) an intrinsic frequency decline from corpus to the pylorus and from greater curvature to the lesser curvature, (2) entrainment of all coupled oscillators at a frequency close to the highest intrinsic frequency, and (3) distally decreasing phase lags between the entrained oscillators. A simulated circumferential transection caused the formation of another frequency plateau aboral to the transection. The frequency of the orad plateau remained unaffected while that of the aborad plateau was decreased. This is consistent with the observed experimental data.

The Electrogastrogram

In a similar manner to other electrophysiological measures such as the electrocardiogram (EKG) and the electroencephalogram (EEG), the electrogastrogram (EGG) was identified [Stern and Koch, 1985; Chen and McCallum, 1994]. The EGG is the signal obtained from cutaneous recording of the gastric myoelectrical activity by using surface electrodes placed on the abdomen over the stomach. Although the first EGG was recorded in the early 1920s [Alvarez, 1922], progress *vis-à-vis* clinical applications has been relatively slow, in particular when compared to the progress made in EKG, which also started in the early 1920s. Despite many attempts made over the decades, visual inspection of the EGG signal has not led to the identification of waveform characteristics that would help the clinician to diagnose functional or organic diseases of the stomach. Even the development of techniques such as time-frequency analysis [Qiao et al., 1998] and artificial neural network-based feature extraction [Liang et al., 1997; Wang et al., 1999] for computer analysis of the EGG did not provide *clinically relevant* information about gastric motility disorders. It has been demonstrated that increased EGG frequencies (1) were seen in perfectly healthy subjects [Pffafenbach et al., 1995], and (2) did not always correspond to serosally recorded tachygastria in dogs [Mintchev and Bowes, 1997]. As yet, there is no effective method of detecting a change in the direction or velocity of propagation of gastric ECA from the EGG.

6.5 The Small Intestine

Anatomical Features

The small intestine is a long hollow organ which consists of the duodenum, jejunum, and ileum. Its length is about 650 cm in humans and 300 cm in dogs. The duodenum extends from the pylorus to the ligament of Treitz (about 30 cm in humans and dogs). In humans, the duodenum forms a C-shaped pattern, with the ligament of Treitz near the corpus of the stomach. In dogs, the duodenum lies along the right side of the peritoneal cavity, with the ligament of Treitz in the pelvis. The duodenum receives pancreatic exocrine secretions and bile. In both humans and dogs, the jejunum consists of the next one-third whereas the ileum consists of the remaining two-thirds of the intestine. The major differences between the jejunum and ileum are functional in nature, relating to their absorption characteristics and motor control. The majority of sugars, amino acids, lipids, electrolytes, and water are absorbed in the jejunum and proximal ileum, whereas bile acids and vitamin B12 are absorbed in the terminal ileum.

Small Intestinal ECA

In the canine small intestine, the ECA is not entrained throughout the entire length [Diamant and Bortoff, 1969a; Sarna et al., 1971]. However, the ECA exhibits a plateau of constant frequency in the proximal region whereby there is a distal increase in phase lag. The frequency plateau (of about 20 cpm) extends over the entire duodenum and part of the jejunum. There is a marked intrinsic frequency gradient in the longitudinal direction with the highest intrinsic frequency being less than the plateau frequency. When the small intestine was transected *in vivo* into small segments (15 cm long), the intrinsic frequency of the ECA in adjacent segments tended to decrease aborally in an exponential manner [Sarna et al.,

1971]. A single transection of the duodenum caused the formation of another frequency plateau aboral to the transection. The ECA frequency in the orad plateau was generally unaffected, while that in the aborad plateau was decreased [Diamant and Bortoff, 1969b; Sarna et al., 1971]. The frequency of the aborad plateau was either higher than or equal to the highest intrinsic frequency distal to the transection, depending on whether the transection of the duodenum was either above or below the region of the bile duct [Diamant and Bortoff, 1969b].

The ECA in canine small intestine was modeled using a chain of 16 bidirectionally coupled relaxation oscillators [Sarna et al., 1971]. Coupling was not uniform along the chain, since the proximal oscillators were strongly coupled and the distal oscillators were weakly coupled. The model featured (1) an exponential intrinsic frequency decline along the chain, (2) a frequency plateau which is higher than the highest intrinsic frequency, and (3) a temporal variation of the frequencies distal to the frequency plateau region. A simulated transection in the frequency plateau region caused the formation of another frequency plateau aboral to the transection, such that the frequency of the orad plateau was unchanged whereas the frequency of the aborad plateau decreased.

The ECA in human small intestine was modeled using a chain of 100 bidirectionally coupled relaxation oscillators [Robertson-Dunn and Linkens, 1976]. Coupling was nonuniform and asymmetrical. The model featured (1) a piecewise linear decline in intrinsic frequency along the chain, (2) a piecewise linear decline in coupling similar to that of the intrinsic frequency, (3) forward coupling which is stronger than backward coupling, and (4) a frequency plateau in the proximal region which is higher than the highest intrinsic frequency in the region.

Small Intestinal MMC

The MMCs in canine small intestine have been observed in intrinsically isolated segments [Sarna et al., 1981, 1983], even after the isolated segment has been stripped of all extrinsic innervation [Sarr and Kelly, 1981] or removed in continuity with the remaining gut as a Thiry Vella loop [Itoh et al., 1981]. This intrinsic mechanism is able to function independently of extrinsic innervation since vagotomy [Weisbrodt et al., 1975; Ruckebusch and Bueno, 1977] does not hinder the initiation of the MMC. The initiation of the small intestinal MMC is controlled by integrative networks within the intrinsic plexuses utilizing nicotinic and muscarinic cholinergic receptors [Ormsbee et al., 1979; El-Sharkawy et al., 1982].

When the canine small intestine was transected into four equal strips [Sarna et al., 1981, 1983], it was found that each strip was capable of generating an independent MMC that would appear to propagate from the proximal to the distal part of each segment. This suggested that the MMC can be modeled by a chain of coupled relaxation oscillators. The average intrinsic periods of the MMC for the four segments were reported to be 106.2, 66.8, 83.1, and 94.8 min, respectively. The segment containing the duodenum had the longest period, while the subsequent segment containing the jejunum had the shortest period. However, in the intact small intestine, the MMC starts in the duodenum and not the jejunum. Bardakjian et al. [1981, 1984] have demonstrated that both the intrinsic frequency gradients and resting level gradients have major roles in the entrainment of a chain of coupled oscillators. In modeling the small intestinal MMC with a chain of four coupled oscillators, it was necessary to include a gradient in the intrinsic resting levels of the MMC oscillators (with the proximal oscillator having the lowest resting level) in order to entrain the oscillators and allow the proximal oscillator to behave as the leading oscillator [Bardakjian and Ahmed, 1992].

6.6 The Colon

Anatomical Features

In humans, the colon is about 100 cm in length. The ileum joins the colon approximately 5 cm from its end, forming the cecum which has a worm-like appendage, the appendix. The colon is sacculated, and the longitudinal smooth muscle is concentrated in three bands (the taeniae). It lies in front of the small intestine against the abdominal wall and it consists of the ascending (on the right side), transverse (across the lower stomach), and descending (on the left side) colon. The descending colon becomes the sigmoid colon in the pelvis as it runs down and forward to the rectum. Major functions of the colon are (1) to absorb water, certain electrolytes, short chain fatty acids, and bacterial metabolites; (2) to slowly propel its luminal contents in the caudad direction; (3) to store the residual matter in the distal region; and (4) to rapidly move its contents in the caudad direction during mass movements [Sarna, 1991]. In dogs, the colon is about 45 cm in length and the cecum has no appendage. The colon is not sacculated, and the longitudinal smooth muscle coat is continuous around the circumference [Miller et al., 1968]. It lies posterior to the small intestine and it consists mainly of ascending and descending segments with a small transverse segment. However, functionally it is assumed to consist of three regions, each of about 15 cm in length, representing the ascending, transverse, and descending colon, respectively.

Colonic ECA

In the human colon, the ECA is almost completely phase-unlocked between adjacent sites as close as 1 to 2 cm apart, and its frequency (about 3 to 15 cpm) and amplitude at each site vary with time [Sarna et al., 1980]. This results in short duration contractions that are also disorganized in time and space. The disorganization of ECA and its associated contractions is consistent with the colonic function of extensive mixing, kneading, and slow net distal propulsion [Sarna, 1991]. In the canine colon, the reports about the intrinsic frequency gradient were conflicting [Vanasin et al., 1974; Shearin et al., 1978; El-Sharkawy, 1983].

The human colonic ECA was modeled [Bardakjian and Sarna, 1980] using a tubular structure of 99 bidirectionally coupled nonlinear oscillators arranged in 33 parallel rings where each ring contained three oscillators. Coupling was nonuniform and it increased in the longitudinal direction. The model featured (1) no phase-locking in the longitudinal or circumferential directions, (2) temporal and spatial variation of the frequency profile with large variations in the proximal and distal regions and small variations in the middle region, and (3) waxing and waning of the amplitudes of the ECA which was more pronounced in the proximal and distal regions. The model demonstrated that the "silent periods" occurred because of the interaction between oscillators and they did not occur when the oscillators were uncoupled. The model was further refined [Bardakjian et al., 1990] such that when the ECA amplitude exceeded an excitation threshold, a burst of ERA was exhibited. The ERA bursts occurred in a seemingly random manner in adjacent sites because (1) the ECA was not phase-locked and (2) the ECA amplitudes and waveshapes varied in a seemingly random manner.

6.7 Epilogue

The ECA in stomach, small intestine, and colon behaves like the outputs of a population of coupled nonlinear oscillators. The populations in the stomach and the proximal small intestine are entrained, whereas those in the distal small intestine and colon are not entrained. There are distinct intrinsic frequency gradients in the stomach and small intestine but their profile in the colon is ambiguous.

The applicability of modeling of gastrointestinal ECA by coupled nonlinear oscillators has been reconfirmed [Daniel et al., 1994], and a novel nonlinear oscillator, the mapped clock oscillator, was proposed [Bardakjian and Diamant, 1994] for modeling the cellular ECA. The oscillator consists of two coupled components: a clock which represents the interstitial cells of Cajal, and a transformer which represents the smooth muscle transmembrane ionic transport mechanisms [Skinner and Bardakjian, 1991]. Such a model accounts for the mounting evidence supporting the role of the interstitial cells of Cajal as a pacemaker for the smooth muscle transmembrane voltage oscillations [Hara et al., 1986; Suzuki et al., 1986; Barajas-Lopez et al., 1989; Serio et al., 1991; Sanders, 1996].

Modeling of the gastrointestinal ECA by populations of coupled nonlinear oscillators [Bardakjian, 1987] suggests that gastrointestinal motility disorders associated with abnormal ECA can be effectively treated by (1) electronic pacemakers to coordinate the oscillators, (2) surgical interventions to remove regional ectopic foci, and (3) pharmacotherapy to stimulate the oscillators. Electronic pacing has been demonstrated in canine stomach [Kelly and LaForce, 1972; Sarna and Daniel, 1973; Bellahsene et al., 1992] and small intestine [Sarna and Daniel, 1975c; Becker et al., 1983]. Also, pharmacotherapy with prokinetic drugs such as Domperidone and Cisapride has demonstrated improvements in the coordination of the gastric oscillators.

Acknowledgments

The author would like to thank his colleagues Dr. Sharon Chung and Dr. Karen Hall for providing biological insight.

References

Alvarez, W.C. and Mahoney, L.J. 1922. Action current in stomach and intestine. *Am. J. Physiol.*, 58:476-493.

Alvarez, W.C. 1922. The electrogastrogram and what it shows. *J. Am. Med. Assoc.*, 78:1116-1119.

Alvarez, W.C. and Mahoney, L.J. 1923. The relations between gastric and duodenal peristalsis. *Am. J. Physiol.*, 64:371-386.

Barajas-Lopez, C., Berezin, I., Daniel, E.E., and Huizinga, J.D. 1989. Pacemaker activity recorded in interstitial cells of Cajal of the gastrointestinal tract. *Am. J. Physiol.*, 257:C830-C835.

Bardakjian, B.L. and Sarna, S.K. 1980. A computer model of human colonic electrical control activity (ECA). *IEEE Trans. Biomed. Eng.*, 27:193-202.

Bardakjian, B.L. and Sarna, S.K. 1981. Mathematical investigation of populations of coupled synthesized relaxation oscillators representing biological rhythms. *IEEE Trans. Biomed. Eng.*, 28:10-15.

Bardakjian, B.L., El-Sharkawy, T.Y., and Diamant, N.E. 1984. Interaction of coupled nonlinear oscillators having different intrinsic resting levels. *J. Theor. Biol.*, 106:9-23.

Bardakjian, B.L. 1987. Computer models of gastrointestinal myoelectric activity. *Automedica*, 7:261-276.

Bardakjian, B.L., Sarna, S.K., and Diamant, N.E. 1990. Composite synthesized relaxation oscillators: Application to modeling of colonic ECA and ERA. *Gastrointest. J. Motil.*, 2:109-116.

Bardakjian, B.L. and Ahmed, K. 1992. Is a peripheral pattern generator sufficient to produce both fasting and postprandial patterns of the migrating myoelectric complex (MMC)? *Dig. Dis. Sci.*, 37:986.

Bardakjian, B.L. and Diamant, N.E. 1994. A mapped clock oscillator model for transmembrane electrical rhythmic activity in excitable cells. *J. Theor. Biol.*, 166:225-235.

Bass, P. 1965. Electric activity of smooth muscle of the gastrointestinal tract. *Gastroenterology*, 49:391-394.

Beck, I.T., McKenna, R.D., Peterfy, G., Sidorov, J., and Strawczynski, H. 1965. Pressure studies in the normal human jejunum. *Am. J. Dig. Dis.*, 10:437-448.

Becker, J.M., Sava, P., Kelly, K.A., and Shturman, L. 1983. Intestinal pacing for canine postgastrectomy dumping. *Gastroenterology*, 84:383-387.

Bellahsene, B.E., Lind, C.D., Schirmer, B.D., et al. 1992. Acceleration of gastric emptying with electrical stimulation in a canine model of gastroparesis. *Am. J. Physiol.*, 262:G826-G834.

Boldireff, W.N. 1905. Le travail periodique de l'appareil digestif en dehors de la digestion. *Arch. Des. Sci. Biol.*, 11:1-157.

Bozler, E. 1938. Action potentials of visceral smooth muscle. *Am. J. Physiol.*, 124:502-510.

Bozler, E. 1939. Electrophysiological studies on the motility of the gastrointestinal tract. *Am. J. Physiol.*, 127:301-307.

Bozler, E. 1941. Action potentials and conduction of excitation in muscle. *Biol. Symp.*, 3:95-110.

Bulbring, E., Burnstock G., and Holman, M.E. 1958. Excitation and conduction in the smooth muscle of the isolated taenia coli of the guinea pig. *J. Physiol.*, 142:420-437.

Burnstock, G., Holman, M.E., and Prosser, C.L. 1963. Electrophysiology of smooth muscle. *Physiol. Rev.*, 43:482-527.

Cannon, W.B. and Washburn, A.L. 1912. An explanation of hunger. *Am. J. Physiol.*, 29:441-454.

Carlson, G.M., Bedi, B.S., and Code, C.F. 1972. Mechanism of propagation of intestinal interdigestive myoelectric complex. *Am. J. Physiol.*, 222:1027-1030.

Chen, J.Z. and McCallum, R.W. 1994. *Electrogastrography: Principles and Applications*. Raven Press, New York.

Christensen, J. 1975. Myoelectric control of the colon. *Gastroenterology*, 68:601-609.

Code, C.F. and Marlett, J.A. 1975. The interdigestive myoelectric complex of the stomach and small bowel of dogs. *J. Physiol.*, 246:289-309.

Daniel, E.E. and Chapman, K.M. 1963. Electrical activity of the gastrointestinal tract as an indication of mechanical activity. *Am. J. Dig. Dis.*, 8:54-102.

Daniel, E.E. 1975. Electrophysiology of the colon. *Gut*, 16:298-329.

Daniel, E.E. and Sakai, Y. 1984. Structural basis for function of circular muscle of canine corpus. *Can. J. Physiol. Pharmacol.*, 62:1304-1314.

Daniel, E.E., Bardakjian, B.L., Huizinga, J.D., and Diamant, N.E. 1994. Relaxation oscillators and core conductor models are needed for understanding of GI electrical activities. *Am. J. Physiol.*, 266:G339-G349.

Diamant, N.E. and Bortoff, A. 1969a. Nature of the intestinal slow wave frequency gradient. *Am. J. Physiol.*, 216:301-307.

Diamant, N.E. and Bortoff, A. 1969b. Effects of transection on the intestinal slow wave frequency gradient. *Am. J. Physiol.*, 216:734-743.

Douglas, D.M. 1949. The decrease in frequency of contraction of the jejunum after transplantation to the ileum. *J. Physiol.*, 110:66-75.

Duthie, H.L. 1974. Electrical activity of gastrointestinal smooth muscle. *Gut*, 15:669-681.

El-Sharkawy, T.Y., Markus, H., and Diamant, N.E. 1982. Neural control of the intestinal migrating myoelectric complex: A pharmacological analysis. *Can. J. Physiol. Pharm.*, 60:794-804.

El-Sharkawy, T.Y. 1983. Electrical activity of the muscle layers of the canine colon. *J. Physiol.*, 342:67-83.

Fleckenstein, P. 1978. Migrating electrical spike activity in the fasting human small intestine. *Dig. Dis. Sci.*, 23:769-775.

Gillespie, J.S. 1962. The electrical and mechanical responses of intestinal smooth muscle cells to stimulation of their extrinsic parasympathetic nerves. *J. Physiol.*, 162:76-92.

Grivel, M.L. and Ruckebusch, Y. 1972. The propagation of segmental contractions along the small intestine. *J. Physiol.*, 277:611-625.

Hara, Y.M., Kubota, M., and Szurszewski, J.H. 1986. Electrophysiology of smooth muscle of the small intestine of some mammals. *J. Physiol.*, 372:501-520.

Itoh, Z., Honda, R., Aizawa, I., Takeuchi, S., Hiwatashi, K., and Couch, E.F. 1978. Interdigestive motor activity of the lower esophageal sphincter in the conscious dog. *Dig. Dis. Sci.*, 23:239-247.

Itoh, Z., Aizawa, I., and Takeuchi, S. 1981. Neural regulation of interdigestive motor activity in canine jejunum. *Am. J. Physiol.*, 240:G324-G330.

Jacoby, H.I., Bass, P., and Bennett, D.R. 1963. *In vivo* extraluminal contractile force transducer for gastrointestinal muscle. *J. Appl. Physiol.*, 18:658-665.

Kelly, K.A. and LaForce, R.C. 1972. Pacing the canine stomach with electric stimulation. *Am. J. Physiol.*, 222:588-594.

Kerlin, P. and Phillips, S. 1982. The variability of motility of the ileum and jejunum in healthy humans. *Gastroenterology*, 82:694-700.

Liang, J., Cheung, J.Y., and Chen, J.D.Z. 1997. Detection and deletion of motion artifacts in electrogastrogram using feature analysis and neural networks. *Ann. Biomed. Eng.*, 25:850-857.

Linkens, D.A., Taylor, I., and Duthie, H.L. 1976. Mathematical modeling of the colorectal myoelectrical activity in humans. *IEEE Trans. Biomed. Eng.*, 23:101-110.

Milton, G.W. and Smith, A.W.M. 1956. The pacemaking area of the duodenum. *J. Physiol.*, 132:100-114.

Miller, M.E., Christensen, G.C., and Evans, H.E. 1968. *Anatomy of the Dog*, Saunders, Philadelphia.

Mintchev, M.P. and Bowes, K.L. 1997. Do increased electrogastrographic frequencies always correspond to internal tachygastria? *Ann. Biomed. Eng.*, 25:1052-1058.

Morat, J.P. 1882. Sur l'innervation motrice de l'estomac. *Lyon. Med.*, 40:289-296.

Morat, J.P. 1893. Sur quelques particularites de l'innervation motrice de l'estomac et de l'intestin. *Arch. Physiol. Norm. Path.*, 5:142-153.

Nelson, T.S. and Becker, J.C. 1968. Simulation of the electrical and mechanical gradient of the small intestine. *Am. J. Physiol.*, 214:749-757.

Ormsbee, H.S., Telford, G.L., and Mason, G.R. 1979. Required neural involvement in control of canine migrating motor complex. *Am. J. Physiol.*, 237:E451-E456.

Pffafenbach, B., Adamek, R.J., Kuhn, K., and Wegener, M. 1995. Electrogastrography in healthy subjects. Evaluation of normal values: influence of age and gender. *Dig. Dis. Sci.*, 40:1445-1450.

Pick, T.P. and Howden, R. 1977. *Gray's Anatomy*, Bounty Books, New York.

Puestow, C.B. 1933. Studies on the origins of the automaticity of the intestine: the action of certain drugs on isolated intestinal transplants. *Am. J. Physiol.*, 106:682-688.

Qiao, W., Sun, H.H., Chey, W.Y., and Lee, K.Y. 1998. Continuous wavelet analysis as an aid in the representation and interpretation of electrogastrographic signals. *Ann. Biomed. Eng.*, 26:1072-1081.

Rees, W.D.W., Malagelada, J.R., Miller, L.J., and Go, V.L.W. 1982. Human interdigestive and postprandial gastrointestinal motor and gastrointestinal hormone patterns. *Dig. Dis. Sci.*, 27:321-329.

Reinke, D.A., Rosenbaum, A.H., and Bennett, D.R. 1967. Patterns of dog gastrointestinal contractile activity monitored *in vivo* with extraluminal force transducers. *Am. J. Dig. Dis.*, 12:113-141.

Robertson-Dunn, B. and Linkens, D.A. 1974. A mathematical model of the slow wave electrical activity of the human small intestine. *Med. Biol. Eng.*, 12:750-758.

Ruckebusch, Y. and Fioramonti, S. 1975. Electrical spiking activity and propulsion in small intestine in fed and fasted states. *Gastroenterology*, 68:1500-1508.

Ruckebusch, Y. and Bueno, L. 1976. The effects of feeding on the motility of the stomach and small intestine in the pig. *Br. J. Nutr.*, 35:397-405.

Ruckebusch, Y. and Bueno, L. 1977. Migrating myoelectrical complex of the small intestine. *Gastroenterology*, 73:1309-1314.

Sanders, K.M. 1996. A case for interstitial cells of Cajal as pacemakers and mediators of neurotransmission in the gastrointestinal tract. *Gastroenterology*, 111(2):492-515.

Sarna, S.K., Daniel, E.E., and Kingma, Y.J. 1971. Simulation of slow wave electrical activity of small intestine. *Am. J. Physiol.*, 221:166-175.

Sarna, S.K., Daniel, E.E., and Kingma, Y.J. 1972. Simulation of the electrical control activity of the stomach by an array of relaxation oscillators. *Am. J. Dig. Dis.*, 17:299-310.

Sarna, S.K. and Daniel, E.E. 1973. Electrical stimulation of gastric electrical control activity. *Am. J. Physiol.*, 225:125-131.

Sarna, S.K. 1975a. Models of smooth muscle electrical activity. In *Methods in Pharmacology*, E.E. Daniel and D.M. Paton, Eds., Plenum Press, New York, 519-540.

Sarna, S.K. 1975b. Gastrointestinal electrical activity: terminology. *Gastroenterology*, 68:1631-1635.

Sarna, S.K. and Daniel, E.E. 1975c. Electrical stimulation of small intestinal electrical control activity. *Gastroenterology*, 69:660-667.

Sarna, S.K., Bardakjian, B.L., Waterfall, W.E., and Lind, J.F. 1980. Human colonic electrical control activity (ECA). *Gastroenterology*, 78:1526-1536.

Sarna, S.K., Stoddard, C., Belbeck, L., and McWade, D. 1981. Intrinsic nervous control of migrating myoelectric complexes. *Am. J. Physiol.*, 241:G16-G23.

Sarna, S., Condon, R.E., and Cowles, V. 1983. Enteric mechanisms of initiation of migrating myoelectric complexes in dogs. *Gastroenterology*, 84:814-822.

Sarna, S.K. 1991. Physiology and pathophysiology of colonic motor activity. *Dig. Dis. Sci.*, 6:827-862.

Sarr M.G. and Kelly, K.A. 1981. Myoelectric activity of the autotransplanted canine jejunoileum. *Gastroenterology*, 81:303-310.

Serio, R., Barajas-Lopez, C., Daniel, E.E., Berezin, I., and Huizinga, J.D. 1991. Pacemaker activity in the colon: Role of interstitial cells of Cajal and smooth muscle cells. *Am. J. Physiol.*, 260:G636-G645.

Shearin, N.L., Bowes, K.L. and Kingma, Y.J. 1978. *In vitro* electrical activity in canine colon. *Gut,* 20:780-786.

Stanciu, C. and Bennett, J.R. 1975. The general pattern of gastroduodenal motility: 24 hour recordings in normal subjects. *Rev. Med. Chir. Soc. Med. Nat. Iasi.,* 79:31-36.

Skinner, F.K. and Bardakjian, B.L. 1991. A barrier kinetic mapping unit. Application to ionic transport in gastric smooth muscle. *Gastrointest. J. Motil.,* 3:213-224.

Stern, R.M. and Koch, K.L. 1985. *Electrogastrography: Methodology, Validation, and Applications.* Praeger, New York.

Summers, R.W., Anuras, S., and Green, J. 1982. Jejunal motility patterns in normal subjects and symptomatic patients with partial mechanical obstruction or pseudo-obstruction. In *Motility of the Digestive Tract,* M. Weinbeck, Ed., Raven Press, New York, 467-470.

Suzuki, N., Prosser, C.L., and Dahms, V., 1986. Boundary cells between longitudinal and circular layers: Essential for electrical slow waves in cat intestine. *Am. J. Physiol.,* 280:G287-G294.

Szurszewski, J.H. 1969. A migrating electric complex of the canine small intestine. *Am. J. Physiol.,* 217:1757-1763.

Szurszewski, J.H. 1987. Electrical basis for gastrointestinal motility. In *Physiology of the Gastrointestinal Tract,* L.R. Johnson, Ed., Raven Press, New York, chap. 12.

Thompson, D.G., Wingate, D.L., Archer, L., Benson, M.J., Green, W.J., and Hardy, R.J. 1980. Normal patterns of human upper small bowel motor activity recorded by prolonged radiotelemetry. *Gut,* 21:500-506.

Vanasin, B., Ustach, T.J., and Schuster, M.M. 1974. Electrical and motor activity of human and dog colon in vitro. *Johns Hopkins Med. J.,* 134:201-210.

Vantrappen, G., Janssens, J.J., Hellemans, J., and Ghoos, Y. 1977. The interdigestive motor complex of normal subjects and patients with bacterial overgrowth of the small intestine. *J. Clin. Invest.,* 59:1158-1166.

Wang, Z., He, Z., and Chen, J.D.Z. 1999. Filter banks and neural network-based feature extraction and automatic classification of electrogastrogram. *Ann. Biomed. Eng.,* 27:88-95.

Weisbrodt, N.W., Copeland, E.M., Moore, E.P., Kearly, K.W., and Johnson, L.R. 1975. Effect of vagotomy on electrical activity of the small intestine of the dog. *Am. J. Physiol.,* 228:650-654.

Wheelon, H. and Thomas, J.E. 1921. Rhythmicity of the pyloric sphincter. *Am. J. Physiol.,* 54:460-473.

Wheelon, H. and Thomas, J.E. 1922. Observations on the motility of the duodenum and the relation of duodenal activity to that of the pars pylorica. *Am. J. Physiol.,* 59:72-96.

7

Respiratory System

Arthur T. Johnson
University of Maryland

Christopher G. Lausted
University of Maryland

Joseph D. Bronzino
Trinity College/The Biomedical Engineering Alliance and Consortium (BEACON)

As functioning units, the lung and heart are usually considered a single complex organ, but because these organs contain essentially two compartments — one for blood and one for air — they are usually separated in terms of the tests conducted to evaluate heart or pulmonary function. This chapter focuses on some of the physiologic concepts responsible for normal function and specific measures of the lung's ability to supply tissue cells with enough oxygen while removing excess carbon dioxide.

7.1 Respiration Anatomy

The respiratory system consists of the lungs, conducting airways, pulmonary vasculature, respiratory muscles, and surrounding tissues and structures (Fig. 7.1). Each plays an important role in influencing respiratory responses.

Lungs

There are two lungs in the human chest; the right lung is composed of three incomplete divisions called *lobes,* and the left lung has two, leaving room for the heart. The right lung accounts for 55% of total gas volume and the left lung for 45%. Lung tissue is spongy because of the very small (200 to 300 $\times 10^{-6}$ m diameter in normal lungs at rest) gas-filled cavities called *alveoli,* which are the ultimate structures for gas exchange. There are 250 million to 350 million alveoli in the adult lung, with a total alveolar surface area of 50 to 100 m^2 depending on the degree of lung inflation [Johnson, 1991].

Conducting Airways

Air is transported from the atmosphere to the alveoli beginning with the oral and nasal cavities, through the pharynx (in the throat), past the glottal opening, and into the trachea or windpipe. Conduction of air begins at the larynx, or voice box, at the entrance to the trachea, which is a fibromuscular tube 10 to 12 cm in length and 1.4 to 2.0 cm in diameter [Kline, 1976]. At a location called the *carina,* the trachea

0-8493-1810-6/03/$0.00+$1.50

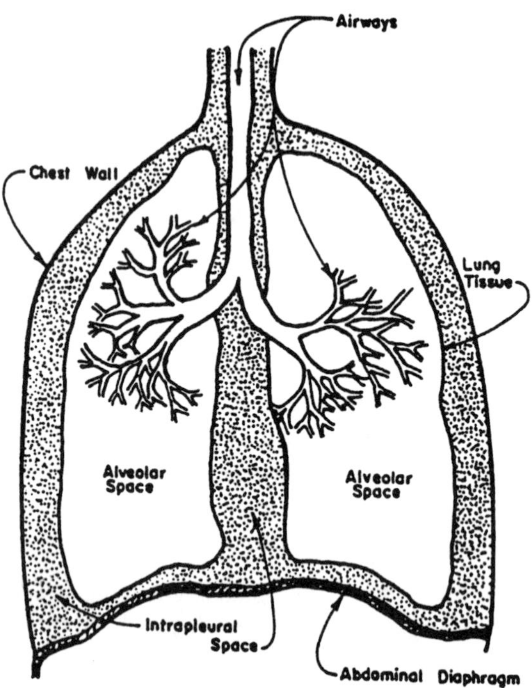

FIGURE 7.1 Schematic representation of the respiratory system.

terminates and divides into the left and right bronchi. Each bronchus has a discontinuous cartilaginous support in its wall. Muscle fibers capable of controlling airway diameter are incorporated into the walls of the bronchi, as well as in those of air passages closer to the alveoli. Smooth muscle is present throughout the respiratory bronchiolus and alveolar ducts but is absent in the last alveolar duct, which terminates in one to several alveoli. The alveolar walls are shared by other alveoli and are composed of highly pliable and collapsible squamous epithelium cells.

The bronchi subdivide into subbronchi, which further subdivide into bronchioli, which further subdivide, and so on, until finally reaching the alveolar level. Table 7.1 provides a description and dimensions of the airways of adult humans. A model of the geometric arrangement of these air passages is presented in Fig. 7.2. It will be noted that each airway is considered to branch into two subairways. In the adult human there are considered to be 23 such branchings, or generations, beginning at the trachea and ending in the alveoli.

Movement of gases in the respiratory airways occurs mainly by bulk flow (convection) throughout the region from the mouth to the nose to the 15th generation. Beyond the 15th generation, gas diffusion is relatively more important. With the low gas velocities that occur in diffusion, dimensions of the space over which diffusion occurs (alveolar space) must be small for adequate oxygen delivery into the walls; smaller alveoli are more efficient in the transfer of gas than are larger ones. Thus animals with high levels of oxygen consumption are found to have smaller-diameter alveoli compared with animals with low levels of oxygen consumption.

Alveoli

Alveoli are the structures through which gases diffuse to and from the body. To ensure gas exchange occurs efficiently, alveolar walls are extremely thin. For example, the total tissue thickness between the inside of the alveolus to pulmonary capillary blood plasma is only about 0.4×10^{-6} m. Consequently, the principal barrier to diffusion occurs at the plasma and red blood cell level, not at the alveolar membrane [Ruch and Patton, 1966].

TABLE 7.1 Classification and Approximate Dimensions of Airways of Adult Human Lung (inflated to about 3/4 of total lung capacity)*

Common Name	Numerical Order of Generation	Number of Each	Diameter, mm	Length, mm	Total Cross-Sectional Area, cm^2	Description and Comment
Trachea	0	1	18	120	2.5	Main cartilaginous airway; partly in thorax
Main bronchus	1	2	12	47.6	2.3	First branching of airway; one to each lung; in lung root; cartilage
Lobar bronchus	2	4	8	19.0	2.1	Named for each lobe; cartilage
Segmental bronchus	3	8	6	7.6	2.0	Named for radiographical and surgical anatomy; cartilage
Subsegmental bronchus	4	16	4	12.7	2.4	Last generally named bronchi; may be referred to as medium-sized bronchi; cartilage
Small bronchi	5–10	1,024†	1.3†	4.6†	13.4†	Not generally named; contain decreasing amounts of cartilage; beyond this level airways enter the lobules as defined by a strong elastic lobular limiting membrane
Bronchioles	11–13	8,192†	0.8†	2.7†	44.5†	Not named; contain no cartilage, mucus-secreting elements, or cilia; tightly embedded in lung tissue
Terminal bronchioles	14–15	32,768†	0.7†	2.0†	113.0†	Generally 2 or 3 orders so designated; morphology not significantly different from orders 11–13
Respiratory bronchioles	16–18	262,144†	0.5†	1.2†	534.0†	Definite class; bronchiolar cuboidal epithelium present, but scattered alveoli are present giving these airways a gas exchange function; order 165 often called first-order respiratory bronchiole; 17, second-order; 18, third-order
Alveolar ducts	19–22	4,194,304†	0.4†	0.8†	5,880.0†	No bronchial epithelium; have no surface except connective tissue framework; open into alveoli
Alveolar sacs	23	8,388,608	0.4	0.6	11,800.0	No reason to assign a special name; are really short alveolar ducts
Alveoli	24	300,000,000	0.2			Pulmonary capillaries are in the septae that form the alveoli

* The number of airways in each generation is based on regular dichotomous branching.

† Numbers refer to last generation in each group.

Source: Used with permission from Staub [1963] and Weibel [1963]; adapted by Comroe [1965].

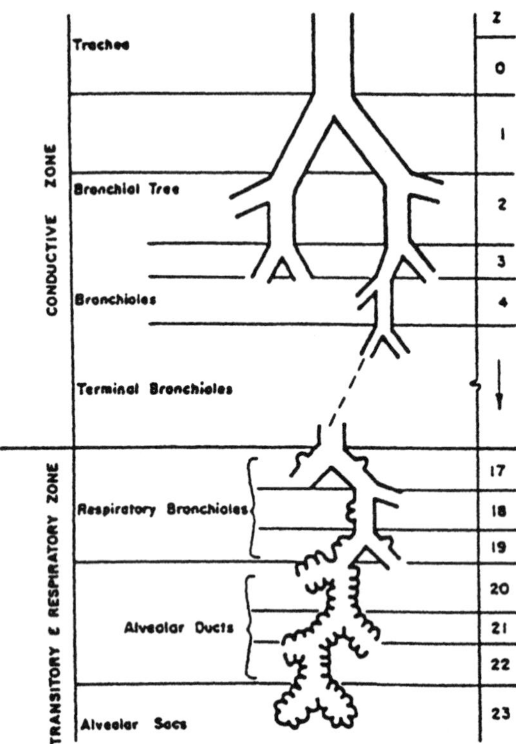

FIGURE 7.2 General architecture of conductive and transitory airways. (Used with permission from Weibel, 1963.) In the conductive zone air is conducted to and from the lungs while in the respiration zone, gas exchange occurs.

Molecular diffusion within the alveolar volume is responsible for mixing of the enclosed gas. Due to small alveolar dimensions, complete mixing probably occurs in less than 10 ms, fast enough that alveolar mixing time does not limit gaseous diffusion to or from the blood [Astrand and Rodahl, 1970].

Of particular importance to proper alveolar operation is a thin surface coating of surfactant. Without this material, large alveoli would tend to enlarge and small alveoli would collapse. It is the present view that surfactant acts like a detergent, changing the stress-strain relationship of the alveolar wall and thereby stabilizing the lung [Johnson, 1991].

Pulmonary Circulation

There is no true pulmonary analogue to the systemic arterioles, since the pulmonary circulation occurs under relatively low pressure [West, 1977]. Pulmonary blood vessels, especially capillaries and venules, are very thin walled and flexible. Unlike systemic capillaries, pulmonary capillaries increase in diameter, and pulmonary capillaries within alveolar walls separate adjacent alveoli with increases in blood pressure or decreases in alveolar pressure. Flow, therefore, is significantly influenced by elastic deformation. Although pulmonary circulation is largely unaffected by neural and chemical control, it does respond promptly to hypoxia.

There is also a high-pressure systemic blood delivery system to the bronchi that is completely independent of the pulmonary low-pressure (~3330 N/m^2) circulation in healthy individuals. In diseased states, however, bronchial arteries are reported to enlarge when pulmonary blood flow is reduced, and some arteriovenous shunts become prominent [West, 1977].

Total pulmonary blood volume is approximately 300 to 500 cm^3 in normal adults, with about 60 to 100 cm^3 in the pulmonary capillaries [Astrand and Rodahl, 1970]. This value, however, is quite variable, depending on such things as posture, position, disease, and chemical composition of the blood [Kline, 1976].

Since pulmonary arterial blood is oxygen poor and carbon dioxide rich, it exchanges excess carbon dioxide for oxygen in the pulmonary capillaries, which are in close contact with alveolar walls. At rest, the transit time for blood in the pulmonary capillaries is computed as

$$t = V_c / \dot{V}_c$$

where t = blood transmit time, s
V_c = capillary blood volume, m^3
$\dot{V}_c$ = total capillary blood flow = cardiac output, m^3/s

and is somewhat less than 1 s, while during exercise it may be only 500 ms or even less.

Respiratory Muscles

The lungs fill because of a rhythmic expansion of the chest wall. The action is indirect in that no muscle acts directly on the lung. The diaphragm, the muscular mass accounting for 75% of the expansion of the chest cavity, is attached around the bottom of the thoracic cage, arches over the liver, and moves downward like a piston when it contracts. The external intercostal muscles are positioned between the ribs and aid inspiration by moving the ribs up and forward. This, then, increases the volume of the thorax. Other muscles are important in the maintenance of thoracic shape during breathing. (For details, see Ruch and Patton [1966] and Johnson [1991]).

Quiet expiration is usually considered to be passive; i.e., pressure to force air from the lungs comes from elastic expansion of the lungs and chest wall. During moderate to severe exercise, the abdominal and internal intercostal muscles are very important in forcing air from the lungs much more quickly than would otherwise occur. Inspiration requires intimate contact between lung tissues, pleural tissues (the pleura is the membrane surrounding the lungs), and chest wall and diaphragm. This is accomplished by reduced intrathoracic pressure (which tends toward negative values) during inspiration.

Viewing the lungs as an entire unit, one can consider the lungs to be elastic sacs within an airtight barrel — the thorax — which is bounded by the ribs and the diaphragm. Any movement of these two boundaries alters the volume of the lungs. The normal breathing cycle in humans is accomplished by the active contraction of the inspiratory muscles, which enlarges the thorax. This enlargement lowers intrathoracic and interpleural pressure even further, pulls on the lungs, and enlarges the alveoli, alveolar ducts, and bronchioli, expanding the alveolar gas and decreasing its pressure below atmospheric. As a result, air at atmospheric pressure flows easily into the nose, mouth, and trachea.

7.2 Lung Volumes and Gas Exchange

Of primary importance to lung functioning is the movement and mixing of gases within the respiratory system. Depending on the anatomic level under consideration, gas movement is determined mainly by diffusion or convection.

Without the thoracic musculature and rib cage, as mentioned above, the barely inflated lungs would occupy a much smaller space than they occupy *in situ*. However, the thoracic cage holds them open. Conversely, the lungs exert an influence on the thorax, holding it smaller than should be the case without the lungs. Because the lungs and thorax are connected by tissue, the volume occupied by both together is between the extremes represented by relaxed lungs alone and thoracic cavity alone. The resting volume V_R, then, is that volume occupied by the lungs with glottis open and muscles relaxed.

Lung volumes greater than resting volume are achieved during inspiration. Maximum inspiration is represented by *inspiratory reserve volume* (IRV). IRV is the maximum additional volume that can be

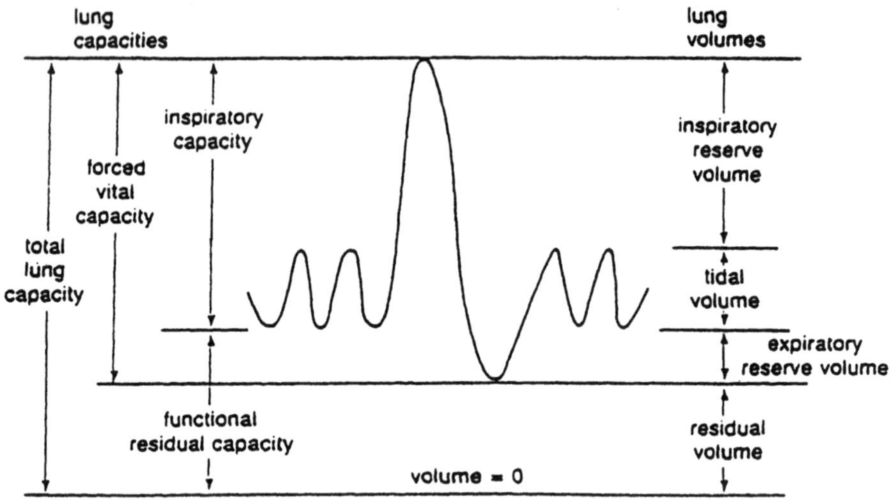

FIGURE 7.3 Lung capacities and lung volumes.

accommodated by the lung at the end of inspiration. Lung volumes less than resting volume do not normally occur at rest but do occur during exhalation while exercising (when exhalation is active). Maximum additional expiration, as measured from lung volume at the end of expiration, is called *expiratory reserve volume* (ERV). *Residual volume* is the amount of gas remaining in the lungs at the end of maximal expiration.

Tidal volume V_T is normally considered to be the volume of air entering the nose and mouth with each breath. Alveolar ventilation volume, the volume of fresh air that enters the alveoli during each breath, is always less than tidal volume. The extent of this difference in volume depends primarily on the *anatomic dead space,* the 150- to 160-ml internal volume of the conducting airway passages. The term *dead* is quite appropriate, since it represents wasted respiratory effort; i.e., no significant gas exchange occurs across the thick walls of the trachea, bronchi, and bronchiolus. Since normal tidal volume at rest is usually about 500 ml of air per breath, one can easily calculate that because of the presence of this dead space, about 340 to 350 ml of fresh air actually penetrates the alveoli and becomes involved in the gas exchange process. An additional 150 to 160 ml of stale air exhaled during the previous breath is also drawn into the alveoli.

The term *volume* is used for elemental differences of lung volume, whereas the term *capacity* is used for combination of lung volumes. Figure 7.3 illustrates the interrelationship between each of the following lung volumes and capacities:

1. *Total lung capacity* (TLC): The amount of gas contained in the lung at the end of maximal inspiration.
2. *Forced vital capacity* (FVC): The maximal volume of gas that can be forcefully expelled after maximal inspiration.
3. *Inspiratory capacity* (IC): The maximal volume of gas that can be inspired from the resting expiratory level.
4. *Functional residual capacity* (FRC): The volume of gas remaining after normal expiration. It will be noted that functional residual capacity (FRC) is the same as the resting volume. There is a small difference, however, between resting volume and FRC because FRC is measured while the patient breathes, whereas resting volume is measured with no breathing. FRC is properly defined only at end-expiration at rest and not during exercise.

TABLE 7.2 Typical Lung Volumes for Normal, Healthy Males

Lung Volume	Normal Values	
Total lung capacity (TLC)	6.0×10^{-3} m³	(6,000 cm³)
Residual volume (RV)	1.2×10^{-3} m³	(1,200 cm³)
Vital capacity (VC)	4.8×10^{-3} m³	(4,800 cm³)
Inspiratory reserve volume (IRV)	3.6×10^{-3} m³	(3,600 cm³)
Expiratory reserve volume (ERV)	1.2×10^{-3} m³	(1,200 cm³)
Functional residual capacity (FRC)	2.4×10^{-3} m³	(2,400 cm³)
Anatomic dead volume (V_D)	1.5×10^{-4} m³	(150 cm³)
Upper airways volume	8.0×10^{-5} m³	(80 cm³)
Lower airways volume	7.0×10^{-5} m³	(70 cm³)
Physiologic dead volume (V_D)	1.8×10^{-4} m³	(180 cm³)
Minute volume ($\dot{V}_e$) at rest	1.0×10^{-4} m³/s	(6,000 cm³/min)
Respiratory period (T) at rest	4s	
Tidal volume (V_T) at rest	4.0×10^{-4} m³	(400 cm³)
Alveolar ventilation volume (V_A) at rest	2.5×10^{-4} m³	(250 cm³)
Minute volume during heavy exercise	1.7×10^{-3} m³/s	(10,000 cm³/min)
Respiratory period during heavy exercise	1.2 s	
Tidal volume during heavy exercise	2.0×10^{-3} m³	(2,000 cm³)
Alveolar ventilation volume during exercise	1.8×10^{-3} m³	(1,820 cm³)

Source: Adapted and used with permission from Forster et al. [1986].

These volumes and specific capacities, represented in Fig. 7.3, have led to the development of specific tests (that will be discussed below) to quantify the status of the pulmonary system. Typical values for these volumes and capacities are provided in Table 7.2.

7.3 Perfusion of the Lung

For gas exchange to occur properly in the lung, air must be delivered to the alveoli via the conducting airways, gas must diffuse from the alveoli to the capillaries through extremely thin walls, and the same gas must be removed to the cardiac atrium by blood flow. This three-step process involves (1) alveolar ventilation, (2) the process of diffusion, and (3) ventilatory perfusion, which involves pulmonary blood flow. Obviously, an alveolus that is ventilated but not perfused cannot exchange gas. Similarly, a perfused alveolus that is not properly ventilated cannot exchange gas. The most efficient gas exchange occurs when ventilation and perfusion are matched.

There is a wide range of ventilation-to-perfusion ratios that naturally occur in various regions of the lung [Johnson, 1991]. Blood flow is somewhat affected by posture because of the effects of gravity. In the upright position, there is a general reduction in the volume of blood in the thorax, allowing for larger lung volume. Gravity also influences the distribution of blood, such that the perfusion of equal lung volumes is about five times greater at the base compared with the top of the lung [Astrand and Rodahl, 1970]. There is no corresponding distribution of ventilation; hence the ventilation-to-perfusion ratio is nearly five times smaller at the top of the lung (Table 7.3). A more uniform ventilation-to-perfusion ratio is found in the supine position and during exercise [Jones, 1984b].

Blood flow through the capillaries is not steady. Rather, blood flows in a halting manner and may even be stopped if intraalveolar pressure exceeds intracapillary blood pressure during diastole. Mean blood flow is not affected by heart rate [West, 1977], but the highly distensible pulmonary blood vessels admit more blood when blood pressure and cardiac output increase. During exercise, higher pulmonary blood pressures allow more blood to flow through the capillaries. Even mild exercise favors more uniform perfusion of the lungs [Astrand and Rodahl, 1970]. Pulmonary artery systolic pressures increases from 2670 N/m² (20 mmHg) at rest to 4670 N/m² (35 mmHg) during moderate exercise to 6670 N/m² (50 mmHg) at maximal work [Astrand and Rodahl, 1970].

TABLE 7.3 Ventilation-to-Perfusion Ratios from the Top to Bottom of the Lung of Normal Man in the Sitting Position

Percent Lung Volume, %	Alveolar Ventilation Rate, cm^3/s	Perfusion Rate, cm^3/s	Ventilation-to-Perfusion Ratio
	Top		
7	4.0	1.2	3.3
8	5.5	3.2	1.8
10	7.0	5.5	1.3
11	8.7	8.3	1.0
12	9.8	11.0	0.90
13	11.2	13.8	0.80
13	12.0	16.3	0.73
13	13.0	19.2	0.68
	Bottom		
13	13.7	21.5	0.63
100	84.9	100.0	

Source: Used with permission from West [1962].

7.4 Gas Partial Pressures

The primary purpose of the respiratory system is gas exchange. In the gas-exchange process, gas must diffuse through the alveolar space, across tissue, and through plasma into the red blood cell, where it finally chemically joins to hemoglobin. A similar process occurs for carbon dioxide elimination.

As long as intermolecular interactions are small, most gases of physiologic significance can be considered to obey the ideal gas law:

$$pV = nRT$$

where p = pressure, N/m^2
V = volume of gas, m^3
n = number of moles, mol
R = gas constant, $(N \times m)/(mol \times K)$
T = absolute temperature, K

The ideal gas law can be applied without error up to atmospheric pressure; it can be applied to a mixture of gases, such as air, or to its constituents, such as oxygen or nitrogen. All individual gases in a mixture are considered to fill the total volume and have the same temperature but reduced pressures. The pressure exerted by each individual gas is called the *partial pressure* of the gas.

Dalton's law states that the total pressure is the sum of the partial pressures of the constituents of a mixture:

$$p = \sum_{i=1}^{N} p_i$$

where p_i = partial pressure of the ith constituent, N/m^2
N = total number of constituents

Dividing the ideal gas law for a constituent by that for the mixture gives

$$\frac{P_i V}{PV} = \frac{n_i R_i T}{nRT}$$

so that

$$\frac{p_i}{p} = \frac{n_i R_i}{nR}$$

which states that the partial pressure of a gas may be found if the total pressure, mole fraction, and ratio of gas constants are known. For most respiratory calculations, p will be considered to be the pressure of 1 atmosphere, 101 kN/m^2. Avogadro's principle states that different gases at the same temperature and pressure contain equal numbers of molecules:

$$\frac{V_1}{V_2} = \frac{nR_1}{nR_2} = \frac{R_1}{R_2}$$

Thus

$$\frac{p_i}{p} = \frac{V_i}{V}$$

where V_i/V is the volume fraction of a constituent in air and is therefore dimensionless. Table 7.4 provides individual gas constants, as well as volume fractions, of constituent gases of air.

Gas pressures and volumes can be measured for many different temperature and humidity conditions. Three of these are body temperature and pressure, saturated (BTPS); ambient temperature and pressure (ATP); and standard temperature and pressure, dry (STPD). To calculate constituent partial pressures at STPD, total pressure is taken as barometric pressure minus vapor pressure of water in the atmosphere:

$$p_i = (V_i/V)(p - pH_2O)$$

where p = total pressure, kN/m^2
pH_2O = vapor pressure of water in atmosphere, kN/m^2

and V_i/V as a ratio does not change in the conversion process.

TABLE 7.4 Molecular Masses, Gas Constants, and Volume Fractions for Air and Constituents

Constituent	Molecular Mass kg/mol	Gas Constant, N·m/(mol·K)	Volume Fraction in Air, m^3/m^3
Air	29.0	286.7	1.0000
Ammonia	17.0	489.1	0.0000
Argon	39.9	208.4	0.0093
Carbon dioxide	44.0	189.0	0.0003
Carbon monoxide	28.0	296.9	0.0000
Helium	4.0	2078.6	0.0000
Hydrogen	2.0	4157.2	0.0000
Nitrogen	28.0	296.9	0.7808
Oxygen	32.0	259.8	0.2095

Note: Universal gas constant is 8314.43 N·m/kg·mol·K.

TABLE 7.5 Gas Partial Pressures (kN/m^2) throughout the Respiratory and Circulatory Systems

Gas	Inspired Air*	Alveolar Air	Expired Air	Mixed Venous Blood	Arterial Blood	Muscle Tissue
H_2O	—	6.3	6.3	6.3	6.3	6.3
CO_2	0.04	5.3	4.2	6.1	5.3	6.7
O_2	21.2	14.0	15.5	5.3	13.3	4.0
N_2[†]	80.1	75.7	75.3	76.4	76.4	76.4
Total	101.3	101.3	101.3	94.1	101.3	93.4

*Inspired air considered dry for convenience.
[†]Includes all other inert components.
Source: Used with permission from Astrand and Rodahl [1970].

Gas volume at STPD is converted from ambient condition volume as

$$V_i = V_{\text{amb}}\left[273/(273+\Theta)\right]\left[(p - pH_2O)/101.3\right]$$

where V_i = volume of gas i corrected to STPD, m^3
V_{amb} = volume of gas i at ambient temperature and pressure, m^3
Θ = ambient temperature, °C
p = ambient total pressure, kN/m^2
pH_2O = vapor pressure of water in the air, kN/m^2

Partial pressures and gas volumes may be expressed in BTPS conditions. In this case, gas partial pressures are usually known from other measurements. Gas volumes are converted from ambient conditions by

$$V_i = V_{\text{amb}}\left[310/(273+\Theta)\right]\left[(p - pH_2O)/p - 6.28\right]$$

Table 7.5 provides gas partial pressure throughout the respiratory and circulatory systems.

7.5 Pulmonary Mechanics

The respiratory system exhibits properties of resistance, compliance, and inertance analogous to the electrical properties of resistance, capacitance, and inductance. Of these, inertance is generally considered to be of less importance than the other two properties.

Resistance is the ratio of pressure to flow:

$$R = p/V$$

where R = resistance, $N \times s/m^5$
P = pressure, N/m^2
V = volume flow rate, m^3/s

Resistance can be found in the conducting airways, in the lung tissue, and in the tissues of the chest wall. Airways exhalation resistance is usually higher than airways inhalation resistance because the surrounding lung tissue pulls the smaller, more distensible airways open when the lung is being inflated. Thus airways inhalation resistance is somewhat dependent on lung volume, and airways exhalation resistance can be very lung volume dependent [Johnson, 1991]. Respiratory tissue resistance varies with frequency, lung volume, and volume history. Tissue resistance is relatively small at high frequencies but increases greatly at low frequencies, nearly proportional to $1/f$. Tissue resistance often exceeds airway resistance below 2 Hz. Lung tissue resistance also increases with decreasing volume amplitude [Stamenovic et al., 1990].

Compliance is the ratio of lung volume to lung pressure:

$$C = V/p$$

where C = compliance, m^5/N
V = lung volume/m^3
P = pressure, N/m^2

As the lung is stretched, it acts as an expanded balloon that tends to push air out and return to its normal size. The static pressure-volume relationship is nonlinear, exhibiting decreased static compliance at the extremes of lung volume [Johnson, 1991]. As with tissue resistance, dynamic tissue compliance does not remain constant during breathing. Dynamic compliance tends to increase with increasing volume and decrease with increasing frequency [Stamenovic et al., 1990].

Two separate approaches can be used to model lung tissue mechanics. The traditional approach places a linear viscoelastic system in parallel with a plastoelastic system. A linear viscoelastic system consists of ideal resistive and compliant elements and can exhibit the frequency dependence of respiratory tissue. A plastoelastic system consists of dry-friction elements and compliant elements and can exhibit the volume dependence of respiratory tissue [Hildebrandt, 1970]. An alternate approach is to utilize a nonlinear viscoelastic system that can characterize both the frequency dependence and the volume dependence of respiratory tissue [Suki and Bates, 1991].

Lung tissue hysteresivity relates resistance and compliance:

$$wR = \eta/C_{\text{dyn}}$$

where ω = frequency, radians/s
R = resistance, $N \times s/m^5$
η = hysteresivity, unitless
C_{dyn} = dynamic compliance, m^5/n

Hysteresivity, analogous to the structural damping coefficient used in solid mechanics, is an empirical parameter arising from the assumption that resistance and compliance are related at the microstructural level. Hysteresivity is independent of frequency and volume. Typical values range from 0.1 to 0.3 [Fredberg and Stamenovic, 1989].

7.6 Respiratory Control

Control of respiration occurs in many different cerebral structures [Johnson, 1991] and regulates many things [Hornbein, 1981]. Respiration must be controlled to produce the respiratory rhythm, ensure adequate gas exchange, protect against inhalation of poisonous substances, assist in maintenance of body pH, remove irritations, and minimize energy cost. Respiratory control is more complex than cardiac control for at least three reasons:

1. Airway airflow occurs in both directions.
2. The respiratory system interfaces directly with the environment outside the body.
3. Parts of the respiratory system are used for other functions, such as swallowing and speaking.

As a result, respiratory muscular action must be exquisitely coordinated; it must be prepared to protect itself against environmental onslaught, and breathing must be temporarily suspended on demand.

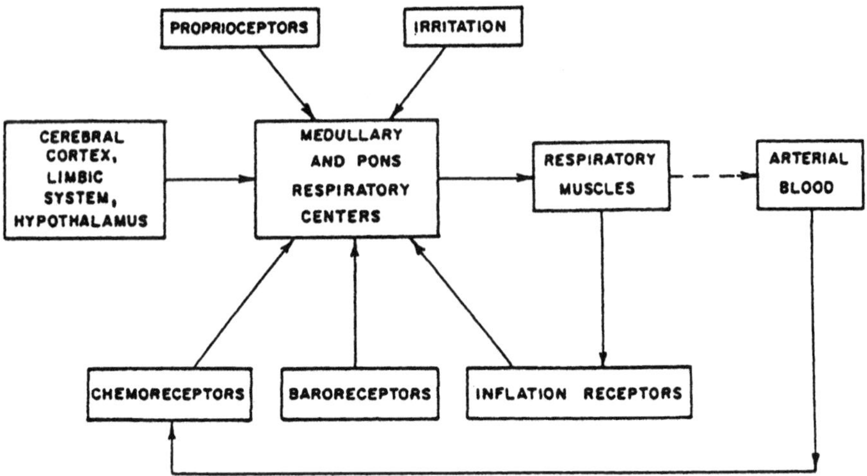

FIGURE 7.4 General scheme of respiratory control.

All control systems require sensors, controllers, and effectors. Figure 7.4 presents the general scheme for respiratory control. There are mechanoreceptors throughout the respiratory system. For example, nasal receptors are important in sneezing, apnea (cessation of breathing), bronchodilation, bronchoconstriction, and the secretion of mucus. Laryngeal receptors are important in coughing, apnea, swallowing, bronchoconstriction, airway mucus secretion, and laryngeal constriction. Tracheobronchial receptors are important in coughing, pulmonary hypertension, bronchoconstriction, laryngeal constriction, and mucus production. Other mechanoreceptors are important in the generation of the respiratory pattern and are involved with respiratory sensation.

Respiratory chemoreceptors exist peripherally in the aortic arch and carotic bodies and centrally in the ventral medulla oblongata of the brain. These receptors are sensitive to partial pressures of CO_2 and O_2 and to blood pH.

The respiratory controller is located in several places in the brain. Each location appears to have its own function. Unlike the heart, the basic respiratory rhythm is not generated within the lungs but rather in the brain and is transmitted to the respiratory muscles by the phrenic nerve.

Effector organs are mainly the respiratory muscles, as described previously. Other effectors are muscles located in the airways and tissues for mucus secretion. Control of respiration appears to be based on two criteria: (1) removal of excess CO_2 and (2) minimization of energy expenditure. It is not the lack of oxygen that stimulates respiration but increased CO_2 partial pressure that acts as a powerful respiratory stimulus. Because of the buffering action of blood bicarbonate, blood pH usually falls as more CO_2 is produced in the working muscles. Lower blood pH also stimulates respiration.

A number of respiratory adjustments are made to reduce energy expenditure during exercise: Respiration rate increases, the ratio of inhalation time to exhalation time decreases, respiratory flow waveshapes become more trapezoidal, and expiratory reserve volume decreases. Other adjustments to reduce energy expenditure have been theorized but not proved [Johnson, 1991].

7.7 The Pulmonary Function Laboratory

The purpose of a pulmonary function laboratory is to obtain clinically useful data from patients with respiratory dysfunction. The pulmonary function tests (PFTs) within this laboratory fulfill a variety of functions. They permit (1) quantification of a patient's breathing deficiency, (2) diagnosis of different types of pulmonary diseases, (3) evaluation of a patient's response to therapy, and (4) preoperative screening to determine whether the presence of lung disease increases the risk of surgery.

Although PFTs can provide important information about a patient's condition, the limitations of these tests must be considered. First, they are nonspecific in that they cannot determine which portion of the lungs is diseased, only that the disease is present. Second, PFTs must be considered along with the medical history, physical examination, x-ray examination, and other diagnostic procedures to permit a complete evaluation. Finally, the major drawback to *some* PFTs is that they require a full patient cooperation and for this reason cannot be conducted on critically ill patients. Consider some of the most widely used PFTs: spirometry, body plethysmography, and diffusing capacity.

Spirometry

The simplest PFT is the spirometry maneuver. In this test, the patient inhales to total lung capacity (TLC) and exhales forcefully to residual volume. The patient exhales into a displacement bell chamber that sits on a water seal. As the bell rises, a pen coupled to the bell chamber inscribes a tracing on a rotating drum. The spirometer offers very little resistance to breathing; therefore, the shape of the spirometry curve (Fig. 7.5) is purely a function of the patient's lung compliance, chest compliance, and airway resistance. At high lung volumes, a rise in intrapleural pressure results in greater expiratory flows. However, at intermediate and low lung volumes, the expiratory flow is independent of effort after a certain intrapleural pressure is reached.

Measurements made from the spirometry curve can determine the degree of a patient's ventilatory obstruction. Forced vital capacity (FVC), forced expiratory volumes (FEV), and forced expiratory flows (FEF) can be determined. The FEV indicates the volume that has been exhaled from TLC for a particular time interval. For example, $FEV_{0.5}$ is the volume exhaled during the first half-second of expiration, and $FEV_{1.0}$ is the volume exhaled during the first second of expiration; these are graphically represented in Fig. 7.5. Note that the more severe the ventilatory obstruction, the lower are the timed volumes ($FEV_{0.5}$ and $FEV_{1.0}$). The FEF is a measure of the average flow (volume/time) over specified portions of the spirometry curve and is represented by the slope of a straight line drawn between volume levels. The average flow over the first quarter of the forced expiration is the $FEF_{0-25\%}$, whereas the average flow over the middle 50% of the FVC is the $FEF_{25-75\%}$. These values are obtained directly from the spirometry curves. The less steep curves of obstructed patients would result in lower values of $FEF_{0-25\%}$ and $FEF_{25-75\%}$ compared with normal values, which are predicted on the basis of the patient's sex, age, and height.

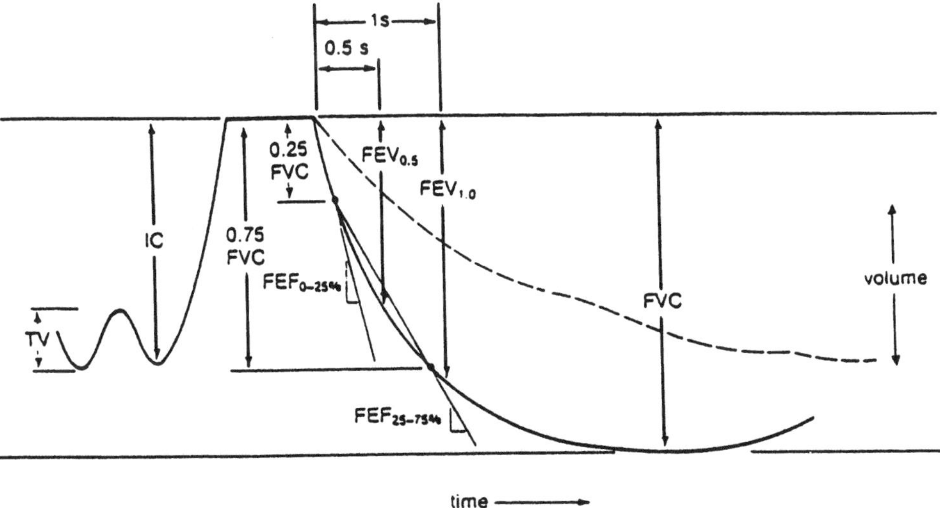

FIGURE 7.5 Typical spirometry tracing obtained during testing; inspiratory capacity (IC), tidal volume (TV), forced vital capacity (FVC), forced expiratory volume (FEV), and forced expiratory flows. Dashed line represents a patient with obstructive lung disease; solid line represents a normal, healthy individual.

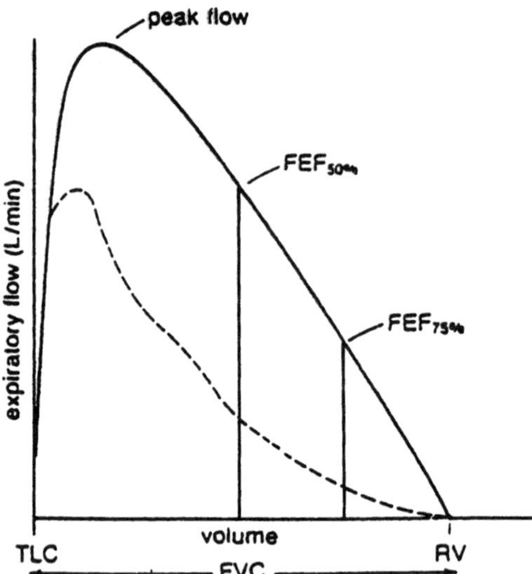

FIGURE 7.6 Flow-volume curve obtained from a spirometry maneuver. Solid line is a normal curve; dashed line represents a patient with obstructive lung disease.

Equations for normal values are available from statistical analysis of data obtained from a normal population. Test results are then interpreted as a percentage of normal.

Another way of presenting a spirometry curve is as a flow-volume curve. Figure 7.6 represents a typical flow-volume curve. The expiratory flow is plotted against the exhaled volume, indicating the maximum flow that may be reached at each degree of lung inflation. Since there is no time axis, a time must mark the $FEV_{0.5}$ and $FEV_{1.0}$ on the tracing. To obtain these flow-volume curves in the laboratory, the patient usually exhales through a *pneumotach.* The most widely used pneumotach measures a pressure drop across a flow-resistive element. The resistance to flow is constant over the measuring range of the device; therefore, the pressure drop is proportional to the flow through the tube. This signal, which is indicative of flow, is then integrated to determine the volume of gas that has passed through the tube.

Another type of pneumotach is the heated-element type. In this device, a small heated mass responds to airflow by cooling. As the element cools, a greater current is necessary to maintain a constant temperature. This current is proportional to the airflow through the tube. Again, to determine the volume that has passed through the tube, the flow signal is integrated.

The flow-volume loop in Fig. 7.7 is a dramatic representation displaying inspiratory and expiratory curves for both normal breathing and maximal breathing. The result is a graphic representation of the patient's reserve capacity in relation to normal breathing. For example, the normal patient's tidal breathing loop is small compared with the patient's maximum breathing loop. During these times of stress, this tidal breathing loop can be increased to the boundaries of the outer ventilatory loop. This increase in ventilation provides the greater gas exchange needed during the stressful situation. Compare this condition with that of the patient with obstructive lung disease. Not only is the tidal breathing loop larger than normal, but the maximal breathing loop is smaller than normal. The result is a decreased ventilatory reserve, limiting the individual's ability to move air in and out of the lungs. As the disease progresses, the outer loop becomes smaller, and the inner loop becomes larger.

The primary use of spirometry is in detection of obstructive lung disease that results from increased resistance to flow through the airways. This can occur in several ways:

1. Deterioration of the structure of the smaller airways that results in early airways closure.
2. Decreased airway diameters caused by bronchospasm or the presence of secretions increases the airway's resistance to airflow.
3. Partial blockage of a large airway by a tumor decreases airway diameter and causes turbulent flow.

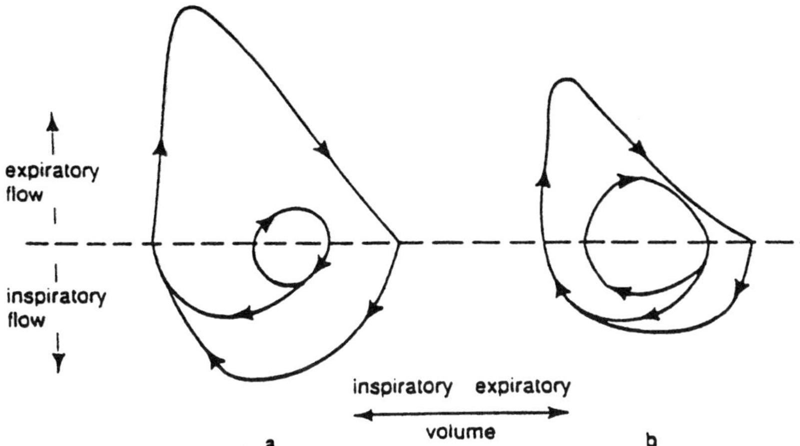

FIGURE 7.7 Typical flow-volume loops. (a) Normal flow-volume loop. (b) Flow-volume loop of patient with obstructive lung disease.

Spirometry has its limitations, however. It can measure only ventilated volumes. It cannot measure lung capacities that contain the residual volume. Measurements of TLC, FRC, and RV have diagnostic value in defining lung overdistension or restrictive pulmonary disease; the body plethysmograph can determine these absolute lung volumes.

Body Plethysmography

In a typical plethysmograph, the patient is put in an airtight enclosure and breathes through a pneumotach. The flow signal through the pneumotach is integrated and recorded as tidal breathing. At the end of a normal expiration (at FRC), an electronically operated shutter occludes the tube through which the patient is breathing. At this time the patient pants lightly against the occluded airway. Since there is no flow, pressure measured at the mouth must equal alveolar pressure. But movements of the chest that compress gas in the lung simultaneously rarify the air in the plethysmograph, and vice versa. The pressure change in the plethysmograph can be used to calculate the volume change in the plethysmograph, which is the same as the volume change in the chest. This leads directly to determination of FRC.

At the same time, alveolar pressure can be correlated to plethysmographic pressure. Therefore, when the shutter is again opened and flow rate is measured, airway resistance can be obtained as the ratio of alveolar pressure (obtainable from plethysmographic pressure) to flow rate [Carr and Brown, 1993]. Airway resistance is usually measured during panting, at a nominal lung volume of FRC and flow rate of ± 1 liter/s.

Airway resistance during inspiration is increased in patients with asthma, bronchitis, and upper respiratory tract infections. Expiratory resistance is elevated in patients with emphysema, since the causes of increased expiratory airway resistance are decreased driving pressures and the airway collapse. Airway resistance also may be used to determine the response of obstructed patients to bronchodilator medications.

Diffusing Capacity

So far the mechanical components of airflow through the lungs have been discussed. Another important parameter is the diffusing capacity of the lung, the rate at which oxygen or carbon dioxide travel from the alveoli to the blood (or vice versa for carbon dioxide) in the pulmonary capillaries. Diffusion of gas across a barrier is directly related to the surface area of the barrier and inversely related to the thickness. Also, diffusion is directly proportional to the solubility of the gas in the barrier material and inversely related to the molecular weight of the gas.

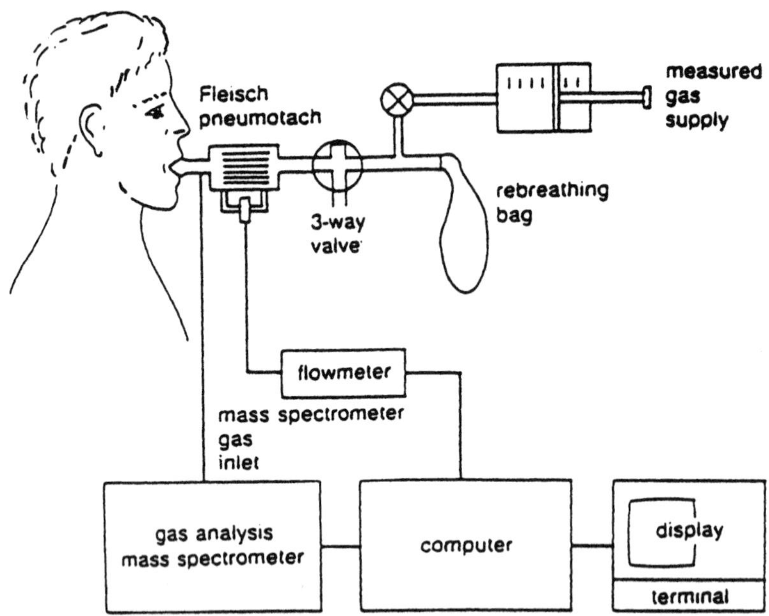

FIGURE 7.8 Typical system configuration for the measurement of rebreathing pulmonary diffusing capacity.

Lung diffusing capacity (D_L) is usually determined for carbon monoxide but can be related to oxygen diffusion. The popular method of measuring carbon monoxide diffusion utilizes a rebreathing technique in which the patient rebreathes rapidly in and out of a bag for approximately 30 s. Figure 7.8 illustrates the test apparatus. The patient begins breathing from a bag containing a known volume of gas consisting of 0.3 to 0.5% carbon monoxide made with heavy oxygen, 0.3 to 0.5% acetylene, 5% helium, 21% oxygen, and a balance of nitrogen. As the patient rebreathes the gas mixture in the bag, a modified mass spectrometer continuously analyzes it during both inspiration and expiration. During this rebreathing procedure, the carbon monoxide disappears from the patient-bag system; the rate at which this occurs is a function of the lung diffusing capacity.

The helium is inert and insoluble in lung tissue and blood and equilibrates quickly in unobstructed patients, indicating the dilution level of the test gas. Acetylene, on the other hand, is soluble in blood and is used to determine the blood flow through the pulmonary capillaries. Carbon monoxide is bound very tightly to hemoglobin and is used to obtain diffusing capacity at a constant pressure gradient across the alveolar-capillary membrane.

Decreased lung diffusing capacity can occur from the thickening of the alveolar membrane or the capillary membrane as well as the presence of interstitial fluid from edema. All these abnormalities increase the barrier thickness and cause a decrease in diffusing capacity. In addition, a characteristic of specific lung diseases is impaired lung diffusing capacity. For example, fibrotic lung tissue exhibits a decreased permeability to gas transfer, whereas pulmonary emphysema results in the loss of diffusion surface area.

Defining Terms

Alveoli: Respiratory airway terminals where most gas exchange with the pulmonary circulation takes place.

BTPS: Body temperature (37°C) and standard pressure (1 atm), saturated (6.28 kN/m^2).

Chemoreceptors: Neural receptors sensitive to chemicals such as gas partial pressures.

Dead space: The portion of the respiratory system that does not take part in gas exchange with the blood.

Diffusion: The process whereby a material moves from a region of higher concentration to a region of lower concentration.

Expiration: The breathing process whereby air is expelled from the mouth and nose. Also called *exhalation.*

Functional residual capacity: The lung volume at rest without breathing.

Inspiration: The breathing process whereby air is taken into the mouth and noise. Also called *inhalation.*

Mass spectrometer: A device that identifies relative concentrations of gases by means of mass-to-charge ratios of gas ions.

Mechanoreceptors: Neural receptors sensitive to mechanical inputs such as stretch, pressure, irritants, etc.

Partial pressure: The pressure that a gas would exert if it were the only constituent.

Perfusion: Blood flow to the lungs.

Plethysmography: Any measuring technique that depends on a volume change.

Pleura: The membrane surrounding the lung.

Pneumotach: A measuring device for airflow.

Pulmonary circulation: Blood flow from the right cardiac ventricle that perfuses the lung and is in intimate contact with alveolar membranes for effective gas exchange.

STPD: Standard temperature (0°C) and pressure (1 atm), dry (moisture removed).

Ventilation: Airflow to the lungs.

References

Astrand PO, Rodahl K. 1970. Textbook of Work Physiology. New York, McGraw-Hill.

Carr JJ, Brown JM. 1993. Introduction to Biomedical Equipment Technology. Englewood Cliffs, NJ, Prentice-Hall.

Fredberg JJ, Stamenovic D. 1989. On the imperfect elasticity of lung tissue. J Appl Physiol 67(6):2408–2419.

Hildebrandt J. 1970. Pressure-volume data of cat lung interpreted by plastoelastic, linear viscoelastic model. J Appl Physiol 28(3):365–372.

Hornbein TF (ed). 1981. Regulation of Breathing. New York, Marcel Dekker.

Johnson AT. 1991. Biomechanics and Exercise Physiology. New York, Wiley.

Jones NL. 1984. Normal values for pulmonary gas exchange during exercise. Am Rev Respir Dis 129:544–546.

Kline J. (ed). 1976. Biologic Foundations of Biomedical Engineering. Boston, Little, Brown.

Parker JF Jr, West VR. (eds). 1973. Bioastronautics Data Book. Washington, NASA.

Ruch TC, Patton HD. (eds). 1966. Physiology Biophysics. Philadelphia, Saunders.

Stamenovic D, Glass GM, Barnas GM, Fredberg JJ. 1990. Viscoplasticity of respiratory tissues. J Appl Physiol 69(3):973–988.

Suki B, Bates JHT. 1991. A nonlinear viscoelastic model of lung tissue mechanics. J Appl Physiol 71(3):826–833.

Weibel ER. 1963. Morphometry of the Human Lung. New York, Academic Press.

West J. 1962. Regional differences in gas exchange in the lung of erect man. J Appl Physiol 17:893–898.

West JB. (ed). 1977. Bioengineering Aspects of the Lung. New York, Marcel Dekker.

Additional References

Fredberg JJ, Jones KA, Nathan A, Raboudi S, Prakash YS, Shore SA, Butler JP, Sieck GC. 1996. Friction in airway smooth muscle: Mechanism, latch, and implications in asthma. J Appl Physiol 81(6):2703–2712.

Hantos Z, Daroczy B, Csendes T, Suki B, Nagy S. 1990. Modeling of low-frequency pulmonary impedance in dogs. J Appl Physiol 68(3):849–860.

Hantos Z, Daroczy B, Suki B, Nagy S. 1990. Low-frequency respiratory mechanical impedance in rats. J Appl Physiol 63(1):36–43.

Hantos Z, Petak F, Adamicza A, Asztalos T, Tolnai J, Fredberg JJ. 1997. Mechanical impedance of the lung periphery. J Appl Physiol 83(5):1595–1601.

Maksym GN, Bates JHT. 1997. A distributed nonlinear model of lung tissue elasticity. J Appl Physiol 82(1):32–41.

Petak F, Hall GL, Sly PD. 1998. Repeated measurements of airway and parenchymal mechanics in rats by using low frequency oscillations. J Appl Physiol 84(5):1680–1686.

Thorpe CW, Bates JHT. 1997. Effect of stochastic heterogeneity on lung impedance during acute bronchoconstriction: A model analysis. J Appl Physiol 82(5):1616–1625.

Yuan H, Ingenito EP, Suki B. 1997. Dynamic properties of lung parenchyma: Mechanical contributions of fiber network and interstitial cells. J Appl Physiol 83(5):1420–1431.

II

Imaging

Karen M. Mudry
The Whitaker Foundation

THE FIELD OF MEDICAL IMAGING has experienced phenomenal growth within the last century. Whereas imaging was the prerogative of the defense and the space science communities in the past, with the advent of powerful, less-expansive computers, new and expanded imaging systems have found their way into the medical field. Systems range from those devoted to planar imaging using x-rays to technologies that are just emerging, such as virtual reality. Some of the systems, such as ultrasound, are relatively inexpensive, while others, such as positron emission tomography (PET) facilities, cost millions of dollars for the hardware and the employment of Ph.D.-level personnel to operate them. Systems that make use of x-rays have been designed to image anatomic structures, while others that make use of radioisotopes provide functional information. The fields of view that can be imaged range from the whole body obtained with nuclear medicine bone scans to images of cellular components using magnetic resonance (MR) microscopy. The design of transducers for the imaging devices to the postprocessing of the data to allow easier interpretation of the images by medical personnel are all aspects of the medical imaging devices field.

Even with the sophisticated systems now available, challenges remain in the medical imaging field. With the increasing emphasis on health care costs, and with medical imaging systems often cited as not only an example of the investment that health care providers must make and consequently recover, but also as a factor contributing to escalating costs, there is increasing emphasis on lowering the costs of new systems. Researchers, for example, are trying to find alternatives to the high-cost superconducting magnets used for magnetic resonance systems. With the decreasing cost of the powerful computers that are currently contained within most imaging systems and with the intense competition among imaging companies, prices for these systems are bound to fall. Other challenges entail presentation of the imaging data. Often multiple modalities are used during a clinical evaluation. If both anatomic and functional information are required, methods to combine and present these data for medical interpretation need to be achieved. The use of medical image data to more effectively execute surgery is a field that is only starting to be explored. How can anatomic data obtained with a tomographic scan be correlated with the surgical field, given that movement of tissues and organs occurs during surgery? Virtual reality is likely to play an important role in this integration of imaging information with surgery. There also are imaging modalities that are just beginning to be intensively explored, such as the detection of impedance and magnetic field data or the use of optical sources and detectors.

Engineers and physical scientists are involved throughout the medical imaging field. They are employed by both large and small companies. The names of the medical imaging giants, such as General Electric, Siemens, Picker, and Acuson are familiar to most. Small startup companies are prevalent. In addition to the medical imaging companies, Ph.D.-trained engineers and scientists are employed by departments of engineering, physics, and chemistry in universities and more and more by radiology departments of research-oriented medical centers. Whereas only a few years ago researchers working in the medical imaging field would submit papers to general scientific journals, such as the *IEEE Transactions on Biomedical Engineering,* now there is a journal, *IEEE Transactions on Medical Imaging,* devoted to the medical imaging field and journals dedicated to certain modalities, such as *Magnetic Resonance in Medicine* and *Journal of Computer Assisted Tomography.* Large scientific meetings for medical imaging, such as the Radiological Society of North America's annual meeting with over 20,000 attendees, are held each year. Modality-specific meetings, such as that of the Society for Magnetic Resonance in Imaging, have thousands of attendees.

Although entire books have been written on each of the medical imaging modalities, this section will provide an overview of the main medical imaging devices and also highlight a few emerging systems. Chapter 8 describes x-ray systems, the backbone of the medical imaging field. X-ray systems are still quite important because of their relatively low system acquisition cost, the low cost of the diagnostic procedures, and the speed with which results are obtained. Chapter 9 describes computed tomographic (CT) systems. This technology became available in the 1970s, with current improvements focused on acquisition speed and data presentations. Chapter 10 highlights magnetic resonance imaging (MRI), a technology that first became available in the 1980s. The technology is rapidly evolving, with major advances recently in the areas of functional and spectroscopic MRI. Nuclear medicine, the subject of Chapter 11, covers both planar and single-photon emission computed tomography (SPECT) systems. Chapter 12 covers ultrasound, the technology that is widely used for obstetrical imaging and vascular

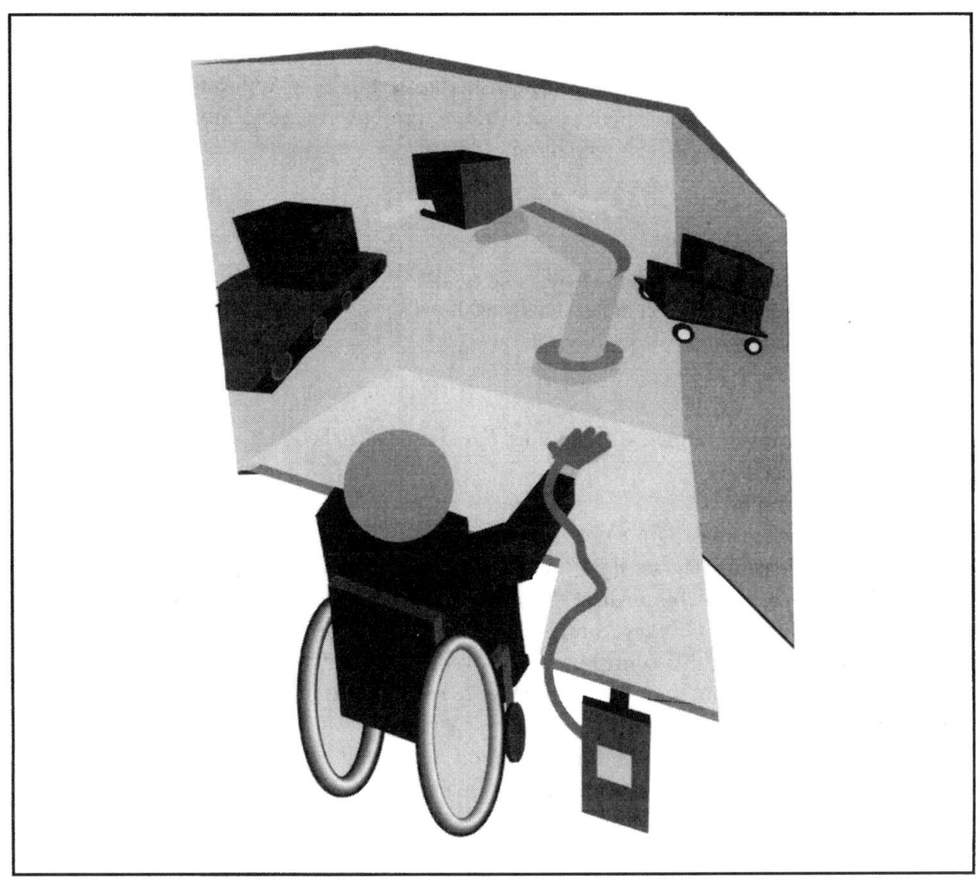

VR system used by the disabled.

flow evaluation. The latest research on linear and two-dimensional transducers, which will be able to provide real-time three-dimensional ultrasound images, is also covered in this chapter. Less prevalent technologies are presented in Chapters 13 to 16. These include the field of MR microscopy, which requires high-field-strength magnets; position emission tomography (PET), which has a tremendous potential for functional imaging; impedance tomography, which is aimed at constructing images based on difference in conductivity between different body tissues; and virtual reality (VR), which provides an overview of the high-tech field of interactive imaging that is bound to become increasingly important as computing power increases.

8

X-Ray

Robert E. Shroy, Jr.
Picker International

Michael S. Van Lysel
University of Wisconsin

Martin J. Yaffe
University of Toronto

8.1 X-Ray Equipment

Robert E. Shroy, Jr.

Conventional x-ray radiography produces images of anatomy that are shadowgrams based on x-ray absorption. The x-rays are produced in a region that is nearly a point source and then are directed on the anatomy to be imaged. The x-rays emerging from the anatomy are detected to form a two-dimensional image, where each point in the image has a brightness related to the intensity of the x-rays at that point. Image production relies on the fact that significant numbers of x-rays penetrate through the anatomy and that different parts of the anatomy absorb different amounts of x-rays. In cases where the anatomy of interest does not absorb x-rays differently from surrounding regions, contrast may be increased by introducing strong x-ray absorbers. For example, barium is often used to image the gastrointestinal tract.

X-rays are electromagnetic waves (like light) having an energy in the general range of approximately 1 to several hundred kiloelectronvolts (keV). In medical x-ray imaging, the x-ray energy typically lies between 5 and 150 keV, with the energy adjusted to the anatomic thickness and the type of study being performed.

X-rays striking an object may either pass through unaffected or may undergo an interaction. These interactions usually involve either the photoelectric effect (where the x-ray is absorbed) or scattering (where the x-ray is deflected to the side with a loss of some energy). X-rays that have been scattered may undergo deflection through a small angle and still reach the image detector; in this case they reduce image contrast and thus degrade the image. This degradation can be reduced by the use of an air gap between the anatomy and the image receptor or by use of an antiscatter grid.

Because of health effects, the doses in radiography are kept as low as possible. However, x-ray quantum noise becomes more apparent in the image as the dose is lowered. This noise is due to the fact that there is an unavoidable random variation in the number of x-rays reaching a point on an image detector. The quantum noise depends on the average number of x-rays striking the image detector and is a fundamental limit to radiographic image quality.

0-8493-1810-6/03/$0.00+$1.50

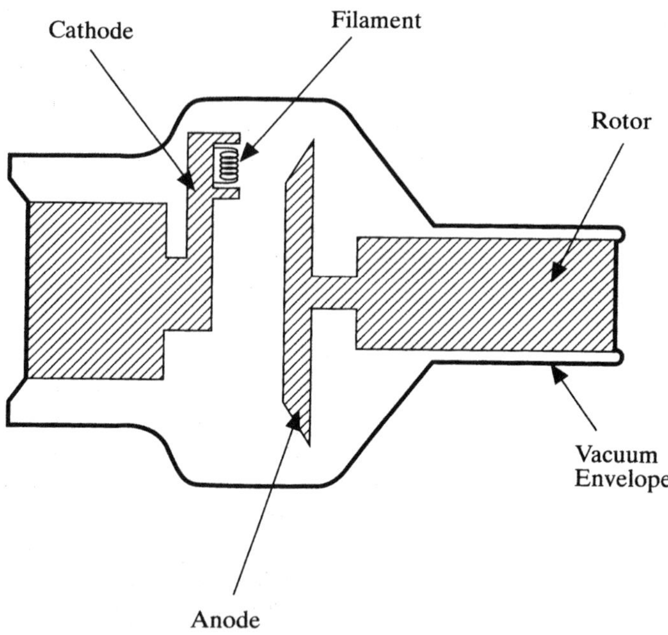

FIGURE 8.1 X-ray tube.

The equipment of conventional x-ray radiography mostly deals with the creation of a desirable beam of x-rays and with the detection of a high-quality image of the transmitted x-rays. These are discussed in the following sections.

Production of X-Rays

X-Ray Tube

The standard device for production of x-rays is the rotating anode x-ray tube, as illustrated in Fig. 8.1. The x-rays are produced from electrons that have been accelerated in vacuum from the cathode to the anode. The electrons are emitted from a filament mounted within a groove in the cathode. Emission occurs when the filament is heated by passing a current through it. When the filament is hot enough, some electrons obtain a thermal energy sufficient to overcome the energy binding the electron to the metal of the filament. Once the electrons have "boiled off" from the filament, they are accelerated by a voltage difference applied from the cathode to the anode. This voltage is supplied by a generator (see below).

After the electrons have been accelerated to the anode, they will be stopped in a short distance. Most of the electrons' energy is converted into heating of the anode, but a small percentage is converted to x-rays by two main methods. One method of x-ray production relies on the fact that deceleration of a charged particle results in emission of electromagnetic radiation, called *bremsstrahlung radiation.* These x-rays will have a wide, continuous distribution of energies, with the maximum being the total energy the electron had when reaching the anode. The number of x-rays is relatively small at higher energies and increases for lower energies.

A second method of x-ray production occurs when an accelerated electron strikes an atom in the anode and removes an inner electron from this atom. The vacant electron orbital will be filled by a neighboring electron, and an x-ray may be emitted whose energy matches the energy change of the electron. The result is production of large numbers of x-rays at a few discrete energies. Since the energy of these characteristic x-rays depends on the material on the surface of the anode, materials are chosen partially to produce x-rays with desired energies. For example, molybdenum is frequently used in anodes of mammography x-ray tubes because of its 20-keV characteristic x-rays.

Low-energy x-rays are undesirable because they increase the dose to the patient but do not contribute to the final image because they are almost totally absorbed. Therefore, the number of low-energy x-rays is usually reduced by use of a layer of absorber that preferentially absorbs them. The extent to which low-energy x-rays have been removed can be quantified by the half-value layer of the x-ray beam.

It is ideal to create x-rays from a point source because any increase in source size will result in blurring of the final image. Quantitatively, the effects of the blurring are described by the focal spot's contribution to the system modulation transfer function (MTF). The blurring has its main effect on edges and small objects, which correspond to the higher frequencies. The effect of this blurring depends on the geometry of the imaging and is worse for larger distances between the object and the image receptor (which corresponds to larger geometric magnifications).

To avoid this blurring, the electrons must be focused to strike a small spot of the anode. The focusing is achieved by electric fields determined by the exact shape of the cathode. However, there is a limit to the size of this focal spot because the anode material will melt if too much power is deposited into too small an area. This limit is improved by use of a rotating anode, where the anode target material is rotated about a central axis and new (cooler) anode material is constantly being rotated into place at the focal spot. To further increase the power limit, the anode is made with an angle surface. This allows the heat to be deposited in a relatively large spot while the apparent spot size at the detector will be smaller by a factor of the sine of the anode angle. Unfortunately, this angle cannot be made too small because it limits the area that can be covered with x-rays. In practice, tubes are usually supplied with two (or more) focal spots of differing sizes, allowing choice of a smaller (sharper, lower-power) spot or a larger (blurrier, higher-power) spot.

The x-ray tube also limits the total number of x-rays that can be used in an exposure because the anode will melt if too much total energy is deposited in it. This limit can be increased by using a more massive anode.

Generator

The voltages and currents in an x-ray tube are supplied by an x-ray generator. This controls the cathode-anode voltage, which partially defines the number of x-rays made because the number of x-rays produced increases with voltage. The voltage is also chosen to produce x-rays with desired energies: Higher voltages make x-rays that generally are more penetrating but give a lower contrast image. The generator also determines the number of x-rays created by controlling the amount of current flowing from the cathode to anode and by controlling the length of time this current flows. This points out the two major parameters that describe an x-ray exposure: the peak kilovolts (peak kilovolts from the anode to the cathode during the exposure) and the milliampere-seconds (the product of the current in milliamperes and the exposure time in seconds).

The peak kilovolts and milliampere-seconds for an exposure may be set manually by an operator based on estimates of the anatomy. Some generators use manual entry of kilovolts and milliamperes but determine the exposure time automatically. This involves sampling the radiation either before or after the image sensor and is referred to as *phototiming.*

The anode-cathode voltage (often 15 to 150 kV) can be produced by a transformer that converts 120 or 220 V ac to higher voltages. This output is then rectified and filtered. Use of three-phase transformers gives voltages that are nearly constant versus those from single-phase transformers, thus avoiding low kilovoltages that produce undesired low-energy x-rays. In a variation of this method, the transformer output can be controlled at a constant voltage by electron tubes. This gives practically constant voltages and, further, allows the voltage to be turned on and off so quickly that millisecond exposure times can be achieved. In a third approach, an ac input can be rectified and filtered to produce a nearly dc voltage, which is then sent to a solid-state inverter that can turn on and off thousands of times a second. This higher-frequency ac voltage can be converted more easily to a high voltage by a transformer. Equipment operating on this principle is referred to as *midfrequency* or *high-frequency generators.*

Image Detection: Screen Film Combinations

Special properties are needed for image detection in radiographic applications, where a few high-quality images are made in a study. Because decisions are not immediately made from the images, it is not necessary to display them instantly (although it may be desirable).

The most commonly used method of detecting such a radiographic x-ray image uses light-sensitive negative film as a medium. Because high-quality film has a poor response to x-rays, it must be used together with x-ray–sensitive screens. Such screens are usually made with $CaWo_2$ or phosphors using rare earth elements such as doped Gd_2O_2S or LaOBr. The film is enclosed in a light-tight cassette in contact with an x-ray screen or between two x-ray screens. When a x-ray image strikes the cassette, the x-rays are absorbed by the screens with high efficiency, and their energy is converted to visible light. The light then exposes a negative image on the film, which is in close contact with the screen.

Several properties have been found to be important in describing the relative performance of different films. One critical property is the *contrast,* which describes the amount of additional darkening caused by an additional amount of light when working near the center of a film's exposure range. Another property, the *latitude* of a film, describes the film's ability to create a usable image with a wide range in input light levels. Generally, latitude and contrast are competing properties, and a film with a large latitude will have a low contrast. Additionally, the modulation transfer function (MTF) of a film is an important property. MTF is most degraded at higher frequencies; this high-frequency MTF is also described by the film's *resolution,* its ability to image small objects.

X-ray screens also have several key performance parameters. It is essential that screens detect and use a large percentage of the x-rays striking them, which is measured as the screen's quantum detection efficiency. Currently used screens may detect 30% of x-rays for images at higher peak kilovolts and as much 60% for lower peak kilovolt images. Such efficiencies lead to the use of two screens (one on each side of the film) for improved x-ray utilization. As with films, a good high-frequency MTF is needed to give good visibility of small structures and edges. Some MTF degradation is associated with blurring that occurs when light spreads as it travels through the screen and to the film. This leads to a compromise on thickness; screens must be thick enough for good quantum detection efficiency but thin enough to avoid excess blurring.

For a film/screen system, a certain amount of radiation will be required to produce a usable amount of film darkening. The ability of the film/screen system to make an image with a small amount of radiation is referred to as its *speed.* The speed depends on a number of parameters: the quantum detection efficiency of the screen, the efficiency with which the screen converts x-ray energy to light, the match between the color emitted by the screen and the colors to which the film is sensitive, and the amount of film darkening for a given amount of light. The number of x-rays used in producing a radiographic image will be chosen to give a viewable amount of exposure to the film. Therefore, patient dose will be reduced by the use of a high-speed screen/film system. However, high-speed film/screen combinations gives a "noisier" image because of the smaller number of x-rays detected in its creation.

Image Detection: X-Ray Image Intensifiers with Televisions

Although screen-film systems are excellent for radiography, they are not usable for fluoroscopy, where lower x-ray levels are produced continuously and many images must be presented almost immediately. Fluoroscopic images are not used for diagnosis but rather as an aid in performing tasks such as placement of catheters in blood vessels during angiography. For fluoroscopy, x-ray image intensifiers are used in conjunction with television cameras. An x-ray image intensifier detects the x-ray image and converts it to a small, bright image of visible light. This visible image is then transferred by lenses to a television camera for final display on a monitor.

The basic structure of an x-ray image intensifier is shown in Fig. 8.2. The components are held in a vacuum by an enclosure made of glass and/or metal. The x-rays enter through a low-absorption window and then strike an input phosphor usually made of doped CsI. As in the x-ray screens described above, the x-rays are converted to light in the CsI. On top of the CsI layer is a photoemitter, which absorbs the

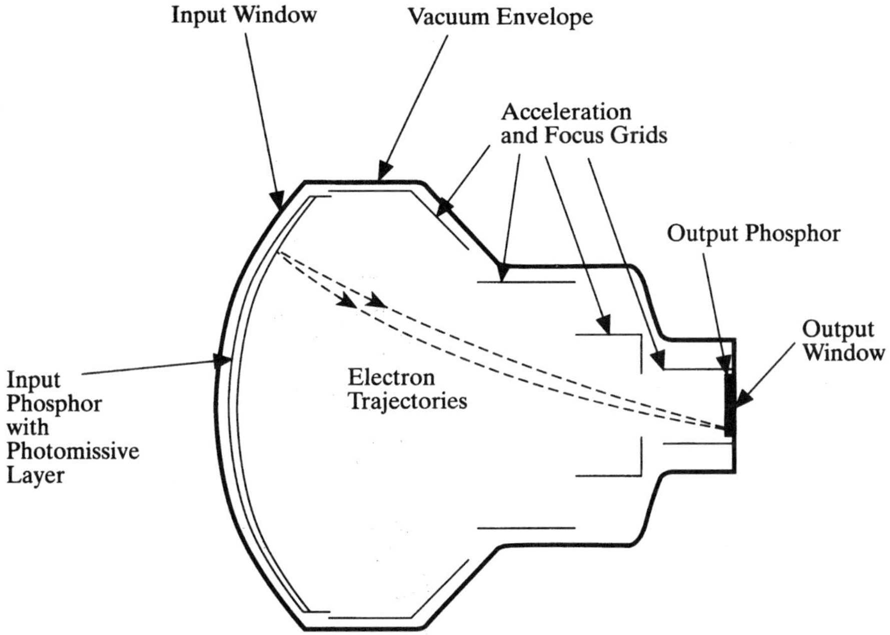

FIGURE 8.2 X-ray image intensifier.

light and emits a number of low-energy electrons that initially spread in various directions. The photoelectrons are accelerated and steered by a set of grids that have voltages applied to them. The electrons strike an output phosphor structure that converts their energy to the final output image made of light. This light then travels through an output window to a lens system. The grid voltages serve to add energy to the electrons so that the output image is brighter. Grid voltages and shapes are also chosen so that the x-ray image is converted to a light image with minimal distortion. Further, the grids must be designed to take photoelectrons that are spreading from a point on the photoemitter and focus them back together at a point on the output phosphor.

It is possible to adjust grid voltages on an image intensifier so that it has different fields of coverage. Either the whole input area can be imaged on the output phosphor, or smaller parts of the input can be imaged on the whole output. Use of smaller parts of the input is advantageous when only smaller parts of anatomy need to be imaged with maximum resolution and a large display. For example, an image intensifier that could cover a 12-in.-diameter input also might be operated so that a 9-in.-diameter or 6-in.-diameter input covers all the output phosphor.

X-ray image intensifiers can be described by a set of performance parameters not unlike those of screen/film combinations. It is important that x-rays be detected and used with a high efficiency; current image intensifiers have quantum detection efficiencies of 60% to 70% for 59-keV x-rays. As with film/screens, a good high-frequency MTF is needed to image small objects and sharp edges without blurring. However, low-frequency MTF also must be controlled carefully in image intensifiers, since it can be degraded by internal scattering of x-rays, photoelectrons, and light over relatively large distances. The amount of intensification depends on brightness and size of the output image for a given x-ray input. This is described either by the gain (specified relative to a standard x-ray screen) or by conversion efficiency [a light output per radiation input measured in $(cd/m^2)/(mR/min)$]. Note that producing a smaller output image is as important as making a light image with more photons because the small image can be handled more efficiently by the lenses that follow. Especially when imaging the full input area, image intensifiers introduce a pincushion distortion into the output image. Thus a square object placed off-center will produce an image that is stretched in the direction away from the center.

Although an image intensifier output could be viewed directly with a lens system, there is more flexibility when the image intensifier is viewed with a television camera and the output is displayed on a monitor. Televisions are currently used with pickup tubes and with CCD sensors.

When a television tube is used, the image is focused on a charged photoconducting material at the tube's input. A number of materials are used, including SbS_3, PbO, and SeTeAs. The light image discharges regions of the photoconductor, converting the image to a charge distribution on the back of the photoconducting layer. Next, the charge distribution is read by scanning a small beam of electrons across the surface, which recharges the photoconductor. The recharging current is proportional to the light intensity at the point being scanned; this current is amplified and then used to produce an image on a monitor. The tube target is generally scanned in an interlaced mode in order to be consistent with broadcast television and allow use of standard equipment.

In fluoroscopy, it is desirable to use the same detected dose for all studies so that the image noise is approximately constant. This is usually achieved by monitoring the image brightness in a central part of the image intensifier's output, since brightness generally increases with dose. The brightness may be monitored by a photomultiplier tube that samples it directly or by analyzing signal levels in the television. However, maintaining a constant detected dose would lead to high patient doses in the case of very absorptive anatomy. To avoid problems here, systems are generally required by federal regulations to have a limit on the maximum patient dose. In those cases where the dose limit prevents the image intensifier from receiving the usual dose, the output image becomes darker. To compensate for this, television systems are often operated with automatic gain control that gives an image on the monitor of a constant brightness no matter what the brightness from the image intensifier.

Image Detection: Digital Systems

In both radiography and fluoroscopy, there are advantages to the use of digital images. This allows image processing for better displayed images, use of lower doses in some cases, and opens the possibility for digital storage with a PACS system or remote image viewing via teleradiology. Additionally, some digital systems provide better image quality because of fewer processing steps, lack of distortion, or improved uniformity.

A common method of digitizing medical x-ray images uses the voltage output from an image-intensifier/TV system. This voltage can be digitized by an analog-to-digital converter at rates fast enough to be used with fluoroscopy as well as radiography.

Another technology for obtaining digital radiographs involves use of photostimulable phosphors. Here the x-rays strike an enclosed sheet of phosphor that stores the x-ray energy. This phorphor can then be taken to a read-out unit, where the phosphor surface is scanned by a small light beam of proper wavelength. As a point on the surface is read, the stored energy is emitted as visible light, which is then detected, amplified, and digitized. Such systems have the advantage that they can be used with existing systems designed for screen/film detection because the phosphor sheet package is the same size as that for screen films.

A new method for digital detection involves use of active-matrix thin-film-transistor technology, in which an array of small sensors is grown in hydrogenated amorphous silicon. Each sensor element includes an electrode for storing charge that is proportional to its x-ray signal. Each electrode is coupled to a transistor that either isolates it during acquisition or couples it to digitization circuitry during readout. There are two common methods for introducing the charge signal on each electrode. In one method, a layer of x-ray absorber (typically selenium) is deposited on the array of sensors; when this layer is biased and x-rays are absorbed there, their energy is converted to electron-hole pairs and the resulting charge is collected on the electrode. In the second method, each electrode is part of the photodiode that makes electron-hole pairs when exposed to light; the light is produced from x-rays by a layer of scintillator (such as CsI) that is deposited on the array.

Use of a digital system provides several advantages in fluoroscopy. The digital image can be processed in real time with edge enhancement, smoothing, or application of a median filter. Also, frame-to-frame averaging can be used to decrease image noise, at the expense of blurring the image of moving objects. Further, digital fluoroscopy with TV system allows the TV tube to be scanned in formats that are optimized for read-out; the image can still be shown in a different format that is optimized for display. Another advantage is that the displayed image is not allowed to go blank when x-ray exposure is ended, but a repeated display of the last image is shown. This last-image-hold significantly reduces doses in those cases where the radiologist needs to see an image for evaluation, but does not necessarily need a continuously updated image.

The processing of some digital systems also allows the use of pulsed fluoroscopy, where the x-rays are produced in a short, intense burst instead of continuously. In this method the pulses of x-rays are made either by biasing the x-ray tube filament or by quickly turning on and off the anode-cathode voltage. This has the advantage of making sharper images of objects that are moving. Often one x-ray pulse is produced for every display frame, but there is also the ability to obtain dose reduction by leaving the x-rays off for some frames. With such a reduced exposure rate, doses can be reduced by a factor of two or four by only making x-rays every second or fourth frame. For those frames with no x-ray pulse, the system repeats a display of the last frame with x-rays.

Defining Terms

Antiscatter grid: A thin structure made of alternating strips of lead and material transmissive to x-rays. Strips are oriented so that most scattered x-rays go through lead sections and are preferentially absorbed, while unscattered x-rays go through transmissive sections.

Focal spot: The small area on the anode of an x-ray tube from where x-rays are emitted. It is the place where the accelerated electron beam is focused.

Half-value layer (HVL): The thickness of a material (often aluminum) needed to absorb half the x-ray in a beam.

keV: A unit of energy useful with x-rays. It is equal to the energy supplied to an electron when accelerated through 1 kilovolt.

Modulation transfer function (MTF): The ratio of the contrast in the output image of a system to the contrast in the object, specified for sine waves of various frequencies. Describes blurring (loss of contrast) in an imaging system for different-sized objects.

Quantum detection efficiency: The percentage of incident x-rays effectively used to create an image.

References

Bushberg JT, Seibert JA, Leidholdt EM, Boone JM. 1994. The Essential Physics of Medical Imaging. Baltimore, Williams & Wilkins.

Curry TS, Dowdey JE, Murry RC. 1984. Christensen's Introduction to the Physics of Diagnostic Radiology. Philadelphia, Lea & Febiger.

Hendee WR, Ritenour R. 1992. Medical Imaging Physics. St. Louis, Mosby-Year Book.

Ter-Pogossian MM. 1969. The Physical Aspects of Diagnostic Radiology. New York, Harper & Row.

Further Information

Medical Physics is a monthly scientific and informational journal published for the American Association of Physicists in Medicine. Papers here generally cover evaluation of existing medical equipment and development of new systems. For more information, contact the American Association of Physicists in Medicine, One Physics Ellipse, College Park, MD 20740-3846.

The Society of Photo-Optical Instrumentation Engineers (SPIE) sponsors numerous conferences and publishes their proceedings. Especially relevant is the annual conference on Medical Imaging. Contact SPIE, P.O. Box 10, Bellham, WA 98277-0010.

Several corporations active in medical imaging work together under the National Electrical Manufacturers Association to develop definitions and testing standards for equipment used in the field. Information can be obtained from NEMA, 2101 L Street, N.W., Washington, DC 20037.

Critical aspects of medical x-ray imaging are covered by rules of the Food and Drug Administration, part of the Department of Health and Human Services. These are listed in the *Code of Federal Regulations*, Title 21. Copies are for sale by the Superintendent of Documents, U.S. Government Printing Office, Washington, DC 20402.

8.2 X-Ray Projection Angiography

Michael S. Van Lysel

Angiography is a diagnostic and, increasingly, therapeutic modality concerned with diseases of the circulatory system. While many imaging modalities (ultrasound, computed tomography, magnetic resonance imaging, angioscopy) are now available, either clinically or for research, to study vascular structures, this section will focus on projection radiography. In this method, the vessel of interest is opacified by injection of a radiopaque contrast agent. Serial radiographs of the contrast material flowing through the vessel are then acquired. This examination is performed in an angiographic suite, a special procedures laboratory, or a cardiac catheterization laboratory.

Contrast material is needed to opacify vascular structures because the radiographic contrast of blood is essentially the same as that of soft tissue. Contrast material consists of an iodine-containing ($Z = 53$) compound, with maximum iodine concentrations of about 350 mg/cm^3. Contrast material is injected through a catheter ranging in diameter roughly from 1 to 3 mm, depending on the injection flow rate to be used. Radiographic images of the contrast-filled vessels are recorded using either film or video.

Digital imaging technology has become instrumental in the acquisition and storage of angiographic images. The most important application of digital imaging is digital subtraction angiography (DSA). Temporal subtraction is a DSA model in which a preinjection image (the mask) is acquired, the injection of contrast agent is then performed, and the sequential images of the opacified vessel(s) are acquired and subtracted from the mask. The result, ideally, is that the fixed anatomy is canceled, allowing contrast enhancement (similar to computed tomographic windowing and leveling) to provide increased contrast sensitivity.

An increasingly important facet of the angiographic procedure is the use of transluminal interventional techniques to effect a therapeutic result. These techniques, including angioplasty, atherectomy, laser ablation, and intraluminal stents, rely on digital angiographic imaging technology to facilitate the precise catheter manipulations necessary for a successful result. In fact, digital enhancement, storage, and retrieval of fluoroscopic images have become mandatory capabilities for digital angiographic systems.

Figure 8.3 is a schematic representation of an angiographic imaging system. The basic components include an x-ray tube and generator, image intensifier, video camera, cine camera (optional for cardiac imaging), and digital image processor.

X-Ray Generation

Angiographic systems require a high-power, sophisticated x-ray generation system in order to produce the short, intense x-ray pulses needed to produce clear images of moving vessels. Required exposure times range from 100 to 200 ms for cerebral studies to 1 to 10 ms for cardiac studies. Angiographic systems use either a constant potential generator, or, increasingly, a medium/high-frequency inverter generator. Power ratings for angiographic generators are generally greater than or equal to 80 kW at 100 kW and must be capable of producing reasonably square x-ray pulses. In most cases (pediatric cardiology being an exception), pulse widths of 5 ms or greater are necessary to keep the x-ray tube potential in the desirable, high-contrast range of 70 to 90 kVp.

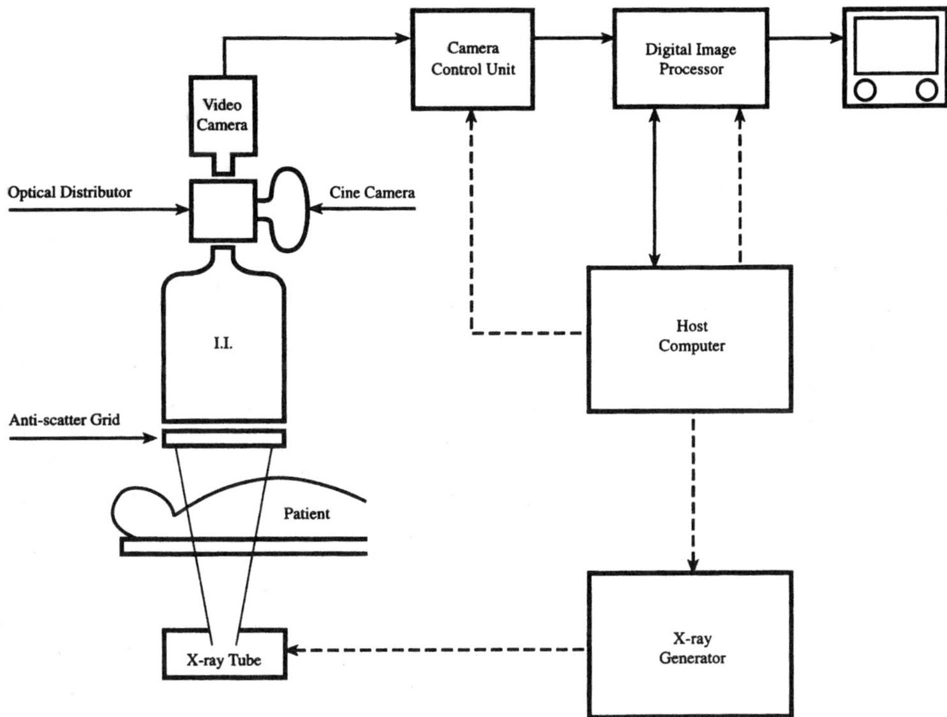

FIGURE 8.3 Schematic diagram of an image intensifier-based digital angiographic and cine imaging system. Solid arrows indicate image signals, and dotted arrows indicate control signals.

The x-ray tube is of the rotating-anode variety. Serial runs of high-intensity x-ray pulses result in high heat loads. Anode heat storage capacities of 1 mega-heat units (MHU) or greater are required, especially in the case of cine angiography. Electronic "heat computers," which calculate and display the current heat load of the x-ray tube, are very useful in preventing damage to the x-ray tube. In a high-throughput angiographic suite, forced liquid cooling of the x-ray tube housing is essential. Angiographic x-ray tubes are of multifocal design, with the focal spot sizes tailored for the intended use. A 0.6-mm (50-kW loading), 1.2-mm (100-kW loading) bifocal insert is common. The specified heat loads for a given focal spot are for single exposures. When serial angiographic exposures are performed, the focal spot load limit must be derated (reduced) to account for the accumulation of heat in the focal spot target during the run. Larger focal spots (e.g., 1.8 mm) can be obtained for high-load procedures. A smaller focal spot [e.g., 0.3 and 0.1 mm (bias)] is needed for magnification studies. Small focal spots have become increasingly desirable for high-resolution fluoroscopic interventional studies performed with 1000-line video systems.

Image Formation

Film

From the 1950s through to the 1980s, the dominant detector system used for recording the angiographic procedure was film/screen angiography using a rapid film changer [Amplatz, 1997]. However, digital angiography, described below, has almost completely replaced this technology. Film provides a higher spatial resolution than digital. However, as the spatial resolution of digital continues to improve, the overwhelming advantages of ease of use and image processing algorithms have prevailed. While film changers can still be found in use, few new film/screen systems are being purchased.

One application where film use is still common is cardiac imaging. *Cine* angiography is performed with a 35-mm motion picture camera optically coupled to the image intensifier output phosphor

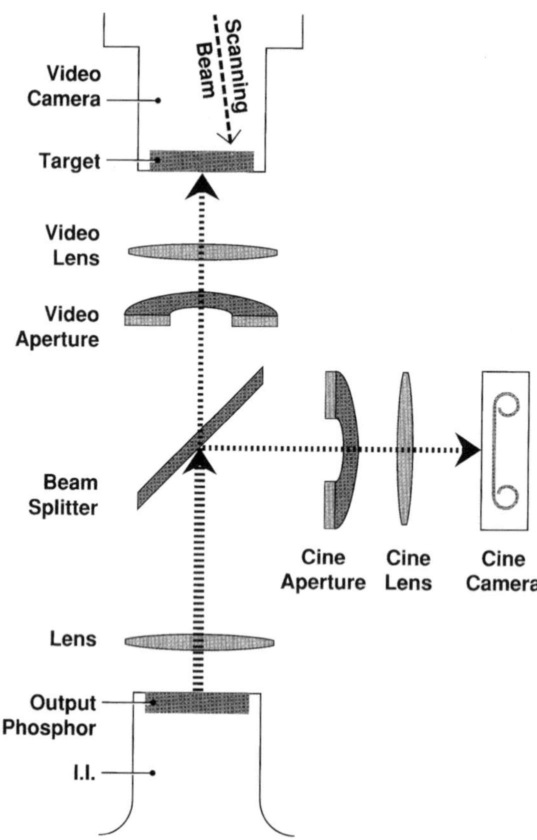

FIGURE 8.4 Schematic diagram of the optical distributor used to couple the image intensifier (I.I.) output phosphor to a video and cine camera. (From Van Lysel MS. Digital angiography. In S Baum (ed), Abrams' Angiography, 4th ed. Boston, Little, Brown, with permission.)

(Fig. 8.4). The primary clinical application is coronary angiography and ventriculography. During cine angiography, x-ray pulses are synchronized both with the cine camera shutter and the vertical retrace of the system video camera. To limit motion blurring, it is desirable to keep the x-ray pulses as short as possible, but no longer than 10 ms.

Imaging runs generally last from 5 to 10 s in duration at a frame rate of 30 to 60 frames/s (fps). Sixty fps is generally used for pediatric studies, where higher heart rates are encountered, while 30 fps is more typical for adult studies ("digital cine," discussed below, generally is performed at 15 fps). Some cine angiographic installations provide biplane imaging in which two independent imaging chains can acquire orthogonal images of the injection sequence. The eccentricity of coronary lesions and the asymmetric nature of cardiac contraction abnormalities require that multiple x-ray projections be acquired. Biplane systems allow this to be done with a smaller patient contrast load. For this reason, biplane systems are considered a requirement for pediatric cath labs. They are relatively uncommon for adult cath labs, however, where the less complicated positioning of a single plane system is often valued over the reduced number of injections possible with a biplane system. The AP and lateral planes of a biplane system are energized out of phase, which results in the potential for image degradation due to detection of the radiation scattered from the opposite plane. Image intensifier *blanking*, which shuts down the accelerating voltage of the non-imaging plane, is used to eliminate this problem.

While film remains in common use for cardiac imaging, here too the medium is being replaced by digital. Digital angiographic systems (described below) were integrated into the cardiac catheterization imaging system beginning in the 1980s, to provide short-term image storage and replay. However, the high resolution and frame rate required for cardiac imaging precluded the use of digital hardware for long-term (greater than 1 day) storage. Film and cine are acquired simultaneously using the beam splitting mirror in the optical distributor (Fig. 8.4). This situation is rapidly changing, as high-speed video servers and the recordable compact disc (CD-R) now provide acceptable performance for this application. Most new cardiac imaging systems are purchased without a cine film camera.

Image Intensifier/Video Camera

The image intensifier (II) is fundamental to the modern angiographic procedure. The purpose of the image intensifier is (1) to produce a light image with sufficient brightness to allow the use of video and film cameras and (2) to produce an output image of small enough size to allow convenient coupling to video and film cameras. The image intensifier provides both real-time imaging capability (fluoroscopy), which allows patient positioning and catheter manipulation, and recording of the angiographic injection (digital angiography, analog video recording, photospot, cine).

Image intensifier output phosphors are approximately 25 mm in diameter, although large (e.g., 50 to 60 mm) output phosphor image intensifiers have been developed to increase spatial resolution. The modulation transfer function (MTF) of the image intensifier is determined primarily by the input and output phosphor stages, so mapping a given input image to a larger output phosphor will improve the MTF of the system. The input phosphor of a modern image intensifier is cesium iodide (CsI). The largest currently available image intensifier input phosphors are approximately 16 in. The effective input phosphor diameter is selectable by the user. For example, an image intensifier designated 9/7/5 allows the user to select input phosphor diameters of 9, 7, or 5 in. These selections are referred to as image intensifier *modes.* The purpose of providing an adjustable input phosphor is to allow the user to trade off between spatial resolution and field of view. A smaller mode provides higher spatial resolution both because the MTF of the image intensifier improves and because it maps a smaller field of view to the fixed size of the video camera target. Generally speaking, angiographic suites designed exclusively for cardiac catheterization use 9-in. image intensifiers, neuroangiography suites use 12-in. intensifiers, while suites that must handle pulmonary, renal, or peripheral angiography require the larger (i.e., 14 to 16 in.) intensifiers.

The brightness gain of the image intensifier derives from two sources: (1) the increase in electron energy produced by the accelerating potential (the *flux* gain) and (2) the decrease in size of the image as it is transferred from the input to the output phosphor (the *minification* gain). The product of these two factors can exceed 5000. However, since the minification gain is a function of the area of the input phosphor exposed to the radiation beam (i.e., the image intensifier mode), the brightness gain drops as smaller image intensifier modes are selected. This is compensated for by a combination of increasing x-ray exposure to maintain the image intensifier light output and opening the video camera aperture. Image intensifier brightness gain declines with age and must be monitored to allow timely replacement. The specification used for this purpose is the image intensifier *conversion factor,* defined as the light output of the image intensifier per unit x-ray exposure input. Modern image intensifiers have a conversion factor of 100 $cd/m^2/mR/s$ or more for the 9-in. mode.

With the increasing emergence of digital angiography as the primary angiographic imaging modality, image intensifier performance has become increasingly important. In the field, the high-spatial-frequency of an image intensifier is assessed by determining the limiting resolution [in the neighborhood of 4 to 5 line-pairs/mm (lp/mm) in the 9-in. mode], while the low-spatial-frequency response is assessed using the contrast ratio (in the neighborhood of 15:1 to 30:1). The National Electrical Manufacturers Association (NEMA) has defined test procedures for measuring the contrast ratio [NEMA, 1992]. The *detective quantum efficiency* (DQE), which is a measure of the efficiency with which the image intensifier utilizes the x-ray energy incident on it, is in the neighborhood of 65% (400 μm phosphor thickness, 60 keV). A tabulation of the specifications of several commercially available image intensifiers has been published by Siedband [1994].

Optical Distributor

The image present at the image intensifier output phosphor is coupled to the video camera, and any film camera present (e.g., cine), by the optical distributor. The components of the distributor are shown in Fig. 8.4. There is an aperture for each camera to allow the light intensity presented to each camera to be adjusted independently. The video camera aperture is usually a motor-driven variable iris, while the film camera aperture is usually fixed. It is important to realize that while the aperture does ensure that the proper light level is presented to the camera, more fundamentally, the aperture determines the x-ray exposure input to the image intensifier. As a result, both the patient exposure and the level of quantum noise in the image are set by the aperture. The noise amplitude in a fluoroscopic or digital angiographic image is inversely proportional to the f-number of the optical system. Because the *quantum sink* of a properly adjusted fluorographic system is at the input of the image intensifier, the aperture diameter is set, for a given type of examination, to provide the desired level of quantum mottle present in the image. The x-ray exposure factors are then adjusted for each patient, by an *automatic exposure control* (AEC) system, to produce the proper postaperture light level. However, some video systems do provide for increasing the video camera aperture during fluoroscopy when the maximum entrance exposure does not provide adequate light levels on a large patient.

The beam-splitting mirror was originally meant to provide a moderate-quality video image simultaneous with cine recording in order to monitor the contrast injection during cardiac studies. More recently, as the importance of digital angiography has mushroomed, precision-quality mirrors with higher transmission have been used in order to provide simultaneous diagnostic-quality cine and video. The latest development has been the introduction of *cine-less* digital cardiac systems, in which the video image is the sole recording means. The introduction of these systems has sometimes been accompanied by the claim that a cine-less system requires less patient exposure due to the fact that light does not have to be provided to the cine camera. However, a conventional cine system operates with an excess of light (i.e., the cine camera aperture is stopped down). Because the image intensifier input is the quantum sink of the system, exposure is determined by the need to limit quantum mottle, not to maintain a given light level at the image intensifier output. Therefore, the validity of this claim is dubious. It should be noted, however, that because of the difference in spatial resolution capabilities of cine and video, the noise power spectrum of images acquired with equal exposure will be different. It is possible that observers accept a lower exposure in a video image than in the higher-resolution film image.

Video System

The video system in an angiographic suite consists of several components, including the camera head, camera control unit (CCU), video monitors, and video recording devices. In addition, a digital image processor is integrated with the video system.

The video camera is responsible for signal generation. Traditionally, pickup-tube based cameras (discussed below) have been used. Recently, high resolution (1024^2), high frame rate (30 fps) charge-coupled device (CCD) video cameras have become available and are replacing tube-based cameras in some angiographic installations. This trend will probably continue. The image quality ramifications are a matter of current research [Blume, 1998]. The advantages of CCD cameras include low-voltage operation, reliability, little required setup tuning, and freedom from geometric distortions. Frame-charge transfer is the preferred CCD read-out scheme, due to the higher optical fill factor of this configuration.

Video camera pickup tubes used for angiography are of the photoconductive *vidicon-style* of construction. This type of tube uses a low-velocity scanning beam and generates a signal from the recharge of the target by the scanning electron beam. There are several types of vidicon-style tubes in use (Plumbicon, Primicon, Saticon, Newvicon) which differ from each other in the material and configuration used for target construction. There is an unfortunate confusion in terminology because the original vidicon-style tube is referred to simply as a *vidicon.* The original vidicon has an antimony trisulfide target (Sb_2S_3) and exhibits such a high degree of lag (image retention) that it is not useful for angiographic work. Even with *low-lag* angiographic cameras, the residual lag can result in artifacts in subtraction images. *Light bias* is often used to further reduce lag by ensuring that the target surface is not driven to a negative potential by energetic electrons in the scanning beam [Sandrik, 1984].

Image noise in a well-designed system is due to x-ray quantum fluctuations and noise related to signal generation in the video camera. When used for digital angiographic purposes, it is important that the video camera exhibit a high signal-to-noise ratio (at least 60 dB) so that video camera noise does not dominate the low-signal (dark) portions of the image. In order to achieve this, the pickup tube must be run at high beam currents (2 to 3 μA). Because long-term operation of the tube at these beam currents can result in damage to the target, beam current is usually either blanked when imaging is not being performed, or the current is held at a low level (e.g., 400 nA) and boosted only when high-quality angiographic images are required. All pickup tubes currently in use for angiographic imaging exhibit a linear response to light input (i.e., $\gamma = 1$, where the relationship between signal current I and image brightness B is described by a relationship of the form $I/I_o = (B/B_o)^{\gamma}$). This has the disadvantage that the range in image brightness presented to the camera often exceeds the camera's dynamic range when a highly transmissive portion of the patient's anatomy (e.g., lung) or unattenuated radiation is included in the image field, either saturating the highlights or forcing the rest of the image to a low signal level, or both. To deal with this problem, it is desirable for the operator to mechanically bolus the bright area with metal filters, saline bags, etc. Specially constructed filters are available for commonly encountered problems, such as the transmissive region between the patient's legs during *runoff* studies of the legs, and most vendors provide a controllable metal filter in the x-ray collimator that the operator can position over bright spots with a joystick.

In addition to mechanical bolusing performed by the laboratory staff, most system vendors have incorporated some form of *gamma curve modification* into the systems. Usually performed using analog processing in the CCU, the technique applies a nonlinear transfer curve to the originally linear data. There are two advantages to this technique. First, the CRT of the display monitor has reduced gain at low signal, so imposing a transfer function with $\gamma \approx 0.5$ via gamma-curve modification provides a better match between the video signal and the display monitor. Second, if the modification is performed prior to digitization, a $\gamma < 1$ results in a more constant ratio between the ADC step size and the image noise amplitude across the full range of the video signal. This results in less contouring in the dark portions of the digital image, especially in images that have been spatially filtered. It is important to note, however, that gamma-curve modification does not eliminate the desirable effects of mechanically bolusing the image field prior to image acquisition. This is so because bolusing allows more photon flux to be selectively applied to the more attenuating regions of the patient, which decreases both quantum and video noise in those regions. Bolusing is especially important for subtraction imaging.

The video system characteristic most apparent to the user is the method employed in scanning the image. Prior to the advent of the digital angiography, EIA RS-170 video (525-line, 30 Hz frames, 2:1 interlace) was the predominant standard used for fluoroscopic systems in the United States. However, this method of scanning has definite disadvantages for angiography, including low resolution and image artifacts related to the interlaced format. The inclusion of a digital image processor in the imaging chain, functioning as an image buffer, allows the scanning mode to be tailored to the angiographic procedure. Many of the important video scanning modes used for angiographic work are dependent on the ability of image processors to perform *scan conversion* operations. Two typical scan conversion operations are progressive-to-interlaced conversion and upscanning. Progressive-to-interlaced scan conversion allows progressive scanning (also referred to as *sequential scanning*) to be used for image acquisition and interlaced scanning for image display. Progressive scanning is a noninterlaced scan mode in which all the lines are read out in a single vertical scan. Progressive scanning is especially necessary when imaging moving arteries, such as during coronary angiography [Seibert et al., 1984]. In noncardiac work, progressive scan acquisition is usually combined with beam blanking. *Beam blanking* refers to the condition in which the pickup tube beam current is blanked (turned off) for one or more integer number of frames. This mode is used in order to allow the image to integrate on the camera target prior to read-out (Fig. 8.5). In this way, x-ray pulses shorter than one frame period can be acquired without scanning artifacts, and x-ray pulses longer than one frame period can be used in order to increase the x-ray quantum statistics

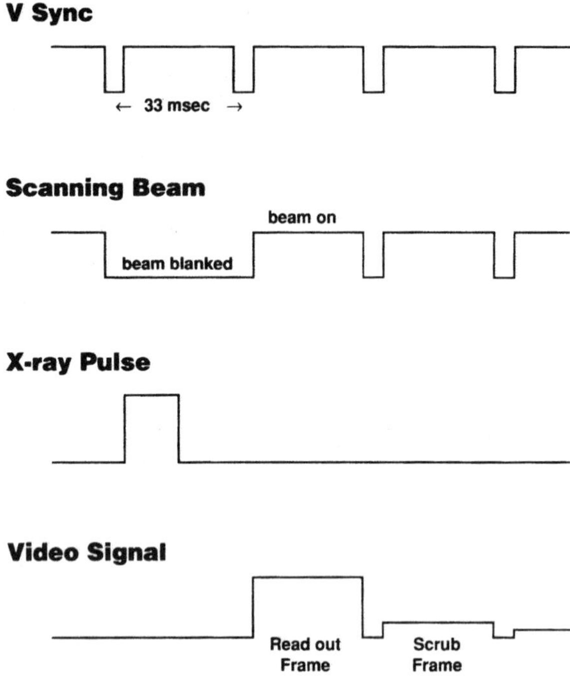

FIGURE 8.5 Timing diagram for image acquisition using the pulsed-progressive mode. (From Van Lysel MS. Digital angiography. In S Baum (ed), Abrams' Angiography, 4th ed. Boston, Little, Brown, with permission.)

of an image. Upscanning refers to the acquisition of data at a low line rate (e.g., 525 lines) and the display of that data at a higher line rate (e.g., 1023 lines) [Holmes et al., 1989]. The extra lines are produced by either replication of the actual data or, more commonly, by interpolation (either linear or spline). Upscanning also can be performed in the horizontal direction as well, but this is less typical. Upscanning is used to decrease the demands on the video camera, system bandwidth, and digital storage requirements while improving display contrast and decreasing interfield flicker.

The image buffering capability of a digital system can provide several operations aimed at reducing patient exposure. If fluoroscopy is performed with pulsed rather than continuous x-rays, then the operator has the freedom to choose the frame rate. During pulsed-progressive fluoroscopy, the digital system provides for display refresh without flicker. Frame rates of less than 30 fps can result in lower patient exposure, though; because of the phenomenon of eye integration, the x-ray exposure per pulse must be increased as the frame rate drops in order to maintain low contrast detectability [Aufrichtig et al., 1994]. *Last image hold,* which stores and displays the last acquired fluoroscopic frame, also can result in an exposure reduction. Combining last image hold with graphic overlays allows collimator shutters and bolus filters to be positioned with the x-rays turned off.

Digital Angiography

Digital imaging technology has quickly replaced film-based recording for most angiographic procedures. Digital image processing provides the ability to manipulate the contrast and spatial-frequency characteristics of the angiographic image, as well as providing immediate access to the image data during the procedure.

The rapid application of digital imaging technology to the angiographic procedure was facilitated by the fact that the image intensifier and video camera imaging chain was already in use when digital imaging appeared. It is a relatively simple matter to digitize the video camera output. Theoretically, additional noise is added to the image due to quantitization errors associated with the digitization process. This additional noise can be kept insignificantly small by using a sufficient number of digital levels so that

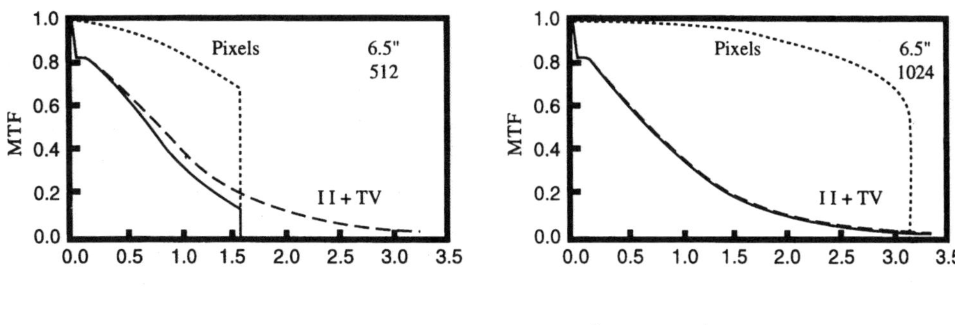

FIGURE 8.6 Detector modulation transfer function, including limits due to the image intensifier (II), video camera (TV), and sampling, including the antialiasing filter (pixels). Figures are for the 6.5-in. image intensifier mode for 512- and 1024-pixel matrices. In both cases, the total detector MTF is given by the solid line. Data used for this figure from Verhoeven [1985].

the amplitude of one digital level is approximately equal to the amplitude of the standard deviation in image values associated with the noise (x-ray quantum and electronic noise) in the image prior to digitization [Kruger et al., 1981]. To meet this condition, most digital angiographic systems employ a 10-bit (1024-level) analog-to-digital convertor (ADC). Those systems which are designed to digitize high-noise (i.e., low x-ray exposure) images exclusively can employ an 8-bit (256-level) ADC. Such systems include those designed for cardiac and fluoroscopic applications.

The spatial resolution of a digital angiographic image is determined by several factors, including the size of the x-ray tube focal spot, the modulation transfer function of the image intensifier-video camera chain, and the size of the pixel matrix. The typical image matrix dimensions for non-cardiac digital angiographic images is 1024 × 1024. Cardiac systems use 512 × 512, 1024(H) × 512(V), or 1024 × 1024. Sampling rates required to digitize 512^2 and 1024^2 matrices in the 33-ms frame period of conventional video are 10 and 40 MHz, respectively. Figure 8.6 shows an example of the detector MTF of a digital angiographic system. The product of the image intensifier and video system MTF constitute the *pre-sampling MTF* [Fujita et al., 1985]. It is seen that the effect of sampling with a 512-pixel matrix is to truncate the high-frequency tail of the presampling MTF, while a 1024-pixel matrix imposes few additional limitations beyond that associated with the analog components (especially for small image intensifier modes) [Verhoeven, 1985]. However, because of blurring associated with the x-ray tube focal spot, the full advantage of the higher density pixel matrix can rarely be realized, clinically (Fig. 8.7).

Digital Image Processor

The digital image processor found in a modern angiographic suite is a dedicated device designed specially to meet the demands of the angiographic procedure. Hardware is structured as a pipeline processor to perform real-time processing at video rates. Image-subtraction, integration, spatial-filtration, and temporal-filtration algorithms are hardwired to meet this requirement. Lookup tables (LUTs) are used to perform intensity transformations (e.g., contrast enhancement and logarithmic transformation). A more general purpose *host* computer is used to control the pipeline processor and x-ray generator, respond to user input, and perform non-real-time image manipulations.

The most clinically important image-processing algorithm is temporal subtraction (DSA). Subtraction imaging is used for most vascular studies. Subtraction allows approximately a factor of 2 reduction in the amount of injected contrast material. As a result, DSA studies can be performed with less contrast load and with smaller catheters than film/screen angiography. The primary limitation of DSA is a susceptibility to misregistration artifacts resulting from patient motion. Some procedures that are particularly susceptible to motion artifacts are routinely performed in a nonsubtracted mode. Unsubtracted digital angiographic studies are usually performed with the same amount of contrast material as

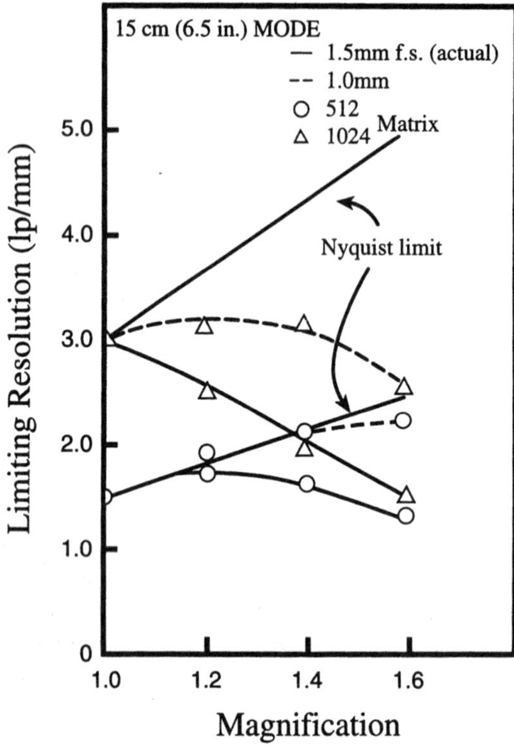

FIGURE 8.7 Experimental determination of the limiting resolution (high-contrast object and high x-ray exposure) for 512- and 1024-pixel matrices, focal spots of actual dimensions 1.0 and 1.5 mm, and a 6.5-in image intensifier mode, as a function of geometric magnification. (From Mistretta CA, Peppler WW. 1988. Digital cardiac x-ray imaging: Fundamental principles. Am J Card Imaging 2:26, with permission.)

film/screen studies. Cardiac angiography is one procedure that is generally performed without subtraction, although in any particular study, if patient and respiratory motion are absent, it is possible to obtain high-quality time subtractions using phase-matched mask subtractions in which the preinjection mask and postinjection contrast images are matched with respect to cardiac phase. In order to do this efficiently, it is necessary to digitize the ECG signal along with the image data.

Additional examples of unsubtracted digital angiographic studies are those in uncooperative patients (e.g., trauma) and digital runoff studies of the vessels in the leg. In a digital runoff study it is necessary to follow the bolus down the legs by moving the patient (or the image gantry). This motion causes difficulties with both mask registration and uniform exposure intensities between the mask and contrast images. The high contrast sensitivity of DSA is valuable for runoff studies, however, because the small vessels and slow flow in the lower extremities can make vessel visualization difficult. Recently, making use of programmed table (or gantry) motion and pixel-shifting strategies, x-ray vendors have begun to offer a viable digital subtraction runoff mode.

In addition to subtraction angiography, two filtration algorithms have become clinically important. The first is high-pass spatial filtration for the purposes of providing edge enhancement. Real-time edge enhancement of fluoroscopy is especially important for interventional procedures, such as angioplasty, where the task requires visualization of high-frequency objects such as vessel edges and guidewires. Because increasing the degree of edge enhancement also increases image noise, operator control of the degree of enhancement (accomplished by adjusting the size and weighing of the convolution kernel) is an important feature.

The second filtration algorithm often available from a digital angiographic system is low-pass temporal filtration (recursive filtering) [Rowlands, 1992]. Temporal filtration is used to reduce quantum noise levels in fluoroscopic images without increasing patient exposure. Recursive filtering is a more desirable method than simple image integration because it requires only two memory planes and because it is a simple matter to turn the filtering algorithm off, on a pixel-by-pixel basis, when motion is detected. Motion-detection circuits monitor the frame-to-frame change in pixel values and assume that an object has moved into or out of the pixel if the change exceeds a preset threshold.

Image Storage

Storage needs during the angiographic procedure are easily met by modern hard drives. These often are configured to provide real-time (i.e., video rate) storage. The immediate access to images provided by real-time disk technology is one of the major advantages of digital angiography over film. Not only is it unnecessary to wait for film to be developed, but review of the image data after the patient's procedure is completed is facilitated by directories and specialized review software. For example, a popular image menu feature is the presentation to users of a low-resolution collage of available images from which they may select a single image or entire run for full-resolution display.

While online storage of recent studies is a strength of digital angiography, long-term (archival) storage is a weakness. Archival devices provided by vendors are generally proprietary devices that make use of various recording media. There is an established communications protocol (ACR-NEMA) [NEMA, 1993] for network transfer of images. For the time being, while large institutions and teaching hospitals are investing in sophisticated digital picture archiving and communications systems (PACS), archival needs at most institutions are met by storage of hardcopy films generated from the digital images. Hardcopy devices include multiformat cameras (laser or video) and video thermal printers. Laser cameras, using either an analog or a digital interface to the digital angiographic unit, can provide diagnostic-quality, large-format, high-contrast, high-resolution films. Multiformat video cameras, which expose the film with a CRT, are a less expensive method of generating diagnostic-quality images but are also more susceptible to drift and geometric distortions. Thermal printer images are generally used as convenient method to generate temporary hardcopy images.

Cardiac angiography labs have long employed a similar method, referred to as *parallel cine*, in which both digital and cine images are recorded simultaneously by use of the semitransparent mirror in the image intensifier optical distributor. Immediate diagnosis would be performed off the digital monitor while the 35-mm film would provide archival storage and the ability to share the image data with other institutions. However, due to the promulgation of an image transfer standard using the recordable CD (CD-R), many laboratories are abandoning cine film. While CD-R cannot replay images at full real-time rates, the read-rate (>1 MB/s) is sufficient to load old data quickly from CD-R to a workstation hard drive for review. Low volume laboratories can use CD-R as an archival storage method. Higher volume labs are installing networked video file servers to provide online or near-line access to archived patient studies.

Summary

For decades, x-ray projection film/screen angiography was the only invasive modality available for the diagnosis of vascular disease. Now several imaging modalities are available to study the cardiovascular system, most of which are less invasive than x-ray projection angiography. However, conventional angiography also has changed dramatically during the last decade. Digital angiography has replaced film/screen angiography in most applications. In addition, the use and capabilities of transluminal interventional techniques have mushroomed, and digital angiographic processor modes have expanded significantly in support of these interventional procedures. As a consequence, while less invasive technologies, such as MR angiography, make inroads into conventional angiography's diagnostic applications, it is likely that x-ray projection angiography will remain an important clinical modality for many years to come.

Defining Terms

Bolus: This term has two, independent definitions: (1) material placed in a portion of the x-ray beam to reduce the sense dynamic range and (2) the injection contrast material.

Digital subtraction angiography (DSA): Methodology in which digitized angiographic images are subtracted in order to provide contrast enhancement of the opacified vasculature. Clinically, temporal subtraction is the algorithm used, though energy subtraction methods also fall under the generic term DSA.

Parallel cine: The simultaneous recording of digital and cine-film images during cardiac angiography. In this mode, digital image acquisition provides diagnostic-quality images.

Picture archiving and communications systems (PACS): Digital system or network for the electronic storage and retrieval of patient images and data.

Progressive scanning: Video raster scan method in which all horizontal lines are read out in a single vertical scan of the video camera target.

Pulsed-progressive fluoroscopy: Method of acquiring fluoroscopic images in which x-rays are produced in discrete pulses coincident with the vertical retrace period of the video camera. The video camera is then read out using progressive scanning. This compares with the older fluoroscopic method of producing x-rays continuously, coupled with interlaced video camera scanning.

Temporal subtraction: Also known as *time subtraction* or *mask-mode subtraction.* A subtraction mode in which an unopacified image (the mask, usually acquired prior to injection) is subtracted from an opacified image.

Upscanning: Scan conversion method in which the number of pixels or video lines displayed is higher (usually by a factor of 2) than those actually acquired from the video camera. Extra display data are produced by either replication or interpolation of the acquired data.

References

Amplatz K. 1997. Rapid film changers. In S Baum (ed), Abrams' Angiography, Chap 6. Boston, Little, Brown.

Aufrichtig R, Xue P, Thomas CW, et al. 1994. Perceptual comparison of pulsed and continuous fluoroscopy. Med Phys 21(2):245.

Blume H. 1998. The imaging chain. In Nickoloff EL, Strauss KJ (eds), Categorical Course in Diagnostic Radiology Physics: Cardiac Catheterization Imaging, pp 83–103. Oak Brook, IL, Radiological Society of North America.

Fujita H, Doi K, Lissak Giger M. 1985. Investigation of basic imaging properties in digital radiography: 6. MTFs of II-TV digital imaging systems. Med Phys 12(6):713.

Holmes DR Jr, Wondrow MA, Reeder GS, et al. 1989. Optimal display of the coronary arterial tree with an upscan 1023-line video display system. Cathet Cardiovasc Diagn 18(3):175.

Kruger RA, Mistretta CA, Riederer SJ. 1981. Physical and technical considerations of computerized fluoroscopy difference imaging. IEEE Trans Nucl Sci 28:205.

National Electrical Manufacturers Association. 1992. Test Standard for the Determination of the System Contrast Ratio and System Veiling Glare Index of an X-ray Image Intensifier System, NEMA Standards Publication No. XR 16. Washington, National Electrical Manufacturers Association.

National Electric Manufacturers Association. 1993. Digital Imaging and Communications in Medicine (DICOM), NEMA Standards Publication PS3.0(1993). Washington, National Electrical Manufacturers Association.

Rowlands JA. 1992. Real-time digital processing of video image sequences for videofluoroscopy. SPIE Proc 1652:294.

Sandrik JM. 1984. The video camera for medical imaging. In GD Fullerton, WR Hendee, JC Lasher, et al. (eds), Electronic Imaging in Medicine, pp 145–183. New York, American Institute of Physics.

Seibert JA, Barr DH, Borger DJ, et al. 1984. Interlaced versus progressive readout of television cameras for digital radiographic acquisitions. Med Phys 11:703.

Siedband MP. 1994. Image intensification and television. In JM Taveras, JT Ferrucci (eds), Radiology: Diagnosis-Imaging-Intervention, Chap 10. Philadelphia, JB Lippincott.

Verhoeven LAJ. 1985. DSA imaging: Some physical and technical aspects. Medicamundi 30:46.

Further Information

Balter S, Shope TB (eds). 1995. A Categorical Course in Physics: Physical and Technical Aspects of Angiography and Interventional Radiology. Oak Brook, IL, Radiological Society of North America.

Baum S (ed). 1997. Abrams' Angiography, 4th ed. Boston, Little, Brown.

Kennedy TE, Nissen SE, Simon R, Thomas JD, Tilkemeier PL. 1997. Digital Cardiac Imaging in the 21st Century: A Primer. Bethesda, MD, The Cardiac and Vascular Information Working Group (American College of Cardiology).

Moore RJ. 1990. Imaging Principles of Cardiac Angiography. Rockville, MD, Aspen Publishers.

Nickoloff EL, Strauss KJ (eds). 1998. Categorical Course in Diagnostic Radiology Physics: Cardiac Catheterization Imaging. Oak Brook, IL, Radiological Society of North America.

Seibert JA, Barnes GT, Gould RG (eds). 1994. Medical Physics Monograph No. 20: Specification, Acceptance Testing and Quality Control of Diagnostic X-Ray Imaging Equipment. Woodbury, NY, American Institute of Physics.

8.3 Mammography

Martin J. Yaffe

Mammography is an x-ray imaging procedure for examination of the breast. It is used primarily for the detection and diagnosis of breast cancer, but also for pre-surgical localization of suspicious areas and in the guidance of needle biopsies.

Breast cancer is a major killer of women. Approximately 179,000 women were diagnosed with breast cancer in the U.S. in 1998 and 43,500 women died of this disease [Landis, 1998]. Its cause is not currently known; however, it has been demonstrated that **survival** is greatly improved if disease is detected at an *early stage* [Tabar, 1993; Smart, 1993]. Mammography is at present the most effective means of detecting early stage breast cancer. It is used both for investigating symptomatic patients (diagnostic mammography) and for **screening** of asymptomatic women in selected age groups.

Breast cancer is detected on the basis of four types of signs on the mammogram:

1. The characteristic morphology of a tumor mass.
2. Certain presentations of mineral deposits as specks called microcalcifications.
3. Architectural distortion of normal tissue patterns caused by the disease.
4. Asymmetry between corresponding regions of images of the left and right breast.

Principles of Mammography

The mammogram is an x-ray shadowgram formed when x-rays from a quasi-point source irradiate the breast and the transmitted x-rays are recorded by an **image receptor**. Because of the spreading of the x-rays from the source, structures are magnified as they are projected onto the image receptor. The signal is a result of differential attenuation of x-rays along paths passing through the structures of the breast.

The essential features of image quality are summarized in Fig. 8.8. This is a one-dimensional profile of x-ray transmission through a simplified computer model of the breast [Fahrig, 1992], illustrated in Fig. 8.9. A region of reduced transmission corresponding to a structure of interest such as a tumor, a calcification, or normal **fibroglandular** tissue is shown. The imaging system must have sufficient *spatial*

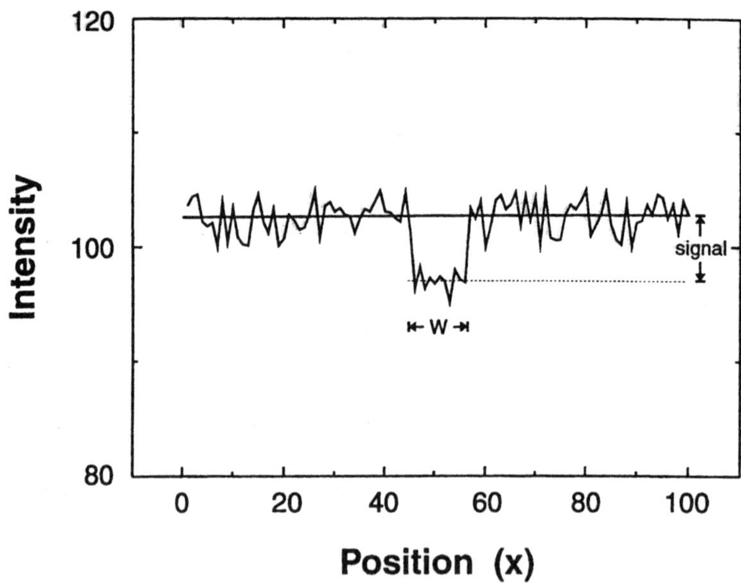

FIGURE 8.8 Profile of a simple x-ray projection image, illustrating the role of contrast, spatial resolution, and noise in mammographic image quality.

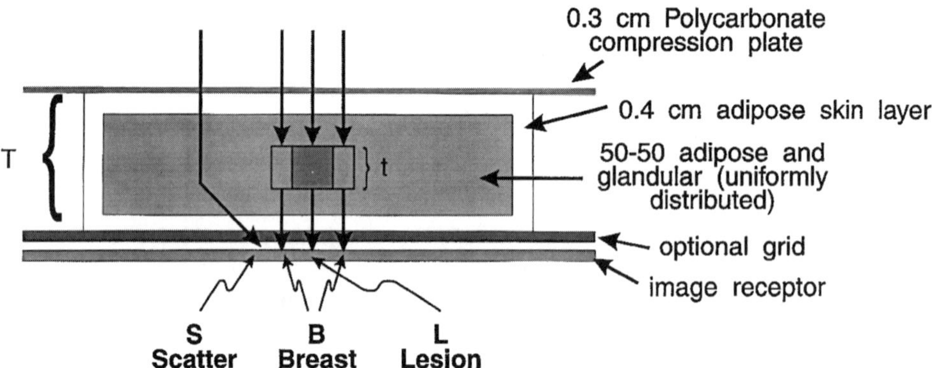

FIGURE 8.9 Simplified computer model of the mammographic image acquisition process.

resolution to delineate the edges of fine structures in the breast. Structural detail as small as 50 μm must be adequately resolved. Variation in x-ray attenuation among tissue structures in the breast gives rise to *contrast*. The detectability of structures providing subtle contrast is impaired, however, by an overall random fluctuation in the profile, referred to as mottle or *noise*. Because the breast is sensitive to ionizing radiation, which at least for high doses is known to cause breast cancer, it is desirable to use the lowest radiation dose compatible with excellent image quality. The components of the imaging system will be described and their design will be related to the imaging performance factors discussed in this section.

Physics of Image Formation

In the model of Fig. 8.9, an "average" breast composed of 50% adipose tissue and 50% fibroglandular tissue is considered. For the simplified case of monoenergetic x-rays of energy, E, the number of x-rays recorded in a fixed area of the image is proportional to

$$N_B = N_0\left(E\right)e^{-\mu T} \qquad (8.1)$$

in the "background" and

$$N_L = N_0\left(E\right)e^{-\left[\mu\left(T-t\right)+\mu' t\right]} \qquad (8.2)$$

in the shadow of the lesion or other structure of interest. In Eqs. (8.1) and (8.2), $N_0(E)$ is the number of x-rays that would be recorded in the absence of tissue in the beam, μ and μ' are the attenuation coefficients of the breast tissue and the lesion, respectively, T is the thickness of the breast, and t is the thickness of the lesion.

The difference in x-ray transmission gives rise to *subject* contrast which can be defined as:

$$C_0 = \frac{N_B - N_L}{N_B + N_L} \qquad (8.3)$$

For the case of monoenergetic x-rays and temporarily ignoring scattered radiation,

$$\frac{1-e^{-\left[\mu'-\mu t\right]}}{1+e^{-\left[\mu'-\mu t\right]}} \qquad (8.4)$$

i.e., contrast would depend only on the thickness of the lesion and the difference between its attenuation coefficient and that of the background material. These are not valid assumptions and in actuality contrast also depends on μ and T.

Shown in Fig. 8.10 are x-ray attenuation coefficients measured vs. energy on samples of three types of materials found in the breast: adipose tissue, normal fibroglandular breast tissue, and infiltrating ductal carcinoma (one type of breast tumor) [Johns, 1987]. Both the attenuation coefficients themselves and

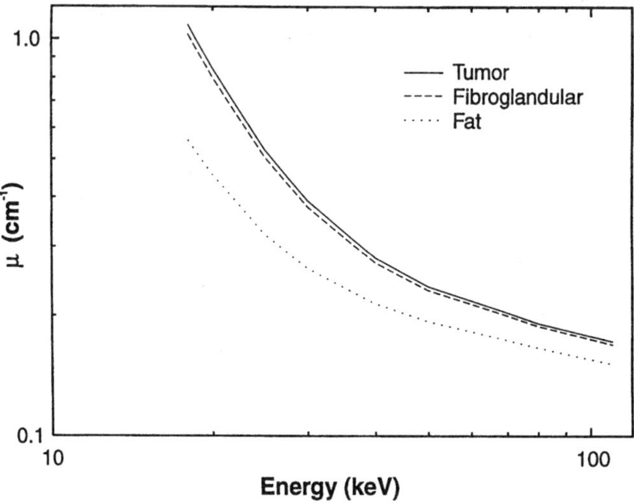

FIGURE 8.10 Measured x-ray linear attenuation coefficients of breast fibroglandular tissue, breast fat, and infiltrating ductal carcinoma plotted vs. x-ray energy.

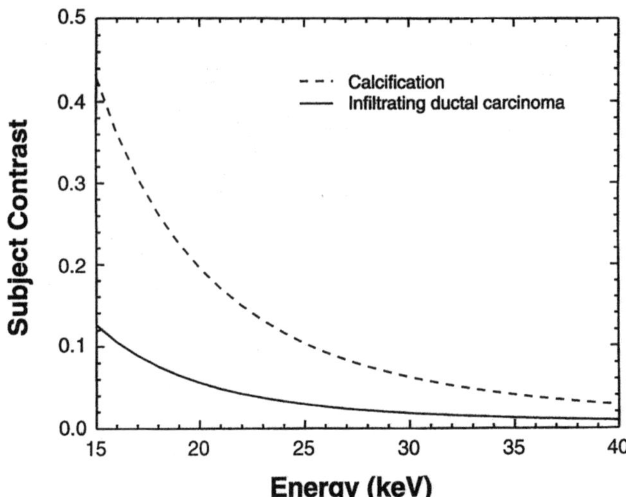

FIGURE 8.11 Dependence of mammographic subject contrast on x-ray energy.

their difference ($\mu' - \mu$) decrease with increasing E. As shown in Fig. 8.11, which is based on Eq. (8.4), this causes C_s to fall as x-ray energy increases. Note that the subject contrast of even small calcifications in the breast is greater than that for a tumor because of the greater difference in attenuation coefficient between calcium and breast tissue.

For a given image recording system (image receptor), a proper exposure requires a specific value of x-ray energy transmitted by the breast and incident on the receptor, i.e., a specific value of N_B. The breast entrance skin exposure[1] (ESE) required to produce an image is, therefore, proportional to

$$N_0 = N_B(E)e^{+\mu T} \tag{8.5}$$

Because μ decreases with energy, the required exposure for constant signal at the image receptor, N_B, will increase if E is reduced to improve image contrast. A better measure of the risk of radiation-induced breast cancer than ESE is the mean glandular dose (MGD) [BEIR V, 1990]. MGD is calculated as the product of the ESE and a factor, obtained experimentally or by Monte Carlo radiation transport calculations, which converts from incident exposure to dose [Wu, 1991, 1994]. The conversion factor increases with E so that MGD does not fall as quickly with energy as does entrance exposure. The trade-off between image contrast and radiation dose necessitates important compromises in establishing mammographic operating conditions.

Equipment

The mammography unit consists of an x-ray tube and an image receptor mounted on opposite sides of a mechanical assembly or gantry. Because the breast must be imaged from different aspects and to accommodate patients of different height, the assembly can be adjusted in a vertical axis and rotated about a horizontal axis as shown in Fig. 8.12.

Most general radiography equipment is designed such that the image field is centered below the x-ray source. In mammography, the system's geometry is arranged as in Fig. 8.13a where a vertical line from the x-ray source grazes the chest wall of the patient and intersects orthogonally with the edge of the image receptor closest to the patient. If the x-ray beam were centered over the breast as in Fig. 8.13b,

[1]Exposure is expressed in roentgens (R) (which is not an SI unit) or in coulombs of ionization collected per kilogram of air.

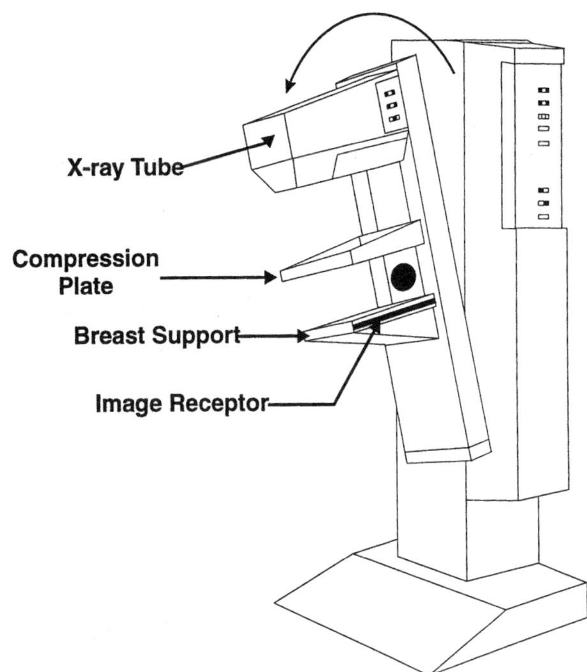

FIGURE 8.12 Schematic diagram of a dedicated mammography machine.

some of the tissue near the chest wall would be projected inside of the patient where it could not be recorded.

Radiation leaving the x-ray tube passes through a metallic spectral-shaping filter, a beam-defining aperture, and a plate which compresses the breast. Those rays transmitted through the breast are incident on an anti-scatter "grid" and then strike the image receptor where they interact and deposit most of their energy locally. A fraction of the x-rays pass through the receptor without interaction and impinge upon a sensor which is used to activate the automatic exposure control mechanism of the unit.

X-Ray Source

Practical monoenergetic x-ray sources are not available and the x-rays used in mammography arise from bombardment of a metal target by electrons in a hot-cathode vacuum tube. The x-rays are emitted from the target over a spectrum of energies, ranging up to the peak kilovoltage applied to the x-ray tube. Typically, the x-ray tube employs a rotating anode design in which electrons from the cathode strike the anode *target* material at a small angle (0 to 16°) from normal incidence (Fig. 8.14). Over 99% of the energy from the electrons is dissipated as heat in the anode. The angled surface and the distribution of the electron bombardment along the circumference of the rotating anode disk allows the energy to be spread over a larger area of target material while presenting a much smaller effective **focal spot** as viewed from the imaging plane. On modern equipment, the typical "nominal" focal spot size for normal contact mammography is 0.3 mm, while the smaller spot used primarily for magnification is 0.1 mm. The specifications for x-ray focal spot size tolerance, established by NEMA (National Electrical Manufacturers Association) or the IEC (International Electrotechnical Commission) allow the *effective focal spot size* to be considerably larger than these nominal sizes. For example, the NEMA specification allows the effective focal spot size to be 0.45 mm in width and 0.65 mm in length for a nominal 0.3 mm spot and 0.15 mm in each dimension for a nominal 0.1 mm spot.

The nominal focal spot size is defined relative to the effective spot size at a "reference axis." As shown in Fig. 8.14, this reference axis, which may vary from manufacturer to manufacturer, is normally specified at some midpoint in the image. The effective size of the focal spot will monotonically increase from the

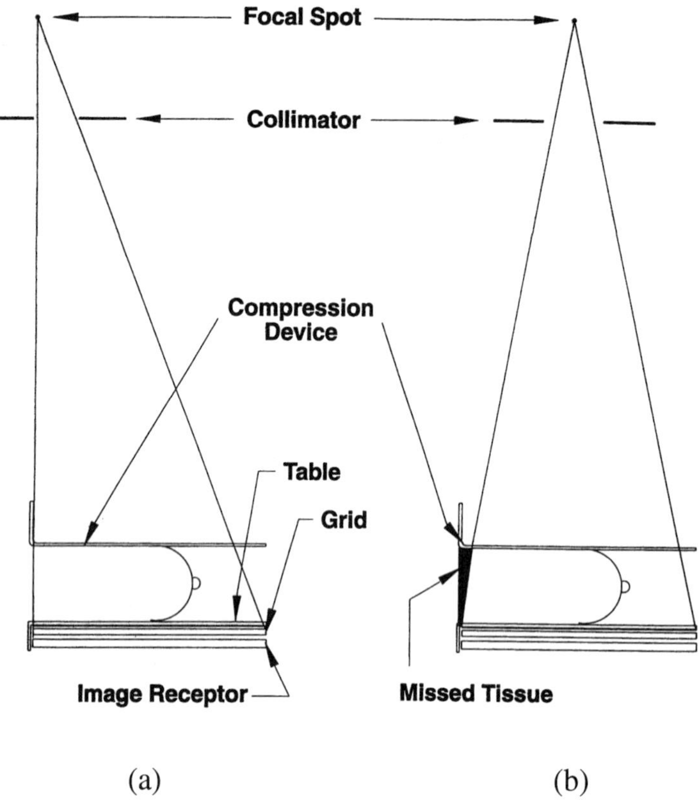

FIGURE 8.13 Geometric arrangement of system components in mammography. (a) Correct alignment provides good tissue coverage, (b) incorrect alignment causes tissue near the chest wall not to be imaged.

anode side to the cathode side of the imaging field. Normally, x-ray tubes are arranged such that the cathode side of the tube is adjacent to the patient's chest wall, since the highest intensity of x-rays is available at the cathode side, and the attenuation of x-rays by the patient is generally greater near the chest wall of the image.

The spatial resolution capability of the imaging system is partially determined by the effective size of the focal spot and by the degree of magnification of the anatomy at any plane in the breast. This is illustrated in Fig. 8.15 where, by similar triangles, the unsharpness region due to the finite size of the focal spot is linearly related to the effective size of the spot and to the ratio of OID to SOD, where SOD is the source-object distance and OID is the object-image receptor distance. Because the breast is a three-dimensional structure, this ratio and, therefore, the unsharpness will vary for different planes within the breast.

The size of the focal spot determines the heat loading capability of the x-ray tube target. For smaller focal spots, the current through the x-ray tube must be reduced, necessitating increased exposure times and the possibility of loss of resolution due to motion of anatomical structures. Loss of geometric resolution can be controlled in part by minimizing OID/SOD, i.e., by designing the equipment with greater source-breast distances, by minimizing space between the breast and the image receptor, and by compressing the breast to reduce its overall thickness.

Magnification is often used intentionally to improve the signal-to-noise ratio of the image. This is accomplished by elevating the breast above the image receptor, in effect reducing SOD and increasing OID. Under these conditions, resolution is invariably limited by focal spot size and use of a small spot for magnification imaging (typically a nominal size of 0.1 mm) is critical.

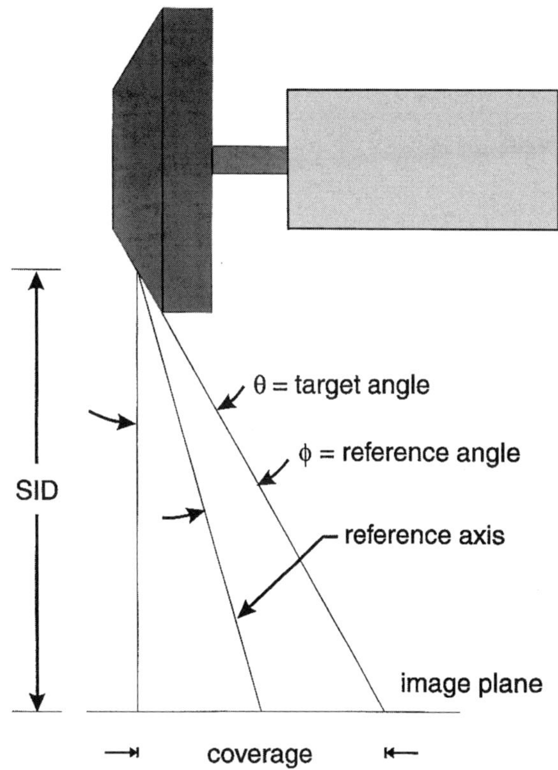

FIGURE 8.14 Angled-target x-ray source provides improved heat loading but causes effective focal spot size to vary across the image.

Since monoenergetic x-rays are not available, one attempts to define a spectrum providing energies which give a reasonable compromise between radiation dose and image contrast. The spectral shape can be controlled by adjustment of the kilovoltage, choice of the target material, and the type and thickness of metallic filter placed between the x-ray tube and the breast.

Based on models of the imaging problem in mammography, it has been suggested that the optimum energy for imaging lies between 18 and 23 keV, depending on the thickness and composition of the breast [Beaman, 1982]. It has been found that for the breast of typical thickness and composition, the characteristic x-rays from molybdenum at 17.4 and 19.6 keV provide good imaging performance. For this reason, molybdenum target x-ray tubes are used on the vast majority of mammography machines.

Most mammography tubes use beryllium exit windows between the evacuated tube and the outside world since glass or other metals used in general purpose tubes would provide excessive attenuation of the useful energies for mammography. Figure 8.16 compares tungsten target and molybdenum target spectra for beryllium window x-ray tubes. Under some conditions, tungsten may provide appropriate image quality for mammography; however, it is essential that the intense emission of L radiation from tungsten be filtered from the beam before it is incident upon the breast, since extremely high doses to the skin would result from this radiation without useful contribution to the mammogram.

Filtration of the X-Ray Beam

In conventional radiology, filters made of aluminum or copper are used to provide selective removal of low x-ray energies from the beam before it is incident upon the patient. In mammography, particularly when a molybdenum anode x-ray tube is employed, a molybdenum filter 20 to 35 μm thick is generally used. This filter attenuates x-rays both at low energies and those above its own K-absorption edge allowing the molybdenum characteristic x-rays from the target to pass through the filter with relatively high

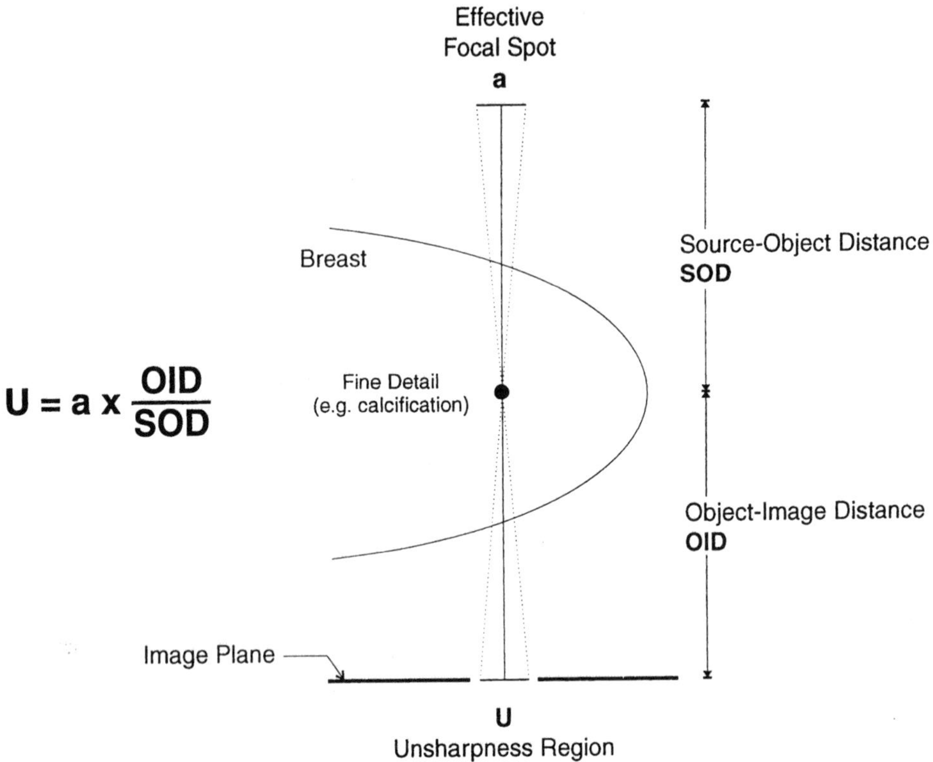

FIGURE 8.15 Dependence of focal spot unsharpness on focal spot size and magnification factor.

efficiency. As illustrated in Fig. 8.17, this K edge filtration results in a spectrum enriched with x-ray energies in the range of 17 to 20 keV.

Although this spectrum is relatively well suited for imaging the breast of average attenuation, slightly higher energies are desirable for imaging dense thicker breasts. Because the molybdenum target spectrum is so heavily influenced by the characteristic x-rays, an increase in the kilovoltage alone does not substantially change the shape of the spectrum. The beam can be "hardened," however, by employing filters of higher atomic number than molybdenum. For example, rhodium (atomic no. 45) has a K absorption edge at 23 keV, providing strong attenuation both for x-rays above this energy and for those at substantially lower energies. Used with a molybdenum target x-ray tube and slightly increased kV, it provides a spectrum with increased penetration (reduced dose) compared to the Mo/Mo combination.

It is possible to go further in optimizing imaging performance, by "tuning" the effective spectral energy by using other target materials in combination with appropriate K-edge filters [Jennings, 1993]. One manufacturer employs an x-ray tube incorporating both molybdenum and rhodium targets, where the electron beam can be directed toward one or the other of these materials [Heidsieck, 1991]. With this system, the filter material (rhodium, molybdenum, etc.) can be varied to suit the target that has been selected. Similarly, work has been reported on K-edge filtration of tungsten spectra [Desponds, 1991], where the lack of pronounced K characteristic peaks provides more flexibility in spectral shaping with filters.

Compression Device

There are several reasons for applying firm (but not necessarily painful) compression to the breast during the examination. Compression causes the different tissues to be spread out, minimizing superposition from different planes and thereby improving a conspicuity of structures. As will be discussed later, scattered radiation can degrade contrast in the mammogram. The use of compression decreases the ratio

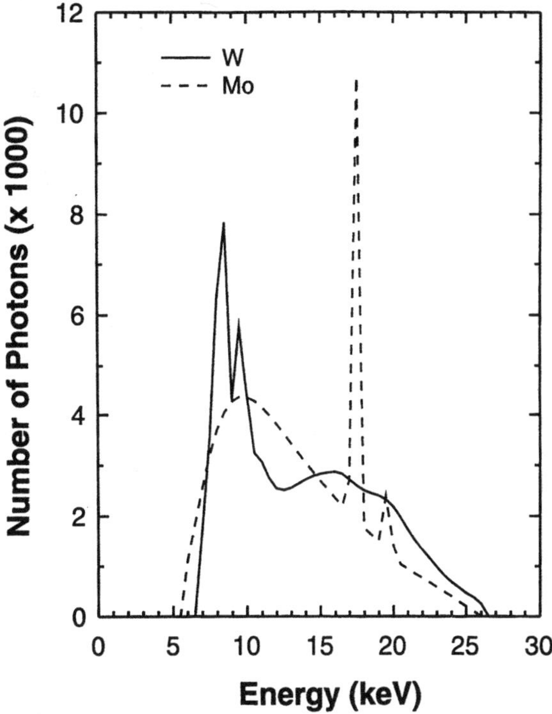

FIGURE 8.16 Comparison of tungsten and molybdenum target x-ray spectra.

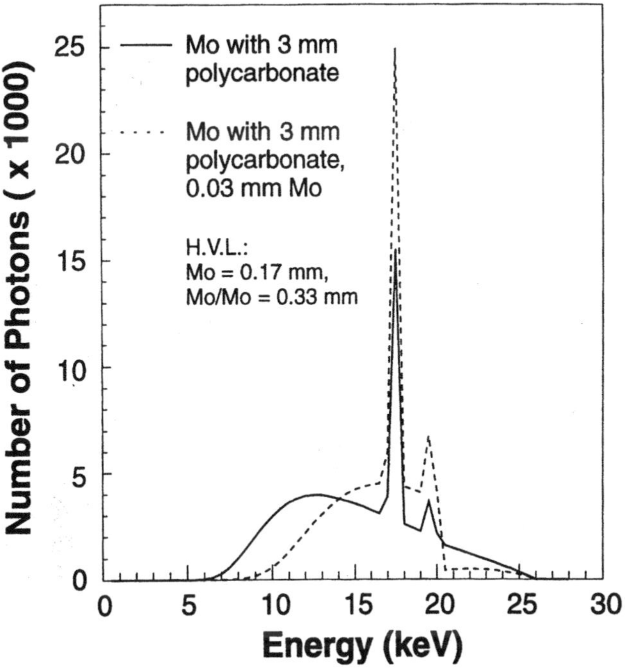

FIGURE 8.17 Molybdenum target spectrum filtered by 0.03 mm Mo foil.

of scattered to directly transmitted radiation reaching the image receptor. Compression also decreases the distance from any plane within the breast to the image receptor (i.e., OID) and in this way reduces geometric unsharpness. The compressed breast provides lower overall attenuation to the incident x-ray beam, allowing the radiation dose to be reduced. The compressed breast also provides more uniform attenuation over the image. This reduces the exposure range which must be recorded by the imaging system, allowing more flexibility in choice of films to be used. Finally, compression provides a clamping action which reduces anatomical motion during the exposure reducing this source of image unsharpness.

It is important that the compression plate allows the breast to be compressed parallel to the image receptor, and that the edge of the plate at the chest wall be straight and aligned with both the focal spot and image receptor to maximize the amount of breast tissue which is included in the image (see Fig. 8.13).

Anti-Scatter Grid

Lower x-ray energies are used for mammography than for other radiological examinations. At these energies, the probability of photoelectric interactions within the breast is significant. Nevertheless, the probability of Compton scattering of x-rays within the breast is still quite high. Scattered radiation recorded by the image receptor has the effect of creating a quasi-uniform haze on the image and causes the subject contrast to be reduced to

$$C_S = \frac{C_0}{1+\mathrm{SPR}} \tag{8.6}$$

where C_0 is the contrast in the absence of scattered radiation, given by Eq. 8.4 and SPR is the scatter-to-primary (directly transmitted) x-ray ratio at the location of interest in the image. In the absence of an anti-scatter device, 37 to 50% of the total radiation incident on the image receptor would have experienced a scattering interaction within the breast; i.e., the scatter-to-primary ratio would be 0.6:1.0. In addition to contrast reduction, the recording of scattered radiation uses up part of the dynamic range of the image receptor and adds statistical noise to the image.

Anti-scatter *grids* have been designed for mammography. These are composed of linear lead (Pb) septa separated by a rigid interspace material. Generally, the grid septa are not strictly parallel but focused (toward the x-ray source). Because the primary x-rays all travel along direct lines from the x-ray source to the image receptor, while the scatter diverges from points within the breast, the grid presents a smaller acceptance aperture to scattered radiation than to primary radiation and thereby discriminates against scattered radiation. Grids are characterized by their *grid ratio* (ratio of the path length through the interspace material to the interseptal width) which typically ranges from 3.5:1 to 5:1. When a grid is used, the SPR is reduced typically by a factor of about 5, leading in most cases to a substantial improvement in image contrast [Wagner, 1991].

On modern mammography equipment, the grid is an integral part of the system, and during x-ray exposure is moved to blur the image of the grid septa to avoid a distracting pattern in the mammogram. It is important that this motion be uniform and of sufficient amplitude to avoid non-uniformities in the image, particularly for short exposures that occur when the breast is relatively lucent.

Because of absorption of primary radiation by the septa and by the interspace material, part of the primary radiation transmitted by the patient does not arrive at the image receptor. In addition, by removing some of the scattered radiation, the grid causes the overall radiation fluence to be reduced from that which would be obtained in its absence. To obtain a radiograph of proper optical density, the entrance exposure to the patient must be increased by a factor known as the *Bucky factor* to compensate for these losses. Typical Bucky factors are in the range of 2 to 3.

A linear grid does not provide scatter rejection for those quanta traveling in planes parallel to the septa. Recently a crossed grid that consists of septa that run in orthogonal directions has been introduced for this purpose. The improved scatter rejection is accomplished at doses comparable to those required

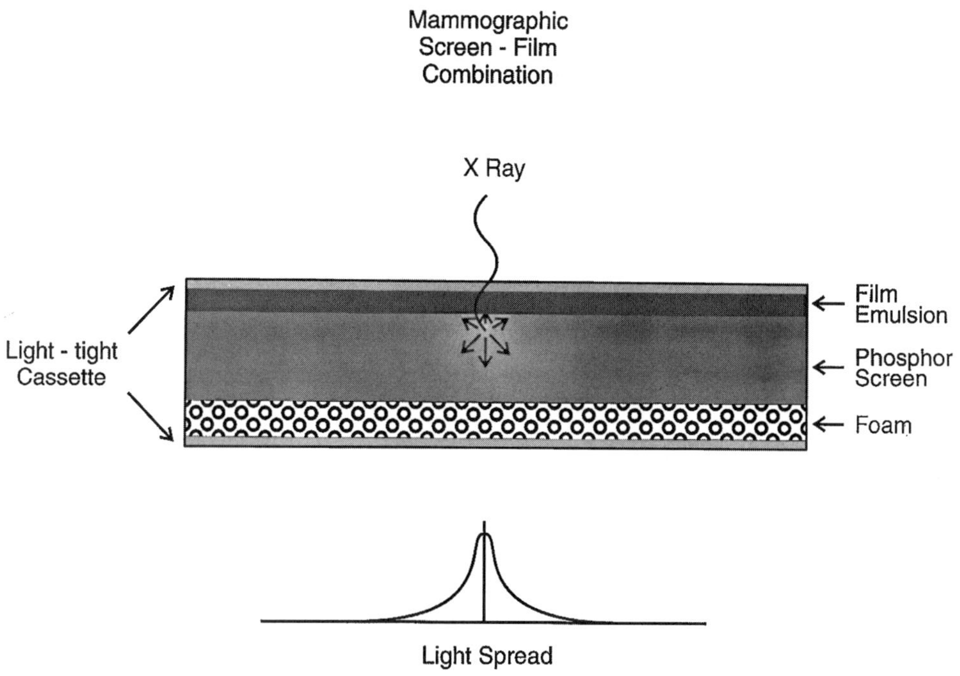

FIGURE 8.18 Design of a screen-film image receptor for mammography.

with a linear grid, because the interspace material of the crossed grid is air rather than solid. To avoid artifacts, the grid is moved in a very precise way during the exposure to ensure a uniform blurring of the image of the grid itself.

Image Receptor

Fluorescent Screens. When first introduced, mammography was carried out using direct exposure radiographic film in order to obtain the high spatial resolution required. Since the mid-1970s, high resolution fluorescent screens have been used to convert the x-ray pattern from the breast into an optical image. These screens are used in conjunction with single-coated radiographic film, and the configuration is shown in Fig. 8.18. With this arrangement, the x-rays pass through the cover of a light-tight cassette and the film to impinge upon the screen. Absorption is exponential, so that a large fraction of the x-rays are absorbed near the entrance surface of the screen. The phosphor crystals which absorb the energy produce light in an isotropic distribution. Because the film emulsion is pressed tightly against the entrance surface of the screen, the majority of the light quanta have only a short distance to travel to reach the film. Light quanta traveling longer distances have an opportunity to spread laterally (see Fig. 8.18), and in this way degrade the spatial resolution. To discriminate against light quanta which travel along these longer oblique paths, the phosphor material of the screen is generally treated with a dye which absorbs much of this light, giving rise to a sharper image. A typical phosphor used for mammography is gadolinium oxysulfide (Gd_2O_2S). Although the K-absorption edge of gadolinium occurs at too high an energy to be useful in mammography, the phosphor material is dense (7.44 g/cm^3) so that the **quantum efficiency** (the fraction of incident x-rays which interact with the screen) is good (about 60%). Also, the **conversion efficiency** of this phosphor (fraction of the absorbed x-ray energy converted to light) is relatively high. The light emitted from the fluorescent screen is essentially linearly dependent upon the total amount of energy deposited by x-rays within the screen.

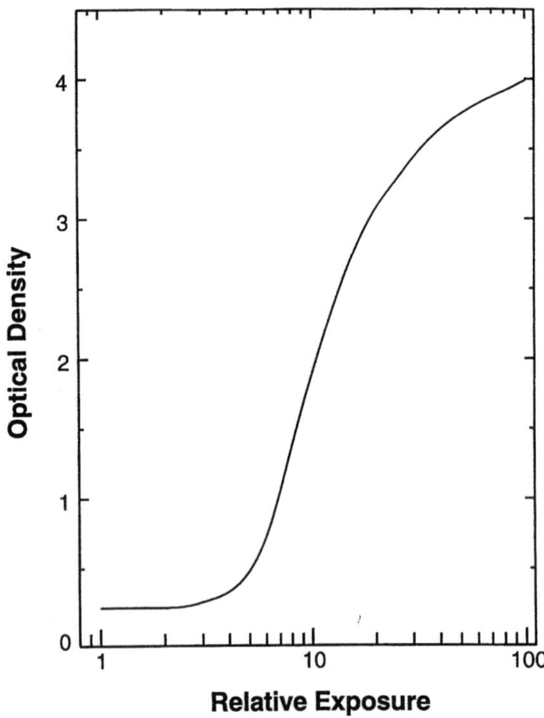

FIGURE 8.19 Characteristic curve of a mammographic screen-film image receptor.

Film. The photographic film emulsion for mammography is designed with a characteristic curve such as that shown in Fig. 8.19, which is a plot of the optical density (blackness) provided by the processed film vs. the logarithm of the x-ray exposure to the screen. Film provides non-linear input-output transfer characteristics. The local gradient of this curve controls the display contrast presented to the radiologist. Where the curve is of shallow gradient, a given increment of radiation exposure provides little change in optical density, rendering structures imaged in this part of the curve difficult to visualize. Where the curve is steep, the film provides excellent image contrast. The range of exposures over which contrast is appreciable is referred to as the *latitude* of the film. Because the film is constrained between two optical density values — the *base + fog* density of the film, where no intentional x-ray exposure has resulted, and the maximum density provided by the emulsion — there is a compromise between maximum gradient of the film and the latitude that it provides. For this reason, some regions of the mammogram will generally be underexposed or overexposed, i.e., rendered with sub-optimal contrast.

Film Processing. Mammography film is processed in an automatic processor similar to that used for general radiographic films. It is important that the development temperature, time, and rate of replenishment of the developer chemistry be compatible with the type of film emulsion used and be designed to maintain good contrast of the film.

Noise and Dose

Noise in mammography results primarily from two sources — the random absorption of x-rays in the detector and the granularity associated with the screen and the film emulsion. The first, commonly known as quantum noise, is governed by Poisson statistics so that for a given area of image the standard deviation in the number of x-rays recorded is equal to the square root of the mean number recorded. In other words, the noise in the image is dependent on both the amount of radiation which strikes the imaging system per unit area, and the quantum efficiency of the imaging system. The quantum efficiency is related to the attenuation coefficient of the phosphor material and the thickness of the screen. In order to maintain high spatial resolution, the screen must be made relatively thin to avoid lateral diffusion of light. The desirability of maintaining a relatively low quantum noise level in the image mandates that the conversion efficiency of the screen material and the sensitivity of the film not be excessively high. With very high conversion efficiency, the image could be produced at low dose but with an inadequate number of quanta contributing to the image. Similarly, film granularity increases as more sensitive films are used, so that again film speed must be limited to maintain high image quality. For current high quality mammographic imaging employing an anti-scatter grid, with films exposed to a mean optical density of at least 1.6, the mean glandular dose to a 5-cm-thick compressed breast consisting of 50% fibroglandular and 50% adipose tissue is in the range of 1 to 2 milligray [Conway, 1992].

Automatic Exposure Control

It is difficult for the technologist to estimate the attenuation of the breast by inspection and, therefore, modern mammography units are equipped with automatic exposure control (AEC). The AEC radiation sensors are located behind the image receptor so that they do not cast a shadow on the image. The sensors measure the x-ray fluence transmitted through both the breast and the receptor and provide a signal which can be used to discontinue the exposure when a certain preset amount of radiation has been received by the image receptor. The location of the sensor must be adjustable so that it can be placed behind the appropriate region of the breast in order to obtain proper image density. AEC devices must be calibrated so that constant image optical density results are independent of variations in breast attenuation, kilovoltage setting, or field size. With modern equipment, automatic exposure control is generally microprocessor-based so that relatively sophisticated corrections can be made during the exposure for the above effects and for *reciprocity law* failure of the film.

Automatic Kilovoltage Control

Many modern mammography units also incorporate automatic control of the kilovoltage or target/filter/kilovoltage combination. Penetration through the breast depends on both breast thickness and composition. For a breast that is dense, it is possible that a very long exposure time would be required to achieve adequate film blackening. This results in high dose to the breast and possibly blur due to anatomical motion. It is possible to sense the compressed breast thickness and the transmitted exposure rate and to employ an algorithm to automatically choose the x-ray target and/or beam filter as well as the kilovoltage.

Quality Control

Mammography is one of the most technically demanding radiographic procedures, and in order to obtain optimal results, all components of the system must be operating properly. Recognizing this, the American College of Radiology implemented and administers a Mammography Accreditation Program [McClelland, 1991], which evaluates both technical and personnel-related factors in facilities applying for accreditation.

In order to verify proper operation, a rigorous quality control program should be in effect. In fact, the U.S. Mammography Quality Standards Act stipulates that a quality control program must be in place in all facilities performing mammography. A program of tests (summarized in Table 8.1) and methods for performing them are contained in the quality control manuals for mammography published by the American College of Radiology [Hendrick, 1999].

Stereotactic Biopsy Devices

Stereoscopic x-ray imaging techniques are currently used for the guidance of needle "core" biopsies. These procedures can be used to investigate suspicious mammographic or clinical findings without the need for surgical excisional biopsies, resulting in reduced patient risk, discomfort, and cost. In these stereotactic biopsies, the gantry of a mammography machine is modified to allow angulated views of the breast (typically ±15° from normal incidence) to be achieved. From measurements obtained from these images, the three-dimensional location of a suspicious lesion is determined and a needle equipped with a spring-

TABLE 8.1 Mammographic Quality Control Minimum Test Frequencies

Test	Performed By:	Minimum Frequency
Darkroom cleanliness	Radiologic technologist	Daily
Processor quality control		Daily
Screen cleanliness		Weekly
Viewboxes and viewing conditions		Weekly
Phantom images		Weekly
Visual check list		Monthly
Repeat analysis		Quarterly
Analysis of fixer retention in film		Quarterly
Darkroom fog		Semi-annually
Screen-film contact		Semi-annually
Compression		Semi-annually
Mammographic unit assembly evaluation	Medical physicist	Annually
Collimation assessment		Annually
Focal spot size performance		Annually
kVp Accuracy/reproducibility		Annually
Beam quality assessment (half-value layer)		Annually
Automatic exposure control (AEC) system performance assessment		Annually
Uniformity of screen speed		Annually
Breast entrance exposure and mean glandular dose		Annually
Image quality — phantom evaluation		Annually
Artifact assessment		Annually
Radiation output rate		Annually
Viewbox luminance and room illuminance		Annually
Compression release mechanism		Annually

Source: Hendrick, R.E. et al., 1999. Mammography Quality Control Manuals (radiologist, radiologic technologist, medical physicist). American College of Radiology, Reston, VA. With permission.

loaded cutting device can be accurately placed in the breast to obtain tissue samples. While this procedure can be performed on an upright mammography unit, special dedicated systems have recently been introduced to allow its performance with the patient lying prone on a table. The accuracy of sampling the appropriate tissue depends critically on the alignment of the system components and the quality of the images produced. A thorough review of stereotactic imaging, including recommended quality control procedures, is given by Hendrick and Parker [1994].

Digital Mammography

There are several technical factors associated with screen-film mammography which limit the ability to display the finest or most subtle details, and produce images with the most efficient use of radiation dose to the patient. In screen-film mammography, the film must act as an image acquisition detector as well as a storage and display device. Because of its sigmoidal shape, the range of x-ray exposures over which the film display gradient is significant, i.e., the image latitude, is limited. If a tumor is located in either a relatively lucent or more opaque region of the breast, then the contrast displayed to the radiologist may be inadequate because of the limited gradient of the film. This is particularly a concern in patients whose breasts contain large amounts of fibroglandular tissue, the so-called dense breast.

Another limitation of film mammography is the effect of structural noise due to the granularity of the film emulsion used to record the image. This impairs the detectibility of microcalcifications and other fine structures within the breast. While Poisson quantum noise is unavoidable, it should be possible to virtually eliminate structural noise by technical improvements. Existing screen-film mammography also suffers because of the inefficiency of grids in removing the effects of scattered radiation and with compromises in spatial resolution vs. quantum efficiency inherent in the screen-film image receptor.

Many of the limitations of conventional mammography can be effectively overcome with a *digital mammography* imaging system (Fig. 8.20), in which image acquisition, display, and storage are performed

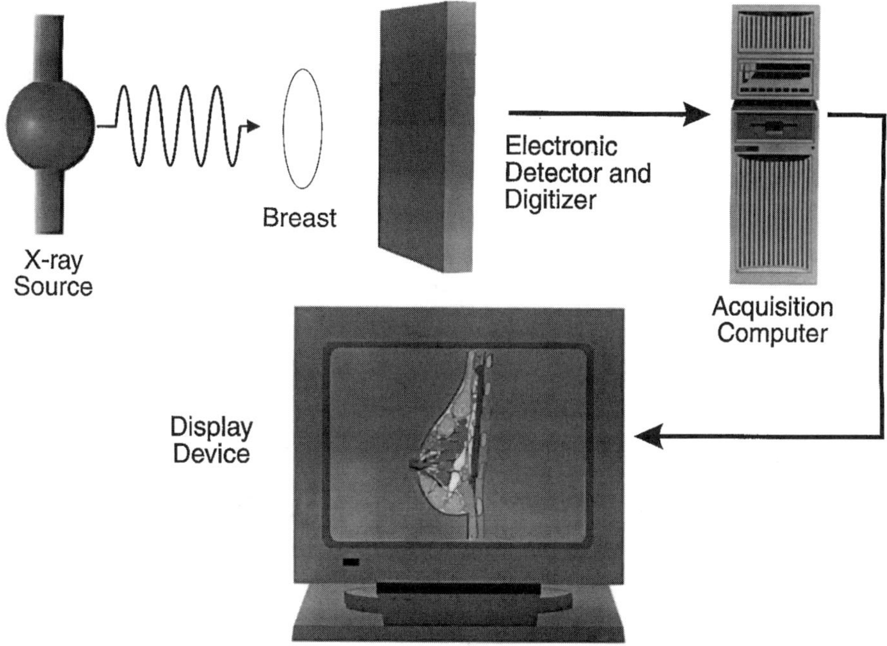

FIGURE 8.20 Schematic representation of a digital mammography system.

independently, allowing optimization of each. For example, acquisition can be performed with low noise, highly linear x-ray detectors, while since the image is stored digitally, it can be displayed with contrast independent of the detector properties and defined by the needs of the radiologist. Whatever image processing techniques are found useful, ranging from simple contrast enhancement to histogram modification and spatial frequency filtering, could conveniently be applied.

The challenges in creating a digital mammography system with improved performance are mainly related to the x-ray detector and the display device. There is active development of high resolution display monitors and hard copy devices to meet the demanding requirements (number of pixels, luminance, speed, multi-image capacity) of displaying digital mammography images, and suitable systems for this purpose should be available in the near future. The detector should have the following characteristics:

1. Efficient absorption of the incident radiation beam
2. Linear response over a wide range of incident radiation intensity
3. Low intrinsic noise
4. Spatial resolution on the order of 10 cycles/mm (50 μm sampling)
5. Can accommodate at least an 18 × 24 cm and preferably a 24 × 30 cm field size
6. Acceptable imaging time and heat loading of the x-ray tube

Two main approaches have been taken in detector development — area detectors and slot detectors. In the former, the entire image is acquired simultaneously, while in the latter only a portion of the image is acquired at one time and the full image is obtained by scanning the x-ray beam and detector across the breast. Area detectors offer convenient, fast image acquisition and could be used with conventional x-ray machines, but may still require a grid, while slot systems are slower and require a scanning x-ray beam, but use relatively simple detectors and have excellent intrinsic efficiency at scatter rejection.

At the time of writing, small-format (5 × 5 cm) digital systems for guidance of stereotactic breast biopsy procedures are in widespread use. These use a lens or a fiber-optic taper to couple a phosphor to

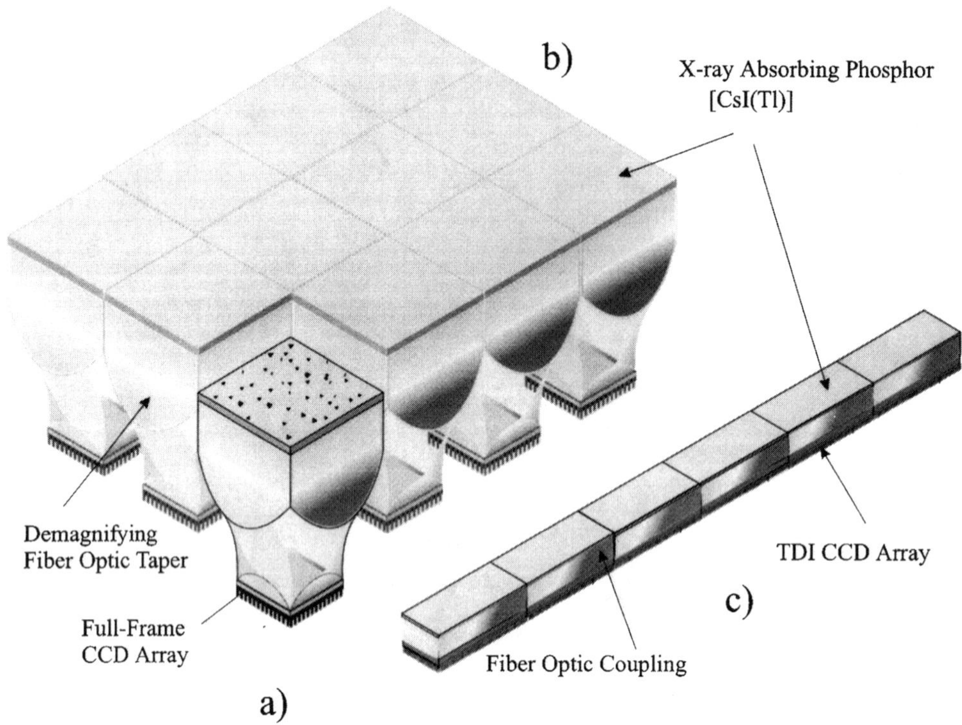

FIGURE 8.21 (a) Small-format detector system for biopsy imaging, (b) full-breast detector incorporating 12 detector modules, (c) slot detector for a full-breast scanning digital mammography system.

a CCD whose format is approximately square and typically provides 1 × 1K images with 50 μm pixels (Fig. 8.21a). Adjustment of display contrast enhances the localization of the lesion while the immediate display of images (no film processing is required) greatly accelerates the clinical procedure.

Four designs of full breast digital mammography systems are undergoing clinical evaluation. Various detector technologies are being developed and evaluated for use in digital mammography. In three of the systems, x-rays are absorbed by a cesium iodide (CsI) phosphor layer and produce light. In one system, the phosphor is deposited directly on a matrix of about 2000^2 photodiodes with thin film transistor switches fabricated on a large area amorphous silicon plate. The electronic signal is read out on a series of data lines as the switches in each row of the array are activated. In another system, the light is coupled through demagnifying fiber-optic tapers to a CCD readout. A mosaic of 3 × 4 detector modules is formed (Fig. 8.21b) to obtain a detector large enough to cover the breast [Cheung, 1998]. A third system also uses fiber-optic coupling of CsI to CCDs; however, the detector is in a slot configuration and is scanned beneath the breast in synchrony with a fan beam of x-rays to acquire the transmitted signal (Fig. 8.21c). The fourth system employs a plate formed of a photostimulable phosphor material. When exposed to x-rays, traps in the phosphor are filled with electrons, the number being related to x-ray intensity. The plate is placed in a reader device and scanned with a red HeNe laser beam which stimulates the traps to release the electrons. The transition of these electrons through energy levels in the phosphor crystal result in the formation of blue light, which is measured as a function of the laser position on the plate to form the image signal.

Other materials in which x-ray energy is directly converted to charge are under development for digital mammography. These materials include lead iodide, amorphous selenium, zinc cadmium telluride, and thallium bromide. A review of the current status of digital mammography is given in Yaffe [1994] and Pisano [1998] and of detectors for digital x-ray imaging in Yaffe [1997].

Summary

Mammography is a technically demanding imaging procedure which can help reduce mortality from breast cancer. To be successful at this purpose, both the technology and technique used for imaging must be optimized. This requires careful system design and attention to quality control procedures. Imaging systems for mammography are still evolving and, in the future, are likely to make greater use of digital acquisition and display methods.

Defining Terms

Conversion efficiency: The efficiency of converting the energy from x-rays absorbed in a phosphor material into that of emitted light quanta.

Fibroglandular tissue: A mixture of tissues within the breast composed of the functional glandular tissue and the fibrous supporting structures.

Focal spot: The area of the anode of an x-ray tube from which the useful beam of x-rays is emitted. Also known as the target.

Grid: A device consisting of evenly spaced lead strips which functions like a venetian blind in preferentially allowing x-rays traveling directly from the focal spot without interaction in the patient to pass through, while those whose direction has been diverted by scattering in the patient strike the slats of the grid and are rejected. Grids improve the contrast of radiographic images at the price of increased dose to the patient.

Image receptor: A device that records the distribution of x-rays to form an image. In mammography, the image receptor is generally composed of a light-tight cassette containing a fluorescent screen, which absorbs x-rays and produces light, coupled to a sheet of photographic film.

Quantum efficiency: The fraction of incident x-rays which interact with a detector or image receptor.

Screening: Examination of asymptomatic individuals to detect disease.

Survival: An epidemiological term giving the fraction of individuals diagnosed with a given disease alive at a specified time after diagnosis, e.g., "10-year survival."

References

Beaman, S.A. and Lillicrap, S.C. 1982. Optimum x-ray spectra for mammography. *Phys. Med. Biol.* 27:1209-1220.

Cheung, L., Bird, R., Ashish, C., Rego A., Rodriguez, C., and Yuen, J. 1998. Initial operating and clinical results of a full-field mammography system.

Conway, B.J., Suleiman, O.H., Rueter, F.G., Antonsen, R.G., Slayton, R.J., and McCrohan, J.L. 1992. Does credentialing make a difference in mammography? *Radiology* 185(P):250.

Desponds, L., Depeursinge, C., Grecescu, M., Hessler, C., Samiri, A., and Valley, J.F. 1991. Image of anode and filter material on image quality and glandular dose for screen-film mammography. *Phys. Med. Biol.* 36:1165-1182.

Fahrig, R., Maidment, A.D.A., and Yaffe, M.J. 1992. Optimization of peak kilovoltage and spectral shape for digital mammography. *Proc. SPIE* 1651:74-83.

Health Effects of Exposure to Low Levels of Ionizing Radiation (BEIR V) 1990. National Academy Press, Washington, D.C., 163-170.

Heidsieck, R., Laurencin, G., Ponchin, A., Gabbay, E., and Klausz, R. 1991. Dual target x-ray tubes for mammographic examinations: Dose reduction with image quality equivalent to that with standard mammographic tubes. *Radiology* 181(P):311.

Hendrick, R.E. et al., 1994. Mammography Quality Control Manuals (radiologist, radiologic technologist, medical physicist). American College of Radiology, Reston, VA.

Hendrick, R.E. and Parker, S.H. 1994. Stereotaxic Imaging. In *A Categorical Course in Physics: Technical Aspects of Breast Imaging*. 3rd ed. A.G. Haus and M.J. Yaffe, Eds., pp 263-274. RSNA Publications, Oak Brook, IL.

Jennings, R.J., Quinn, P.W., Gagne, R.M., and Fewell, T.R. 1993. Evaluation of x-ray sources for mammography. *Proc. SPIE* 1896:259-268.

Johns, P.C. and Yaffe, M.J. 1987. X-ray characterization of normal and neoplastic breast tissues. *Phys. Med. Biol.* 32:675-695.

Karellas, A., Harris, L.J., and D'Orsi, C.J., 1990. Small field digital mammography with a 2048x2048 pixel charge-coupled device. *Radiology* 177:288.

Landis, S.H., Murray, T., Bolden, S., and Wingo, P. 1998. Cancer Statistics, 1998 CA *Cancer J. Clin.* 48:6-29.

McClelland, R., Hendrick, R.E., Zinninger, M.D., and Wilcox, P.W. 1991. The American College of Radiology Mammographic Accreditation Program. *Am. J. Roentgenol.* 157:473-479.

Nishikawa, R.M. and Yaffe, M.J. 1985. Signal-to-noise properties of mammography film-screen systems. *Med. Phys.* 12:32-39.

Pisano, E.D. and Yaffe, M.J. 1998. Digital Mammography. *Contemp. Diagn. Radiol.* 21:1-6.

Smart, C.R., Hartmann, W.H., Beahrs, O.H. et al. 1993. Insights into breast cancer screening of younger women: Evidence from the 14-year follow-up of the Breast Cancer Detection Demonstration Project. *Cancer* 72:1449-1456.

Tabar, L., Duffy, S.W., and Burhenne, L.W. 1993. New Swedish breast cancer detection results for women aged 40-49. *Cancer (suppl.)* 72:1437-1448.

Wagner, A.J. 1991. Contrast and grid performance in mammography. In *Screen Film Mammography: Imaging Considerations and Medical Physics Responsibilities.* G.T. Barnes and G.D. Frey, Eds., pp 115-134. Medical Physics Publishing, Madison, WI.

Wu, X., Barnes, G.T., and Tucker, D.M. 1991 Spectral dependence of glandular tissue dose in screen-film mammography, *Radiology* 179:143-148.

Wu, X., Gingold, E.L., Barnes, G.T., and Tucker, D.M. 1994. Normalized average glandular dose in molybdenum target-rhodium filter and rhodium target-rhodium filter mammography, *Radiology* 193:83-89.

Yaffe, M.J. 1994. Digital mammography. In *A Categorical Course in Physics: Technical Aspects of Breast Imaging*, 3rd ed. A.G. Haus and M.J. Yaffe, Eds., pp 275-286. RSNA Publications, Oak Brook, IL.

Yaffe, M.J. and Rowlands, J.A. 1997. X-ray detectors for digital radiography. *Phys. Med. Biol.* 42:1-39.

Further Information

Yaffe, M.J. et al., 1993. *Recommended Specifications for New Mammography Equipment:* ACR-CDC Cooperative Agreement for Quality Assurance Activities in Mammography, ACR Publications, Reston, VA.

Haus, A.G. and Yaffe, M.J. 1994. *A Categorical Course in Physics: Technical Aspects of Breast Imaging.* RSNA Publications, Oak Brook, IL. In this syllabus to a course presented at the Radiological Society of North America all technical aspects of mammography are addressed by experts and a clinical overview is presented in language understandable by the physicist or biomedical engineer.

Screen Film Mammography: Imaging Considerations and Medical Physics Responsibilities. Eds., G.T Barnes and G.D. Frey. Medical Physics Publishing, Madison, WI. Considerable practical information related to obtaining and maintaining high quality mammography is provided here.

Film Processing in Medical Imaging. A.G. Haus, Ed., Medical Physics Publishing, Madison, WI. This book deals with all aspects of medical film processing with particular emphasis on mammography.

9

Computed Tomography

Ian A. Cunningham
Victoria Hospital, the John P. Robarts Research Institute, and the University of Western Ontario

Philip F. Judy
Brigham and Women's Hospital and Harvard Medical School

9.1 Instrumentation

Ian A. Cunningham

The development of computed tomography (CT) in the early 1970s revolutionized medical radiology. For the first time, physicians were able to obtain high-quality tomographic (cross-sectional) images of internal structures of the body. Over the next 10 years, 18 manufacturers competed for the exploding world CT market. Technical sophistication increased dramatically, and even today, CT continues to mature, with new capabilities being researched and developed.

Computed tomographic images are reconstructed from a large number of measurements of x-ray transmission through the patient (called projection data). The resulting images are tomographic "maps" of the x-ray linear attenuation coefficient. The mathematical methods used to reconstruct CT images from projection data are discussed in the next section. In this section, the hardware and instrumentation in a modern scanner are described.

The first practical CT instrument was developed in 1971 by Dr. G. N. Hounsfield in England and was used to image the brain [Hounsfield, 1980]. The projection data were acquired in approximately 5 min, and the tomographic image was reconstructed in approximately 20 min. Since then, CT technology has developed dramatically, and CT has become a standard imaging procedure for virtually all parts of the body in thousands of facilities throughout the world. Projection data are typically acquired in approximately 1 s, and the image is reconstructed in 3 to 5 s. One special-purpose scanner described below acquires the projection data for one tomographic image in 50 ms. A typical modern CT scanner is shown in Fig. 9.1, and typical CT images are shown in Fig. 9.2.

The fundamental task of CT systems is to make an extremely large number (approximately 500,000) of highly accurate measurements of x-ray transmission through the patient in a precisely controlled geometry. A basic system generally consists of a gantry, a patient table, a control console, and a computer. The gantry contains the x-ray source, x-ray detectors, and the data-acquisition system (DAS).

Data-Acquisition Geometries

Projection data may be acquired in one of several possible geometries described below, based on the scanning configuration, scanning motions, and detector arrangement. The evolution of these geometries

0-8493-1810-6/03/$0.00+$1.50

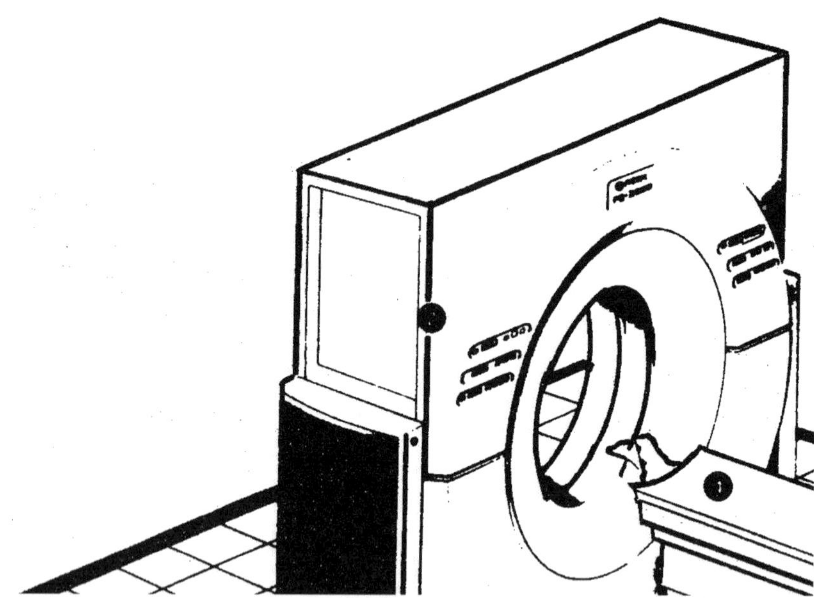

FIGURE 9.1 Schematic drawing of a typical CT scanner installation, consisting of (1) control console, (2) gantry stand, (3) patient table, (4) head holder, and (5) laser imager. (Courtesy of Picker International, Inc.)

is descried in terms of "generations," as illustrated in Fig. 9.3, and reflects the historical development [Newton and Potts, 1981; Seeram, 1994]. Current CT scanners use either third-, fourth-, or fifth-generation geometries, each having its own pros and cons.

First Generation: Parallel-Beam Geometry

Parallel-beam geometry is the simplest technically and the easiest with which to understand the important CT principles. Multiple measurements of x-ray transmission are obtained using a single highly collimated x-ray pencil beam and detector. The beam is translated in a linear motion across the patient to obtain a projection profile. The source and detector are then rotated about the patient isocenter by approximately 1°, and another projection profile is obtained. This translate-rotate scanning motion is repeated until the source and detector have been rotated by 180°. The highly collimated beam provides excellent rejection of radiation scattered in the patient; however, the complex scanning motion results in long (approximately 5-min) scan times. This geometry was used by Hounsfield in his original experiments [Hounsfield, 1980] but is not used in modern scanners.

Second Generation: Fan Beam, Multiple Detectors

Scan times were reduced to approximately 30 s with the use of a fan beam of x-rays and a linear detector array. A translate-rotate scanning motion was still employed; however, a larger rotate increment could be used, which resulted in shorter scan times. The reconstruction algorithms are slightly more complicated than those for first-generation algorithms because they must handle fan-beam projection data.

Third Generation: Fan Beam, Rotating Detectors

Third-generation scanners were introduced in 1976. A fan beam of x-rays is rotated 360° around the isocenter. No translation motion is used; however, the fan beam must be wide enough to completely contain the patient. A curved detector array consisting of several hundred independent detectors is mechanically coupled to the x-ray source, and both rotate together. As a result, these rotate-only motions acquire projection data for a single image in as little as 1 s. Third-generation designs have the advantage that thin tungsten septa can be placed between each detector in the array and focused on the x-ray source to reject scattered radiation.

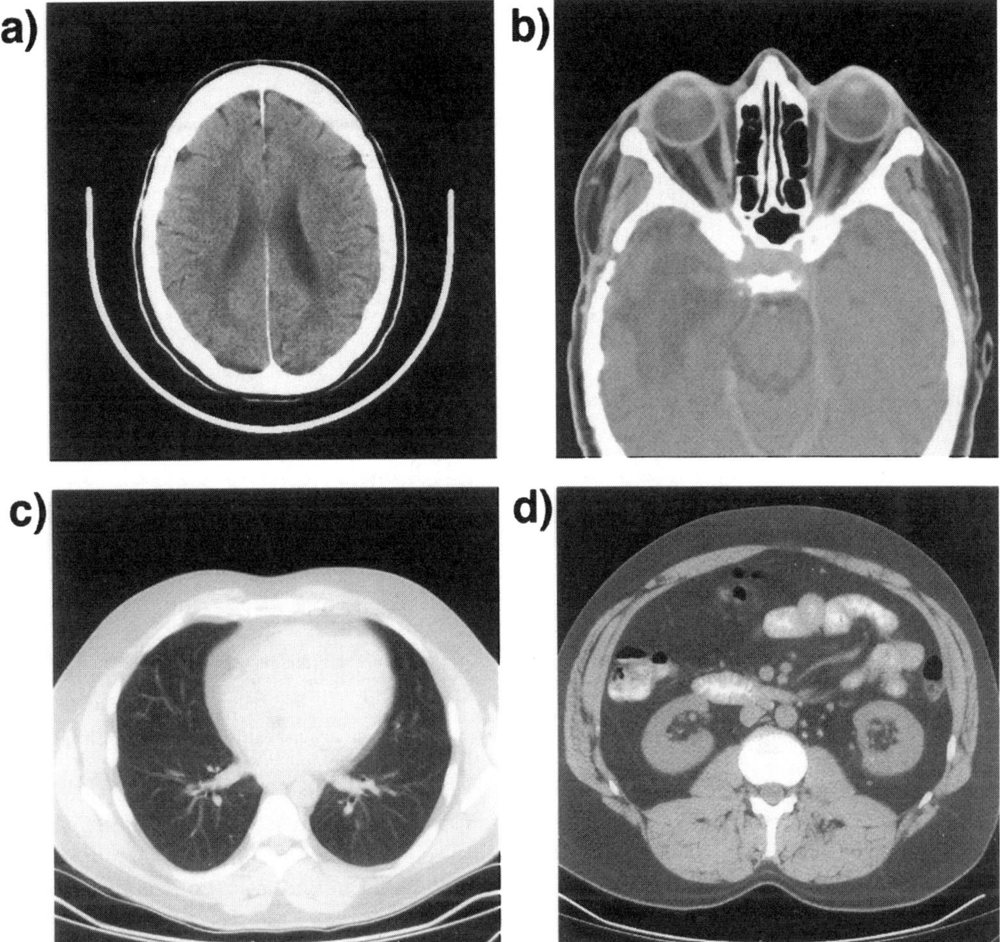

FIGURE 9.2 Typical CT images of (a) brain, (b) head showing orbits, (c) chest showing lungs, and (d) abdomen.

Fourth Generation: Fan Beam, Fixed Detectors

In a fourth-generation scanner, the x-ray source and fan beam rotate about the isocenter, while the detector array remains stationary. The detector array consists of 600 to 4800 (depending on the manufacturer) independent detectors in a circle that completely surrounds the patient. Scan times are similar to those of third-generation scanners. The detectors are no longer coupled to the x-ray source and hence cannot make use of focused septa to reject scattered radiation. However, detectors are calibrated twice during each rotation of the x-ray source, providing a self-calibrating system. Third-generation systems are calibrated only once every few hours.

Two detector geometries are currently used for fourth-generation systems: (1) a rotating x-ray source inside a fixed detector array and (2) a rotating x-ray source outside a nutating detector array. Figure 9.4 shows the major components in the gantry of a typical fourth-generation system using a fixed-detector array. Both third- and fourth-generation systems are commercially available, and both have been highly successful clinically. Neither can be considered an overall superior design.

Fifth Generation: Scanning Electron Beam

Fifth-generation scanners are unique in that the x-ray source becomes an integral part of the system design. The detector array remains stationary, while a high-energy electron beams is electronically swept along a semicircular tungsten strip anode, as illustrated in Fig. 9.5. X-rays are produced at the point

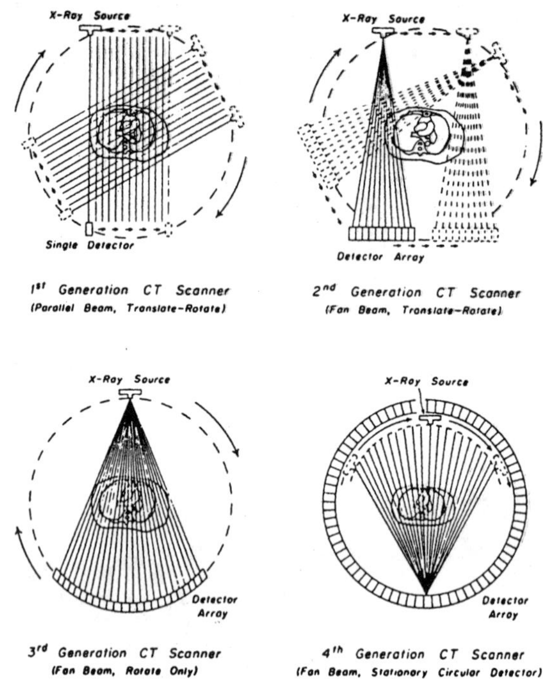

FIGURE 9.3 Four generations of CT scanners illustrating the parallel- and fan-beam geometries [Robb, 1982].

where the electron beam hits the anode, resulting in a source of x-rays that rotates about the patient with no moving parts [Boyd et al., 1979]. Projection data can be acquired in approximately 50 ms, which is fast enough to image the beating heart without significant motion artifacts [Boyd and Lipton, 1983].

An alternative fifth-generation design, called the *dynamic spatial reconstructor (DSR) scanner,* is in use at the Mayo Clinic [Ritman, 1980, 1990]. This machine is a research prototype and is not available commercially. It consists of 14 x-ray tubes, scintillation screens, and video cameras. Volume CT images can be produced in as little as 10 ms.

Spiral/Helical Scanning

The requirement for faster scan times, and in particular for fast multiple scans for three-dimensional imaging, has resulted in the development of spiral (helical) scanning systems [Kalendar et al., 1990]. Both third- and fourth-generation systems achieve this using self-lubricating slip-ring technology (Fig. 9.6) to make the electrical connections with rotating components. This removes the need for power and signal cables which would otherwise have to be rewound between scans and allows for a continuous rotating motion of the x-ray fan beam. Multiple images are acquired while the patient is translated through the gantry in a smooth continuous motion rather than stopping for each image. Projection data for multiple images covering a volume of the patient can be acquired in a single breath hold at rates of approximately one slice per second. The reconstruction algorithms are more sophisticated because they must accommodate the spiral or helical path traced by the x-ray source around the patient, as illustrated in Fig. 9.7.

X-Ray System

The x-ray system consists of the x-ray source, detectors, and a data-acquisition system.

X-Ray Source

With the exception of one fifth-generation system described above, all CT scanners use bremsstrahlung x-ray tubes as the source of radiation. These tubes are typical of those used in diagnostic imaging and

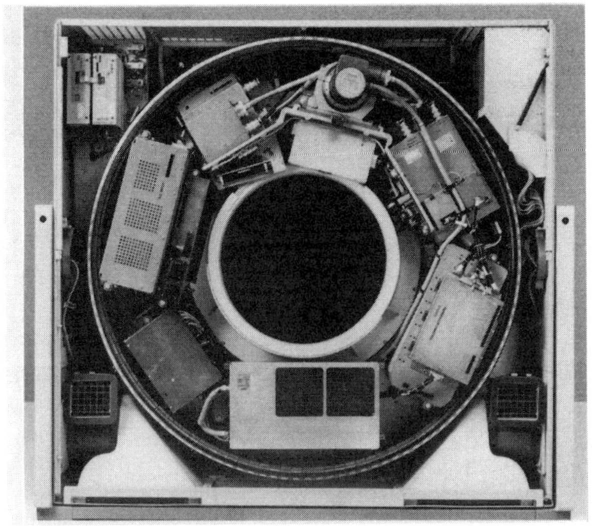

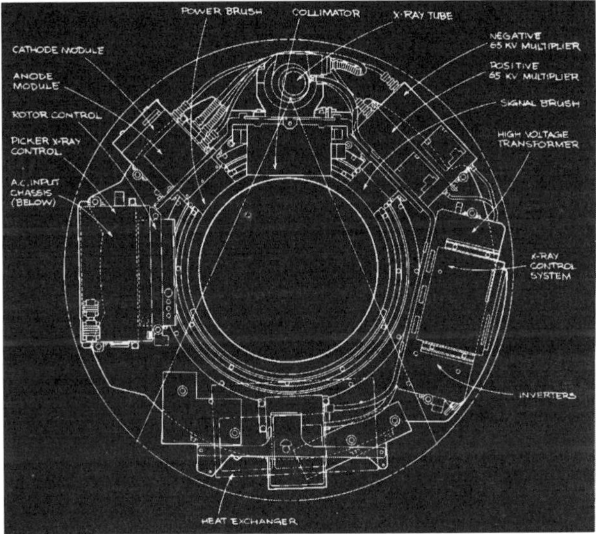

FIGURE 9.4 The major internal components of a fourth-generation CT gantry are shown in a photograph with the gantry cover removed (upper) and identified in the line drawing (lower). (Courtesy of Picker International, Inc.)

produce x-rays by accelerating a beam of electrons onto a target anode. The anode area from which x-rays are emitted, projected along the direction of the beam, is called the focal spot. Most systems have two possible focal spot sizes, approximately 0.5 × 1.5 mm and 1.0 × 2.5 mm. A collimator assembly is used to control the width of the fan beam between 1.0 and 10 mm, which in turn controls the width of the imaged slice.

The power requirements of these tubes are typically 120 kV at 200 to 500 mA, producing x-rays with an energy spectrum ranging between approximately 30 and 120 keV. All modern systems use high-frequency generators, typically operating between 5 and 50 kHz [Brunnett et al., 1990]. Some spiral systems use a stationary generator in the gantry, requiring high-voltage (120-kV) slip rings, while others use a rotating generator with lower-voltage (480-V) slip rings. Production of x-rays in bremsstrahlung tubes is an inefficient process, and hence most of the power delivered to the tubes results in heating of

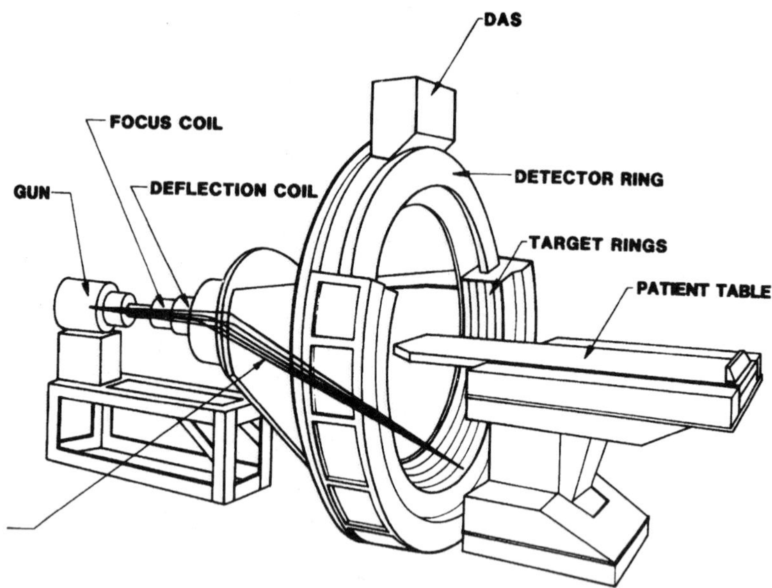

FIGURE 9.5 Schematic illustration of a fifth-generation ultrafast CT system. Image data are acquired in as little as 50 ms, as an electron beam is swept over the strip anode electronically. (Courtesy of Imatron, Inc.)

the anode. A heat exchanger on the rotating gantry is used to cool the tube. Spiral scanning, in particular, places heavy demands on the heat-storage capacity and cooling rate of the x-ray tube.

The intensity of the x-ray beam is attenuated by absorption and scattering processes as it passes through the patient. The degree of attenuation depends on the energy spectrum of the x-rays as well as on the average atomic number and mass density of the patient tissues. The transmitted intensity is given by

$$I_t = I_o e^{-\int_0^L \mu(x)dx} \tag{9.1}$$

where I_o and I_t are the incident and transmitted beam intensities, respectively; L is the length of the x-ray path; and $\mu(x)$ is the x-ray linear attenuation coefficient, which varies with tissue type and hence is a function of the distance x through the patient. The integral of the attenuation coefficient is therefore given by

$$\int_0^L \mu(x)dx = -\frac{1}{L}\ln\left(I_t/I_o\right) \tag{9.2}$$

The reconstruction algorithm requires measurements of this integral along many paths in the fan beam at each of many angles about the isocenter. The value of L is known, and I_o is determined by a system calibration. Hence values of the integral along each path can be determined from measurements of I_t.

X-Ray Detectors

X-ray detectors used in CT systems must (a) have a high overall efficiency to minimize the patient radiation dose, have a large dynamic range, (b) be very stable with time, and (c) be insensitive to temperature variations within the gantry. Three important factors contributing to the detector efficiency are geometric efficiency, quantum (also called *capture*) efficiency, and conversion efficiency [Villafanaet et al., 1987]. *Geometric efficiency* refers to the area of the detectors sensitive to radiation as a fraction of the total exposed area. Thin septa between detector elements to remove scattered radiation, or other

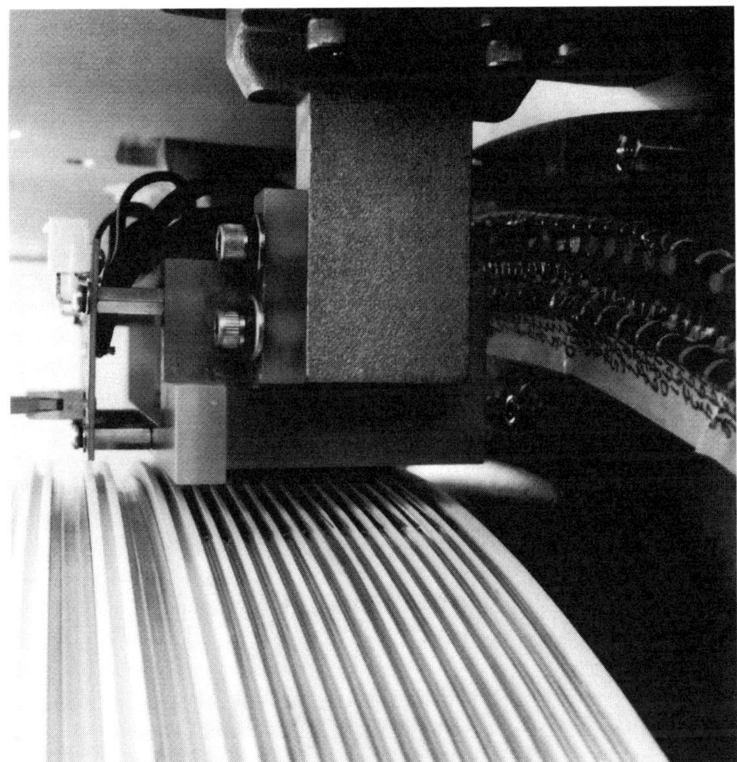

FIGURE 9.6 Photograph of the slip rings used to pass power and control signals to the rotating gantry. (Courtesy of Picker International, Inc.)

insensitive regions, will degrade this value. *Quantum efficiency* refers to the fraction of incident x-rays on the detector that are absorbed and contribute to the measured signal. *Conversion efficiency* refers to the ability to accurately convert the absorbed x-ray signal into an electrical signal (but is not the same as the energy conversion efficiency). *Overall efficiency* is the product of the three, and it generally lies between 0.45 and 0.85. A value of less than 1 indicates a nonideal detector system and results in a required increase in patient radiation dose if image quality is to be maintained. The term *dose efficiency* sometimes has been used to indicate overall efficiency.

Modern commercial systems use one of two detector types: solid-state or gas ionization detectors.

Solid-State Detectors. Solid-state detectors consist of an array of scintillating crystals and photodiodes, as illustrated in Fig. 9.8. The scintillators generally are either cadmium tungstate ($CdWO_4$) or a ceramic material made of rare earth oxides, although previous scanners have used bismuth germanate crystals with photomultiplier tubes. Solid-state detectors generally have very high quantum and conversion efficiencies and a large dynamic range.

Gas Ionization Detectors. Gas ionization detectors, as illustrated in Fig. 9.9, consist of an array of chambers containing compressed gas (usually xenon at up to 30 atm pressure). A high voltage is applied to tungsten septa between chambers to collect ions produced by the radiation. These detectors have excellent stability and a large dynamic range; however, they generally have a lower quantum efficiency than solid-state detectors.

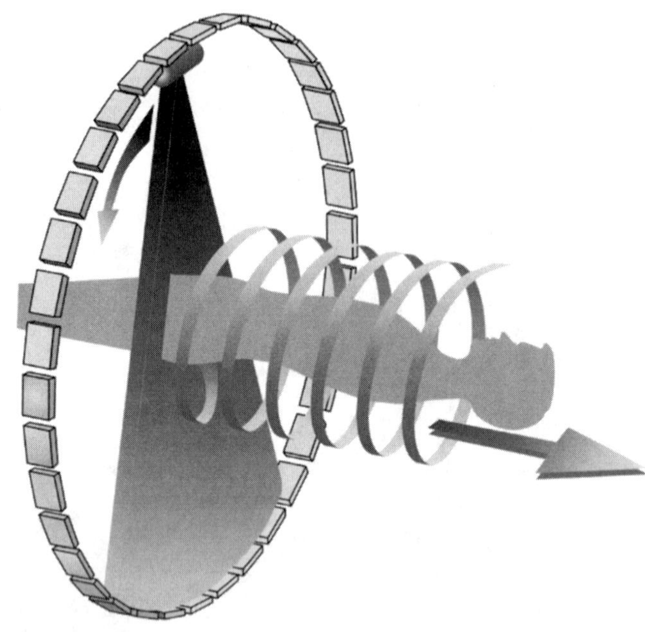

FIGURE 9.7 Spiral scanning causes the focal spot to follow a spiral path around the patient as indicated. (Courtesy of Picker International, Inc.)

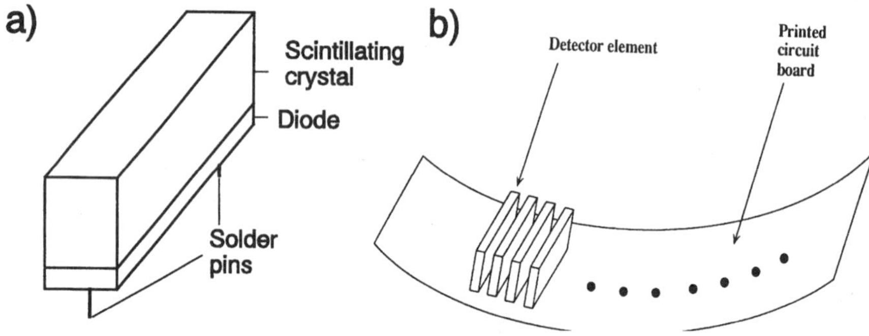

FIGURE 9.8 (a) A solid-state detector consists of a scintillating crystal and photodiode combination. (b) Many such detectors are placed side by side to form a detector array that may contain up to 4800 detectors.

Data-Acquisition System

The transmitted fraction I_t/I_o in Eq. (9.2) through an obese patient can be less than 10^{-4}. Thus it is the task of the data-acquisition system (DAS) to accurately measure I_t over a dynamic range of more than 10^4, encode the results into digital values, and transmit the values to the system computer for reconstruction. Some manufacturers use the approach illustrated in Fig. 9.10, consisting of precision preamplifiers, current-to-voltage converters, analog integrators, multiplexers, and analog-to-digital converters. Alternatively, some manufacturers use the preamplifier to control a synchronous voltage-to-frequency converter (SVFC), replacing the need for the integrators, multiplexers, and analog-to-digital converters [Brunnett et al., 1990]. The logarithmic conversion required in Eq. (9.2) is performed with either an analog logarithmic amplifier or a digital lookup table, depending on the manufacturer.

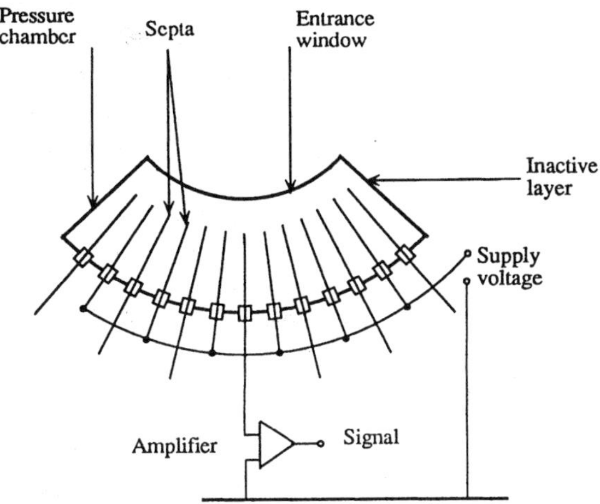

FIGURE 9.9 Gas ionization detector arrays consist of high-pressure gas in multiple chambers separated by thin septa. A voltage is applied between alternating septa. The septa also act as electrodes and collect the ions created by the radiation, converting them into an electrical signal.

Sustained data transfer rates to the computer are as high as 10 Mbytes/s for some scanners. This can be accomplished with a direct connection for systems having a fixed detector array. However, third-generation slip-ring systems must use more sophisticated techniques. At least one manufacturer uses optical transmitters on the rotating gantry to send data to fixed optical receivers [Siemens, 1989].

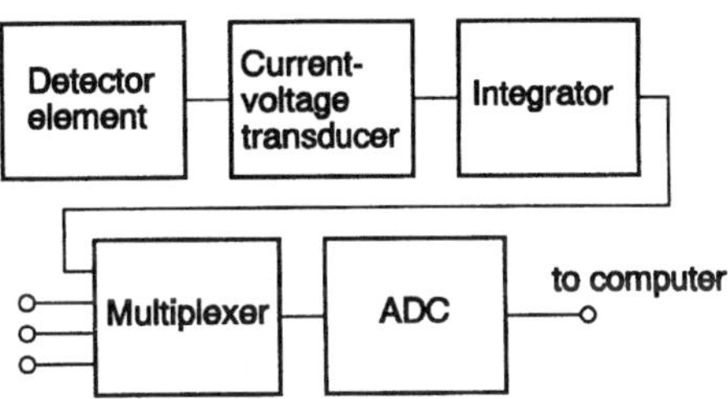

FIGURE 9.10 The data-acquisition system converts the electrical signal produced by each detector to a digital value for the computer.

Computer System

Various computer systems are used by manufacturers to control system hardware, acquire the projection data, and reconstruct, display, and manipulate the tomographic images. A typical system is illustrated in Fig. 9.11, which uses 12 independent processors connected by a 40-Mbyte/s multibus. Multiple custom array processors are used to achieve a combined computational speed of 200 MFLOPS (million floating-point operations per second) and a reconstruction time of approximately 5 s to produce an image on a 1024 × 1024 pixel display. A simplified UNIX operating system is used to provide a multitasking, multiuser environment to coordinate tasks.

Patient Dose Considerations

The patient dose resulting from CT examinations is generally specified in terms of the CT dose index (CTDI) [Felmlee et al., 1989; Rothenberg and Pentlow, 1992], which includes the dose contribution from radiation scattered from nearby slices. A summary of CTDI values, as specified by four manufacturers, is given in Table 9.1.

Summary

Computed tomography revolutionized medical radiology in the early 1970s. Since that time, CT technology has developed dramatically, taking advantage of developments in computer hardware and detector technology. Modern systems acquire the projection data required for one tomographic image in approximately

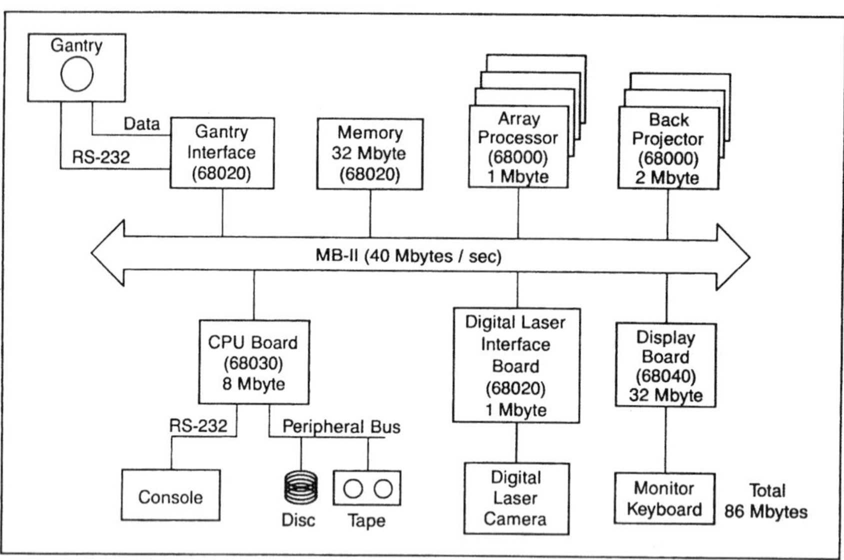

FIGURE 9.11 The computer system controls the gantry motions, acquires the x-ray transmission measurements, and reconstructs the final image. The system shown here uses 12 68000-family CPUs. (Courtesy of Picker International, Inc.)

TABLE 9.1 Summary of the CT Dose Index (CTDI) Values at Two Positions (Center of the Patient and Near the Skin) as Specified by Four CT Manufacturers for Standard Head and Body Scans

Manufacturer	Detector	kVp	mA	Scan Time (s)	CTDI, center (mGy)	CTDI, skin (mGy)
A, head	Xenon	120	170	2	50	48
A, body	Xenon	120	170	2	14	25
A, head	Solid state	120	170	2	40	40
A, body	Solid state	120	170	2	11	20
B, head	Solid state	130	80	2	37	41
B, body	Solid state	130	80	2	15	34
C, head	Solid state	120	500	2	39	50
C, body	Solid state	120	290	1	12	28
D, head	Solid state	120	200	2	78	78
D, body	Solid state	120	200	2	9	16

1 s and present the reconstructed image on a 1024 × 1024 matrix display within a few seconds. The images are high-quality tomographic "maps" of the x-ray linear attenuation coefficient of the patient tissues.

Defining Terms

Absorption: Some of the incident x-ray energy is absorbed in patient tissues and hence does not contribute to the transmitted beam.

Anode: A tungsten bombarded by a beam of electrons to produce x-rays. In all but one fifth-generation system, the anode rotates to distribute the resulting heat around the perimeter. The anode heat-storage capacity and maximum cooling rate often limit the maximum scanning rates of CT systems.

Attenuation: The total decrease in the intensity of the primary x-ray beam as it passes through the patient, resulting from both scatter and absorption processes. It is characterized by the linear attenuation coefficient.

Computed tomography (CT): A computerized method of producing x-ray tomographic images. Previous names for the same thing include *computerized tomographic imaging, computerized axial tomography (CAT), computer-assisted tomography (CAT),* and *reconstructive tomography (RT).*

Control console: The control console is used by the CT operator to control the scanning operations, image reconstruction, and image display.

Cormack, Dr. Allan MacLeod: A physicist who developed mathematical techniques required in the reconstruction of tomographic images. Dr. Cormack shared the Nobel Prize in Medicine and Physiology with Dr. G. N. Hounsfield in 1979 [Cormack, 1980].

Data-acquisition system (DAS): Interfaces the x-ray detectors to the system computer and may consist of a preamplifier, integrator, multiplexer, logarithmic amplifier, and analog-to-digital converter.

Detector array: An array of individual detector elements. The number of detector elements varies between a few hundred and 4800, depending on the acquisition geometry and manufacturer. Each detector element functions independently of the others.

Fan beam: The x-ray beam is generated at the focal spot and so diverges as it passes through the patient to the detector array. The thickness of the beam is generally selectable between 1.0 and 10 mm and defines the slice thickness.

Focal spot: The region of the anode where x-rays are generated.

Focused septa: Thin metal plates between detector elements which are aligned with the focal spot so that the primary beam passes unattenuated to the detector elements, while scattered x-rays which normally travel in an altered direction are blocked.

Gantry: The largest component of the CT installation, containing the x-ray tube, collimators, detector array, DAS, other control electronics, and the mechanical components required for the scanning motions.

Helical scanning: The scanning motions in which the x-ray tube rotates continuously around the patient while the patient is continuously translated through the fan beam. The focal spot therefore traces a helix around the patient. Projection data are obtained which allow the reconstruction of multiple contiguous images. This operation is sometimes called *spiral, volume,* or *three-dimensional* CT scanning.

Hounsfield, Dr. Godfrey Newbold: An engineer who developed the first practical CT instrument in 1971. Dr. Hounsfield received the McRobert Award in 1972 and shared the Nobel Prize in Medicine and Physiology with Dr. A. M. Cormack in 1979 for this invention [Hounsfield, 1980].

Image plane: The plane through the patient that is imaged. In practice, this plane (also called a *slice*) has a selectable thickness between 1.0 and 10 mm centered on the image plane.

Pencil beam: A narrow, well-collimated beam of x-rays.

Projection data: The set of transmission measurements used to reconstruct the image.

Reconstruct: The mathematical operation of generating the tomographic image from the projection data.

Scan time: The time required to acquire the projection data for one image, typically 1.0 s.

Scattered radiation: Radiation that is removed from the primary beam by a scattering process. This radiation is not absorbed but continues along a path in an altered direction.

Slice: See Image plane.

Spiral scanning: See Helical scanning.

Three-dimensional imaging: See Helical scanning.

Tomography: A technique of imaging a cross-sectional slice.

Volume CT: See Helical scanning.

X-ray detector: A device that absorbs radiation and converts some or all of the absorbed energy into a small electrical signal.

X-ray linear attenuation coefficient μ: Expresses the relative rate of attenuation of a radiation beam as it passes through a material. The value of μ depends on the density and atomic number of the material and on the x-ray energy. The units of μ are cm^{-1}.

X-ray source: The device that generates the x-ray beam. All CT scanners are rotating-anode bremsstrahlung x-ray tubes except one fifth-generation system, which uses a unique scanned electron beam and a strip anode.

X-ray transmission: The fraction of the x-ray beam intensity that is transmitted through the patient without being scattered or absorbed. It is equal to I_t/I_o in Eq. (9.2), can be determined by measuring the beam intensity both with (I_t) and without (I_o) the patient present, and is expressed as a fraction. As a rule of thumb, n^2 independent transmission measurements are required to reconstruct an image with an $n \times n$ sized pixel matrix.

References

Body DP, et al. 1979. A proposed dynamic cardiac 3D densitometer for early detection and evaluation of heart disease. IEEE Trans Nucl Sci 2724.

Boyd DP, Lipton MJ. 1983. Cardiac computed tomography. Proc IEEE 198.

Brunnett CJ, Heuscher DJ, Mattson RA, Vrettos CJ. 1990. CT Design Considerations and Specifications. Picker International, CT Engineering Department, Highland Heights, OH.

Cormack AM. 1980. Nobel Award Address: Early two-dimensional reconstruction and recent topics stemming from it. Med Phys 7(4):277.

Felmlee JP, Gray JE, Leetzow ML, Price JC. 1989. Estimated fetal radiation dose from multislice CT studies. Am Roent Ray Soc 154:185.

Hounsfield GN. 1980. Nobel Award Address: Computed medical imaging. Med Phys 7(4):283.

Kalendar WA, Seissler W, Klotz E, et al. 1990. Spiral volumetric CT with single-breath-hold technique, continuous transport, and continuous scanner rotation. Radiology 176:181.

Newton TH, Potts DG (eds). 1981. Radiology of the Skull and Brain: Technical Aspects of Computed Tomography. St. Louis, Mosby.

Picker. 1990. Computed Dose Index PQ2000 CT Scanner. Picker International, Highland Heights, OH.

Ritman EL. 1980. Physical and technical considerations in the design of the DSR, and high temporal resolution volume scanner. AJR 134:369.

Ritman EL. 1990. Fast computed tomography for quantitative cardiac analysis—State of the art and future perspectives. Mayo Clin Proc 65:1336.

Robb RA. 1982. X-ray computed tomography: An engineering synthesis of multiscientific principles. CRC Crit Rev Biomed Eng 7:265.

Rothenberg LN, Pentlow KS. 1992. Radiation dose in CT. RadioGraphics 12:1225.

Seeram E. 1994. Computed Tomography: Physical Principles, Clinical Applications and Quality Control. Philadelphia, WB Saunders.

Siemens. 1989. The Technology and Performance of the Somatom Plus. Siemens Aktiengesellschaft, Medical Engineering Group, Erlangen, Germany.

Villafana T, Lee SH, Rao KCVG (eds). 1987. Cranial Computed Tomography. New York, McGraw-Hill.

Further Information

A recent summary of CT instrumentation and concepts is given by E. Seeram in *Computed Tomography: Physical Principles, Clinical Applications and Quality Control.* The author summarizes CT from the perspective of the nonmedical, nonspecialist user. A summary of average CT patient doses is described by Rothenberg and Pentlow [1992] in *Radiation Dose in CT.* Research papers on both fundamental and practical aspects of CT physics and instrumentation are published in numerous journals, including *Medical Physics, Physics in Medicine and Biology, Journal of Computer Assisted Tomography, Radiology, British Journal of Radiology,* and the IEEE Press. A comparison of technical specifications of CT systems provided by the manufacturers is available from ECRI to help orient the new purchaser in a selection process. Their *Product Comparison System* includes a table of basic specifications for all the major international manufacturers.

9.2 Reconstruction Principles

Philip F. Judy

Computed tomography (CT) is a two-step process: (1) the transmission of an x-ray beam is measured through all possible straight-line paths as in a plane of an object, and (2) the attenuation of an x-ray beam is estimated at points in the object. Initially, the transmission measurements will be assumed to be the results of an experiment performed with a narrow monoenergetic beam of x-rays that are confined to a plane. The designs of devices that attempt to realize these measurements are described in the preceding section. One formal consequence of these assumptions is that the logarithmic transformation of the measured x-ray intensity is proportional to the line integral of attenuation coefficients. In order to satisfy this assumption, computer processing procedures on the measurements of x-ray intensity are necessary even before image reconstruction is performed. These linearization procedures will reviewed after background.

Both analytical and iterative estimations of linear x-ray attenuation have been used for transmission CT reconstruction. Iterative procedures are of historical interest because an iterative reconstruction procedure was used in the first commercially successful CT scanner [EMI, Mark I, Hounsfield, 1973]. They also permit easy incorporation of physical processes that cause deviations from the linearity. Their practical usefulness is limited. The first EMI scanner required 20 min to finish its reconstruction. Using the identical hardware and employing an analytical calculation, the estimation of attenuation values was performed during the 4.5-min data acquisition and was made on a 160×160 matrix. The original iterative procedure reconstructed the attenuation values on an 80×80 matrix and consequently failed to exploit all the spatial information inherent in transmission data.

Analytical estimation, or direct reconstruction, uses a numerical approximation of the inverse Radon transform [Radon, 1917]. The direct reconstruction technique (convolution-backprojection) at present used in x-ray CT was initially applied in other areas such as radio astronomy [Bracewell and Riddle, 1967] and electron microscopy [Crowther et al., 1970; Ramachandran and Lakshminarayana, 1971]. These investigations demonstrated that the reconstructions from the discrete spatial sampling of bandlimited data led to full recovery of the cross-sectional attenuation. The random variation (noise) in x-ray transmission measurements may not be bandlimited. Subsequent investigators [e.g., Chesler and Riederer, 1975; Herman and Roland, 1973; Shepp and Logan, 1974] have suggested various bandlimiting windows that reduce the propagation and amplification of noise by the reconstruction. These issues have been investigated by simulation, and investigators continue to pursue these issues using a computer phantom [e.g., Guedon and Bizais, 1994, and references therein] described by Shepp and Logan. The subsequent investigations of the details of choice of reconstruction parameters have had limited practical impact because real variation of transmission data is bandlimited by the finite size of the focal spot and radiation detector, a straightforward design question, and because random variation of the transmission tends to be uncorrelated. Consequently, the classic procedures suffice.

Image Processing: Artifact and Reconstruction Error

An *artifact* is a reconstruction defect that is obviously visible in the image. The classification of an image feature as an artifact involves some visual criterion. The effect must produce an image feature that is greater than the random variation in image caused by the intrinsic variation in transmission measurements. An artifact not recognized by the physician observer as an artifact may be reported as a lesion. Such false-positive reports could lead to an unnecessary medical procedure, e.g., surgery to remove an imaginary tumor. A *reconstruction error* is a deviation of the reconstruction value from its expected value.

Reconstruction errors are significant if the application involves a quantitative measurement, not a common medical application. The reconstruction errors are characterized by identical material at different points in the object leading to different reconstructed attenuation values in the image which are not visible in the medical image.

Investigators have used computer simulation to investigate artifact [Herman, 1980] because image noise limits the visibility of their visibility. One important issue investigated was required spatial sampling of transmission slice plane [Crawford and Kak, 1979; Parker et al., 1982]. These simulations provided a useful guideline in design. In practice, these aliasing artifacts are overwhelmed by random noise, and designers tend to oversample in the slice plane. A second issue that was understood by computer simulation was the partial volume artifact [Glover and Pelc, 1980]. This artifact would occur even for mononergetic beams and finite beam size, particularly in the axial dimension. The axial dimension of the beams tend to be greater (about 10 mm) than their dimensions in the slice plane (about 1 mm). The artifact is created when the variation of transmission within the beam varies considerably, and the exponential variation within the beam is summed by the radiation detector. The logarithm transformation of the detected signal produces a nonlinear effect that is propagated throughout the image by the reconstruction process. Simulation was useful in demonstrating that isolated features in the same cross section act together to produce streak artifacts. Simulations have been useful to illustrate the effects of patient motion during the data-acquisition streaks off high-contrast objects.

Projection Data to Image: Calibrations

Processing of transmission data is necessary to obtain high-quality images. In general, optimization of the projection data will optimize the reconstructed image. Reconstruction is a process that removes the spatial correlation of attenuation effects in the transmitted image by taking advantage of completely sampling the possible transmissions. Two distinct calibrations are required: registration of beams with the reconstruction matrix and linearization of the measured signal.

Without loss of generalization, a projection will be considered a set of transmissions made along parallel lines in the slice plane of the CT scanner. *Without loss of generalization* means that essential aspects of all calibration and reconstruction procedures required for fan-beam geometries are captured by the calibration and reconstruction procedures described for parallel projections. One line of each projection is assumed to pass through the center of rotation of data collection. Shepp et al. [1979] showed that errors in the assignment of that center-of-rotation point in the projections could lead to considerable distinctive artifacts and that small errors (0.05 mm) would produce these effects. The consequences of these errors have been generalized to fan-beam collection schemes, and images reconstructed from 180° projection sets were compared with images reconstructed from 360° data sets [Kijewski and Judy, 1983]. A simple misregistration of the center of rotation was found to produce blurring of image without the artifact. These differences may explain the empirical observation that most commercial CT scanners collect a full 360° data set even though 180° of data will suffice.

The data-acquisition scheme that was designed to overcome the limited sampling inherent in third-generation fan-beam systems by shifting detectors a quarter sampling distance while opposite 180° projection is measured, has particularly stringent registration requirements. Also, the fourth-generation scanner does not link the motion of the x-ray tube and the detector; consequently, the center of rotation is determined as part of a calibration procedure, and unsystematic effects lead to artifacts that mimic noise besides blurring the image.

Misregistration artifacts also can be mitigated by *feathering*. This procedure requires collection of redundant projection data at the end of the scan. A single data set is produced by linearly weighting the redundant data at the beginning and end of the data collection [Parker et al., 1982]. These procedures have be useful in reducing artifacts from gated data collections [Moore et al., 1987].

The other processing necessary before reconstruction of project data is *linearization*. The formal requirement for reconstruction is that the line integrals of some variable be available; this is the variable that ultimately is reconstructed. The logarithm of x-ray transmission approximates this requirement. There are physical effects in real x-ray transmissions that cause deviations from this assumption. X-ray beams of sufficient intensity are composed of photons of different energies. Some photons in the beam interact with objects and are scattered rather than absorbed. The spectrum of x-ray photons of different attenuation coefficients means the logarithm of the transmission measurement will not be proportional to the line integral of the attenuation coefficient along that path, because an attenuation coefficient cannot even be defined. An effective attenuation coefficient can only be defined uniquely for a spectrum for a small mass of material that alters that intensity. It has to be small enough not to alter the spectrum [McCullough, 1979].

A straightforward approach to this nonunique attenuation coefficient error, called *hardening*, is to assume that the energy dependence of the attenuation coefficient is constant and that differences in attenuation are related to a generalized density factor that multiplies the spectral dependence of attenuation. The transmission of an x-ray beam then can be estimated for a standard material, typically water, as a function of thickness. This assumption is that attenuations of materials in the object, the human body, differ because specific gravities of the materials differ. Direct measurements of the transmission of an actual x-ray beam may provide initial estimates that can be parameterized. The inverse of this function provides the projection variable that is reconstructed. The parameters of the function are usually modified as part of a calibration to make the CT image of a uniform water phantom flat.

Such a calibration procedure does not deal completely with the hardening effects. The spectral dependence of bone differs considerably from that of water. This is particularly critical in imaging of the brain, which is contained within the skull. Without additional correction, the attenuation values of brain are lower in the center than near the skull.

The detection of scattered energy means that the reconstructed attenuation coefficient will differ from the attenuation coefficient estimated with careful narrow-beam measurements. The x-rays appear more penetrating because scattered x-rays are detected. The zero-ordered scatter, a decrease in the attenuation coefficient by some constant amount, is dealt with automatically by the calibration that treats hardening. First-order scattering leads to a widening of the x-ray beam and can be dealt with by a modification of the reconstruction kernel.

Projection Data to Image: Reconstruction

The impact of CT created considerable interest in the formal aspects of reconstruction. There are many detailed descriptions of direct reconstruction procedures. Some are presented in textbooks used in graduate courses for medical imaging [Barrett and Swindell, 1981; Cho et al., 1993]. Herman [1980] published a textbook that was based on a two-semester course that dealt exclusively with reconstruction principles, demonstrating the reconstruction principles with simulation.

The standard reconstruction method is called *convolution-backprojection*. The first step in the procedure is to convolve the projection, a set of transmissions made along parallel lines in the slice plane, with a reconstruction kernel derived from the inverse Radon transform. The choice of kernel is dictated by bandlimiting issues [Chesler and Riederer, 1975; Herman and Roland, 1973; Shepp and Logan, 1974]. It can be modified to deal with the physical aperture of the CT system [Bracewell, 1977], which might include the effects of scatter. The convolved projection is then backprojected onto a two-dimensional image matrix. Backprojection is the opposite of projection; the value of the projection is added to each point along the line of the projection. This procedure makes sense in the continuous description, but in the discrete world of the computer, the summation is done over the image matrix.

Consider a point of the image matrix; very few, possibly no lines of the discrete projection data intersect the point. Consequently, to estimate the projection value to be added to that point, the procedure must interpolate between two values of sampled convolve projection. The linear interpolation scheme is a significant improvement over nearest project nearest to the point. More complex schemes get confounded with choices of reconstruction kernel, which are designed to accomplish standard image processing in the image, e.g., edge enhancement.

Scanners have been developed to acquire a three-dimensional set of projection data [Kalender et al., 1990]. The motion of the source defines a spiral motion relative to the patient. The spiral motion defines an axis. Consequently, only one projection is available for reconstruction of the attenuation values in the plane. This is the backprojection problem just discussed; no correct projection value is available from the discrete projection data set. The solution is identical: a projection value is interpolated from the existing projection values to estimate the necessary projections for each plane to be reconstructed. This procedure has the advantage that overlapping slices can be reconstructed without additional exposure, and this eliminates the risk that a small lesion will be missed because it straddles adjacent slices. This data-collection scheme is possible because systems that continuously rotate have been developed. The spiral scan motion is realized by moving the patient through the gantry. Spiral CT scanners have made possible the acquisition of an entire data set in a single breath hold.

References

Barrett HH, Swindell W. 1981. Radiological Imaging: The Theory and Image Formation, Detection, and Processing, vol 2. New York, Academic Press.

Bracewell RN, Riddle AC. 1976. Inversion of fan-beam scans in radio astronomy. Astrophys J 150:427–434.

Chesler DA, Riederer SJ. 1975. Ripple suppression during reconstruction in transverse tomography. Phys Med Biol 20(4):632–636.

Cho Z, Jones JP, Singh M. 1993. Foundations of medical imaging. New York, Wiley & Sons.

Crawford CR, Kak AC. 1979. Aliasing artifacts in computerized tomography. Appl Opt 18:3704–3711.

Glover GH, Pelc NJ. 1980. Nonlinear partial volume artifacts in x-ray computed tomography. Med Phys 7:238–248.

Guedon J-P, Bizais. 1994. Bandlimited and harr filtered back-projection reconstruction. IEEE Trans Med Imaging 13(3):430–440.

Herman GT, Rowland SW. 1973. Three methods for reconstruction objects for x-rays—a comparative study. Comp Graph Imag Process 2:151–178.

Herman GT. 1980. Image Reconstruction from Projection: The Fundamentals of Computerized Tomography. New York, Academic Press.

Hounsfield, GN. 1973. Computerized transverse axial scanning (tomography): Part I. Br J Radiol 46:1016–1022.

Kalender WA, Weissler, Klotz E, et al. 1990. Spiral volumetric CT with single-breath-hold technique, continuous transport, and continuous scanner rotation. Radiology 176:181–183.

Kijewski MF, Judy PF. 1983. The effect of misregistration of the projections on spatial resolution of CT scanners. Med Phys 10:169–175.

McCullough EC. 1979. Specifying and evaluating the performance of computed tomographic (CT) scanners. Med Phys 7:291–296.

Moore SC, Judy PF, Garnic JD, et al. 1983. The effect of misregistration of the projections on spatial resolution of CT scanners. Med Phys 10:169–175.

10

Magnetic Resonance Imaging

Steven Conolly
Stanford University

Albert Macovski
Stanford University

John Pauly
Stanford University

John Schenck
General Electric Corporate Research and Development Center

Kenneth K. Kwong
Massachusetts General Hospital and Harvard University Medical School

David A. Chesler
Massachusetts General Hospital and Harvard University Medical School

Xiaoping Hu
Center for Magnetic Resonance Research and the University of Minnesota Medical School

Wei Chen
Center for Magnetic Resonance Research and the University of Minnesota Medical School

Maqbool Patel
Center for Magnetic Resonance Research and the University of Minnesota Medical School

Kamil Ugurbil
Center for Magnetic Resonance Research and the University of Minnesota Medical School

10.1 Acquisition and Processing

Steven Conolly, Albert Macovski, and John Pauly

Magnetic resonance imaging (MRI) is a clinically important medical imaging modality due to its exceptional soft-tissue contrast. MRI was invented in the early 1970s [1]. The first commercial scanners appeared about 10 years later. Noninvasive MRI studies are now supplanting many conventional invasive procedures. A 1990 study [2] found that the principal applications for MRI are examinations of the head (40%), spine (33%), bone and joints (17%), and the body (10%). The percentage of bone and joint studies was growing in 1990.

Although typical imaging studies range from 1 to 10 min, new fast imaging techniques acquire images in less than 50 ms. MRI research involves fundamental trade-offs between resolution, imaging time, and signal-to-noise ratio (SNR). It also depends heavily on both gradient and receiver coil hardware innovations.

In this section we provide a brief synopsis of basic nuclear magnetic resonance (NMR) physics. We then derive the *k*-space analysis of MRI, which interprets the received signal as a scan of the Fourier

0-8493-1810-6/03/$0.00+$1.50

transform of the image. This powerful formalism is used to analyze the most important imaging sequences. Finally, we discuss the fundamental contrast mechanisms for MRI.

Fundamentals of MRI

Magnetic resonance imaging exploits the existence of induced nuclear magnetism in the patient. Materials with an odd number of protons or neutrons possess a weak but observable nuclear magnetic moment. Most commonly protons (^1H) are imaged, although carbon (^{13}C), phosphorus (^{31}P), sodium (^{23}Na), and fluorine (^{19}F) are also of significant interest. The nuclear moments are normally randomly oriented, but they align when placed in a strong magnetic field. Typical field strengths for imaging range between 0.2 and 1.5 T, although spectroscopic and functional imaging work is often performed with higher field strengths. The nuclear magnetization is very weak; the ratio of the induced magnetization to the applied fields is only 4×10^{-9}. The collection of nuclear moments is often referred to as magnetization or spins.

The static nuclear moment is far too weak to be measured when it is aligned with the strong static magnetic field. Physicists in the 1940s developed resonance techniques that permit this weak moment to be measured. The key idea is to measure the moment while it oscillates in a plane perpendicular to the static field [3,4]. First one must tip the moment away from the static field. When perpendicular to the static field, the moment feels a torque proportional to the strength of the static magnetic field. The torque always points perpendicular to the magnetization and causes the spins to oscillate or precess in a plane perpendicular to the static field. The frequency of the rotation ω_0 is proportional to the field:

$$\omega_0 = -\gamma B_0$$

where γ, the gyromagnetic ratio, is a constant specific to the nucleus, and B_0 is the magnetic field strength. The direction of B_0 defines the z axis. The precession frequency is called the Larmor frequency. The negative sign indicates the direction of the precession.

Since the precessing moments constitute a time-varying flax, they produce a measurable voltage in a loop antenna arranged to receive the x and y components of induction. It is remarkable that in MRI we are able to directly measure induction from the precessing nuclear moments of water protons.

Recall that to observe this precession, we first need to tip the magnetization away from the static field. This is accomplished with a weak rotating radiofrequency (RF) field. It can be shown that a rotating RF field introduces a fictitious field in the z direction of strength ω/γ. By tuning the frequency of the RF field to ω_0, we effectively delete the B_0 field. The RF slowly nutates the magnetization away from the z axis. The Larmor relation still holds in this "rotating frame," so the frequency of the nutation is γB_1, where B_1 is the amplitude of the RF field. Since the coils receive x and y (transverse) components of induction, the signal is maximized by tipping the spins completely into the transverse plane. This is accomplished by a $\pi/2$ RF pulse, which requires $\gamma B_1 \tau = \pi/2$, where τ is the duration of the RF pulse. Another useful RF pulse rotates spins by π radians. This can be used to invert spins. It also can be used to refocus transverse spins that have dephased due to B_0 field inhomogeneity. This is called a spin echo and is widely used in imaging.

NMR has been used for decades in chemistry. A complex molecule is placed in a strong, highly uniform magnetic field. Electrónic shielding produces microscopic field variations within the molecule so that geometrically isolated nuclei rotate about distinct fields. Each distinct magnetic environment produces a peak in the spectra of the received signal. The relative size of the spectral peaks gives the ratio of nuclei in each magnetic environment. Hence the NMR spectrum is extremely useful for elucidating molecular structure.

The NMR signal from a human is due predominantly to water protons. Since these protons exist in identical magnetic environments, they all resonate at the same frequency. Hence the NMR signal is simply proportional to the volume of the water. They key innovation for MRI is to impose spatial variations on the magnetic field to distinguish spins by their location. Applying a magnetic field gradient causes each region of the volume to oscillate at a distinct frequency. The most effective nonuniform field is a linear gradient where the field and the resulting frequencies vary linearly with distance along the object being studied. Fourier analysis of the signal obtains a map of the spatial distribution of spins. This argument is formalized below, where we derive the powerful *k*-space analysis of MRI [5,6].

k-Space Analysis of Data Acquisition

In MRI, we receive a volume integral from an array of oscillators. By ensuring that the phase "signature" of each oscillator is unique, one can assign a unique location to each spin and thereby reconstruct an image. During signal reception, the applied magnetic field points in the z direction. Spins precess in the xy plane at the Larmor frequency. Hence a spin at position $\mathbf{r} = (x,y,z)$ has a unique phase θ that describes its angle relative to the y axis in the xy plane:

$$\theta(\mathbf{r},t) = -\gamma \int_0^t B_z(\mathbf{r},\tau)\,d\tau \tag{10.1}$$

where $B_z(\mathbf{r},t)$ is the z component of the instantaneous, local magnetic flux density. This formula assumes there are no x and y field components.

A coil large enough to receive a time-varying flux uniformly from the entire volume produces an EMF proportional to

$$s(t) \propto \frac{d}{dt} \int_V M(\mathbf{r}) e^{-i\theta(\mathbf{r},t)} dr \tag{10.2}$$

where $M(\mathbf{r})$ represents the equilibrium moment density at each point $\mathbf{r}$.

The key idea for imaging is to superimpose a linear field gradient on the static field B_0. This field points in the direction z, and its magnitude varies linearly with a coordinate direction. For example, an x gradient points in the z direction and varies along the coordinate x. This is described by the vector field $xG_x\hat{\mathbf{z}}$, where $\hat{\mathbf{z}}$ is the unit vector in the z direction. In general, the gradient is $(xG_x + yG_y + zG_z)\,\hat{\mathbf{z}}$, which can be written compactly as the dot product $\mathbf{G}\cdot\mathbf{r}\,\hat{\mathbf{z}}$. These gradient field components can vary with time, so the total z field is

$$B_z(\mathbf{r},t) = B_0 + \mathbf{G}(t)\cdot\mathbf{r} \tag{10.3}$$

In the presence of this general time-varying gradient, the received signal is

$$s(t) \propto \frac{d}{dt} \int_V e^{-i\gamma B_0 t} M(\mathbf{r}) e^{-i\gamma \int_0^t \mathbf{G}(\tau)\cdot\mathbf{r}\,d\tau} dr \tag{10.4}$$

The center frequency γB_0 is always much larger than the bandwidth of the signal. Hence the derivative operation is approximately equivalent to multiplication by $-i\omega_0$. The signal is demodulated by the waveform $e^{i\gamma B_0 t}$ to obtain the "baseband" signal:

$$s(t) \propto -i\omega_0 \int_V M(\mathbf{r}) e^{-i\gamma \int_0^t \mathbf{G}(\tau)\cdot\mathbf{r}\,d\tau} dr \tag{10.5}$$

It will be helpful to define the term $\mathbf{k}(t)$:

$$\mathbf{k}(t) = \gamma \int_0^t \mathbf{G}(\tau)\,d\tau \tag{10.6}$$

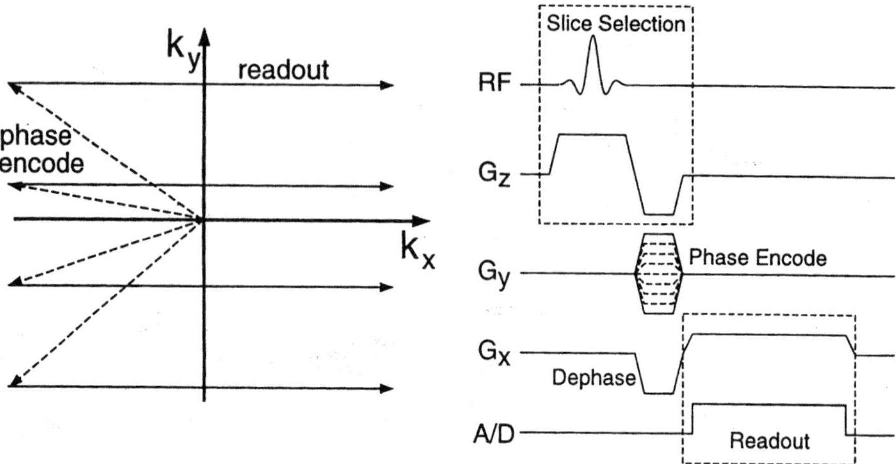

FIGURE 10.1 The drawing on the left illustrates the scanning pattern of the 2D Fourier transform imaging sequence. On the right is a plot of the gradient and RF waveforms that produce this pattern. Only four of the N_y horizontal k-space lines are shown. The phase-encode period initiates each acquisition at a different k_y and at $-k_x(\max)$. Data are collected during the horizontal traversals. After all N_y k-space lines have been acquired, a 2D FFT reconstructs the image. Usually 128 or 256 k_y lines are collected, each with 256 samples along k_x. The RF pulse and the z gradient waveform together restrict the image to a particular slice through the subject.

Then we can rewrite the received baseband signal as

$$S(t) \propto \int_V M(\mathbf{r}) e^{-i\mathbf{k}(t)\cdot\mathbf{r}}\, dr \tag{10.7}$$

which we can now identify as *the spatial Fourier transform of* $M(\mathbf{r})$ *evaluated at* $\mathbf{k}(t)$. That is, $S(t)$ scans the spatial frequencies of the function $M(\mathbf{r})$. This can be written explicitly as

$$S(t) \propto \mathcal{M}(\mathbf{k}(t)) \tag{10.8}$$

where $\mathcal{M}(\mathbf{k})$ is the three-dimensional Fourier transform of the object distribution $M(\mathbf{r})$. Thus we can view MRI with linear gradients as a "scan" of k-space or the spatial Fourier transform of the image. After the desired portion of k-space is scanned, the image $M(\mathbf{r})$ is reconstructed using an inverse Fourier transform.

2D Imaging. Many different gradient waveforms can be used to scan k-space and to obtain a desired image. The most common approach, called *two-dimensional Fourier transform imaging* (**2D FT**), is to scan through k-space along several horizontal lines covering a rectilinear grid in 2D k-space. See Fig. 10.1 for a schematic of the k-space traversal. The horizontal grid lines are acquired using 128 to 256 excitations separated by a time *TR*, which is determined by the desired contrast, RF flip angle, and the T_1 of the desired components of the image. The horizontal-line scans through k-space are offset in k_y by a variable area y-gradient pulse, which happens before data acquisition starts. These variable offsets in k_y are called *phase encodes* because they affect the phase of the signal rather than the frequency. Then for each k_y phase encode, signal is acquired while scanning horizontally with a constant x gradient.

Resolution and Field of View. The fundamental image characteristics of resolution and field of view (FOV) are completely determined by the characteristics of the k-space scan. The extent of the coverage of k-space determines the resolution of the reconstructed image. The resolution is inversely proportional to the highest spatial frequency acquired:

$$\frac{1}{\Delta x} = \frac{k_x(\max)}{\pi} = \frac{\gamma G_x T}{2\pi} \tag{10.9}$$

$$\frac{1}{\Delta y} = \frac{k_y(\max)}{\pi} = \frac{\gamma G_y T_{\text{phase}}}{\pi} \tag{10.10}$$

where G_x is the readout gradient amplitude and T is the readout duration. The time T_{phase} is the duration of the phase-encode gradient G_y. For proton imaging on a 1.5-T imaging system, a typical gradient strength is $G_x = 1$ G/cm. The signal is usually read for about 8 ms. For water protons, $\gamma = 26{,}751$ rad/s/G, so the maximum excursion in k_x is about 21 rad/mm. Hence we cannot resolve an object smaller than 0.3 mm in width. From this one might be tempted to improve the resolution dramatically using very strong gradients or very long readouts. But there are severe practical obstacles, since higher resolution increases the scan time and also degrades the image SNR.

In the phase-encode direction, the k-space data are sampled discretely. This discrete sampling in k-space introduces replication in the image domain [7]. If the sampling in k-space is finer than 1/FOV, then the image of the object will not fold back on itself. When the k-space sampling is coarser than 1/FOV, the image of the object does fold back over itself. This is termed *aliasing*. Aliasing is prevented in the readout direction by the sampling filter.

Perspective. For most imaging systems, diffraction limits the resolution. That is, the resolution is limited to the wavelength divided by the angle subtended by the receiver aperture, which means that the ultimate resolution is approximately the wavelength itself. This is true for imaging systems based on optics, ultrasound, and x-rays (although there are other important factors, such as quantum noise, in x-ray).

MRI is the only imaging system for which the resolution is independent of the wavelength. In MRI, the wavelength is often many meters, yet submillimeter resolution is routinely achieved. The basic reason is that no attempt is made to focus the radiation pattern to the individual pixel or voxel (volume element), as is done in all other imaging modalities. Instead, the gradients create spatially varying magnetic fields so that individual pixels emit unique waveform signatures. These signals are decoded and assigned to unique positions. An analogous problem is isolating the signals from two transmitting antenna towers separated by much less than a wavelength. Directive antenna arrays would fail because of diffraction spreading. However, we can distinguish the two signals if we use the a priori knowledge that the two antennas transmit at different frequencies. We can receive both signals with a wide-angle antenna and then distinguish the signals through frequency-selective filtering.

SNR Considerations. The signal strength is determined by the EMF induced from each voxel due to the processing moments. The magnetic moment density is proportional to the polarizing field B_0. Recall that the EMF is proportional to the rate of change of the coil flux. The derivative operation multiplies the signal by the Larmor frequency, which is proportional to B_0, so the received signal is proportional to B_0^2 times the volume of the voxel V_v.

In a well-designed MRI system, the dominant noise source is due to thermally generated currents within the conductive tissues of the body. These currents create a time-varying flux which induces noise voltages in the receiver coil. Other noise sources include the thermal noise from the antenna and from the first amplifier. These subsystems are designed so that the noise is negligible compared with the noise from the patient. The noise received is determined by the total volume seen by the antenna pattern V_n and the effective resistivity and temperature of the conductive tissue. One can show [8] that the standard deviation of the noise from conductive tissue varies linearly with B_0. The noise is filtered by an integration over the total acquisition time T_{acq}, which effectively attenuates the noise standard deviation by $\sqrt{T_{acq}}$. Therefore, the SNR varies as

$$\text{SNR} \propto \frac{B_0^2 V_v}{B_0 V_n / \sqrt{T_{acq}}} = B_0 \sqrt{T_{acq}} \left(V_v / V_n \right) \tag{10.11}$$

The noise volume V_n is the effective volume based on the distribution of thermally generated currents. For example, when imaging a spherical object of radius r, the noise standard deviation varies as $r^{5/2}$ [9]. The effective resistance depends strongly on the radius because currents near the outer radius contribute more to the noise flux seen by the receiver coil.

To significantly improve the SNR, most systems use *surface coils*, which are simply small coils that are just big enough to see the desired region of the body. Such a coil effectively maximizes the voxel-volume to noise-volume ratio. The noise is significantly reduced because these coils are sensitive to currents from a smaller part of the body. However, the field of view is somewhat limited, so "phased arrays" of small coils are now being offered by the major manufacturers [10]. In the phased array, each coil sees a small noise volume, while the combined responses provide the wide coverage at a greatly improved SNR.

Fast Imaging. The 2D FT scan of k-space has the disadvantage that the scan time is proportional to the number of phase encodes. It is often advantageous to trade off SNR for a shorter scan time. This is especially true when motion artifacts dominate thermal noise. To allow for a flexible trade-off of SNR for imaging time, more than a single line in k-space must be covered in a single excitation. The most popular approach, called *echo-planar imaging* (EPI), traverses k-space back and forth on a single excitation pulse. The k-space trajectory is drawn in Fig. 10.2.

It is important that the trade-off be flexible so that one can maximize the imaging time given the motion constraints. For example, patients can hold their breath for about 12 s. So a scan of 12 s duration gives the best SNR given the breath-hold constraint. The EPI trajectory can be *interleaved* to take full advantage of the breath-hold interval. If each acquisition takes about a second, 12 interleaves can be collected. Each interleaf acquires every 12th line in k-space.

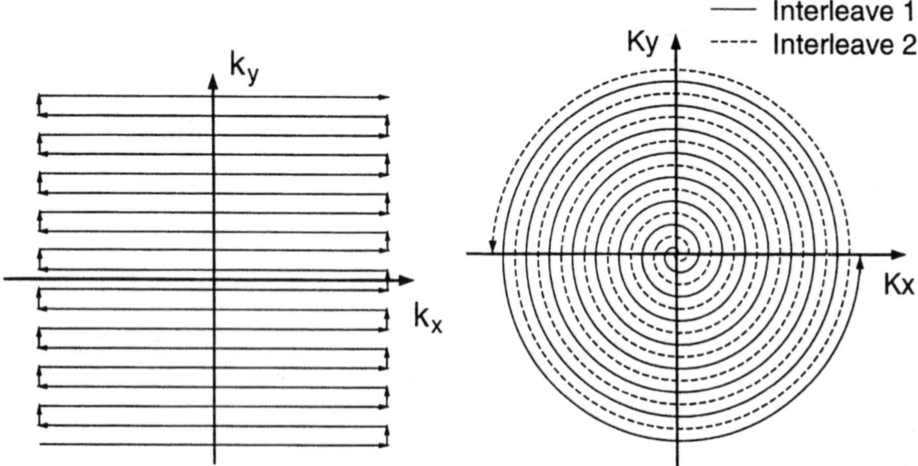

FIGURE 10.2 Alternative methods for the rapid traversal of k-space. On the left is the echo planar trajectory. Data are collected during the horizontal traversals. When all N_y horizontal lines in k-space have been acquired, the data are sent to a 2D FFT to reconstruct the image. On the right is an interleaved spiral trajectory. The data are interpolated to a 2D rectilinear grid and then Fourier transformed to reconstruct the image. These scanning techniques allow for imaging within a breath hold.

Another trajectory that allows for a flexible trade-off between scan time and SNR is the spiral trajectory. Here the trajectory starts at the origin in *k*-space and spirals outward. Interleaving is accomplished by rotating the spirals. Figure 10.2 shows two interleaves in a spiral format. Interleaving is very helpful for reducing the hardware requirements (peak amplitude, peak slew rate, average dissipation, etc.) for the gradients amplifiers. For reconstruction, the data are interpolated to a 2D rectilinear grid and then Fourier-transformed. Our group has found spiral imaging to be very useful for imaging coronary arteries within a breath-hold scan [11]. The spiral trajectory is relatively immune to artifacts due to the motion of blood.

Contrast Mechanisms

The tremendous clinical utility of MRI is due to the great variety of mechanisms that can be exploited to create image contrast. If magnetic resonance images were restricted to water density, MRI would be considerably less useful, since most tissues would appear identical. Fortunately, many different MRI contrast mechanisms can be employed to distinguish different tissues and disease processes.

The primary contrast mechanisms exploit *relaxation* of the magnetization. The two types of relaxations are termed spin-lattice relaxation, characterized by a relaxation time T_1, and spin-spin relaxation, characterized by a relaxation time T_2.

Spin-lattice relaxation describes the rate of recovery of the z component of magnetization toward equilibrium after it has been disturbed by RF pulses. The recovery is given by

$$M_z(t) = M_0\left(1 - e^{-t/T_1}\right) + M_z(0)e^{-t/T_1} \tag{10.12}$$

where M_0 is the equilibrium magnetization. Differences in the T_1 time constant can be used to produce image contrast by exciting all magnetization and then imaging before full recovery has been achieved. This is illustrated on the left in Fig. 10.3. An initial $\pi/2$ RF pulse destroys all the longitudinal magnetization. The plots show the recovery of two different T_1 components. The short T_1 component recovers faster and produces more signal. This gives a T_1-weighted image.

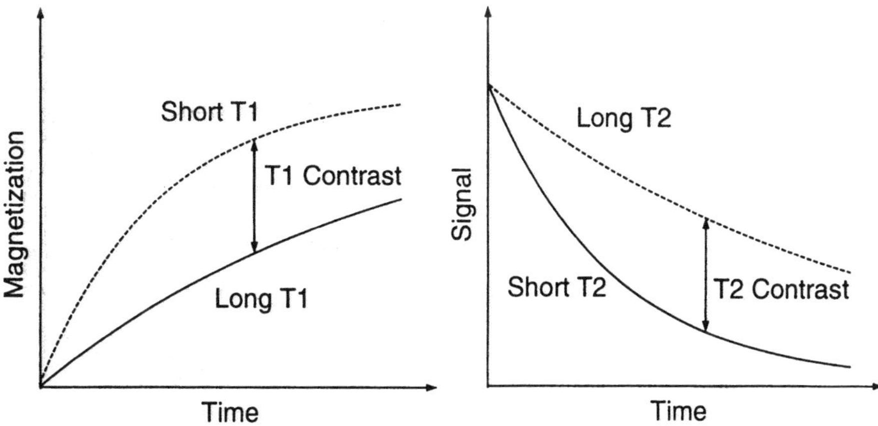

FIGURE 10.3 The two primary MRI contrast mechanisms, T_1 and T_2. T_1, illustrated on the left, describes the rate at which the equilibrium M_{zk} magnetization is restored after it has been disturbed. T_1 contrast is produced by imaging before full recovery has been obtained. T_2, illustrated on the right, describes the rate at which the MRI signal decays after it has been created. T_2 contrast is produced by delaying data acquisition, so shorter T_2 components produce less signal.

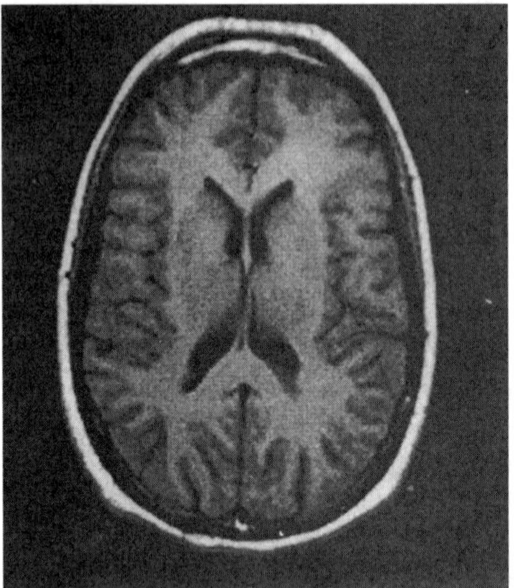
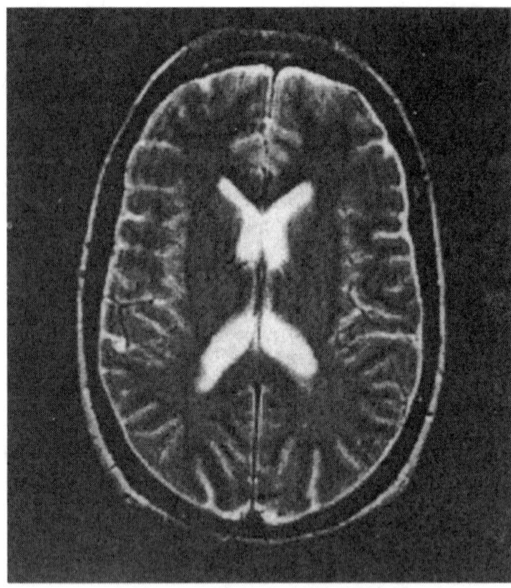

FIGURE 10.4 Example images of a normal volunteer demonstrating T_1 contrast on the left and T_2 contrast on the right.

Spin-spin relaxation describes the rate at which the NMR signal decays after it has been created. The signal is proportional to the transverse magnetization and is given by

$$M_{xy}(t) = M_{xy}(0)e^{-t/T_2} \tag{10.13}$$

Image contrast is produced by delaying the data acquisition. The decay of two different T_2 species is plotted on the right in Fig. 10.3. The signal from the shorter T_2 component decays more rapidly, while that of the longer T_2 component persists. At the time of data collection, the longer T_2 component produces more signal. This produces a T_2-weighted image.

Figure 10.4 shows examples of these two basic types of contrast. These images are of identical axial sections through the brain of a normal volunteer. The image of the left was acquired with an imaging method that produces T_1 contrast. The very bright ring of subcutaneous fat is due to its relatively short T_1. White matter has a shorter T_1 than gray matter, so it shows up brighter in this image. The image on the right was acquired with an imaging method that produces T_2 contrast. Here the cerebrospinal fluid in the ventricles is bright due to its long T_2. White matter has a shorter T_2 than gray matter, so it is darker in this image.

There are many other contrast mechanisms that are important in MRI. Different chemical species have slightly different resonant frequencies, and this can be used to image one particular component. It is possible to design RF and gradient waveforms so that the image shows only moving spins. This is of great utility in MR angiography, allowing the noninvasive depiction of the vascular system. Another contrast mechanism is called T_2^*. This relaxation parameter is useful for functional imaging. It occurs when there is a significant spread of Larmor frequencies within a voxel. The superposition signal is attenuated faster than T_2 due to destructive interference between the different frequencies.

In addition to the intrinsic tissue contrast, artificial MRI contrast agents also can be introduced. These are usually administered intravenously or orally. Many different contrast mechanisms can be exploited, but the most popular agents decrease both T_1 and T_2. One agent approved for clinical use is gadolinium DPTA. Decreasing T_1 causes faster signal recovery and a higher signal on a T_1-weighted image. The contrast-enhanced regions then show up bright relative to the rest of the image.

Defining Terms

Gyromagnetic ratio γ: An intrinsic property of a nucleus. It determines the Larmor frequency through the relation $\omega_0 = -\gamma B_0$.

***k*-space:** The reciprocal of object space, *k*-space describes MRI data acquisition in the spatial Fourier transform coordinate system.

Larmor frequency ω_0: The frequency of precession of the spins. It depends on the product of the applied flux density B_0 and on the gyromagnetic ratio γ. The Larmor frequency is $\omega_0 = -\gamma B_0$.

Magnetization *M*: The macroscopic ensemble of nuclear moments. The moments are induced by an applied magnetic field. At body temperatures, the amount of magnetization is linearly proportional ($M_0 = 4 \times 10^{-9} H_0$) to the applied magnetic field.

Precession: The term used to describe the motion of the magnetization about an applied magnetic field. The vector locus traverses a cone. The precession frequency is the frequency of the magnetization components perpendicular to the applied field. The precession frequency is also called the *Larmor frequency* ω_0.

Spin echo: The transverse magnetization response to a π RF pulse. The effects of field inhomogeneity are refocused at the middle of the spin echo.

Spin-lattice relaxation T_1: The exponential rate constant describing the decay of the *z* component of magnetization toward the equilibrium magnetization. Typical values in the body are between 300 and 3000 ms.

Spin-spin relaxation T_2: The exponential rate constant describing the decay of the transverse components of magnetization (M_x and M_y).

Spins M: Another name for magnetization.

2D FT: A rectilinear trajectory through *k*-space. This popular acquisition scheme requires several (usually 128 to 256) excitations separated by a time *TR*, which is determined by the desired contrast, RF flip angle, and the T_1 of the desired components of the image.

References

1. Lauterbur PC. 1973. Nature 242:190.
2. Evens RG, Evens JRG. 1991. AJR 157:603.
3. Bloch F, Hansen WW, Packard ME. 1946. Phys Rev 70:474.
4. Bloch F. 1946. Phys Rev 70:460.
5. Twieg DB. 1983. Med Phys 10:610.
6. Ljunggren S. 1983. J Magn Reson 54:338.
7. Bracewell RN. 1978. The Fourier Transform and Its Applications. New York, McGraw-Hill.
8. Hoult DI, Lauterbur PC. 1979. J Magn Reson 34:425.
9. Chen CN, Hoult D. 1989. Biomedical Magnetic Resonance Technology. New York, Adam Hilger.
10. Roemer PB, Edelstein WA, Hayes CE, et al. 1990. Magn Reson Med 16:192.
11. Meyer CH, Hu BS, Nishimura DG, Macovski A. 1992. Magn Reson Med 28(2):202.

10.2 Hardware/Instrumentation

John Schenck

This section describes the basic components and the operating principles of MRI scanners. Although scanners capable of making diagnostic images of the human internal anatomy through the use of magnetic resonance imaging (MRI) are now ubiquitous devices in the radiology departments of hospitals in the U.S. and around the world, as recently as 1980 such scanners were available only in a handful of research institutions. Whole-body superconducting magnets became available in the early 1980s and greatly increased the clinical acceptance of this new imaging modality. Market research data indicate that between

1980 and 1996 more than 100 million clinical MRI scans were performed worldwide. By 1996 more than 20 million MRI scans were being performed each year.

MRI scanners use the technique of nuclear magnetic resonance (NMR) to induce and detect a very weak radiofrequency signal that is a manifestation of nuclear magnetism. The term *nuclear magnetism* refers to weak magnetic properties that are exhibited by some materials as a consequence of the nuclear spin that is associated with their atomic nuclei. In particular, the proton, which is the nucleus of the hydrogen atom, possesses a nonzero nuclear spin and is an excellent source of NMR signals. The human body contains enormous numbers of hydrogen atoms—especially in water (H_2O) and lipid molecules. Although biologically significant NMR signals can be obtained from other chemical elements in the body, such as phosphorus and sodium, the great majority of clinical MRI studies utilize signals originating from protons that are present in the lipid and water molecules within the patient's body.

The patient to be imaged must be placed in an environment in which several different magnetic fields can be simultaneously or sequentially applied to elicit the desired NMR signal. Every MRI scanner utilizes a strong static field magnet in conjunction with a sophisticated set of gradient coils and radiofrequency coils. The gradients and the radiofrequency components are switched on and off in a precisely timed pattern, or pulse sequence. Different pulse sequences are used to extract different types of data from the patient. MR images are characterized by excellent contrast between the various forms of soft tissues within the body. For patients who have no ferromagnetic foreign bodies within them, MRI scanning appears to be perfectly safe and can be repeated as often as necessary without danger [Shellock and Kanal, 1998]. This provides one of the major advantages of MRI over conventional x-ray and computed tomographic (CT) scanners. The NMR signal is not blocked at all by regions of air or bone within the body, which provides a significant advantage over ultrasound imaging. Also, unlike the case of nuclear medicine scanning, it is not necessary to add radioactive tracer materials to the patient.

Fundamentals of MRI Instrumentation

Three types of magnetic fields—main fields or static fields (B_2), gradient fields, an radiofrequency (RF) fields (B_1)—are required in MRI scanners. In practice, it is also usually necessary to use coils or magnets that produce shimming fields to enhance the spatial uniformity of the static field B_0. Most MRI hardware engineering is concerned with producing and controlling these various forms of magnetic fields. The ability to construct NMR instruments capable of examining test tube-sized samples has been available since shortly after World War II. The special challenge associated with the design and construction of medical scanners was to develop a practical means of scaling these devices up to sizes capable of safely and comfortably accommodating an entire human patient. Instruments capable of human scanning first became available in the late 1970s. The successful implementation of MRI requires a two-way flow of information between analog and digital formats (Fig. 10.5). The main magnet, the gradient and RF coils, and the gradient and RF power supplies operate in the analog domain. The digital domain is centered on a general-purpose computer (Fig. 10.6) that is used to provide control information (signal timing and amplitude) to the gradient and RF amplifiers, to process time-domain MRI signal data returning from the receiver, and to drive image display and storage systems. The computer also provides miscellaneous control functions, such as permitting the operator to control the position of the patient table.

Static Field Magnets

The main field magnet [Thomas, 1993] is required to produce an intense and highly uniform, static magnetic field over the entire region to be imaged. To be useful for imaging purposes, this field must be extremely uniform in space and constant in time. In practice, the spatial variation of the main field of a whole-body scanner must be less than about 1 to 10 parts per million (ppm) over a region approximately 40 cm in diameter. To achieve these high levels of homogeneity requires careful attention to magnet design and to manufacturing tolerances. The temporal drift of the field strength is normally required to be less than 0.1 ppm/h.

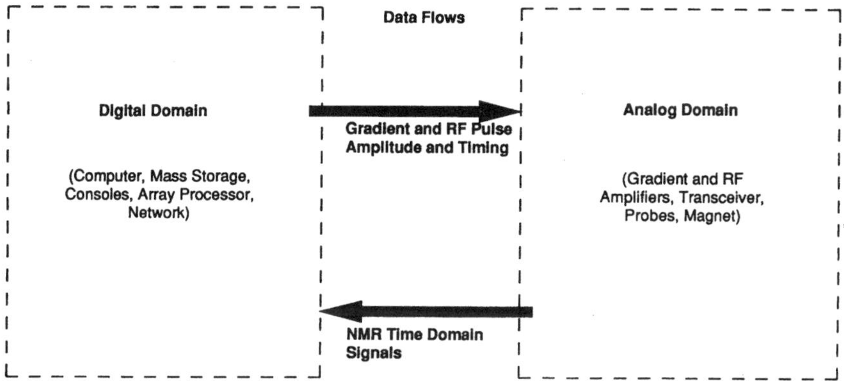

FIGURE 10.5 Digital and analog domains for MRI imaging. MRI involves the flow of data and system commands between these two domains. (Courtesy of WM Leue. Reprinted with permission from Schenck and Leue, 1991.)

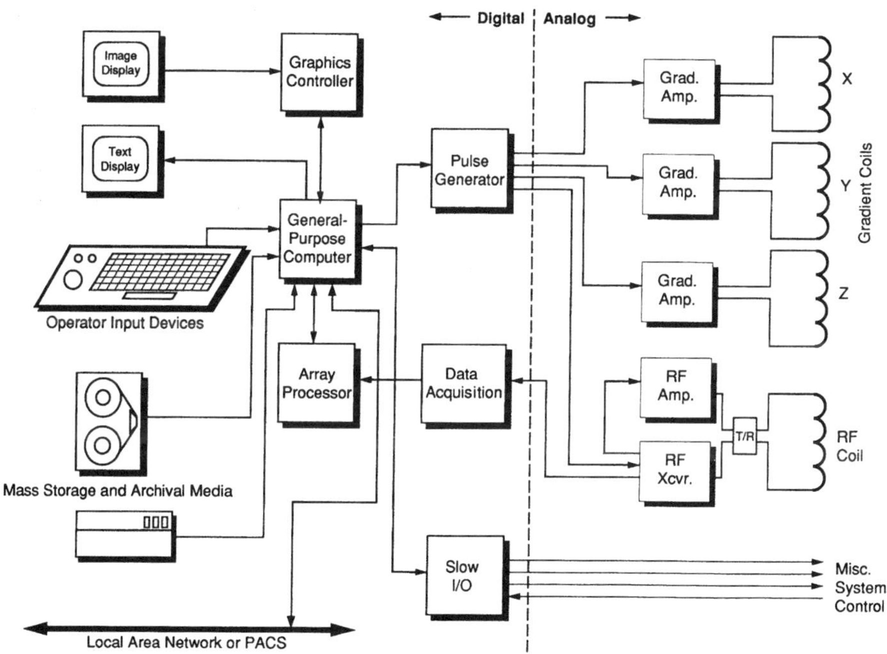

FIGURE 10.6 Block diagram for an MRI scanner. A general-purpose computer is used to generate the commands that control the pulse sequence and to process data during MR scanning. (Courtesy of WM Leue. Reprinted with permission from Schenck and Leue, 1991.)

Two units of magnetic field strength are now in common use. The gauss (G) has a long historical usage and is firmly embedded in the older scientific literature. The tesla (T) is a more recently adopted unit, but is a part of the SI system of units and, for this reason, is generally preferred. The tesla is a much larger unit than the gauss—1 T corresponds to 10,000 G. The magnitude of the earth's magnetic field is about 0.05 mT (5000 G). The static magnetic fields of modern MRI scanners arc most commonly in the range of from 0.5 to 1.5 T; useful scanners, however, have been built using the entire range from 0.02 to 8 T. The signal-to-noise ration (SNR) is the ratio of the NMR signal voltage to the ever-present noise voltages that arise within the patient and within the electronic components of the receiving system. The

SNR is one of the key parameters that determine the performance capabilities of a scanner. The maximum available SNR increases linearly with field strength. The improvement in SNR as the field strength is increased is the major reason that so much effort has gone into producing high-field magnets for MRI systems.

Magnetic fields can be produced by using either electric currents or permanently magnetized materials as sources. In either case, the field strength falls off rapidly away from the source, and it is not possible to create a highly uniform magnetic field on the outside of a set of sources. Consequently, to produce the highly uniform field required for MRI, it is necessary to more or less surround the patient with a magnet. The main field magnet must be large enough, therefore, to effectively surround the patient; in addition, it must meet other stringent performance requirements. For these reasons, the main field magnet is the most important determinant of the cost, performance, and appearance of an MRI scanner. Four different classes of main magnets—(1) permanent magnets, (2) electromagnets, (3) resistive magnets, and (4) superconducting magnets—have been used in MRI scanners.

Permanent Magnets and Electromagnets

Both these magnet types use magnetized materials to produce the field that is applied to the patient. In a permanent magnet, the patient is placed in the gap between a pair of permanently magnetized pole faces. Electromagnets use a similar configuration, but the pole faces are made of soft magnetic materials, which become magnetized only when subjected to the influence of electric current coils that are wound around them. Electromagnets, but not permanent magnets, require the use of an external power supply. For both types of magnets, the magnetic circuit is completed by use of a soft iron yoke connecting the pole faces to one another (Fig. 10.7). The gap between the pole faces must be large enough to contain the patient as well as the gradient and RF coils. The permanent magnet materials available for use in MRI scanners include high-carbon iron, alloys such as Alnico, ceramics such as barium ferrite, and rare earth alloys such as samarium cobalt.

Permanent magnet scanners have some advantages: They produce a relatively small fringing field and do not require power supplies. However, they tend to be very heavy (up to 100 tons) can produce only

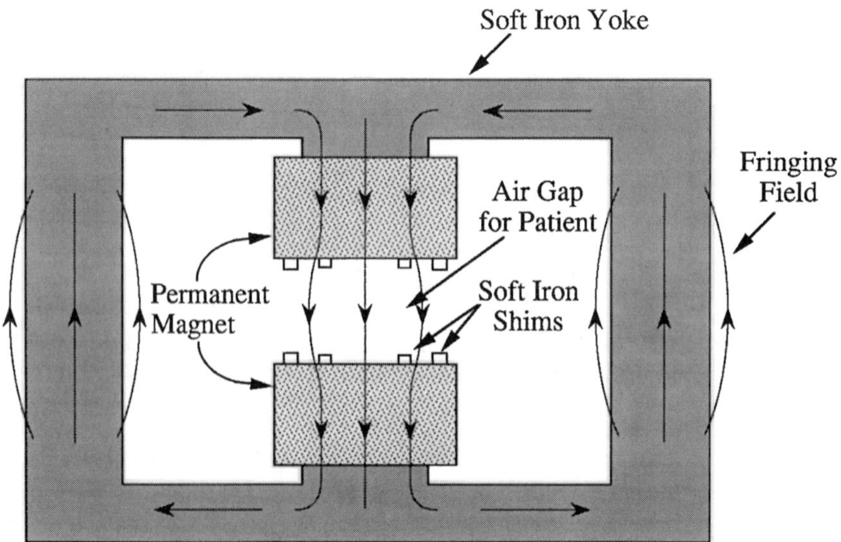

FIGURE 10.7 Permanent magnet. The figure shows a schematic cross section of a typical permanent magnet configuration. Electromagnets have a similar construction but are energized by current-carrying coils wound around the iron yoke. Soft magnetic shims are used to enhance the homogeneity of the field. (Reprinted with permission from Schenck and Leue, 1991.)

relatively low fields—on the order of 0.3 T or less. They are also subject to temporal field drift caused by temperature changes. If the pole faces are made from an electrically conducting material, eddy currents induced in the pole faces by the pulsed gradient fields can limit performance as well. A recently introduced alloy of neodymium, boron, and iron (usually referred to as *neodymium iron*) has been used to make lighter-weight permanent magnet scanners.

Resistive Magnets

The first whole-body scanners, manufactured in the late 1970s and early 1980s, used four to six large coils of copper or aluminum wire surrounding the patient. These coils are energized by powerful (40 to 100 kW) direct-current (dc) power supplies. The electrical resistance of the coils leads to substantial joule heating, and the use of cooling water flowing through the coils is necessary to prevent overheating. The heat dissipation increases rapidly with field strength, and it is not feasible to build resistive magnets operating at fields much higher than 0.15 to 0.3 T. At present, resistive magnets are seldom used except for very low field strength (0.02 to 0.06 T) applications.

Superconducting Magnets

Since the early 1980s, the use of cryogenically cooled superconducting magnets [Wilson, 1983] has been the most satisfactory solution to the problem of producing the static magnet field for MRI scanners. The property of exhibiting absolutely no electrical resistance near absolute zero has been known as an exotic property of some materials since 1911. Unfortunately, the most common of these materials, such as lead, tin, and mercury, exhibit a phase change back to the normal state at relatively low magnetic field strengths and cannot be used to produce powerful magnetic fields. In the 1950s, a new class of materials (type II superconductors) was discovered. These materials retain the ability to carry loss-free electric currents in very high fields. One such material, an alloy of niobium and titanium, has been used in most of the thousands of superconducting whole-body magnets that have been constructed for use in MRI scanners (Fig. 10.8). The widely publicized discovery in 1986 of another class of materials which remain superconducting at much higher temperatures than any previously known material has not yet led to any material capable of carrying sufficient current to be useful in MRI scanners.

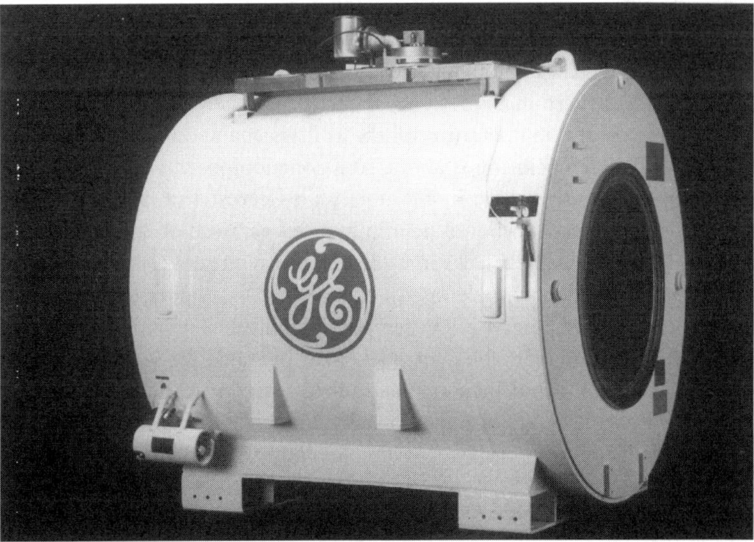

FIGURE 10.8 Superconducting magnet. This figure shows a 1.5-T whole-body superconducting magnet. The nominal warm bore diameter is 1 m. The patient to be imaged, as well as the RF and gradient coils, are located within this bore. (Courtesy of General Electric Medical Systems. Reprinted with permission from Schenck and Leue, 1991.)

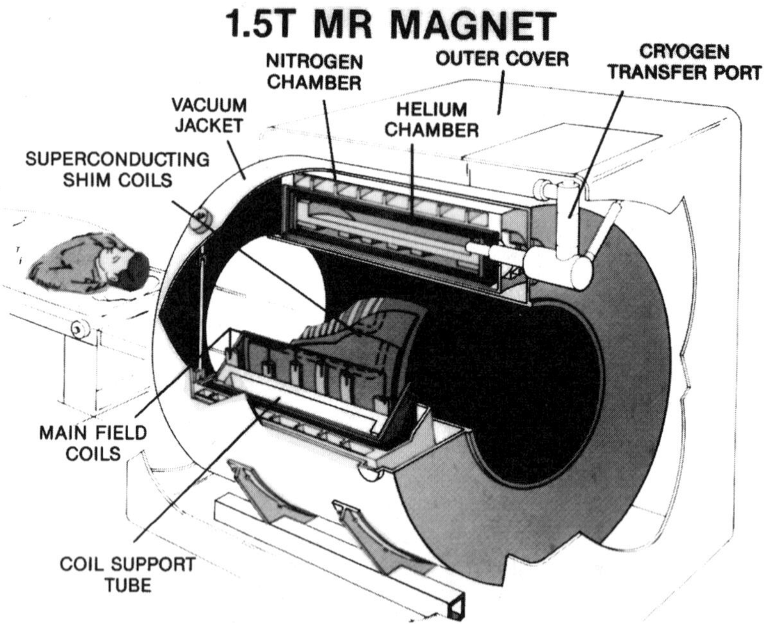

FIGURE 10.9 Schematic drawing of a superconducting magnet. The main magnet coils and the superconducting shim coils are maintained at liquid helium temperature. A computer-controlled table is used to advance the patient into the region of imaging. (Reprinted with permission from Schenck and Leue, 1991.)

Figure 10.9 illustrates the construction of a typical superconducting whole-body magnet. In this case, six coils of superconducting wire are connected in a series and carry an intense current—on the order of 200 A—to produce the 1.5-T magnetic field at the magnet's center. The diameter of the coils is about 1.3 m, and the total length of wire is about 65 km (40 miles). The entire length of this wire must be without any flaws—such as imperfect welds—that would interrupt the superconducting properties. If the magnet wire has no such flaws, the magnet can be operated in the persistent mode—that is, once the current is established, the terminals may be connected together, and a constant persistent current flow indefinitely so long as the temperature of the coils is maintained below the superconducting transition temperature. This temperature is about 10 K for niobium–titanium wire. The coils are kept at this low temperature by encasing them in a double-walled cryostat (analogous to a Thermos bottle) that permits them to be immersed in liquid helium at a temperature of 4.2 K. The gradual boiling of liquid helium caused by inevitable heat leaks into the cryostat requires that the helium be replaced on a regular schedule. Many magnets now make use of cryogenic refrigerators that reduce or eliminate the need for refilling the liquid helium reservoir. The temporal stability of superconducting magnets operating in the persistent mode is truly remarkable—magnets have operated for years completely disconnected from power supplies and maintained their magnetic field constant to within a few parts per million. Because of their ability to achieve very strong and stable magnetic field strengths without undue power consumption, superconducting magnets have become the most widely used source of the main magnetic fields for MRI scanners.

Magnetic Field Homogeneity

The necessary degree of spatial uniformity of the field can be achieved only by carefully placing the coils at specific spatial locations. It is well known that a single loop of wire will produce, on its axis, a field that is directed along the coil axis and that can be expressed as a sum of spherical harmonic fields. The first term in this sum is constant in space and represents the desired field that is completely independent of position. The higher-order terms represent contaminating field inhomogeneities that spoil the field uniformity. More than a century ago, a two-coil magnet system—known as the *Helmholtz pair*—was developed which produced a much more homogeneous field at its center than is produced by a single current loop. This design is based on the mathematical finding that when two coaxial coils of the same radius are separated by a distance equal to their radius, the first nonzero contaminating term in the harmonic expansion is of the fourth order. This results in an increased region of the field homogeneity, which, although it is useful in many applications, is far too small to be useful in MRI scanners. However, the principle of eliminating low-order harmonic fields can be extended by using additional coils. This is the method now used to increase the volume of field homogeneity to values that are useful for MRI. For example, in the commonly used six-coil system, it is possible to eliminate all the error fields through the 12th order.

In practice, manufacturing tolerances and field perturbations caused by extraneous magnetic field sources—such as steel girders in the building surrounding the magnet—produce additional inhomogeneity in the imaging region. These field imperfections are reduced by the use of shimming fields. One approach—*active shimming*—uses additional coils (either resistive coils, superconducting coils, or some of each) which are designed to produce a magnetic field corresponding to a particular term in the spherical harmonic expansion. When the magnet is installed, the magnetic field is carefully mapped, and the currents in the shim coils are adjusted to cancel out the terms in the harmonic expansion to some prescribed high order. The alternative approach—*passive shimming*—utilizes small permanent magnets that are placed at the proper locations along the inner walls of the magnet bore to cancel out contaminating fields. If a large object containing magnetic materials—such as a power supply—is moved in the vicinity of superconducting magnets, it may be necessary to reset the shimming currents or magnet locations to account for the changed pattern of field inhomogeneity.

Fringing Fields

A large, powerful magnet produces a strong magnetic field in the region surrounding it as well as in its interior. This fringing field can produce undesirable effects such as erasing magnetic tapes (and credit cards). It is also a potential hazard to people with implanted medical devices such as cardiac pacemakers. For safety purposes, it is general practice to limit access to the region where the fringing field becomes intense. A conventional boundary for this region is the "5-gaussline," which is about 10 to 12 m from the center of an unshielded 1.5-T magnet. Magnetic shielding—in the form of iron plates (passive shielding) or external coils carrying current in the direction opposite to the main coil current (active shielding)—is frequently used to restrict the region in which the fringing field is significant.

Gradient Coils

Three gradient fields, one each for the *x*, *y*, and *z* directions of a Cartesian coordinate system, are used to code position information into the MRI signal and to permit the imaging of thin anatomic slices [Thomas, 1993]. Along with their larger size, it is the use of these gradient coils that distinguishes MRI scanners from the conventional NMR systems such as those used in analytical chemistry. The direction of the static field, along the axis of the scanner, is conventionally taken as the z direction, and it is only the Cartesian component of the gradient field in this direction that produces a significant contribution to the resonant behavior of the nuclei. Thus, the three relevant gradient fields are $B_z = G_x X$, $B_z = G_y y$, and $B_z = G_z Z$. MRI scans are carried out by subjecting the spin system to a sequence of pulsed gradient and RF fields. Therefore, it is necessary to have three separate coils—one for each of the relevant gradient fields—each with its own power supply and under independent computer control. Ordinarily, the most practical method for constructing the gradient coils is to wind them on a cylindrical coil form that surrounds the patient and is located inside the warm bore of the magnet. The *z* gradient field can be produced by sets of circular coils wound around the cylinder with the current direction reversed for coils on the opposite sides of the magnet center ($z = 0$). To reduce deviations from a perfectly linear B_z gradient field, a spiral winding can be used with the direction of the turns reversed at $z = 0$ and the spacing

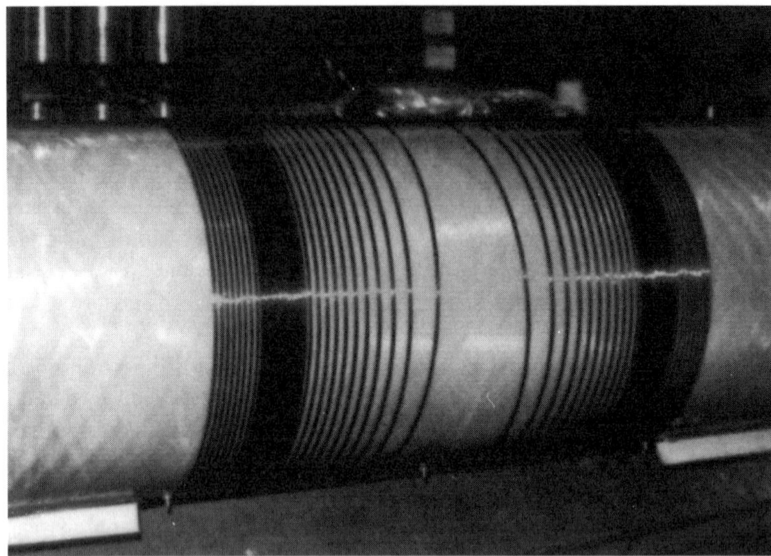

FIGURE 10.10 *Z*-gradient coil. The photograph shows a spiral coil wound on a cylindrical surface with an overwinding near the end of the coil. (Courtesy of R. J. Dobberstein, General Electric Medical Systems. Reprinted with permission from Schenck and Leue, 1991.)

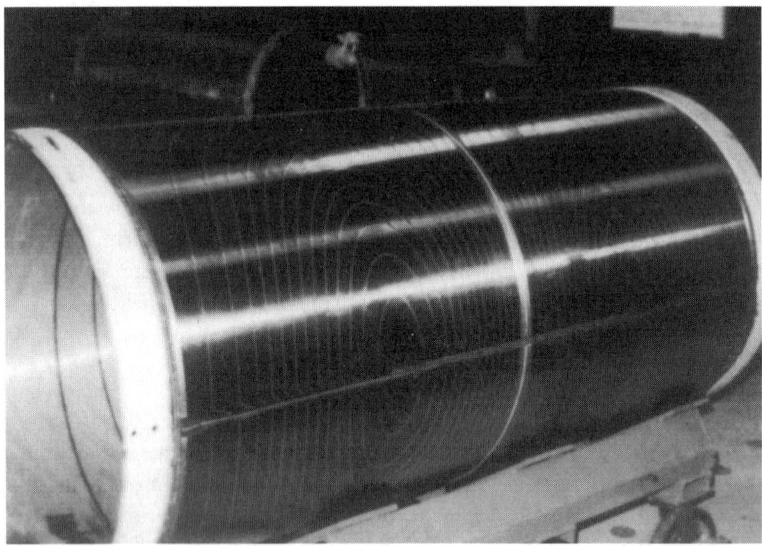

FIGURE 10.11 Transverse gradient coil. The photograph shows the outer coil pattern of an actively shielded transverse gradient coil. (Courtesy of R. J. Dobberstien, General Electric Medical Systems. Reprinted with permission from Schenck and Leue, 1991.)

between windings decreasing away from the coil center (Fig. 10.10). A more complex current pattern is required to produce the transverse (x and y) gradients. As indicated in Fig. 10.11, transverse gradient fields are produced by windings which utilize a four-quadrant current pattern.

The generation of MR images requires that a rapid sequence of time-dependent gradient fields (on all three axes) be applied to the patient. For example, the commonly used technique of spin-warp imaging [Edelstein et al., 1980] utilizes a slice-selection gradient pulse to select the spins in a thin (3 to 10 mm) slice of the patient and then applies readout and phase-encoding gradients in the two orthogonal directions to encode two-dimensional spatial information into the NMR signal. This, in turn, requires that the currents in the three gradient coils be rapidly switched by computer-controlled power supplies. The rate at which gradient currents can be switched is an important determinant of the imaging capabilities of a scanner. In typical scanners, the gradient coils have an electrical resistance of about 1 Ω and an inductance of about 1 mH, and the gradient field can be switched from 0 to 10 mT/m (1 G/cm) in about 0.5 ms. The current must be switched from 0 to about 100 A in this interval, and the instantaneous voltage on the coils, $L\, di/dt$, is on the order of 200 V. The power dissipation during the switching interval is about 20 kW. In more demanding applications, such as are met in cardiac MRI, the gradient field may be as high as 4 to 5 mT/m and switched in 0.2 ms or less. In this case, the voltage required during gradient switching is more than 1 kV. In many pulse sequences, the switching duty cycle is relatively low, and coil heating is not significant. However, fast-scanning protocols use very rapidly switched gradients at a high duty cycle. This places very strong demands on the power supplies, and it is often necessary to use water cooling to prevent overheating the gradient coils.

Radiofrequency Coils

Radiofrequency (RF) coils are components of every scanner and are used for two essential purposes—transmitting and receiving signals at the resonant frequency of the protons within the patient [Schenck, 1993]. The precession occurs at the Larmor frequency of the protons, which is proportional to the static magnetic field. At IT this frequency is 42.58 MHz. Thus in the range of field strengths currently used in whole-body scanners, 0.02 to 4 T, the operating frequency ranges from 0.85 to 170.3 MHz. For the commonly used 1.5-T scanners, the operating frequency is 63.86 MHz. The frequency of MRI scanners overlaps the spectral region used for radio and television broadcasting. As an example, the frequency of a 1.5-T scanner is within the frequency hand 60 to 66 MHz, which is allocated to television channel 3. Therefore, it is not surprising that the electronic components in MRI transmitter and receiver chains closely resemble corresponding components in radio and television circuitry. An important difference between MRI scanners and broadcasting systems is that the transmitting and receiving antennas of broadcast systems operate in the far field of the electromagnetic wave. These antennas are separated by many wavelengths. On the other hand, MRI systems operate in the near field, and the spatial separation of the sources and receivers is much less than a wavelength. In far-field systems, the electromagnetic energy is shared equally between the electric and magnetic components of the wave. However, in the near field of magnetic dipole sources, the field energy is almost entirely in the magnetic component of the electromagnetic wave. This difference accounts for the differing geometries that are most cost effective for broadcast and MRI antenna structures.

Ideally, the RF field is perpendicular to the static field, which is in the z direction. Therefore, the RF field can be linearly polarized in either the x or y direction. However, the most efficient RF field results from quadrature excitation, which requires a coil that is capable of producing simultaneous x and y fields with a 90° phase shift between them. Three classes of RF coils—body coils, head coils, and surface coils — are commonly used in MRI scanners. These coils are located in the space between the patient and the gradient coils. Conducting shields just inside the gradient coils are used to prevent electromagnetic coupling between the RF coils and the rest of the scanner. Head and body coils are large enough to surround the legion being imaged and are designed to produce an RF magnetic field that is uniform across the region to be imaged. Body coils are usually constructed on cylindrical coil forms and have a large enough diameter (50 to 60 cm) to entirely surround the patient's body. Coils are designed only for head imaging (Fig. 10.12) have a smaller diameter (typically 28 cm). Surface coils are smaller coils designed to image a restricted region of the patient's anatomy. They come in a wide variety of shapes and sizes. Because they can be closely applied to the region of interest, surface coils can provide SNR advantages over head and body coils for localized regions, but because of their asymmetric design, they do not have uniform sensitivity.

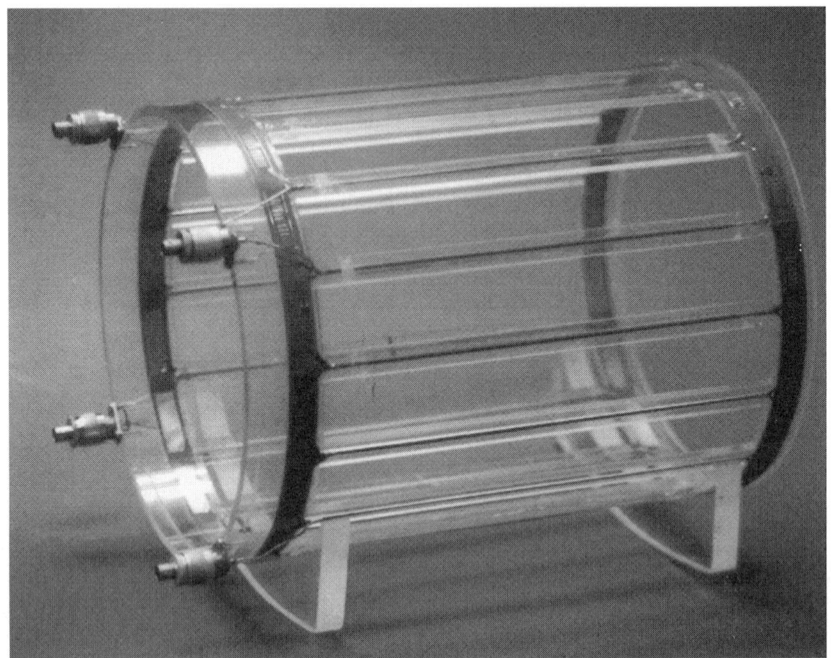

FIGURE 10.12 Birdcage resonator. This is a head coil designed to operate in a 4-T scanner at 170 MHz. Quadrature excitation and receiver performance are achieved by using two adjacent ports with a 90° phase shift between them. (Reprinted with permission from Schenck and Leue, 1991.)

A common practice is to use separate coils for the transmitter and receiver functions. This permits the use of a large coil—such as the body coil—with a uniform excitation pattern as the transmitter and a small surface coil optimized to the anatomic region—such as the spine—being imaged. When this two-coil approach is used, it is important to provide for electronically decoupling of the two coils because they are tuned at the same frequency and will tend to have harmful mutual interactions.

Digital Data Processing

A typical scan protocol calls for a sequence of tailored RF and gradient pulses with duration controlled in steps of 0.1 ms. To achieve sufficient dynamic range in control of pulse amplitudes, 12- to 16-bit digital-to-analog converters are used. The RF signal at the Larmor frequency (usually in the range from 1 to 200 MHz) is mixed with a local oscillator to produce a baseband signal which typically has a bandwidth of 16 to 32 kHz. The data-acquisition system must digitize the baseband signal at the Nyquist rate, which requires sampling the detected RF signal at a rate one digital data point every 5 to 20 ms. Again, it is necessary to provide sufficient dynamic range. Analog-to-digital converters with 16 to 18 bits are used to produce the desired digitized signal data. During the data acquisition, information is acquired at a rate on the order of 800 kilobytes per second, and each image can contain up to a megabyte of digital data. The array processor (AP) is a specialized computer that is designed for the rapid performance of specific algorithms, such as the fast Fourier transform (FFT), which are used to convert the digitized time-domain data to image data. Two-dimensional images are typically displayed as 256 × 128, 256 × 256, or 512 × 512 pixel arrays. The images can be made available for viewing within about 1 s after data acquisition. Three-dimensional imagining data, however, require more computer processing, and this results in longer delays between acquisition and display.

A brightness number, typically containing 16 bits of gray-scale information, is calculated for each pixel element of the image, and this corresponds to the signal intensity originating in each voxel of the object. To make the most effective use of the imaging information, sophisticated display techniques, such as multi-image displays, rapid sequential displays (cine loop), and three-dimensional renderings of anatomic surfaces, are frequently used. These techniques are often computationally intensive and require the use of specialized computer hardware. Interfaces to microprocessor-based workstations are frequently used to provide such additional display and analysis capabilities. MRI images are available as digital data; therefore, there is considerable utilization of local arena networks (LANs) to distribute information throughout the hospital, and long-distance digital transmission of the images can be used for purposes of teleradiology.

Current Trends in MRI

At present, there is a substantial effort directed at enhancing the capabilities and cost-effectiveness of MR imagers. The activities include efforts to reduce the cost of these scanners, improve image quality, reduce scan times, and increase the number of useful clinical applications. Examples of these efforts include the development of high-field scanners, the advent of MRI-guided therapy, and the development of niche scanners that are designed for specific anatomical and clinical applications. Scanners have been developed that are dedicated to low-field imaging of the breast and other designs are dedicated to orthopedic applications such as the knees, wrists, and elbows. Perhaps the most promising incipient application of MRI is to cardiology. Scanners are now being developed to permit studies of cardiac wall motion, cardiac perfusion, and the coronary arteries in conjunction with cardiac stress testing. These scanners emphasize short magnet configurations to permit close monitoring and interaction with the patient, and high strength rapidly switched gradient fields.

Conventional spin-warp images typically require several minutes to acquire. The fast spin echo (FSE) technique can reduce this to the order of 20 s, and gradient-echo techniques can reduce this time to a few seconds. The echo-planar technique (EPI) [Cohen and Weisskoff, 1991; Wehrli, 1990] requires substantially increased gradient power and receiver bandwidth but can produce images in 40 to 60 ms. Scanners with improved gradient hardware that are capable of handling higher data-acquisition rates are now available.

For most of the 1980s and 1990s, the highest field strength commonly used in MRI scanners was 1.5 T. To achieve better SNRs, higher-field scanners, operating at fields up to 4 T, were studied experimentally. The need for very high-field scanners has been enhanced by the development of functional brain MRI. This technique utilizes magnetization differences between oxygenated and deoxygenated hemoglobin, and this difference is enhanced at higher field strengths. It has now become possible to construct 3- and 4-T and even 8-T [Robitaille et al., 1998], whole-body scanners of essentially the same physical size (or footprint) as conventional 1.5-T systems. Along with the rapidly increasing clinical interest in functional MRI, this is resulting in a considerable increase in the use of high-field systems.

For the first decade or so after their introduction, MRI scanners were used almost entirely to provide diagnostic information. However, there is now considerable interest in systems capable of performing image-guided, invasive surgical procedures. Because MRI is capable of providing excellent soft-tissue contrast and has the potential for providing excellent positional information with submillimeter accuracy, it can be used for guiding biopsies and stereotactic surgery. The full capabilities of MRI-guided procedures can only be achieved if it is possible of provide surgical access to the patient simultaneously with the MRI scanning. This has led to the development of new system designs, including the introduction of a scanner with a radically modified superconducting magnet system that permits the surgeon to operate at the patient's side within the scanner (Fig. 10.13) [Schenck et al., 1995; Black et al., 1997]. These systems have led to the introduction of magnetic field-compatible surgical instruments, anesthesia stations, and patient monitoring equipment [Schenck, 1996].

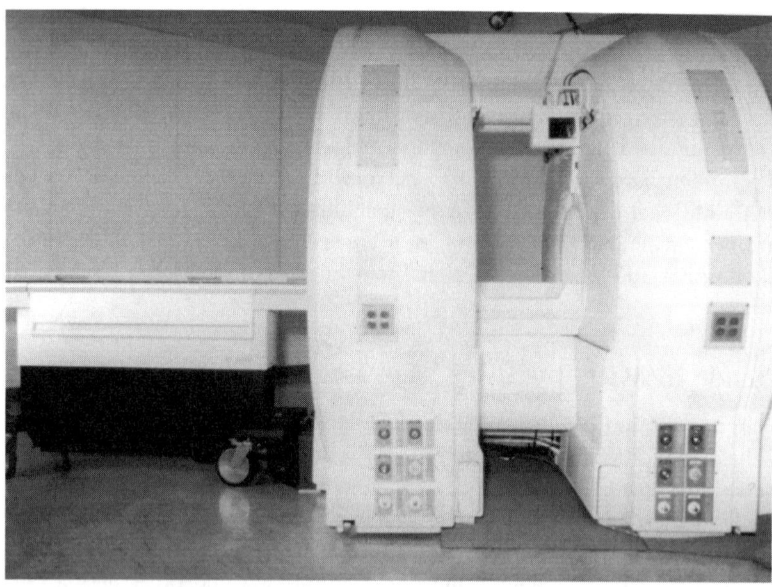

FIGURE 10.13 Open magnet for MRI-guided therapy. This open-geometry superconducting magnet provides a surgion with direct patient access and the ability to interactively control the MRI scanner. This permits imaging to be performed simultaneously with surgical interventions.

Defining Terms

Bandwidth: The narrow frequency range, approximately 32 kHz, over which the MRI signal is transmitted. The bandwidth is proportional to the strength of the readout gradient field.

Echo-planar imaging (EPI): A pulse sequence used to produce very fast MRI scans. EPI times can be as short as 50 ms.

Fast Fourier transform (FFT): A mathematical technique used to convert data sampled from the MRI signal into image data. This version of the Fourier transform can be performed with particular efficiency on modern array processors.

Gradient coil: A coil designed to produce a magnetic field for which the field component B varies linearly with position. Three gradient coils, one each for the x, y, and z directions, are required for MRI. These coils are used to permit slice selection and to encode position information into the MRI signal.

Larmor frequency: The rate at which the magnetic dipole moment of a particle precesses in an applied magnetic field. It is proportional to the field strength and is 42.58 MHz for protons in a 1-T magnetic field.

Magnetic resonance imaging (MRI): A technique for obtaining images of the internal anatomy based on the use of nuclear magnetic resonance signals. During the 1980s, it became a major modality for medical diagnostic imaging.

Nuclear magnetic resonance (NMR): A technique for observing and studying nuclear magnetism. It is based on partially aligning the nuclear spins by use of a strong, static magnetic field, stimulating these spins with a radiofrequency field oscillating at the Larmor frequency, and detecting the signal that is induced at this frequency.

Nuclear magnetism: The magnetic properties arising from the small magnetic dipole moments possessed by the atomic nuclei of some materials. This form of magnetism is much weaker than the more familiar form that originates from the magnetic dipole moments of the atomic electrons.

Pixel: A single element or a two-dimensional array of image data.

Pulse sequence: A series of gradient and radiofrequency pulses used to organize the nuclear spins into a pattern that encodes desired imaging information into the NMR signal.

Quadrature excitation and detection: The use of circularly polarized, rather than linearly polarized, radiofrequency fields to excite and detect the NMR signal. It provides a means of reducing the required excitation power by $^1/_2$ and increasing the signal-to-noise ratio by 2.

Radiofrequency (RF) **coil:** A coil designed to excite and/or detect NMR signals. These coils can usually be tuned to resonate at the Larmor frequency of the nucleus being studied.

Spin: The property of a particle, such as an electron or nucleus, that leads to the presence of an intrinsic angular momentum and magnetic moment.

Spin-warp imagining: The pulse sequence used in the most common method of MRI imaging. It uses a sequence of gradient field pulses to encode position information into the NMR signal and applies Fourier transform mathematics to this signal to calculate the image intensity value for each pixel.

Static magnetic field: The field of the main magnet that is used to magnetize the spins and to drive their Larmor precession.

Voxel: The volume element associated with a pixel. The voxel volume is equal to the pixel area multiplied by the slice thickness.

References

Black PMcL, Moriarty T, Alexander E III, et al. 1997. Development and implementation of intraoperative magnetic resonance imaging and its neurosurgical applications. Neurosurgery 41:831.

Cohen MS, Weisskoff RM. 1991. Ultra-fast imaging. Magn Reson Imaging 9:1.

Edelstein WA, Hutchinson JMS, Johnson G, Redpath TW. 1980. Spin-warp NMR imaging and applications to human whole-body imaging. Phys Med Biol 25:751.

Robitaille P-ML, Abdujalil AM, Kangarlu A, et al. 1998. Human magnetic resonance imaging at 8 T. NMR Biomed 11:263.

Schenck JF, Leue WM. 1996. Instrumentation: Magnets coils and hardware. In SW Atlas (ed), Magnetic Resonance Imaging of the Brain and Spine, 2nd ed. pp 1–27. Philadelphia, Lippincott-Raven.

Schenck JF. 1993. Radiofrequency coils: Types and characteristics. In MI Bronskill, P Sprawls (eds), The Physics of MRI, Medical Physics Monograph No. 21, pp 98–134. Woodbury, NY, American Institute of Physics.

Schenck JF, Jolesz A, Roemer PB, et al. 1995. Superconducting open-configuration MR imaging system for image-guided therapy. Radiology 195:805.

Schenck JF. 1996. The role of magnetic susceptibility in magnetic resonance imaging: magnetic field compatibility of the first and second kinds. Med Phys 23:815.

Shellock FG, Kanal E. 1998. Magnetic Resonance: Bioeffects, Safety and Patient Management, 2nd ed. Philadelphia, Saunders.

Thomas SR. 1993. Magnet and gradient coils: Types and characteristics. In MJ Bronskill, P Sprawls (eds), The Physics of MRI, Medical Physics Monograph No. 21, pp 56–97. Woodbury, NY, American Institute of Physics.

Wehrli FW. 1990. Fast scan magnetic resonance: Principles and applications. Magn Reson Q 6:165.

Wilson MN. 1983. Superconducting Magnets. Oxford, Clarendon Press.

Further Information

There are several journals devoted entirely to MR imaging. These include *Magnetic Resonance in Medicine*, *JMRI—Journal of Magnetic Resonance Imaging*, and *NMR in Biomedicine*, all three of which are published by Wiley-Liss, 605 Third Avenue, New York, NY 10158. Another journal dedicated to this field is *Magnetic Resonance Imaging* (Elsevier Publishing, 655 Avenue of the Americas, New York, NY 10010). The clinical aspects of MRI are covered extensively in *Radiology* (Radiological Society of North America, 2021 Spring

Road, Suite 600, Oak Brook, IL 60521), *The American Journal of Radiology* (American Roentgen Ray Society, 1891 Preston White Drive, Reston, VA 20191), as well as in several other journals devoted to the practice of radiology. There is a professional society, now known as the International Society for Magnetic Resonance in Medicine (ISMRM), devoted to the medical aspects of magnetic resonance. The main offices of this society are at 2118 Milvia, Suite 201, Berkeley, CA 94704. This society holds an annual meeting that includes displays of equipment and the presentation of approximately 2800 technical papers on new developments in the field. The annual *Book of Abstracts* of this meeting provides an excellent summary of current activities in the field. Similarly, the annual meeting of the Radiological Society of North America (RSNA) provides extensive coverage of MRI that is particularly strong on the clinical applications. The RSNA is located at 2021 Spring Road, Suite 600, Oak Brook, IL 60521.

Several book-length accounts of MRI instrumentation and techniques are available. *Biomedical Magnetic Resonance Technology* (Adam Higler, Bristol, 1989) by Chen and D. I. Hoult, *The Physics of MRI* (Medical Physics Monograph 21, American Institute of Physics, Woodbury, NY, 1993), edited by M. J. Bronskill and P. Sprawls, and *Electromagnetic Analysis and Design in Magnetic Resonance Imaging* (CRC Press, Boca Raton, FL, 1998) by J. M. Jin each contain thorough accounts of instrumentation and the physical aspects of MRI. There are many books that cover the clinical aspects of MRI. Of particular interest are *Magnetic Resonance Imaging*, 3rd edition (Mosby, St. Louis, 1999), edited by D. D. Stark and W. G. Bradley, Jr., and *Magnetic Resonance Imaging of the Brain and Spine*, 2nd ed. (Lippincott-Raven, Philadelphia, 1996), edited by S. W. Atlas.

10.3 Functional MRI

Kenneth K. Kwong and David A. Chesler

Functional magnetic resonance imaging (fMRI), a technique that images intrinsic blood signal change with magnetic resonance (MR) imagers, has in the last 3 years become one of the most successful tools used to study blood flow and perfusion in the brain. Since changes in neuronal activity are accompanied by focal changes in cerebral blood flow (CBF), blood volume (CBV), blood oxygenation, and metabolism, these physiologic changes can be used to produce functional maps of mental operations.

There are two basic but completely different techniques used in fMRI to measure CBF. The first one is a classic steady-state perfusion technique first proposed by Detre et al. [1], who suggested the use of saturation or inversion of incoming blood signal to quantify absolute blood flow [1–5]. By focusing on blood flow *change* and not just steady-state blood flow, Kwong et al. [6] were successful in imaging brain visual functions associated with quantitative perfusion change. There are many advantages in studying blood flow change because many common baseline artifacts associated with MRI absolute flow techniques can be subtracted out when we are interested only in changes. And one obtains adequate information in most functional neuroimaging studies with information of flow change alone.

The second technique also looks at change of a blood parameter—blood oxygenation *change* during neuronal activity. The utility of the change of blood oxygenation characteristics was strongly evident in Turner's work [7] with cats with induced hypoxia. Turner et al. found that with hypoxia, the MRI signal from the cats' brains went down as the level of deoxyhemoglobin rose, a result that was an extension of an earlier study by Ogawa et al. [8,9] of the effect of deoxyhemoglobin on MRI signals in animals' veins. Turner's new observation was that when oxygen was restored, the cats' brain signals climbed up and went *above* their baseline levels. This was the suggestion that the vascular system overcompensated by bringing more oxygen, and with more oxygen in the blood, the MRI signal would rise beyond the baseline.

Based on Turner's observation and the perfusion method suggested by Detre et al., movies of human visual cortex activation utilizing both the perfusion and blood oxygenation techniques were successfully acquired in May 1991 (Fig. 10.14) at the Massachusetts General Hospital with a specially equipped superfast 1.5-T system known as an *echo-planar imaging* (EPI) MRI system [10]. fMRI results using intrinsic blood contrast were first presented in public at the Tenth Annual Meeting of the Society of Magnetic Resonance in Medicine in August 1991 [6,11]. The visual cortex activation work was carried

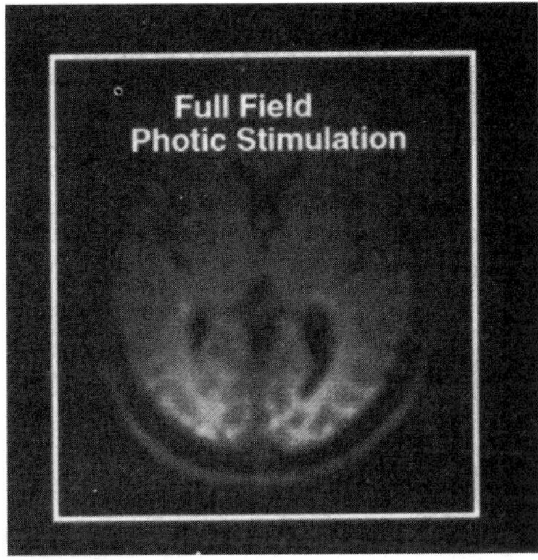

FIGURE 10.14 Functional MR image demonstrating activation of the primary visual cortex (V1). Image acquired on May 9, 1991 with a blood oxygenation–sensitive MRI gradient-echo (GE) technique.

out with flickering goggles, a photic stimulation protocol employed by Belliveau et al. [12] earlier to acquire the MRI functional imaging of the visual cortex with the injection of the contrast agent gadolinium-DTPA. The use of an external contrast agent allows the study of change in blood volume. The intrinsic blood contrast technique, sensitive to blood flow and blood oxygenation, uses no external contrast material. Early model calculation showed that signal due to blood perfusion change would only be around 1% above baseline, and the signal due to blood oxygenation change also was quite small. It was quite a pleasant surprise that fMRI results turned out to be so robust and easily detectable.

The blood oxygenation–sensitive MRI signal change, coined *blood oxygenation level dependent* (BOLD) by Ogawa et al. [8,9,13], is in general much larger than the MRI perfusion signal change during brain activation. Also, while the first intrinsic blood contrast fMRI technique was demonstrated with a superfast EPI MRI system, most centers doing fMRI today are only equipped with conventional MRI systems, which are really not capable of applying Detre's perfusion method. Instead, the explosive growth of MR functional neuroimaging [14–33] in the last 3 years relies mainly on the measurement of blood oxygenation change, utilizing a MR parameter called T_2^*. Both high speed echo planar (EPI) and conventional MR have now been successfully employed for functional imaging in MRI systems with magnet field strength ranging from 1.5 to 4.0 T.

Advances in Functional Brain Mapping

The popularity of fMRI is based on many factors. It is safe and totally noninvasive. It can be acquired in single subjects for a scanning duration of several minutes, and it can be repeated on the same subjects as many times as necessary. The implementation of the blood oxygenation–sensitive MR technique is universally available. Early neuroimaging, work focused on time-resolved MR topographic mapping of human primary visual (VI) (Figs. 10.15, 10.16), motor (MI), somatosensory (S1), and auditory (A1) cortices during task activation. Today, with BOLD technique combined with EPI, one can acquire 20 or more contiguous brain slices covering the whole head (3 × 3 mm in plane and 5 mm slice thickness) every 3 s for a total duration of several minutes. Conventional scanners can only acquire a couple of slices at a time. The benefits of whole-head imaging are many. Not only can researchers identify and test their hypotheses on known brain activation centers, they can also search for previously unknown or unsuspected sites. High resolution work done with EPI has a resolution of 1.5 × 1.5 mm in plane and a slice thickness of 3 mm. Higher spatial resolution has been reported in conventional 1.5-T MR systems [34].

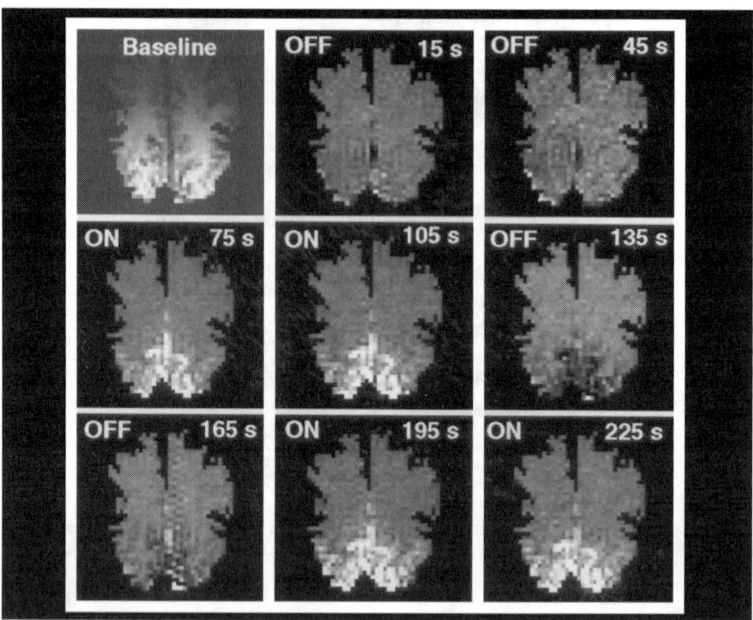

FIGURE 10.15 Movie of fMRI mapping of primary visual cortex (V1) activation during visual stimulation. Images are obliquely aligned along the calcarine fissures with the occipital pole at the bottom. Images were acquired at 3-s intervals using a blood oxygenation–sensitive MRI sequence (80 images total). A baseline image acquired during darkness (*upper left*) was subtracted from subsequent images. Eight of these subtraction images are displayed, chosen when the image intensities reached a steady-state signal level during darkness (OFF) and during 8-Hz photic stimulation (ON). During stimulation, local increases in signal intensity are detected in the posteromedial regions of the occipital lobes along the calcarine fissures.

Of note with Fig. 10.16 is that with blood oxygenation–sensitive MR technique, one observers an undershoot [6,15,35] in signal in V1 when the light stimulus is turned off. The physiologic mechanism underlying the undershoot is still not well understood.

The data collected in the last 3 years have demonstrated that fMRI maps of the visual cortex correlate well with known retinotopic organization [24,36]. Higher visual regions such as V5/MT [37] and motor-cortex organization [6,14,27,38] have been explored successfully. Preoperative planning work (Fig. 10.17) using motor stimulation [21,39,40] has helped neurosurgeons who attempt to preserve primary areas from tumors to be resected. For higher cognitive functions, several fMRI language studies have already demonstrated known language-associated regions [25,26,41,42] (Fig. 10.18). There is more detailed modeling work on the mechanism of functional brain mapping by blood-oxygenation change [43–46]. Postprocessing techniques that would help to alleviate the serious problem of motion/displacement artifacts are available [47].

Mechanism

Flow-sensitive images show increased perfusion with stimulation, while blood oxygenation–sensitive images show changes consistent with an increase in venous blood oxygenation. Although the precise biophysical mechanisms responsible for the signal changes have yet to be determined, good hypotheses exist to account for our observations.

Two fundamental MRI relaxation rates, T_1 and T_2^*, are used to describe the fMRI signal. T_1 is the rate at which the nuclei approach thermal equilibrium, and perfusion change can be considered as an additional T_1 change. T_2^* represents the rate of the decay of MRI signal due to magnetic field inhomogeneities, and the change of T_2^* is used to measure blood-oxygenation change.

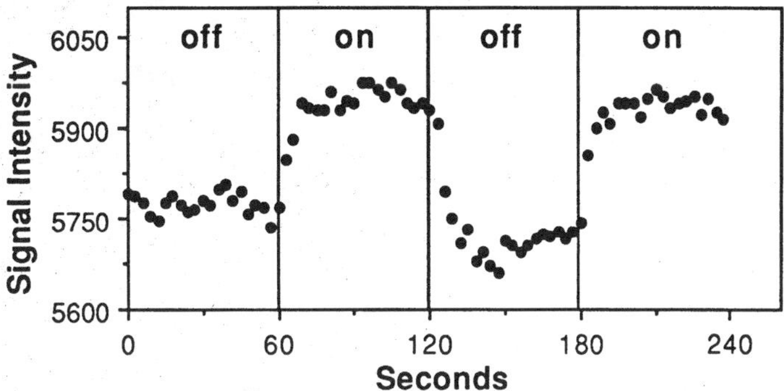

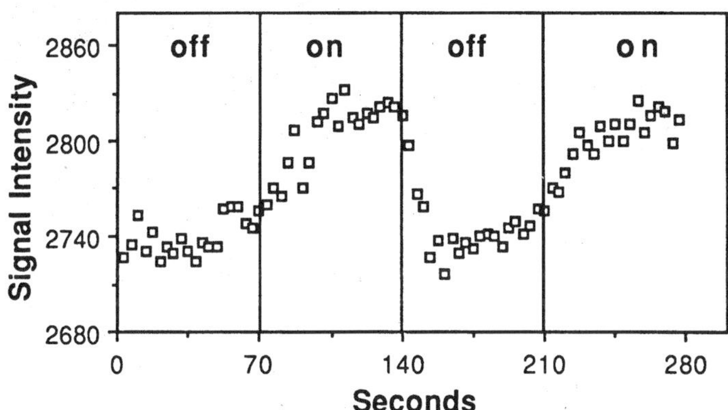

FIGURE 10.16 Signal intensity changes for a region of interest (~60 mm^2) within the visual cortex during darkness and during 8-Hz photic stimulation. Results using oxygenation-sensitive (*top graph*) and flow-sensitive (*bottom graph*) techniques are shown. The flow-sensitive data were collected once every 3.5 s, and the oxygenation-sensitive data were collected once every 3 s. Upon termination of photic stimulation, an undershoot in the oxygenation-sensitive signal intensity is observed.

T_2^* changes reflect the interplay between changes in cerebral blood flow, volume, and oxygenation. As hemoglobin becomes deoxygenated, it becomes more paramagnetic than the surrounding tissue [48] and thus creates a magnetically inhomogeneous environment. The observed *increased* signal on T_2^*-weighted images during activation reflects a decrease in deoxyhemoglobin content, i.e., an increase in venous blood oxygenation. Oxygen delivery, cerebral blood flow, and cerebral blood volume all increase with neuronal activation. Because CBF (and hence oxygen-delivery) changes exceed CBV changes by two to four times [49], while blood-oxygen extraction increases only slightly [50,51], the total paramagnetic blood deoxyhemoglobin content within brain tissue voxels will decrease with brain activation. The resulting decrease in the tissue-blood magnetic susceptibility difference leads to less intravoxel dephasing within brain tissue voxels and hence *increased* signal on T_2^*-weighted images [6,14,15,17]. These results independently confirm PET observations that activation-induced changes in blood flow and volume are accompanied by little or no increases in tissue oxygen consumption [50–52].

Since the effect of volume susceptibility difference $\Delta\chi$ is more pronounced at high field strength [53], higher-field imaging magnets [17] will increase the observed T_2^* changes.

Signal changes can also be observed on T_1-weighted MR images. The relationship between T_1 and regional blood flow was characterized by Detre et al. [1]:

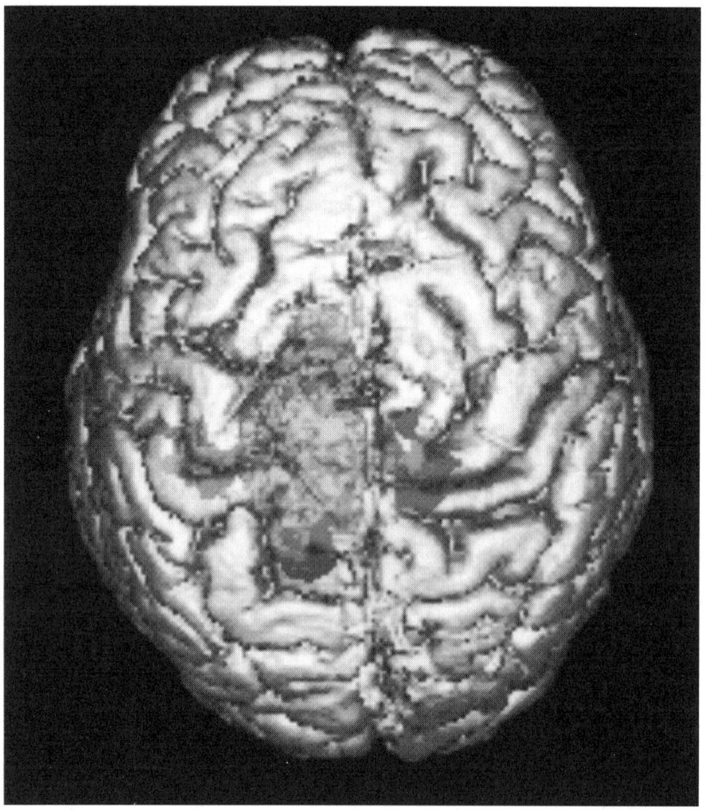

FIGURE 10.17 Functional MRI mapping of motor cortex for preoperative planning. This three-dimensional rendering of the brain represents fusion of functional and structural anatomy. Brain is viewed from the top. A tumor is shown in the left hemisphere, near the midline. The other areas depict sites of functional activation during movement of the right hand, right foot, and left foot. The right foot cortical representation is displaced by tumor mass effect from its usual location. (Courtesy of Dr. Brad Buchbinder.)

$$\frac{dM}{dt} = \frac{M_0 - M}{T_1} + fM_b - \frac{f}{\lambda}M \tag{10.14}$$

where M is tissue magnetization and M_b is incoming blood signal. M_0 is proton density, f is the flow in ml/gm/unit time, and λ is the brain-blood partition coefficient of water (~0.95 ml/gm). From this equation, the brain tissue magnetization M relaxes with an apparent T_1 time constant $T_{1\,\mathrm{app}}$ given by

$$\frac{f}{\lambda} = \frac{1}{T_{1\,\mathrm{app}}} - \frac{1}{T_1} \tag{10.15}$$

where the $T_{1\,\mathrm{app}}$ is the observed (apparent) longitudinal relaxation time with flow effects included. T_1 is the true tissue longitudinal relaxation time in the absence of flow. If we assume that the true tissue T_1 remains constant with stimulation, a change in blood flow Δf will lead to a change in the observed $T_{1\,\mathrm{app}}$:

$$\Delta\frac{1}{T_{1\,\mathrm{app}}} = \Delta\frac{f}{\lambda} \tag{10.16}$$

Thus the MRI signal change can be used to estimate the change in blood flow.

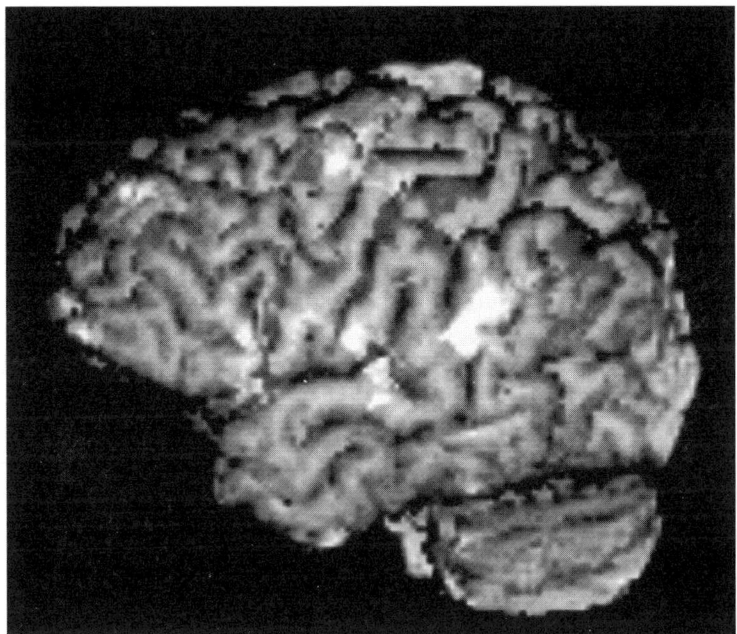

FIGURE 10.18 Left hemisphere surface rendering of functional data (EPI, gradient-echo, 10 oblique coronal slices extending to posterior sylvian fissure) and high-resolution anatomic image obtained on a subject (age 33 years) during performance of a same-different (visual matching) task of pairs of words or nonwords (false font strings). Foci of greatest activation for this study are located in dominant perisylvian cortex, i.e., inferior frontal gyrus (Broca's area), superior temporal gyrus (Wernicke's area), and inferior parietal lobule (angular gyrus). Also active in this task are sensorimotor cortex and prefrontal cortex. The perisylvian sites of activation are known to be key nodes in a left hemisphere language network. Prefrontal cortex probably plays a more general, modulatory role in attentional aspects of the task. Sensorimotor activation is observed in most language studies despite the absence of overt vocalization. (Courtesy of Dr. Randall Benson.)

From Eq. (10.14), if the magnetization of blood and tissue always undergoes a similar T_1 relaxation, the flow effect would be minimized. This is a condition that can be approximated by using a flow-nonsensitive T_1 technique inverting *all* the blood coming into the imaged slice of interest. This flow-nonsensitive sequence can be subtracted from a flow-sensitive T_1 technique to provide an index of CBF without the need of external stimulation [54,55] (Fig. 10.19). Initial results with tumor patients show that such flow-mapping techniques are useful for mapping out blood flow of tumor regions [55].

Other flow techniques under investigation include the continuous inversion of incoming blood at the carotid level [1] or the use of a single inversion pulse at the carotid level (EPIstar) inverting the incoming blood [56,57]. Compared with the flow-nonsensitive and flow-sensitive methods, the blood-tagging techniques at the carotid level are basically similar concepts except that the MRI signal of tagged blood is expected to be smaller by a factor that depends on the time it takes blood to travel from the tagged site to the imaged slice of interest [55]. The continuous-inversion technique also has a significant problem of magnetization transfer [1] that contaminates the flow signal with a magnetization transfer signal that is several times larger. On the other hand, the advantage of the continuous inversion is that it can under optimal conditions provide a flow contrast larger than all the other methods by a factor of e [55].

Problems and Artifacts in fMRI: The Brain-Vein Problem? The Brain-Inflow Problem?

The artifacts arising from large vessels pose serious problems to the interpretation of oxygenation sensitive fMRI data. It is generally believed that microvascular changes are specific to the underlying region of

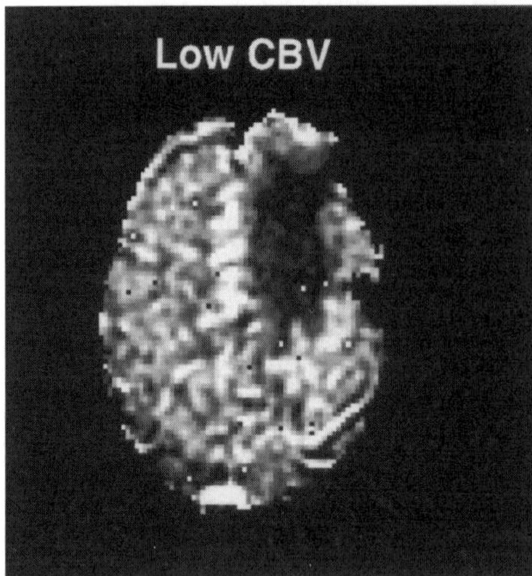

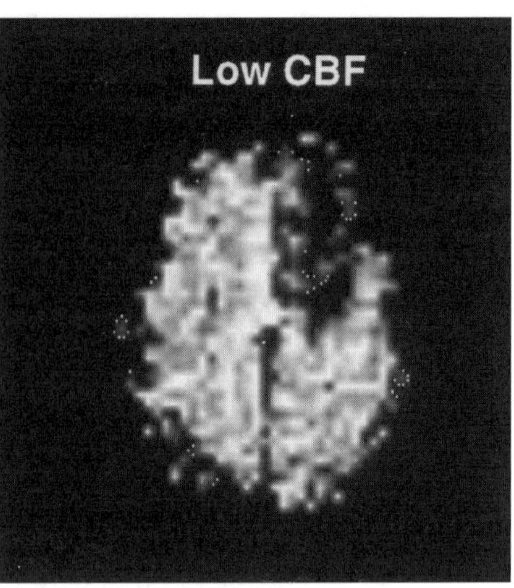

FIGURE 10.19 Functional MRI cerebral blood flow (CBF) index (*right*) of a low-flow brain tumor (dark region right of the midline) generated by the subtraction of a flow-nonsensitive image from a flow-sensitive image. This low-flow region matches well with a cerebral blood volume (CBV) map (*left*) of the tumor region generated by the injection of a bolus of MRI contrast agent Gd-DTPA, a completely different and established method to measure hemodynamics with MRI.

neuronal activation. However, MRI gradient echo (GE) is sensitive to vessels of all dimensions [46,58], and there is concern that macrovascular changes distal to the site of neuronal activity can be induced [20]. This has been known as the *brain-vein problem.* For laboratories not equipped with EPI, GE sensitive to variations in T_2^* and magnetic susceptibility are the only realistic sequences available for fMRI acquisition, so the problem is particularly acute.

In addition, there is a non-deoxyhemoglobin-related problem, especially acute in conventional MRI. This is the inflow problem of fresh blood that can be time-locked to stimulation [28,29,59]. Such nonparenchymal and macrovascular responses can introduce error in the estimate of activated volumes.

Techniques to Reduce the Large Vessel Problems

In dealing with the inflow problems, EPI has special advantages over conventional scanners. The use of long repetition times (2 to 3 s) in EPI significantly reduces the brain-inflow problem. Small-flip-angle methods in conventional MRI scanners can be used to reduce inflow effect [59]. Based on inflow modeling, one observes that at an angle smaller than the Ernst angle [60], the inflow effect drops much faster than the tissue signal response to activation. Thus one can effectively remove the inflow artifacts with small-flip-angle techniques.

A new exciting possibility is to add small additional velocity-dephasing gradients to suppress slow in-plane vessel flow [60,61]. Basically, moving spins lose signals, while stationary spins are unaffected. The addition of these velocity-dephasing gradients drops the overall MRI signal (Fig. 10.20). The hypothesis that large vessel signals are suppressed while tissue signals remain intact is a subject of ongoing research.

Another advantage with EPI is that another oxygenation-sensitive method such as the EPI T_2-weighted spin-echo (T2SE) is also available. T2SE methods are sensitive to the MRI parameter T_2, which is affected by microscopic susceptibility and hence blood oxygenation. Theoretically, T2SE methods are far less sensitive to large vessel signals [1,6,46,58]. For conventional scanners, T2SE methods take too long to perform and therefore are not practical options.

The flow model [1] based on T_1-weighted sequences and independent of deoxyhemoglobin is also not so prone to large vessel artifacts, since the T_1 model is a model of perfusion at the tissue level.

Based on the study of volunteers, the average T_2^*-weighted GE signal percentage change at V1 was $2.5 \pm 0.8\%$. The average oxygenation-weighted T2SE signal percentage change was $0.7 \pm 0.3\%$. The

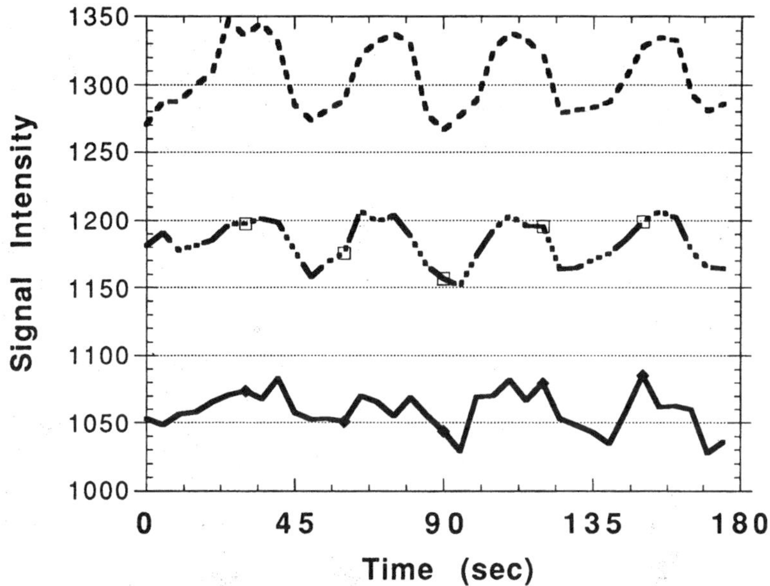

FIGURE 10.20 The curves represent time courses of MRI response to photic stimulation (off-on-off-on ...) with different levels of velocity-dephasing gradients turned on to remove MRI signals coming from the flowing blood of large vessels. The top curve had no velocity-dephasing gradients turned on. The bottom curve was obtained with such strong velocity-dephasing gradients turned on that all large vessel signals were supposed to have been eliminated. The middle curve represents a moderate amount of velocity-dephasing gradients, a trade-off between removing large vessel signals and retaining a reasonable amount of MRI signal to noise.

average perfusion-weighted and T_1-weighted MRI signal percentage change was 1.5 ± 0.5%. These results demonstrate that T2SE and T_1 methods, despite their ability to suppress large vessels, are not competitive with T_2^* effect at 1.5 T. However, since the microscopic effect detected by T2SE scales up with field strength [62], we expect the T2SE to be a useful sequence at high field strength such as 3 or 4 T. Advancing field strength also should benefit T_1 studies due to better signal-to-noise and to the fact that T_1 gets longer at higher field strength.

While gradient-echo sequence has a certain ambiguity when it comes to tissue versus vessels, its sensitivity at current clinical field strength makes it an extremely attractive technique to identify activation sites. By using careful paradigms that rule out possible links between the primary activation site and secondary sites, one can circumvent many of the worries of "signal from the primary site draining down to secondary sites." A good example is as follows: Photic stimulation activates both the primary visual cortex and the extrastriates. To show that the extrastriates are not just a drainage from the primary cortex, one can utilize paradigms that activate the primary visual cortex but not the extrastriate, and vice versa. There are many permutations of this [37]. This allows us to study the higher-order functions umambiguously even if we are using gradient-echo sequences.

The continuous advance of MRI mapping techniques utilizing intrinsic blood-tissue contrast promises the development of a functional human neuroanatomy of unprecedented spatial and temporal resolution.

References

1. Detre J, Leigh J, Williams D, Koretsky A. 1992. Magn Reson Med 23:37.
2. Williams DS, Detre JA, Leigh JS, Koretsky AP. 1992. Proc Natl Acad Sci USA 89:212.
3. Zhang W, Williams DS, Detre JA. 1992. Magn Reson Med 25:362.
4. Zhang W, Williams DS, Koretsky AP. 1993. Magn Reson Med 29:416.
5. Dixon WT, Du LN, Faul D, et al. 1986. Magn Reson Med 3:454.

6. Kwong KK, Belliveau JW, Chesler DA, et al. 1992. Proc Natl Acad Sci USA 89:5675.
7. Turner R, Le Bihan D, Moonen CT, et al. 1991. Magn Reson Med 22:159.
8. Ogawa S, Lee TM, Kay AR, Tank DW. 1990. Proc Natl Acad Sci USA 87:9868.
9. Ogawa S, Lee TM. 1990. Magn Reson Med 16:9.
10. Cohen MS, Weisskoff RM. 1991. Magn Reson Imaging 9:1.
11. Brady TJ, Society of Magnetic Resonance in Medicine, San Francisco, CA 2, 1991.
12. Belliveau JW, Kennedy DN Jr, McKinstry RC, et al. 1991. Science 254:716.
13. Ogawa S, Lee TM, Nayak AS, Glynn P. 1990. Magn Reson Med 14:68.
14. Bandettini PA, Wong EC, Hinks RS, et al. 1992. Magn Reson Med 25:390.
15. Ogawa S, Tank DW, Menon R, et al. 1992. Proc Natl Acad Sci USA 89:5951.
16. Frahm J, Bruhn H, Merboldt K, Hanicke W. 1992. J Magn Reson Imaging 2:501.
17. Turner R, Jezzard P, Wen H, et al. 1992. Society of Magnetic Resonance in Medicine Eleventh Annual Meeting, Berlin.
18. Blamire A, Ogawa S, Ugurbil K, et al. 1992. Proc Natl Acad Sci USA 89:11069.
19. Menon R, Ogawa S, Tank D, Ugurbil K. 1993. Magn Reson Med 30:380.
20. Lai S, Hopkins A, Haacke E, et al. 1993. Magn Reson Med 30:387.
21. Cao Y, Towle VL, Levin DN, et al. 1993. Society of Magnetic Resonance in Medicine Meeting.
22. Connelly A, Jackson GD, Frackowiak RSJ, et al. 1993. Radiology 125.
23. Kim SG, Ashe J, Georgopouplos AP, et al. 1993. J Neurophys 69:297.
24. Schneider W, Noll DC, Cohen JD. 1993. Nature 365:150.
25. Hinke RM, Hu X, Stillman AE, et al. 1993. Neurol Rep 4:675.
26. Binder JR, Rao SM, Hammeke TA, et al. 1993. Neurology (suppl 2):189.
27. Rao SM, Binder JR, Bandettini PA, et al. 1993. Neurology 43:2311.
28. Gomiscek G, Beisteiner R, Hittmair K, et al. 1993. MAGMA 1:109.
29. Duyn J, Moonen C, de Boer R, et al. 1993. Society of Magnetic Resonance in Medicine, 12th Annual Meeting, New York.
30. Hajnal JV, Collins AG, White SJ, et al. 1993. Magn Reson Med 30:650.
31. Hennig J, Ernst T, Speck O, et al. 1994. Magn Reson Med 31:85.
32. Constable RT, Kennan RP, Puce A, et al. 1994. Magn Reson Med 31:686.
33. Binder JR, Rao SM, Hammeke TA, et al. 1994. Ann Neurol 35:662.
34. Frahm J, Merboldt K, Hänicke W. 1993. Magn Reson Med 29:139.
35. Stern CE, Kwong KK, Belliveau JW, et al. 1992. Society of Magnetic Resonance in Medicine Annual Meeting, Berlin, Germany.
36. Belliveau JW, Kwong KK, Baker JR, et al. 1992. Society of Magnetic Resonance in Medicine Annual Meeting, Berlin, Germany.
37. Tootell RBH, Kwong KK, Belliveau JW, et al. 1993. Investigative Ophthalmology and Visual Science, p 813.
38. Kim S-G, Ashe J, Hendrich K, et al. 1993. Science 261:615.
39. Buchbinder BR, Jiang HJ, Cosgrove GR, et al. 1994. ASNR 162.
40. Jack CR, Thompson RM, Butts RK, et al. 1994. Radiology 190:85.
41. Benson RR, Kwong KK, Belliveau JW, et al. 1993. Soc Neurosci.
42. Benson RR, Kwong KK, Buchbinder BR, et al. 1994. Society of Magnetic Resonance, San Francisco.
43. Ogawa S, Menon R, Tank D, et al. 1993. Biophys J 64:803.
44. Ogawa S, Lee TM, Barrere B. 1993. Magn Reson Med 29:205.
45. Kennan RP, Zhong J, Gore JC. 1994. Magn Reson Med 31:9.
46. Weisskoff RM, Zuo CS, Boxerman JL, Rosen BR. 1994. Magn Reson Med 31:601.
47. Bandettini PA, Jesmanowicz A, Wong EC, Hyde JS. 1993. Magn Reson Med 30:161.
48. Thulborn KR, Waterton JC, Matthews PM, Radda GK. 1982. Biochim Biophys Acta 714:265.
49. Grubb RL, Raichle ME, Eichling JO, Ter-Pogossian MM. 1974. Stroke 5:630.
50. Fox PT, Raichle ME, 1986. Proc Natl Acad Sci USA 83:1140.

51. Fox PT, Raichle ME, Mintun MA, Dence C. 1988. Science 241:462.
52. Prichard J, Rothman D, Novotny E, et al. 1991. Proc Natl Acad Sci USA 88:5829.
53. Brooks RA, Di Chiro G. 1987. Med Phys 14:903.
54. Kwong K, Chesler D, Zuo C, et al. 1993. Society of Magnetic Resonance in Medicine, 12th Annual Meeting, New York, p 172.
55. Kwong KK, Chesler DA, Weisskoff RM, Rosen BR. 1994. Society of Magnetic Resonance, San Francisco.
56. Edelman R, Sievert B, Wielopolski P, et al. 1994. JMRI 4(P).
57. Warach S, Sievert B, Darby D, et al. 1994. JMRI 4(**P**):S8.
58. Fisel CR, Ackerman JL, Buxton RB, et al. 1991. Magn Reson Med 17:336.
59. Frahm J, Merboldt K, Hanicke W. 1993. Society of Magnetic Resonance in Medicine, 12th Annual Meeting, New York, p 1427.
60. Kwong KK, Chesler DA, Boxerman JL, et al. 1994. Society of Magnetic Resonance, San Francisco.
61. Song W, Bandettini P, Wong E, Hyde J. 1994. Personal communication.
62. Zuo C, Boxerman J, Weisskoff R. 1992. Society of Magnetic Resonance in Medicine, 11th Annual Meeting, Berlin, p 866.

10.4 Chemical-Shift Imaging: An Introduction to Its Theory and Practice

Xiaoping Hu, Wei Chen, Maqbool Patel, and Kamil Ugurbil

Over the past two decades, there has been a great deal of development in the application of nuclear magnetic resonance (NMR) to biomedical research and clinical medicine. Along with the development of magnetic resonance imaging [1], *in vivo* magnetic resonance spectroscopy (MRS) is becoming a research tool for biochemical studies of humans as well as a potentially more specific diagnostic tool, since it provides specific information on individual chemical species in living systems. Experimental studies in animals and humans have demonstrated that MRS can be used to study the biochemical basis of disease and to follow the treatment of disease.

Since biologic subjects (e.g., humans) are heterogeneous, it is necessary to spatially localize the spectroscopic signals to a well-defined volume or region of interest (VOI or ROI, respectively) in the intact body. Toward this goal, various localization techniques have been developed (see Ref. [2] for a recent review). Among these techniques, chemical-shift imaging (CSI) or spectroscopic imaging [3–6] is an attractive technique, since it is capable of producing images reflecting the spatial distribution of various chemical species of interest. Since the initial development of CSI in 1982 [3], further developments have been made to provide better spatial localization and sensitivity, and the technique has been applied to numerous biomedical problems.

In this section we will first present a qualitative description of the basic principles of chemical-shift imaging and subsequently present some practical examples to illustrate the technique. Finally, a summary is provided in the last subsection.

General Methodology

In an NMR experiment, the subject is placed in a static magnetic field B_0. Under the equilibrium condition, nuclear spins with nonzero magnetic moment are aligned along B_0, giving rise to an induced bulk magnetization. To observe the bulk magnetization, it is tipped to a direction perpendicular to B_0 (transverse plane) with a radiofrequency (RF) pulse that has a frequency corresponding to the resonance frequency of the nuclei. The resonance frequency is determined by the product of the gyromagnetic ratio of the nucleus γ and the strength of the static field, i.e., γB_0, and is called the *Larmor frequency.* The Larmor frequency also depends on the chemical environment of the nuclei, and this dependency gives rise to chemical shifts that allow one to identify different chemical species in an NMR spectrum. Upon excitation, the magnetization in the transverse plane (perpendicular to the main B_0 field direction) oscillates with the Larmor frequencies of all the different chemical species and induces a signal in a receiving RF coil; the signal is also termed the *free induction decay* (FID). The FID can be Fourier-transformed with respect to time to produce a spectrum in frequency domain.

In order to localize an NMR signal from an intact subject, spatially selective excitation and/or spatial encoding are usually utilized. Selective excitation is achieved as follows: In the excitation, an RF pulse with a finite bandwidth is applied in the presence of a linear static magnetic field gradient. With the application of the gradient, the Larmor frequency of spins depends linearly on the spatial location along the direction of the gradient. Consequently, only the spins in a slice whose resonance frequency falls into the bandwidth of the RF pulse are excited.

The RF excitation rotates all or a portion of the magnetization to the transverse plane, which can be detected by a receiving RF coil. Without spatial encoding, the signal detected is the integral of the signals over the entire excited volume. In CSI based on Fourier imaging, spatial discrimination is achieved by phase encoding. Phase encoding is accomplished by applying a gradient pulse after the excitation and before the data acquisition. During the gradient pulse, spins precess at Larmor frequencies that vary linearly along the direction of the gradient and accrue a phase proportional to the position along the phase-encoding gradient as well as the strength and the duration of the gradient pulse. This acquired spatially encoded phase is typically expressed as $\vec{k}\cdot\vec{r} = \int \gamma\, \vec{g}(t)\cdot\vec{r}\, dt$, where γ is the gyromagnetic ratio; $\vec{r}$ is the vector designating spatial location; $\vec{g}(t)$ defines the magnitude, the direction, and the time dependence of the magnetic field gradient applied during the phase-encoding; and the integration is performed over time when the phase-encoding gradient is on. Thus, in one-dimensional phase encoding, if the phase encoding is along, for example, the y axis, the phase acquired becomes $k \times y = \int \gamma g_y(t) \times y\, dt$. The acquired signal $S(t)$ is the integral of the spatially distributed signals modulated by a spatially dependent phase, given by the equation

$$S(t) = \int \rho(\vec{r},t)\, e^{(i\vec{k}\cdot\vec{r})}\, d^3r \tag{10.17}$$

where ρ is a function that describes the spatial density and the time evolution of the transverse magnetization of all the chemical species in the sample. This signal mathematically corresponds to a sample of the Fourier transform along the direction of the gradient. The excitation and detection process is repeated with various phase-encoding gradients to obtain many phase-encoded signals that can be inversely Fourier-transformed to resolve an equal number of pixels along this direction. Taking the example of one-dimensional phase-encoding along the y axis to obtain a one-dimensional image along this direction of n pixels, the phase encoding gradient is incremented n times so that n FIDs are acquired, each of which is described as

$$S(t,n) = \int \rho^*(y,t)\, e^{(ink_0 y)}\, dy \tag{10.18}$$

where ρ^* is already integrated over the x and z directions, and k_0 is the phase-encoding increment; the latter is decided on using the criteria that the full field of view undergo a 360° phase difference when $n = 1$, as dictated by the sampling theorem. The time required for each repetition (TR), which is dictated by the longitudinal relaxation time, is usually on the order of seconds.

In CSI, phase encoding is applied in one, two, or three dimensions to provide spatial localization. Meanwhile, selective excitation also can be utilized in one or more dimensions to restrict the volume to be resolved with the phase encodings. For example, with selective excitation in two dimensions, CSI in one spatial dimension can resolve voxels within the selected column. In multidimensional CSI, all the phase-encoding steps along one dimension need to be repeated for all the steps along the others. Thus, for three dimensions with *M, N,* and *L* number of phase encoding steps, one must acquire $M \times N \times L$ number of FIDS:

$$S(t,m,n,l) = \int \rho(\vec{r},t) e^{i(mkx_0 x + nky_0 y + lkz_0 z)} d^3\vec{r} \tag{10.19}$$

where *m, n,* and *l* must step through *M, N,* and *L* in integer steps, respectively. As a result, the time needed for acquiring a chemical-shift image is proportional to the number of pixels desired and may be very long. In practice, due to the time limitation as well as the signal-to-noise ratio (SNR) limitation, chemical-shift imaging is usually performed with relatively few spatial encoding steps, such as 16×16 or 32×32 in a two-dimensional experiment.

The data acquired with the CSI sequence need to be properly processed before the metabolite information can be visualized and quantitated. The processing consists of spatial reconstruction and spectral processing. Spatial reconstruction is achieved by performing discrete inverse Fourier transformation, for each of the spatial dimensions, with respect to the phase-encoding steps. The spatial Fourier transform is applied for all the points of the acquired FID. For example, for a data set from a CSI in two spatial dimensions with 32×32 phase-encoding steps and 1024 sampled data points for each FID, a 32×32 two-dimensional inverse Fourier transform is applied to each of the 1024 data points. Although the nominal spatial resolution achieved by the spatial reconstruction is determined by the number of phase-encoding steps and the field of view (FOV), it is important to note that due to the limited number of phase-encoding steps used in most CSI experiments, the spatial resolution is severely degraded by the truncation artifacts, which results in signal "bleeding" between pixels. Various methods have been developed to reduce this problem [7–14].

The localized FIDs derived from the spatial reconstruction are to be further processed by spectral analysis. Standard procedures include Fourier transformation, filtering, zero-filling, and phasing. The localized spectra can be subsequently presented for visualization or further processed to produce quantitative metabolite information. The presentation of the localized spectra in CSI is not a straightforward task because there can be thousands of spectra. In one-dimensional experiments, localized spectra are usually presented in a stack plot. In two-dimensional experiments, localized spectra are plotted in small boxes representing the extent of the pixels, and the plots can be overlaid on corresponding anatomic images for reference. Spectra from three-dimensional CSI experiments are usually presented slice by slice, each displaying the spectra as in the two-dimensional case.

To derive metabolite maps, peaks corresponding to the metabolites of interest need to be quantified. In principle, the peaks can be quantified using the standard methods developed for spectral quantification [15–17]. The most straightforward technique is to calculate the peak areas by integrating the spectra over the peak of interest if it does not overlap with other peaks significantly. In integrating all the localized spectra, spectral shift due to B_0 inhomogeneity should be taken into account. A more robust approach is to apply spectral fitting programs to each spectrum to obtain various parameters of each peak. The fitted area for the peak of interest can then be used to represent the metabolite signal. The peak areas are then used to generate metabolite maps, which are images with intensities proportional to the localized peak area. The metabolite map can be displayed by itself as a gray-scale image or color-coded image or overlaid on a reference anatomic image.

Practical Examples

To illustrate the practical utility of CSI, we present two representative CSI studies in this section. The sequence for the first study is shown in Fig. 10.21. This is a three-dimensional sequence in which phase encoding is applied in all three directions and no slice selection is used. Such a sequence is usually used with a surface RF coil whose spatial extent of sensitivity defines the field of view. In this sequence, the FID is acquired immediately after the application of the phase-encoding gradient to minimize the decay

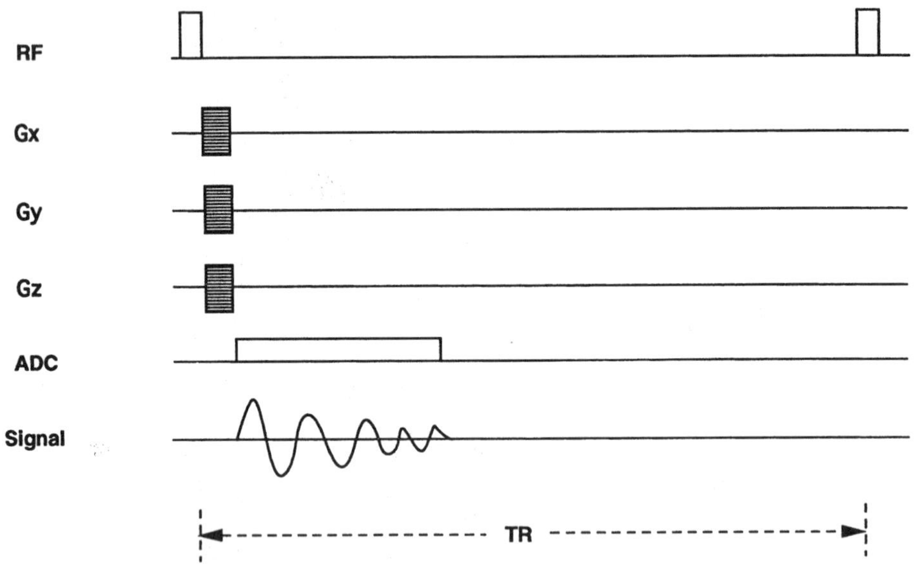

FIGURE 10.21 Sequence diagram for a three-dimensional chemical shift imaging sequence using a nonselective RF pulse.

of the transverse magnetization, and the sequence is suitable for imaging metabolites with short transverse relaxation time (e.g., ATP).

With the sequence shown in Fig. 10.21, a phosphorus-31 CSI study of the human brain was conducted using a quadrature surface coil. A nonselective RF pulse with an Ernest angle (40°) optimized for the repetition time was used for the excitation. Phase-encoding gradients were applied for a duration of 500 μs; the phase-encoding gradients were incremented according to a FOV of $25 \times 25 \times 20$ cm^3. Phase-encoded FIDs were acquired with 1024 complex data points over a sampling window of 204.8 ms; the corresponding spectral width was 5000 Hz. To reduce intervoxel signal contamination, a technique that utilizes variable data averaging to introduce spatial filtering during the data acquisition for optimal signal-to-noise ratio is employed [7–10], resulting in spherical voxels with diameter of 3 cm (15 cc volume). The data were acquired with a *TR* of 1 s, and the total acquisition time was approximately 28 min.

The acquired data were processed to generate three-dimensional voxels, each containing a localized phosphorus spectrum, in a $17 \times 13 \times 17$ matrix. In Fig. 10.22A–C, spectra in three slices of the three-dimensional CSI are presented; these spectra are overlaid on the corresponding anatomic images obtained with a T_1-weighted imaging sequence. One representative spectrum of the brain is illustrated in Fig. 10.22D, where the peaks corresponding to various metabolites are labeled. It is evident that the localized phosphorus spectra contain a wealth of information about several metabolites of interest, including adenosine triphosphate (ATP), phosphocreatine (PCr), phosphomonoester (PME), inorganic phosphate (P_i), and phosphodiester (PDE). In pathologic cases, focal abnormalities in phosphorus metabolites have been detected in patients with tumor, epilepsy, and other diseases [18–25].

The second study described below is performed with the sequence depicted in Fig. 10.23. This is a two-dimensional spin-echo sequence in which a slice is selectively excited by a 90° excitation pulse. The 180° refocusing pulse is selective with a slightly broader slice profile. Here the phase-encoding gradients are applied before the refocusing pulse; they also can be placed after the 180° pulse or split to both sides of the 180° pulse. This sequence was used for a proton CSI experiment. In proton CSI, a major problem arises from the strong water signal that overwhelms that of the metabolites. In order to suppress the water signal, many techniques have been devised [26–29]. In this study, a three-pulse CHESS [26] technique

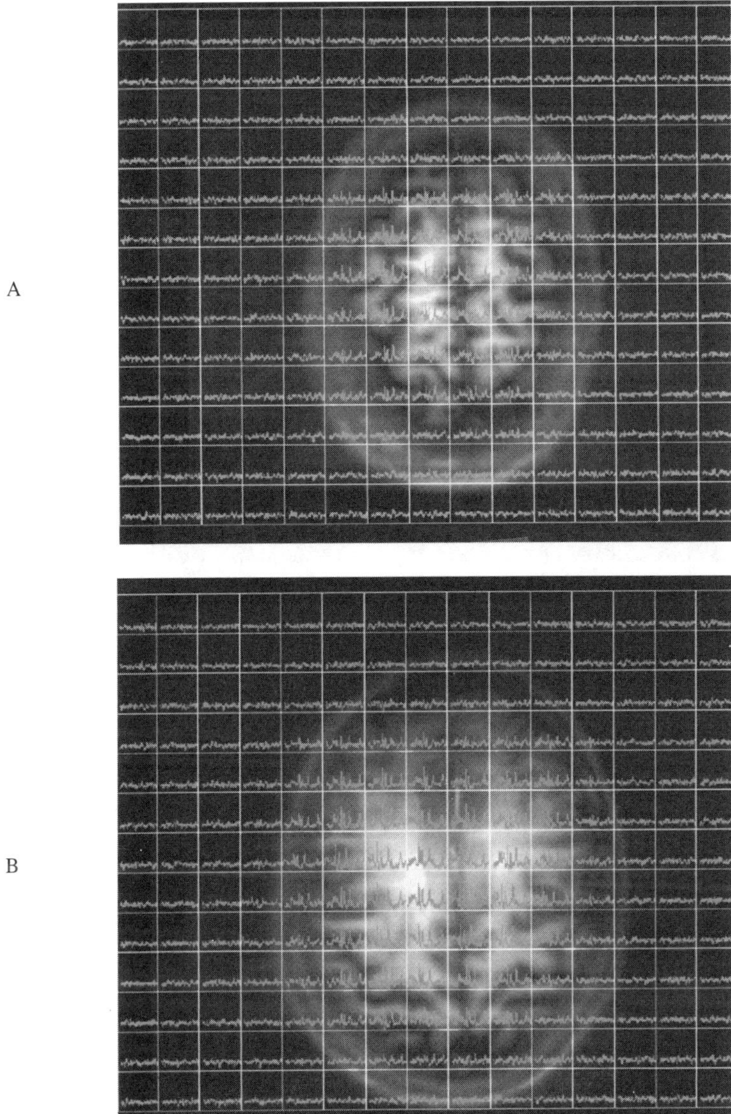

FIGURE 10.22 (A–C) Boxed plot of spectra in three slices from the three-dimensional ^{31}P CSI experiment overlaid on corresponding anatomic images. The spectral extent displayed is from 10 to –20 ppm. A 20-Hz line broadening is applied to all the spectra. (D) Representative spectrum from the three-dimensional ^{31}P CSI shown in (B). Metabolite peaks are labeled. *(Continued next page.)*

was applied before the application of the excitation pulse as shown in Fig. 10.23. The CSI experiment was performed on a 1.4-cm slice with 32 × 32 phase encodings over a 22 × 22 cm^2 FOV. The second half of the spin-echo was acquired with 512 complex data points over a sampling window of 256 ms, corresponding to a spectral width of 2000 Hz. Each phase-encoding FID was acquired twice for data averaging. The repetition time (*TR*) and the echo time (*TE*) used were 1.2 s and 136 ms, respectively. The total acquisition time was approximately 40 min.

C

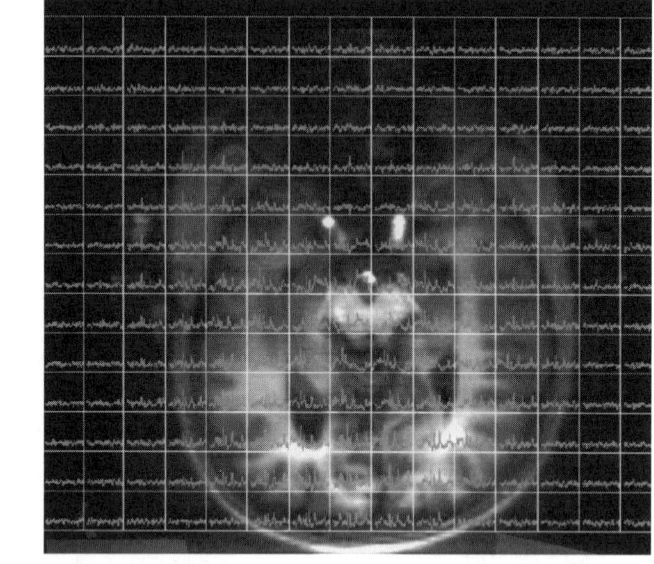

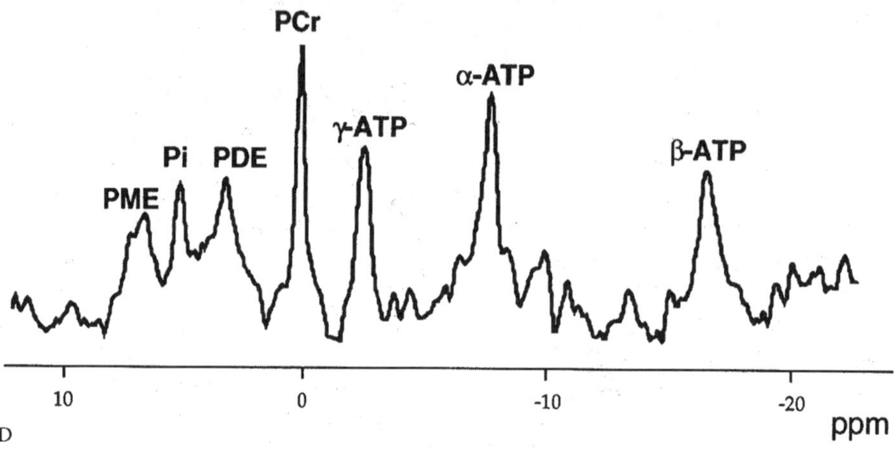

D

FIGURE 10.22 (continued)

Another major problem in proton CSI study of the brain is that the signal from the subcutaneous lipid usually is much stronger than those of the metabolites, and this strong signal leaks into pixels within the brain due to truncation artifacts. To avoid lipid signal contamination, many proton CSI studies of the brain are performed within a selected region of interest excluding the subcutaneous fat [30–34]. Recently, several techniques have been proposed to suppress the lipid signal and consequently suppress the lipid signal contamination. These include the use of WEFT [27] and the use of outer-volume signal suppression [34]. In the example described below, we used a technique that utilizes the spatial location of the lipid to extrapolate data in the *k*-space to reduce the signal contamination due to truncation [35].

In Fig. 10.24, the results from the proton CSI study are presented. In panel (*a*), the localized spectra are displayed. Note that the spectra in the subcutaneous lipid are ignored because they are all off the scale. The nominal spatial resolution is approximately 0.66 cc. A spectrum from an individual pixel in this study is presented in Fig. 10.24*b* with metabolite peaks indicated. Several metabolite peaks, such as those corresponding to the *N*-acetyl aspartate (NAA), creatine/phosphocreatine (Cr/PCr), and choline

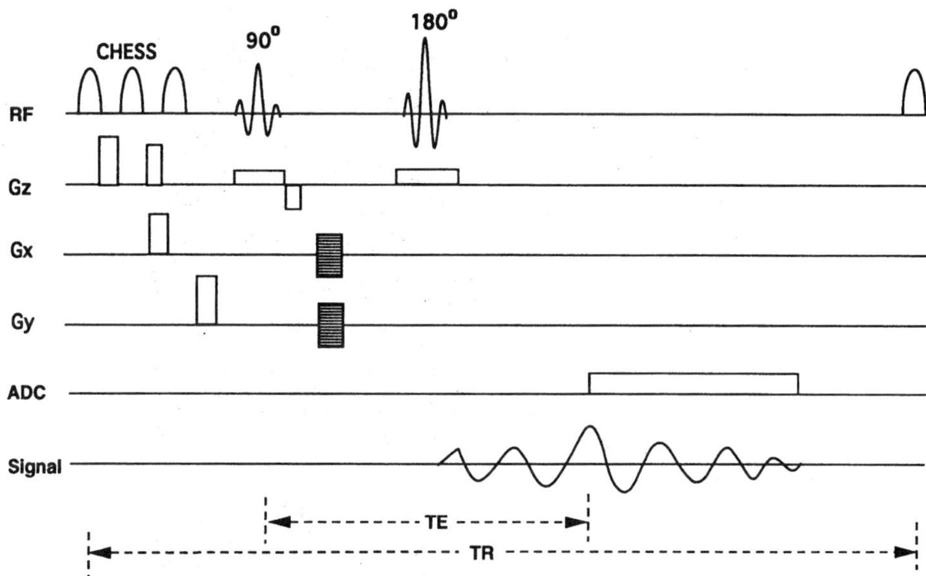

FIGURE 10.23 A two-dimensional spin-echo CSI sequence with chemical selective water suppression (CHESS) for proton study.

(Cho), are readily identified. In addition, there is still a noticeable amount of residual lipid signal contamination despite the use of the data extrapolation technique. Without the lipid suppression technique, the brain spectra would be severely contaminated by the lipid signal, making the detection of the metabolite peaks formidable. The peak of NAA in these spectra is fitted to generate the metabolite map shown in panel (*c*). Although the metabolite map is not corrected for coil sensitivity and other factors and only provides a relative measure of the metabolite concentration in the brain, it is a reasonable measure of the NAA distribution in the brain slice. The spatial resolution of the CSI study can be appreciated from the brain structure present in the map. In biomedical research, proton CSI is potentially the most promising technique, since it provides best sensitivity and spatial resolution. Various *in vivo* applications of proton spectroscopy can be found in the literature [36].

Summary

CSI is a technique for generating localized spectra that provide a wealth of biochemical information that can be used to study the metabolic activity of living systems and to detect disease associated biochemical changes. This section provides an introduction to the technique and illustrates it by two representative examples. More specific topics concerning various aspects of CSI can be found in the literature.

Acknowledgments

The authors would like to thank Dr. Xiao-Hong Zhu for assisting data acquisition and Mr. Gregory Adriany for hardware support. The studies presented here are supported by the National Institutes of Health (RR08079).

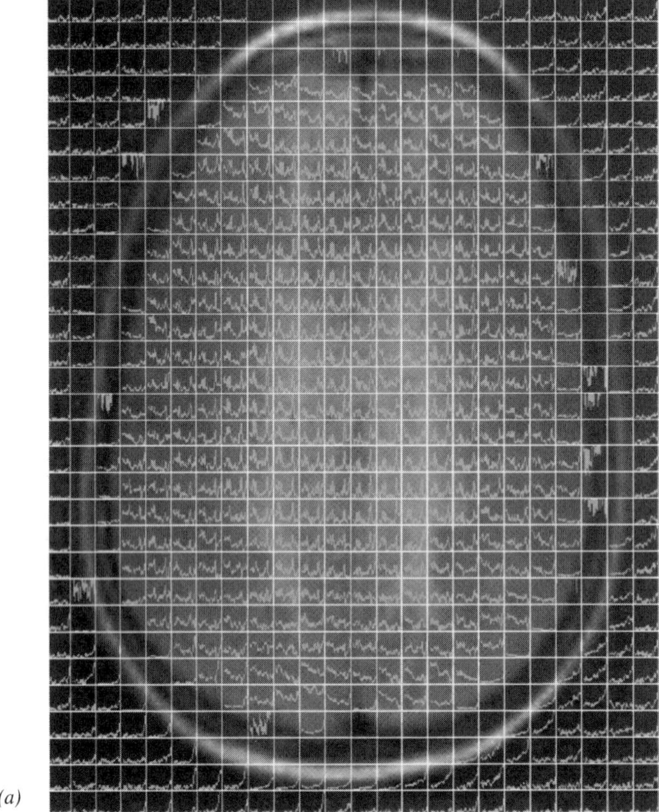

(a)

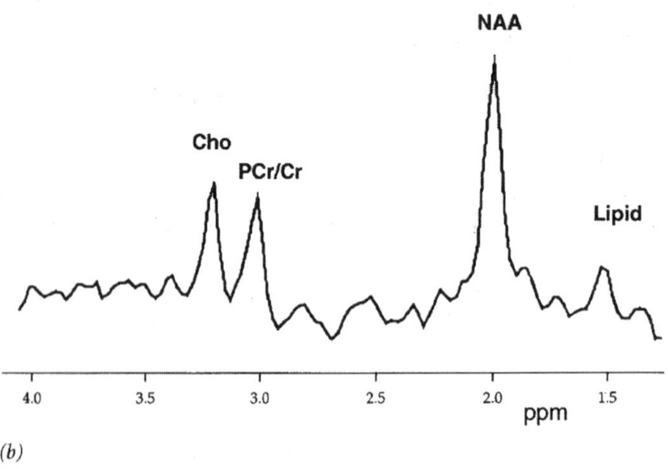

(b)

FIGURE 10.24 (*a*) Boxed plot of spectra for the two-dimensional proton study overlaid on the anatomic image. A spectral range of 1.7 to 3.5 ppm is used in the plot to show Cho, PCr/Cr, and NAA. A 5-Hz line broadening is applied in the spectral processing. (*b*) A representative spectrum from the two-dimensional CSI in panel (*a*). Peaks corresponding to Cho, PCr/Cr, and NAA are indicated. (*c*) A map of the area under the NAA peak obtained by spectral fitting. The anatomic image is presented along with the metabolite map for reference. The spatial resolution of the metabolite image can be appreciated from the similarities between the two images. The lipid suppression technique has successfully eliminated the signal contamination from the lipid in the skull.

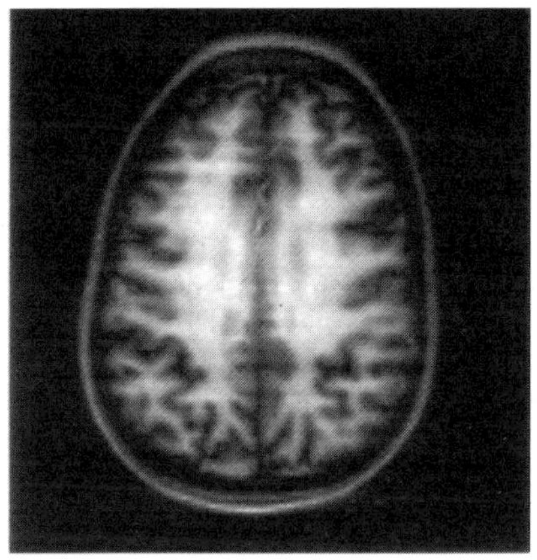

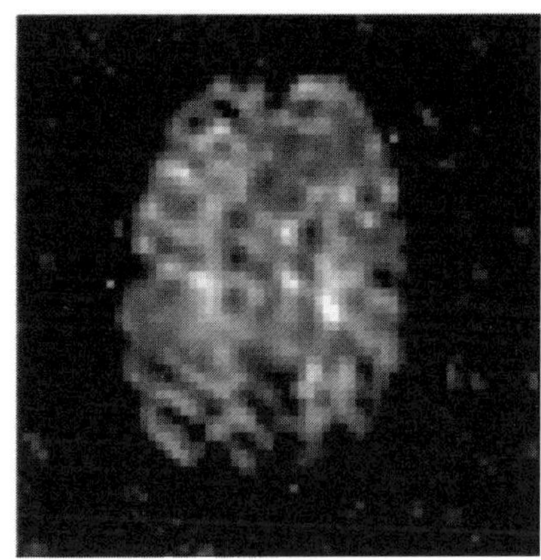

(c)

FIGURE 10.24 (continued)

References

1. Lauterbur PC. 1973. Image formation by induced local interactions: Examples employing nuclear magnetic resonance. Nature 242:190.
2. Alger JR. 1994. Spatial localization for in vivo magnetic resonance spectroscopy: Concepts and commentary. In RJ Gillies (ed), NMR in Physiology and Biomedicine, pp 151–168. San Diego, Academic Press.
3. Brown TR, Kincaid MB, Ugurbil K. 1982. NMR chemical shift imaging in three dimensions. Proc Natl Acad Sci USA 79:3523.
4. Maudsley AA, Hilal SK, Simon HE, Perman WH. 1983. Spatially resolved high resolution spectroscopy by "four dimensional" NMR. J Magn Reson 51:147.
5. Haselgrove JC, Subramanian VH, Leigh JS Jr, et al. 1983. In vivo one-dimensional imaging of phosphorous metabolites by phosphorus-31 nuclear magnetic resonance. Science 220:1170.
6. Maudsley AA, Hilal SK, Simon HE, Wittekoek S. 1984. In vivo MR spectroscopic imaging with P-31. Radiology 153:745.
7. Garwood M, Schleich T, Ross BD, et al. 1985. A modified rotating frame experiment based on a Fourier window function: Application to in vivo spatially localized NMR spectroscopy. J Magn Reson 65:239.
8. Garwood M, Robitalle PM, Ugurbil K. 1987. Fourier series windows on and off resonance using multiple coils and longitudinal modulation. J Magn Reson 75:244.
9. Mareci TH, Brooker HR. 1984. High-resolution magnetic resonance spectra from a sensitive region defined with pulsed gradients. J Magn Reson 57:157.
10. Brooker HR, Mareci TH, Mao JT. 1987. Selective Fourier transform localization. Magn Reson Med 5:417.
11. Hu X, Levin DN, Lauterbur PC. Spraggins TA. 1988. SLIM: Spectral localization by imaging. Magn Reson Med 8:314.
12. Liang ZP, Lauterbur PC. 1991. A generalized series approach to MR spectroscopic imaging. IEEE Trans Med Imag MI-10:132.
13. Hu X, Stillman AE. 1991. Technique for reduction of truncation artifact in chemical shift images. IEEE Trans Med Imag MI-10(3):290.
14. Hu X, Patel MS, Ugurbil K. 1993. A new strategy for chemical shift imaging. J Magn Reson B103:30.

15. van den Boogaart A, Ala-Korpela M, Jokisaari J, Griffiths JR. 1994. Time and frequency domain analysis of NMR data compared: An application to 1D ^{1}H spectra of lipoproteins. Magn Reson Med 31:347.
16. Ernst T, Kreis R, Ross B. 1993. Absolute quantification of water and metabolites in human brain: I. Compartments and water. J Magn Reson 102:1.
17. Kreis R, Ernst T, Ross B. 1993. Absolute quantification of water and metabolites in human brain. II. Metabolite concentration. J Magn Reson 102:9.
18. Lenkinski RE, Holland GA, Allman T, et al. 1988. Integrated MR imaging and spectroscopy with chemical shift imaging of P-31 at 1.5 T: Initial clinical experience. Radiology 169:201.
19. Hugg JW, Matson GB, Twieg DB, et al. ^{31}P MR spectroscopic imaging of normal and pathological human brains. Magn Reson Imaging 10:227.
20. Vigneron DB, Nelson SJ, Murphy-Boesch J, et al. 1990. Chemical shift imaging of human brain: Axial, sagittal, and coronal ^{31}P metabolite images. Radiology 177:643.
21. Hugg JW, Laxer KD, Matson GB, et al. 1992. Lateralization of human focal epilepsy by ^{31}P magnetic resonance spectroscopic imaging. Neurology 42:2011.
22. Meyerhoff DJ, Maudsley AA, Schafer S, Weiner MW. 1992. Phosphorous-31 magnetic resonance metabolite imaging in the human body. Magn Reson Imaging 10:245.
23. Bottomley PA, Hardy C, Boemer P. 1990. Phosphate metabolite imaging and concentration measurements in human heart by nuclear magnetic resonance. Magn Reson Med 14:425.
24. Robitaille PM, Lew B, Merkle H, et al. 1990. Transmural high energy phosphate distribution and response to alterations in workload in the normal canine myocardium as studied with spatially localized ^{31}P NMR spectroscopy. Magn Reson Med 16:91.
25. Ugurbil K, Garwood M, Merkle H, et al. 1989. Metabolic consequences of coronary stenosis: Transmurally heterogeneous myocardial ischemia studied by spatially localized ^{31}P NMR spectroscopy. NMR Biomed 2:317.
26. Hasse A, Frahm J, Hanicker H, Mataei D. 1985. ^{1}H NMR chemical shift selective (CHESS) imaging. Phys Med Biol 30(4):341.
27. Patt SL, Sykes BD. 1972. T_1 water eliminated Fourier transform NMR spectroscopy. Chem Phys 56:3182.
28. Moonen CTW, van Zijl PCM. 1990. Highly effective water suppression for in vivo proton NMR spectroscopy (DRYSTEAM). J Magn Reson 88:28.
29. Ogg R, Kingsley P, Taylor JS. 1994. WET: A T_1 and B_1 insensitive water suppression method for in vivo localized ^{1}H NMR spectroscopy. B104:1.
30. Lampman DA, Murdoch JB, Paley M. 1991. In vivo proton metabolite maps using MESA 3D technique. Magn Reson Med 18:169.
31. Luyten PR, Marien AJH, Heindel W, et al. 1990. Metabolic imaging of patients with intracranial tumors: ^{1}H MR spectroscopic imaging and PET. Radiology 176:791.
32. Arnold DL, Matthews PM, Francis GF, et al. 1992. Proton magnetic resonance spectroscopic imaging for metabolite characterization of demyelinating plaque. Ann Neurol 31:319.
33. Duijin JH, Matson GB, Maudsley AA, et al. 1992. Human brain infarction: Proton MR spectroscopy. Radiology 183:711.
34. Duyn JH, Gillen J, Sobering G, et al. 1993. Multisection proton MR spectroscopic imaging of the brain. Radiology 188:277.
35. Patel MS, Hu X. 1994. Selective data extrapolation for chemical shift imaging. Soc Magn Reson Abstr 3:1168.
36. Rothman DL. 1994. ^{1}H NMR studies of human brain metabolism and physiology. In RJ Gillies (ed), NMR in Physiology and Biomedicine, pp 353–372. San Diego, Academic Press.

11

Nuclear Medicine

Barbara Y. Croft
National Institutes of Health

Benjamin M.W. Tsui
University of North Carolina at Chapel Hill

11.1 Instrumentation

Barbara Y. Croft

Nuclear medicine can be defined as the practice of making patients radioactive for diagnostic and therapeutic purposes. The radioactivity is injected intravenously, rebreathed, or ingested. It is the internal circulation of radioactive material that distinguishes nuclear medicine from diagnostic radiology and radiation oncology in most of its forms. This section will examine only the diagnostic use and will concentrate on methods for detecting the radioactivity from outside the body without trauma to the patient. Diagnostic nuclear medicine is successful for two main reasons: (1) It can rely on the use of very small amounts of materials (picomolar concentrations in chemical terms) and thus usually not have any effect on the processes being studied, and (2) the radionuclides being used can penetrate tissue and be detected outside the patient. Thus the materials can trace processes or "opacify" organs without affecting their function.

Parameters for Choices in Nuclear Medicine

Of the various kinds of emanations from radioactive materials, photons alone have a range in tissue great enough to escape so that they can be detected externally. Electrons or beta-minus particles of high energy can create bremsstrahlung in interactions with tissue, but the radiation emanates from the site of the interaction, not the site of the beta ray's production. Positrons or beta-plus particles annihilate with electrons to create gamma rays so that they can be detected (see Chap. 14). For certain radionuclides, the emanation being detected is x-rays, in the 50- to 100-keV energy range.

The half-lives of materials in use in nuclear medicine range from a few minutes to weeks. The half-life must be chosen with two major points in mind: the time course of the process being studied and the radiation dose to the target organ, i.e., that organ with the highest concentration over the longest time (the cumulated activity or area underneath the activity versus time curve). In general, it is desired to stay under 5 rad to the target organ.

0-8493-1810-6/03/$0.00+$1.50

TABLE 11.1 Gamma Ray Detection

Type of Sample	Activity	Energy	Type of Instrument
Patient samples, e.g., blood, urine	0.001 μCi	20–5000 keV	Gamma counter with annular NaI(TI) detector, 1 or 2 PMTs, external Pb shielding
Small organ function <30 cm field of view at 60 cm distance	5–200 μCi	20–1500 keV	2–4-in. NaI(TI) detector with flared Pb collimator
Static image of body part, e.g., liver, lung	0.2–30 mCi	50–650 keV	Rectilinear scanner with focused Pb collimator
Dynamic image of body part, e.g., xenon in airways	2–30 mCi	80–300 keV	Anger camera and parallel-hole Pb collimator
Static tomographic image of body part			

The choice of the best energy range to use is also based on two major criteria: the energy that will penetrate tissue but can be channeled by heavy metal shielding and collimation and that which will interact in the detector to produce a pulse. Thus the ideal energy is dependent on the detector being used and the kind of examination being performed. Table 11.1 describes the kinds of gamma-ray detection, the activity and energy ranges, and an example of the kind of information to be gained. The lesser amounts of activity are used in situations of lesser spatial resolution and/or of greater sensitivity. Positron imaging is omitted because it is treated elsewhere.

Radiation dose is affected by all the emanations of a radionuclide, not just the desirable ones, thus constricting the choice of nuclide further. There can be no alpha radiation used in diagnosis; the use of materials with primary beta radiation should be avoided because the beta radiation confers a radiation dose without adding to the information being gained. For imaging, in addition, even if there is a primary gamma ray in the correct energy window for the detector, there should be no large amount of radiation, either of primary radiation of higher energy, because it interferes with the image collimation, or of secondary radiation of a very similar energy, because it interferes with the perception of the primary radiation emanating from the site of interest.

For imaging using heavy-metal collimation, the energy range is constrained to be that which will emanate from the human body and which the collimation can contain, or about 50 to 500 keV.

Detectors must be made from materials that exhibit some detectable change when ionizing radiation is absorbed and that are of a high enough atomic number and density to make possible stopping large percentages of those gamma rays emanating (high sensitivity). In addition, because the primary gamma rays are not the only rays emanating from the source—a human body and therefore a distributed source accompanied by an absorber—there must be energy discrimination in the instrument to prevent the formation of an image of the scattered radiation. To achieve pulse size proportional to energy, and therefore to achieve identification of the energy and source of the energy, the detector must be a proportional detector. This means that Geiger-Muller detection, operating in an all-or-none fashion, is not acceptable.

Gaseous detectors are not practical because their density is not great enough. Liquid detectors (in which any component is liquid) are not practical because the liquid can spill when the detector is positioned; this problem can be compensated for if absolutely necessary, but it is better to consider it from the outset. Another property of a good detector is its ability to detect large numbers of gamma rays per time unit. With detection capabilities to separate 100,000 counts per second or a dead time of 2 μs, the system is still only detecting perhaps 1000 counts per square centimeter per second over a 10 × 10 cm area. The precision of the information is governed by Poisson statistics, so the imprecision in information collected for 1 s in a square centimeter is ±3% at the 1 standard deviation level. Since we would hope for better spatial resolution than 1 cm^2, the precision is obviously worse than this. This points to the need for fast detectors, in addition to the aforementioned sensitivity. The more detector that surrounds the patient, the more sensitive the system will be. Table 11.2 lists in order from least sensitive to most sensitive some of the geometries used for imaging in nuclear medicine. This generally is also a listing from the older methods to the more recent.

TABLE 11.2 Ways of Imaging Using Lead Collimation

Moving probe; rectilinear scanner
Array of multiple crystals; autofluoroscope, "fly-eye" camera
Two moving probes: dual-head rectilinear scanner
Large single-crystal system: Anger camera
Two crystals on opposite sides of patient for two views using Anger logic
Large multiple-crystal systems using Anger logic SPECT
Other possibilities

For the purposes of this section, we shall consider that the problems of counting patient and other samples and of detecting the time course of activity changes in extended areas with probes are not our topic and confine ourselves to the attempts made to image distributions of gamma-emitting radionuclides in patients and research subjects. The previous section treats the three-dimensional imaging of these distributions; this section will treat detection of the distribution in a planar fashion or the image of the projection of the distribution onto a planar detector.

Detection of Photon Radiation

Gamma rays are detected when atoms in a detector are ionized and the ions are collected either directly as in gaseous or semiconductor systems or by first conversion of the ionized electrons to light and subsequent conversion of the light to electrons in a photomultiplier tube (P-M tube or PMT). In all cases there is a voltage applied across some distance that causes a pulse to be created when a photon is absorbed.

The gamma rays are emitted according to Poisson statistics because each decaying nucleus is independent of the others and has an equal probability of decaying per unit time. Because the uncertainty in the production of gamma rays is therefore on the order of magnitude of the square root of the number of gamma rays, the more gamma rays that are detected, the less the proportional uncertainty will be. Thus sensitivity is a very important issue for the creation of images, since the rays will be detected by area. To get better resolution, one must have the numbers of counts and the apparatus to resolve them spatially. Having the large numbers of counts also means the apparatus must resolve them temporally.

The need for energy resolution carries its own burden. Depending on the detector, the energy resolution may be easily achieved or not (Table 11.3). In any case, the attenuation and scattering inside the body means that there will be a range of gamma rays emitted, and it will be difficult to tell those scattered through very small angles from those not scattered at all. This affects the spatial resolution of the instrument.

The current practice of nuclear medicine has defined the limits of the amount of activity that can be administered to a patient by the amount of radiation dose. Since planar imaging with one detector allows only 2 pi detection at best and generally a view of somewhat less because the source is in the patient and the lead collimation means that only rays that are directed from the decay toward the crystal will be detected, it is of utmost importance to detect every ray possible. To the extent that no one is ever satisfied with the resolution of any system and always wishes for better, there is the need to be able to get spatial resolution better than the intrinsic 2 mm currently achievable. Some better collimation system, such as

TABLE 11.3 Detector Substances and Size Considerations, Atomic Number of the Attenuator, Energy Resolution Capability

PMT connected
NaI(TI): up to 50 cm across; 63; 5–10%
Plastic scintillators: unlimited; 6; only Compton absorption for gamma rays used in imaging
CsI(TI): <3 cm × 3 cm; 53, 55; poorer than NaI(TI)
BiGermanate: <3 cm × 3 cm; 83; poorer than NaI(TI)
Semiconductors: Liquid nitrogen operation and liquid nitrogen storage
GeLi: <3 cm × 3 cm; 32; <1%
SiLi: <3 cm × 3 cm; 14; <1%

TABLE 11.4 Calculation of Number of Counts Achieved with Anger Camera

	cpm	cps
Activity		
mCi/cm^3	0.001	
counts/s		3.7×10^7
counts/min	2.22×10^9	
2π geometry	1.11×10^9	1.85×10^7
Attenuated by tissue of 0.12/cm attenuation and 3 cm thick	7.44×10^8	1.29×10^7
X Camera efficiency of 0.0006	4.64×10^5	7744
Good uptake in liver = 5 mCi/1000 g = 0.005 mCi/g	2.32×10^6	3.8×10^4
Thyroid uptake of Tc-99m = (2 mCi/37 g) * 2% = 0.001 mCi/G	4.6×10^5	7.7×10^3

envisioned in a coincidence detection system like that used in PET, might make it possible to avoid stopping so many of the rays with the collimator.

We have now seen that energy resolution, sensitivity, and resolving time of the detector are all bound up together to produce the spatial resolution of the instrument as well as the more obvious temporal resolution. The need to collimate to create an image rather than a blush greatly decreases the numbers of counts and makes Poisson statistics a major determinant of the appearance of nuclear medical images.

Table 11.4 shows a calculation for the NaI(TI)-based Anger camera showing 0.06% efficiency for the detection system. Thus the number of counts per second is not high and so is well within the temporal resolving capabilities of the detector system. The problem is the 0.06% efficiency, which is the effect of both the crystal thickness being optimized for imaging rather than for stopping all the gamma rays, and the lead collimation. Improvements in nuclear medicine imaging resolution can only come if both these factors are addressed.

Various Detector Configurations

The detectors in clinical nuclear medicine are NaI(TI) crystals. In research applications, other substances are employed, but the engineering considerations for the use of other detectors are more complex and have been less thoroughly explored (Table 11.3).

The possibilities for configuring the detectors have been increasing, although the older methods tend to be discarded as the new ones are exploited (see Table 11.2). This is in part because each laboratory cannot afford to have one of every kind of instrument, although there are tasks for which each one is ideally suited.

The first instruments possible for plane-projection imaging consisted of a moving single crystal probe, called a *rectilinear scanner.* The probe consisted of a detector [beginning with NaI(TI) but later incorporating small semiconductors] that was collimated by a focused lead collimator of appreciable thickness (often 2 in. of lead or more) with hole sizes and thicknesses of septa consonant with the intended energy and organ size and depth to be imaged. The collimated detector was caused to move across the patient at a constant speed; the pulses from the detector were converted to visible signals either by virtue of markings on a sheet or of light flashes exposing a film. This detector could see only one spot at a time, so only slow temporal changes in activity could be appreciated. A small organ such as the thyroid could be imaged in this fashion very satisfactorily. Bone imaging also could be done with the later versions of this instrument.

To enlarge the size of the detector, several probes, each with its own photomultiplier tube and collimator, could be used. Versions of this idea were used to create dual-probe instruments to image both sides of the patient simultaneously, bars of probes to sweep down the patient and create a combined image, etc.

To go further with the multiple crystals to create yet larger fields of view, the autofluoroscope (Fig. 11.1) combined crystals in a rectangular array. For each to have its own photomultiplier tube required too

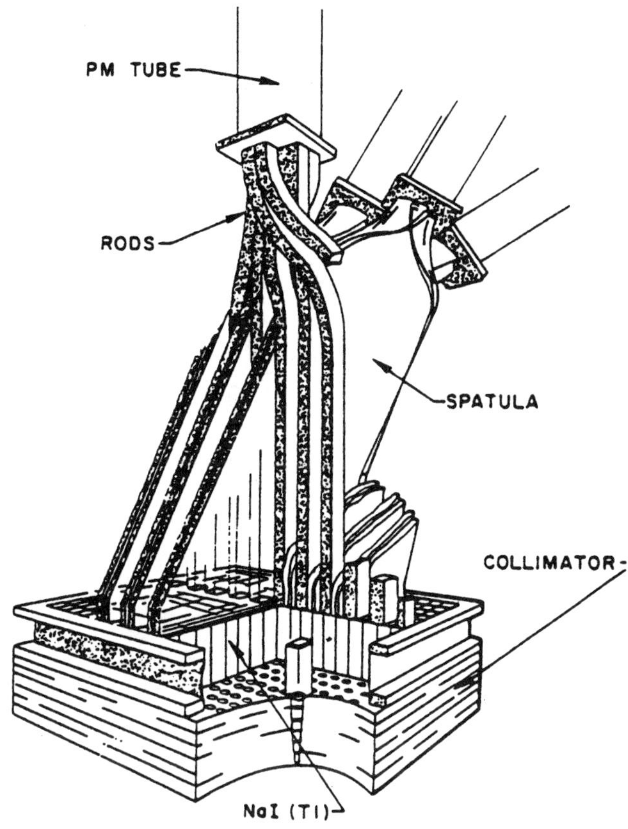

FIGURE 11.1 The Bender-Blau autofluoroscope is a multicrystal imager with a rectangular array of crystals connected to PMTs by plastic light guides. There is a PMT for each row of crystals and a PMT for each column of crystals, so an N by M array would have $(N + M)$ PMTs.

many PMTs, so the instrument was designed with a light pipe to connect each crystal with a PMT to indicate its row and a second one to indicate its column. The crystals are separated by lead septa to prevent scattered photons from one crystal affecting the next. Because of the large number of crystals and PMTs, the instrument is very fast, but because of the size of the crystals, the resolution is coarse. To improve the resolution, the collimator is often jittered so that each crystal is made to see more than one field of view to create a better resolved image. For those dynamic examinations in which temporal resolution is more important than spatial resolution, the system has a clear advantage. It has not been very popular for general use, however. In its commercial realization, the field of view was not large enough to image either lungs or livers or bones in any single image fashion.

As large NaI(TI) crystals became a reality, new ways to use them were conceived. The Anger camera (Fig. 11.2) is one of the older of these methods. The idea is to use a single crystal of diameter large enough to image a significant part of the human body and to back the crystal by an array of photomultiplier tubes to give positional sensitivity. Each PMT is assigned coordinates (Fig. 11.3). When a photon is absorbed by the crystal, a number of PMTs receive light and therefore emit signals. The X and Y signal values for the emanation are determined by the strength of the signal from each of the tubes and its x and y position, and the energy of the emanation (which determines if it will be used to create the image) is the sum of all the signals (the Z pulse). If the discriminator passes the Z pulse, then the X and Y signals are sent to whatever device is recording the image, be it an oscilloscope and film recording system or the analog-to-digital (A/D) converters of a computer system. More recently, the A/D conversion is done earlier in the system so that the X and Y signals are themselves digital. The Anger camera is the major

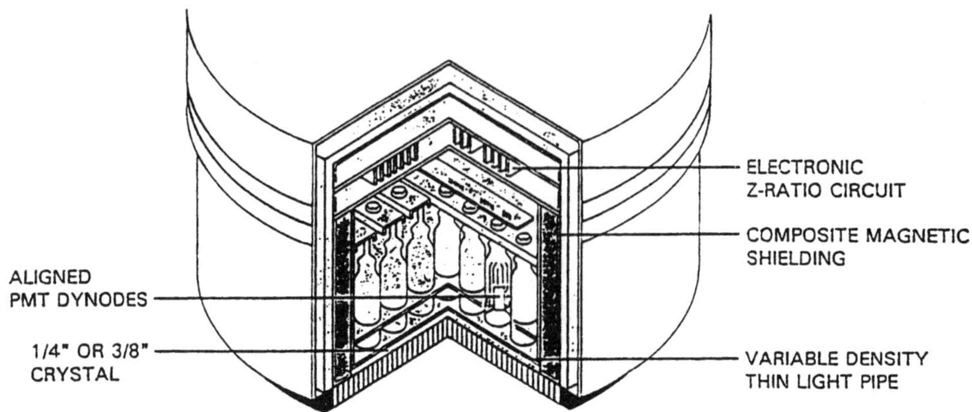

FIGURE 11.2 Anger camera detector design. This figure shows a cross section through the camera head. The active surface is pointed down. Shielding surrounds the assembly on the sides and top.

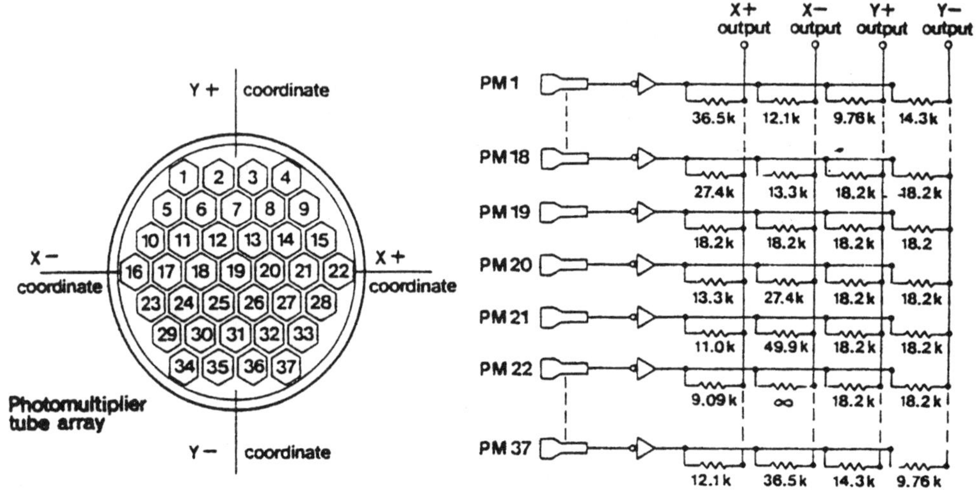

FIGURE 11.3 An array of PMTs in the Anger camera showing the geometric connection between the PMTs and the X and Y output.

instrument in use in nuclear medicine today. It has been optimized for use with the 140-keV radiation from Tc-99m, although collimators have been designed for lower and higher energies, as well as optimized for higher sensitivity and higher resolution. The early systems used circular crystals, while the current configuration is likely to be rectangular or square.

A combination of the Anger positional logic and the focused collimator in a scanner produced the PhoCon instrument, which, because of the design of its collimators, had planar tomographic capabilities (the instrument could partially resolve activity in different planes, parallel to the direction of movement of the detector).

Ancillary Electronic Equipment for Detection

The detectors used in nuclear medicine are attached to preamplifiers, amplifiers, and pulse shapers to form a signal that can be examined for information about the energy of the detected photon (Fig. 11.4). The energy discriminator has lower and upper windows that are set with reference radionuclides so that

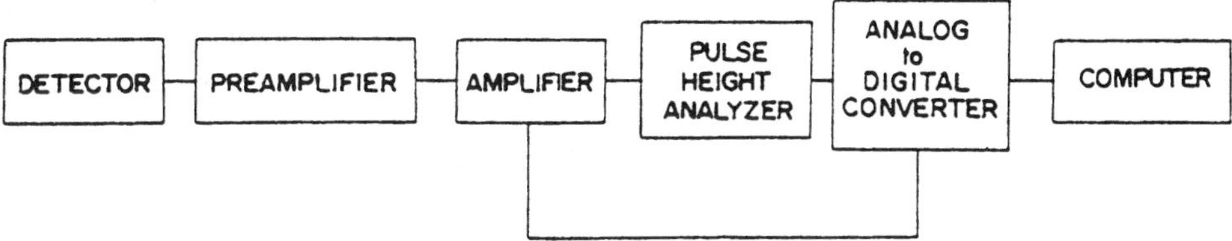

FIGURE 11.4 Schematic drawing of a generalized detector system. There would be a high-voltage power supply for the detector in an NaI(TI)-PMT detector system.

typically the particular nuclide in use can be dialed in along with the width of the energy window. A photon with an energy that falls in the selected range will cause the creation of a pulse of a voltage that falls in between the levels; all other photon energies will cause voltages either too high or too low. If only gross features are being recorded, any of the instruments may be used as probe detectors and the results recorded on strip-chart recordings of activity versus time.

The PMT "multiplies" photons (Fig. 11.5) because it has a quartz entrance window which is coated to release electrons when it absorbs a light photon and there is a voltage drop; the number of electrons released is proportional to the amount of light that hits the coating. The electrons are guided through a hole and caused to hit the first dynode, which is coated with a special substance to allow it to release electrons when it is hit by an electron. There are a series of dynodes each with a voltage that pulls the electrons from the last dynodes toward it. The surface coating not only releases electrons but also

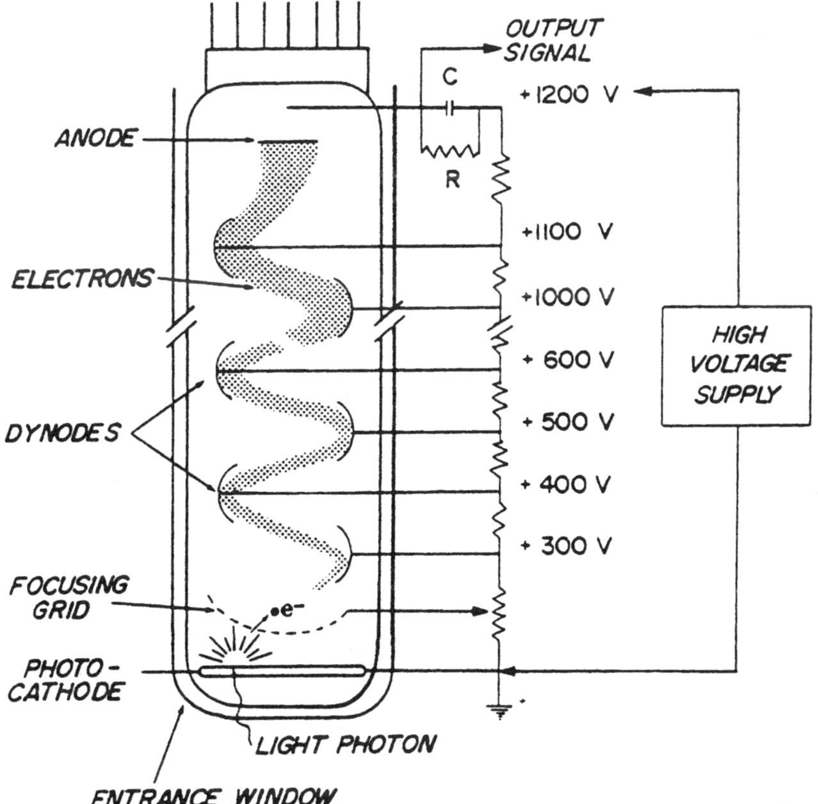

FIGURE 11.5 Schematic drawing of a photomultiplier tube (PMT). Each of the dynodes and the anode is connected to a separate pin in the tube socket. The inside of the tube is evacuated of all gas. Dynodes are typically copper with a special oxidized coating for electron multiplication.

multiplies the electron shower. In a cascade through 10 to 12 dynodes, there is a multiplication of approximately 10^6, so that pulses of a few electrons become currents of the order of 10^{-12} amps. The PMTs must be protected from other influences, such as stray radioactivity or strong magnetic fields, which might cause extraneous electron formation or curves in the electron path. Without the voltage drop from one dynode to the next, there is no cascade of electrons and no counting.

For imaging, the x and y positions of those photons in the correct energy range will be recorded in the image because they have a Z pulse. Once the pulse has been accepted and the position determined, that position may be recorded to make an image either in analog or digital fashion; a spot may be made on an oscilloscope screen and recorded on film or paper, or the position may be digitized and stored in a computer file for later imaging on an oscilloscope screen and/or for photography. In general, the computers required are very similar to those used for other imaging modalities, except for the hardware that allows the acceptance of the pulse. The software is usually specifically created for nuclear medicine because of the unique needs for determination of function.

The calibration of the systems follows a similar pattern, no matter how simple or complex the instrument. Most probe detectors must be "peaked," which means that the energy of the radioactivity must be connected with some setting of the instrument, often meant to read in kiloelectronvolts. This is accomplished by counting a sample with the instrument, using a reasonably narrow energy window, while varying the high voltage until the count rate reading is a maximum. The window is then widened for counting samples to encompass all the energy peak being counted. The detector is said to be linear if it can be set with one energy and another energy can be found where it should be on the kiloelectronvolt scale.

To ensure that the images of the radioactivity accurately depict the distribution in the object being imaged, the system must be initialized correctly and tested at intervals. The several properties that must be calibrated and corrected are sensitivity, uniformity, energy pulse shape, and linearity.

These issues are addressed in several ways. The first is that all the PMTs used in an imaging system must be chosen to have matched sensitivities and energy spectra. Next, during manufacture, and at intervals during maintenance, the PMTs' response to voltage is matched so that the voltage from the power supply causes all the tubes to have maximum counts at the same voltage. The sensitivities of all the tubes are also matched during periodic maintenance. Prior to operation, usually at the start of each working day, the user will check the radioactive peak and then present the instrument with a source of activity to give an even exposure over the whole crystal. This uniform "flood" is recorded. The image may be used by the instrument for calibration; recalibration is usually performed at weekly intervals. The number of counts needed depends on the use the instrument is to be put to, but generally the instrument must be tested and calibrated with numbers of counts at least equal to those being emitted by the patients and other objects being imaged.

Because the PMT placement means that placement of the x and y locations is not perfect over the face of the crystal but has the effect of creating wiggly lines that may be closer together over the center of the PMT and farther apart at the interstices between tubes, the image may suffer from spatial nonlinearity. This can be corrected for by presenting the system with a lead pattern in straight-line bars or holes in rows and using a hard-wired or software method to position the X and Y signals correctly. This is called a *linearity correction.* In addition, there may be adjustments of the energy spectra of each tube to make them match each other so that variations in the number of kiloelectronvolts included in the window (created by varying the discriminator settings) will not create variations in sensitivity. This is called an *energy correction.*

Place of Planar Imaging in Nuclear Medicine Today: Applications and Economics

There are various ways of thinking about diagnostic imaging and nuclear medicine. If the reason for imaging the patient is to determine the presence of disease, then there are at least two possible strategies. One is to do the most complicated examination that will give a complete set of results on all patients.

The other is to start with a simple examination and hope to categorize patients, perhaps into certain abnormals and all others, or even into abnormals, indeterminates, and normals. Then a subsequent, more complex examination is used to determine if there are more abnormals, or perhaps how abnormal they are. If the reason for imaging the patient is to collect a set of data that will be compared with results from that patient at a later time and with a range of normal results from all patients, then the least complex method possible for collecting the information should be used in a regular and routine fashion so that the comparisons are possible.

In the former setting, where the complexity of the examination may have to be changed after the initial results are seen, in order to take full advantage of the dose of radioactive material that has been given to the patient, it is sensible to have the equipment available that will be able to perform the more complex examination and not to confine the equipment available to that capable of doing only the simple first examination. For this reason and because for some organs, such as the brain, the first examination is a SPECT examination, the new Anger cameras being sold today are mostly capable of doing rotating SPECT. The added necessities that SPECT brings to the instrument specifications are of degree: better stability, uniformity, and resolution. Thus they do not obviate the use of the equipment for planar imaging but rather enhance it. In the setting of performing only the examination necessary to define the disease, the Anger SPECT camera can be used for plane projection imaging and afterward for SPECT to further refine the examination. There are settings in which a planar camera will be purchased because of the simplicity of all the examinations (as in a very large laboratory that can have specialized instruments, a thyroid practice, or in the developing countries), but in the small- to medium-sized nuclear medicine practice, the new cameras being purchased are all SPECT-capable.

Nuclear medicine studies are generally less expensive than x-ray computed tomography or magnetic resonance imaging and more so than planar x-ray or ultrasound imaging. The general conduct of a nuclear medicine laboratory is more complex than these others because of the radioactive materials and the accompanying regulations. The specialty is practice both in clinics and in hospitals, but again, the complication imposed by the presence of the radioactive materials tips the balance of the practices toward the hospital. In that setting the practitioners may be imagers with a broad range of studies offered or cardiologists with a concentration on cardiac studies. Thus the setting also will determine what kind of instrument is most suitable.

Defining Terms

Energy resolution: Full width at half maximum of graph of detected counts versus energy, expressed as a percentage of the energy.

Poisson statistics: Expresses probability in situations of equal probability for an event per unit of time, such as radioactive decay or cosmic-ray appearance. The standard deviation of a mean number of counts is the square root of the mean number of counts, which is a decreasing fraction of the number of counts when expressed as a fraction of the number of counts.

rad: The unit of radiation energy absorption (dose) in matter, defined as the absorption of 100 ergs per gram of irradiated material. The unit is being replaced by the gray, an SI unit, where 1 gray (Gy) = 100 rad.

Further Information

A good introduction to nuclear medicine, written as a text for technologists, is *Nuclear Medicine Technology and Techniques,* edited by D. R. Bernier, J. K. Langan, and L. D. Wells. A treatment of many of the nuclear medicine physics issues is given in L. E. Williams' *Nuclear Medicine Physics,* published in three volumes. Journals that publish nuclear medicine articles include the monthly *Journal of Nuclear Medicine,* the *European Journal of Nuclear Medicine, Clinical Nuclear Medicine, IEEE Transactions in Nuclear Science, IEEE Transactions in Medical Imaging,* and *Medical Physics.* Quarterly and annual publications include *Seminars in Nuclear Medicine, Yearbook of Nuclear Medicine,* and *Nuclear Medicine Annual.*

The Society of Nuclear Medicine holds an annual scientific meeting that includes scientific papers, continuing education which could give the novice a broad introduction, poster sessions, and a large equipment exhibition. Another large meeting, devoted to many radiologic specialties, is the Radiologic Society of North America's annual meeting, held just after Thanksgiving.

11.2 SPECT (Single-Photon Emission Computed Tomography)

Benjamin M. W. Tsui

During the last three decades, there has been much excitement in the development of diagnostic radiology. The development is fueled by inventions and advances made in a number of exciting new medical imaging modalities, including ultrasound (US), x-ray CT (computed tomography), PET (positron emission tomography), SPECT (single-photon emission computed tomography), and MRI (magnetic resonance imaging). These new imaging modalities have revolutionized the practice of diagnostic radiology, resulting in substantial improvement in patient care.

Single-photon emission computed tomography (SPECT) is a medical imaging modality that combines conventional nuclear medicine (NM) imaging techniques and CT methods. Different from x-ray CT, SPECT uses radioactive-labeled pharmaceuticals, i.e., radiopharmaceuticals, that distribute in different internal tissues or organs instead of an external x-ray source. The spatial and uptake distributions of the radiopharmaceuticals depend on the biokinetic properties of the pharmaceuticals and the normal or abnormal state of the patient. The gamma photons emitted from the radioactive source are detected by radiation detectors similar to those used in conventional nuclear medicine. The CT method requires projection (or planar) image data to be acquired from different views around the patient. These projection data are subsequently reconstructed using image reconstruction methods that generate cross-sectional images of the internally distributed radiopharmaceuticals. The SPECT images provide much improved contrast and detailed information about the radiopharmaceutical distribution as compared with the planar images obtained from conventional nuclear medicine methods.

As an emission computed tomographic (ECT) method, SPECT differs from PET in the types of radionuclides used. PET uses radionuclides such as C-11, N-13, O-15, and F-18 that emit positrons with subsequent emission of two coincident 511 keV annihilation photons. These radionuclides allow studies of biophysiologic functions that cannot be obtained from other means. However, they have very short half-lives, often requiring an on-site cyclotron for their production. Also, detection of the annihilation photons requires expensive imaging systems. SPECT uses standard radionuclides normally found in nuclear medicine clinics and which emit individual gamma-ray photons with energies that are much lower than 511 keV. Typical examples are the 140-keV photons from Tc-99m and the ~70-keV photons from TI-201. Subsequently, the costs of SPECT instrumentation and of performing SPECT are substantially less than PET.

Furthermore, substantial advances have been made in the development of new radiopharmaceuticals, instrumentation, and image processing and reconstruction methods for SPECT. The results are much improved quality and quantitative accuracy of SPECT images. These advances, combined with the relatively lower costs, have propelled SPECT to become an increasingly more important diagnostic tool in nuclear medicine clinics.

This section will present the basic principles of SPECT and the instrumentation and image processing and reconstruction methods that are necessary to reconstruct SPECT images. Finally, recent advances and future development that will continue to improve the diagnostic capability of SPECT will be discussed.

Basic Principles of SPECT

Single-photon emission computed tomography (SPECT) is a medical imaging technique that is based on the conventional nuclear medicine imaging technique and tomographic reconstruction methods.

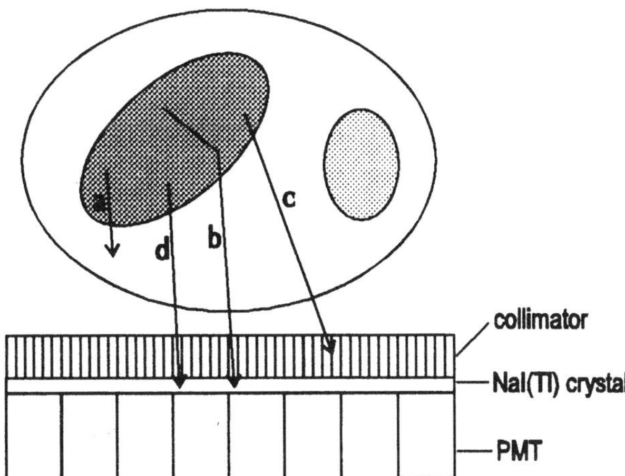

FIGURE 11.6 The conventional nuclear medicine imaging process. Gamma-ray photons emitted from the internally distributed radioactivity may experience photoelectric (a) or scatter (b) interactions. Photons that are not traveling in the direction within the acceptance analog of the collimator (c) will be intercepted by the lead collimator. Photons that experience no interaction and travel within the acceptance angle of the collimator will be detected (d).

General review of the basic principles, instrumentation, and reconstruction technique for SPECT can be found in a few review articles [Barrett, 1986; Jaszczak et al., 1980; Jaszczak and Coleman, 1985a; Jaszczak and Tsui, 1994].

The SPECT Imaging Process

The imaging process of SPECT can be simply depicted as in Fig. 11.6. Gamma-ray photons emitted from the internal distributed radiopharmaceutical penetrate through the patient's body and are detected by a single or a set of collimated radiation detectors. The emitted photons experience interactions with the intervening tissues through basic interactions of radiation with matter [Evans, 1955]. The photoelectric effect absorbs all the energy of the photons and stops their emergence from the patient's body. The other major interaction is Compton interaction, which transfers part of the photon energy to free electrons. The original photon is scattered into a new direction with reduced energy that is dependent on the scatter angle. Photons that escape from the patient's body include those that have not experienced any interactions and those which have experienced Compton scattering. For the primary photons from the commonly used radionuclides in SPECT, e.g., 140-keV of TC-99m and ~70-keV of TI-201, the probability of pair production is zero.

Most of the radiation detectors used in current SPECT systems are based on a single or multiple NaI(TI) scintillation detectors. The most significant development in nuclear medicine is the scintillation camera (or Anger camera) that is based on a large-area (typically 40 cm in diameter) NaI(TI) crystal [Anger, 1958, 1964]. An array of photomultiplier tubes (PMTs) is placed at the back of the scintillation crystal. When a photon hits and interacts with the crystal, the scintillation generated will be detected by the array of PMTs. An electronic circuitry evaluates the relative signals from the PMTs and determines the location of interaction of the incident photon in the scintillation crystal. In addition, the scintillation cameras have built-in energy discrimination electronic circuitry with finite energy resolution that provides selection of the photons that have not been scattered or been scattered within a small scattered angle. The scintillation cameras are commonly used in commercial SPECT systems.

Analogous to the lens in an optical imaging system, a scintillation camera system consists of a collimator placed in front of the NaI(TI) crystal for the imaging purpose. The commonly used collimator is made of a large number of parallel holes separated by lead septa [Anger, 1964; Keller, 1968; Tsui, 1988]. The geometric dimensions, i.e., length, size, and shape of the collimator apertures, determine the directions of photons that will be detected by the scintillation crystals or the geometric response of the collimator.

The width of the geometric response function increases (or the spatial resolution worsens) as the source distance from the collimator increases. Photons that do not pass through the collimator holes properly will be intercepted and absorbed by the lead septal walls of the collimator. In general, the detection efficiency is approximately proportional to the square of the width of the geometric response function of the collimator. This trade-off between detection efficiency and spatial resolution is a fundamental property of a typical SPECT system using conventional collimators.

The amount of radioactivity that is used in SPECT is restricted by the allowable radiation dose to the patient. Combined with photon attenuation within the patient, the practical limit on imaging time, and the trade-off between detection efficiency and spatial resolution of the collimator, the number of photons that are collected by a SPECT system is limited. These limitations resulted in SPECT images with relatively poor spatial resolution and high statistical noise fluctuations as compared with other medical imaging modalities. For example, currently a typical brain SPECT image has a total of about 500K counts per image slice and a spatial resolution in the order of approximately 8 mm. A typical myocardial SPECT study using TI-201 has about 150K total count per image slice and a spatial resolution of approximately 15 mm.

In SPECT, projection data are acquired from different views around the patient. Similar to x-ray CT, image processing and reconstruction methods are used to obtain transaxial or cross-sectional images from the multiple projection data. These methods consist of preprocessing and calibration procedures before further processing, mathematical algorithms for reconstruction from projections, and compensation methods for image degradation due to photon attenuation, scatter, and detector response.

The biokinetics of the radiopharmaceutical used, anatomy of the patient, instrumentation for data acquisition, preprocessing methods, image reconstruction techniques, and compensation methods have important effects on the quality and quantitative accuracy of the final SPECT images. A full understanding of SPECT cannot be accomplished without clear understanding of these factors. The biokinetics of radiopharmaceuticals and conventional radiation detectors have been described in the previous section on conventional nuclear medicine. The following subsections will present the major physical factors that affect SPECT and a summary review of the instrumentation, image reconstruction techniques, and compensation methods that are important technological and engineering aspects in the practice of SPECT.

Physical and Instrumentation Factors That Affect SPECT Images

There are several important physical and instrumentation factors that affect the measured data and subsequently the SPECT images. The characteristics and effects of these factors can be found in a few review articles [Jaszczak et al., 1981; Jaszczak and Tsui, 1994; Tsui et al., 1994a, 1994b]. As described earlier, gamma-ray photons that emit from an internal source may experience photoelectric absorption within the patient without contributing to the acquired data, Compton scattering with change in direction and loss of energy, or no interaction before exiting the patient's body. The exiting photons will be further selected by the geometric response of the collimator-detector. The photoelectric and Compton interactions and the characteristics of the collimator-detector have significant effects on both the quality and quantitative accuracy of SPECT image.

Photon attenuation is defined as the effect due to photoelectric and Compton interactions resulting in a reduced number of photons that would have been detected without them. The degree of attenuation is determined by the linear attenuation coefficient, which is a function of photon energy and the amount and types of materials contained in the attenuating medium. For example, the attenuation coefficient for the 140-keV photon emitted from the commonly used Tc-99m in water or soft tissue is 0.15 cm^{-1}. This gives rise to a half-valued layer, the thickness of material that attenuates half the incident photons, or 4.5 cm H_2O for the 140-keV photon. Attenuation is the most important factor that affects the quantitative accuracy of SPECT images.

Attenuation effect is complicated by the fact that within the patient the attenuation coefficient can be quite different in various organs. The effect is most prominent in the thorax, where the attenuation coefficients range from as low as 0.05 cm^{-1} in the lung to as high as 0.18 cm^{-1} in the compact bone for the 140-keV photons. In x-ray CT, the attenuation coefficient distribution is the target for image reconstruction.

In SPECT, however, the wide range of attenuation coefficient values and the variations of attenuation coefficient distributions among patients are major difficulties in obtaining quantitative accurate SPECT images. Therefore, compensation for attenuation is important to ensure good image quality and quantitatively high accuracy in SPECT. Review of different attenuation methods that have been used in SPECT is a subject of discussion later in this chapter.

Photons that have been scattered before reaching the radiation detector provide misplaced spatial information about the origin of the radioactive source. The results are inaccurate quantitative information and poor contrast in the SPECT images. For radiation detectors with perfect energy discrimination, scattered photons can be completely rejected. In a typical scintillation camera system, however, the energy resolution is in the order of 10% at 140 keV. With this energy resolution, the ratio of scattered to scattered total photons detected by a typical scintillation detector is about 20% to 30% in brain and about 30% to 40% in cardiac and body SPECT studies for 140-keV photons. Furthermore, the effect of scatter depends on the distribution of the radiopharmaceutical, the proximity of the source organ to the target organ, and the energy window used in addition to the photon energy and the energy resolution of the scintillation detector. The compensation of scatter is another important aspect of SPECT to ensure good image quality and quantitative accuracy.

The advances in SPECT can be attributed to simultaneous development of new radiopharmaceuticals, instrumentation, reconstruction methods, and clinical applications. Most radiopharmaceuticals that are developed for conventional nuclear medicine can readily be used in SPECT, and review of these developments is beyond the scope of this chapter. Recent advances include new agents that are labeled with iodine and technetium for blood perfusion for brain and cardiac studies. Also, the use of receptor agents and labeled antibiotics is being investigated. These developments have resulted in radiopharmaceuticals with improved uptake distribution, biokinetics properties, and potentially new clinical applications. The following subsections will concentrate on the development of instrumentation and image reconstruction methods that have made substantial impact on SPECT.

SPECT Instrumentation

Review of the advances in SPECT instrumentation can be found in several recent articles [Jaszczak et al., 1980; Rogers and Ackermann, 1992; Jaszczak and Tsui, 1994]. A typical SPECT system consists of a single or multiple units of radiation detectors arranged in a specific geometric configuration and a mechanism for moving the radiation detector(s) or specially designed collimators to acquire data from different projection views. In general, SPECT instrumentation can be divided into three general categories: (1) arrays of multiple scintillation detectors, (2) one or more scintillation cameras, and (3) hybrid scintillation detectors combining the first two approaches. In addition, special collimator designs have been proposed for SPECT for specific purposes and clinical applications. The following is a brief review of these SPECT systems and special collimators.

Multidetector SPECT System

The first fully functional SPECT imaging acquisition system was designed and constructed by Kuhl and Edwards [Kuhl and Edwards, 1963, 1964, 1968] in the 1960s, well before the conception of x-ray CT. As shown in Fig. 11.7a, the MARK IV brain SPECT system consisted of four linear arrays of eight discrete NaI(TI) scintillation detectors assembled in a square arrangement. Projection data were obtained by rotating the square detector array around the patient's head. Although images from the pioneer MARK IV SPECT system were unimpressive without the use of proper reconstruction methods that were developed in later years, the multidetector design has been the theme of several other SPECT systems that were developed. An example is the Gammatom-1 developed by Cho et al. [1982]. The design concept also was used in a dynamic SPECT system [Stokely et al., 1980] and commercial multidetector SPECT systems marketed by Medimatic, A/S (Tomomatic-32). Recently, the system design was extended to a multislice SPECT system with the Tomomatic-896, consisting of eight layers of 96 scintillation detectors. Also, the system allows both body and brain SPECT imaging by varying the aperture size.

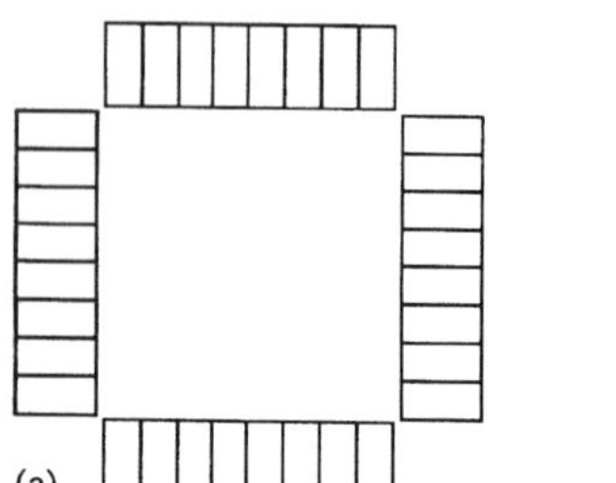

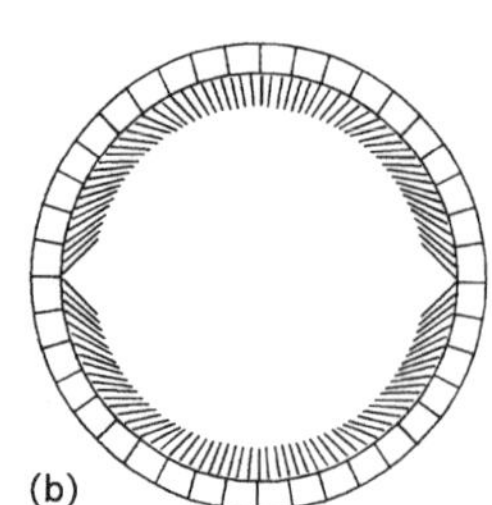

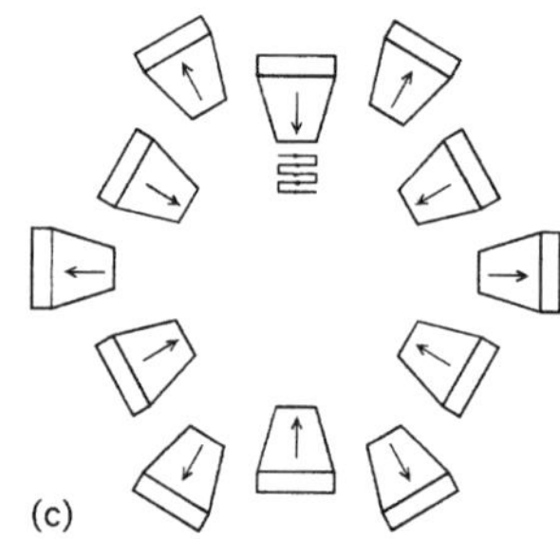

FIGURE 11.7 Examples of multidetector-based SPECT systems. (a) The MARK IV system consists of four arrays of eight individual NaI(TI) detectors arranged in a square configuration. (b) The Headtome-II system consists of a circular ring of detectors. A set of collimator vanes that swings in front of the discrete detector is used to collect projection data from different views. (c) A unique Cleon brain SPECT system consists of 12 detectors that scan both radially and tangentially.

Variations of the multiple-detectors arrangement have been proposed for SPECT system designs. Figure 11.7b shows the Headtome-II system by Shimadzu Corporation [Hirose et al., 1982], which consists of a stationary array of scintillation detectors arranged in a circular ring. Projection data are obtained by a set of collimator vanes that swings in front of the discrete detectors. A unique Cleon brain SPECT system (see Fig. 11.7c), originally developed by Union Carbide Corporation in the 1970s, consists of 12 detectors that scan both radially and tangentially [Stoddart and Stoddart, 1979]. Images from the original system were unimpressive due to inadequate sampling, poor axial resolution, and a reconstruction algorithm that did not take full advantage of the unique system design and data acquisition strategy. A much improved version of the system with a new reconstruction method [Moore et al., 1984] is currently marketed by Strichman Corporation.

The advantages of multidetector SPECT systems are their high sensitivity per image slice and high counting rate capability resulting from the array of multidetectors fully surrounding the patient. However, disadvantages of multidetector SPECT systems include their ability to provide only one or a few noncontiguous cross-sectional image slices. Also, these systems are relatively more expensive compared with camera-based SPECT systems described in the next subsection. With the advance of multicamera SPECT systems, the disadvantages of multidetector SPECT systems outweigh their advantages. As a result, they are less often found in nuclear medicine clinics.

Camera-Based SPECT Systems

The most popular SPECT systems are based on single or multiple scintillation cameras mounted on a rotating gantry. The successful design was developed almost simultaneously by three separate groups [Budinger and Gullberg, 1977; Jaszczak et al., 1977; Keyes et al., 1977]. In 1981, General Electric Medical Systems offered the first commercial SPECT system based on a single rotating camera and brought SPECT to clinical use. Today, there are more than ten manufacturers (e.g., ADAC, Elscint, General Electric, Hitachi, Picker, Siemens, Sopha, Toshiba, Trionix) offering an array of commercial SPECT systems in the marketplace.

An advantage of camera-based SPECT systems is their use of off-the-shelf scintillation cameras that have been widely used in conventional nuclear medicine. These systems usually can be used in both conventional planar and SPECT imaging. Also, camera-based SPECT systems allow truly three-dimensional (3D) imaging by providing a large set of contiguous transaxial images that cover the entire organ of interest. They are easily adaptable for SPECT imaging of the brain or body by simply changing the radius of rotation of the camera.

A disadvantage of a camera-based SPECT system is its relatively low counting rate capability. The dead time of a typical state-of-the-art scintillation camera gives rise to a loss of 20% of its true counts at about 80K counts per second. A few special high-count-rate systems give the same count rate loss at about

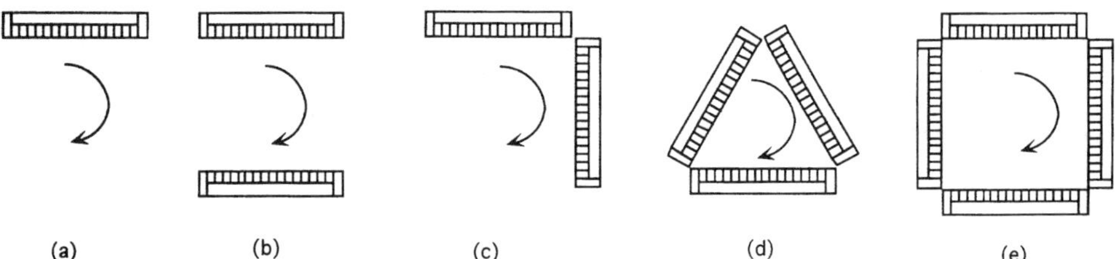

FIGURE 11.8 Examples of camera-based SPECT systems. (a) Single-camera system. (b) Dual-camera system with the two cameras placed at opposing sides of patient during rotation. (c) Dual-camera system with the two cameras placed at right angles. (d) Triple-camera system. (e) Quadruple-camera system.

150K counts per second. For SPECT systems using a single scintillation camera, the sensitivity per image slice is relative low compared with a typical multidetector SPECT system.

Recently, SPECT systems based on multiple cameras became increasingly more popular. Systems with two [Jaszczak et al., 1979a], three [Lim et al., 1980, 1985], and four cameras provide increased sensitivity per image slice that is proportional to the number of cameras. Figure 11.8 shows the system configurations of these camera-based SPECT systems. The dual-camera systems with two opposing cameras (Fig. 11.8b) can be used for both whole-body scanning and SPECT, and those with two right-angled cameras (Fig. 11.8c) are especially useful for 180° acquisition in cardiac SPECT. The use of multicameras has virtually eliminated the disadvantages of camera-based SPECT systems as compared with multidetector SPECT systems. The detection efficiency of camera-based SPECT systems can be further increased by using converging-hole collimators such as fan, cone, and astigmatic collimators at the cost of a smaller field of view. The use of converging-hole collimators in SPECT will be described in a later subsection.

Novel SPECT System Designs

There are several special SPECT systems designs that do not fit into the preceding two general categories. The commercially available CERESPECT (formerly known as ASPECT) [Genna and Smith, 1988] is a dedicated brain SPECT system. As shown in Fig. 11.9a, it consists of a single fixed-annular NaI(TI) crystal that completely surrounds the patient's head. Similar to a scintillation camera, an array of PMTs and electronics circuitry are placed behind the crystal to provide positional and energy information about photons that interact with the crystal. Projection data are obtained by rotating a segmented annular collimator with parallel holes that fits inside the stationary detector. A similar system is also being developed by Larsson et al. [1991] in Sweden.

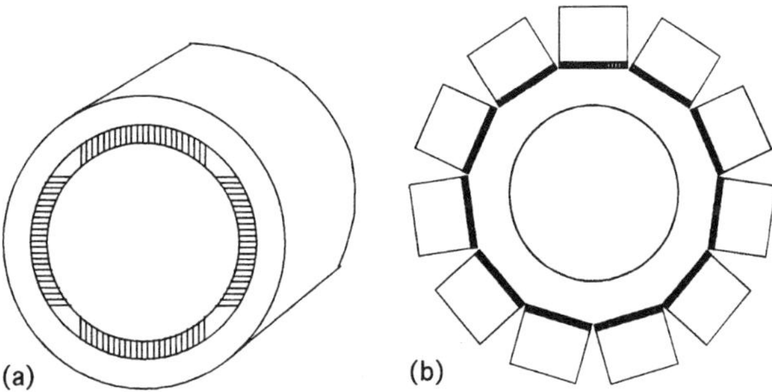

FIGURE 11.9 Examples of novel SPECT system designs. (a) The CERESPECT brain SPECT system consists of a single fixed annular NaI(TI) crystal and a rotating segmented annular collimator. (b) The SPRINT II brain SPECT system consists of 11 detector modules and a rotating lead ring with slit opening.

Several unique SPECT systems are currently being developed in research laboratories. They consist of modules of small scintillation cameras that surround the patient. The hybrid designs combine the advantage of multidetector and camera-based SPECT systems with added flexibility in system configuration. An example is the SPRINT II brain SPECT system developed at the University of Michigan [Rogers et al., 1988]. As shown in Fig. 11.9b, the system consists of 11 detector modules arranged in a circular ring around the patient's head. Each detector module consists of 44 one-dimensional bar NaI(TI) scintillation cameras. Projection data are required through a series of narrow slit openings on a rotating lead ring that fits inside the circular detector assemblies. A similar system was developed at the University of Iowa [Chang et al., 1990] with 22 detector modules, each consisting of four bar detectors. A set of rotating focused collimators is used to acquire projection data necessary for image reconstruction. At the University of Arizona, a novel SPECT system is being developed that consists of 20 small modular scintillation cameras [Milster et al., 1990] arranged in a hemispherical shell surrounding the patient's head [Rowe et al., 1992]. Projection data are acquired through a stationary hemispherical array of pinholes that are fitted inside the camera array. Without moving parts, the system allows acquisition of dynamic 3D SPECT data.

Special Collimator Designs for SPECT Systems

Similar to conventional nuclear medicine imaging, parallel-hole collimators (Fig. 11.10a) are commonly used in camera-based SPECT systems. As described earlier, the trade-off between detection efficiency and

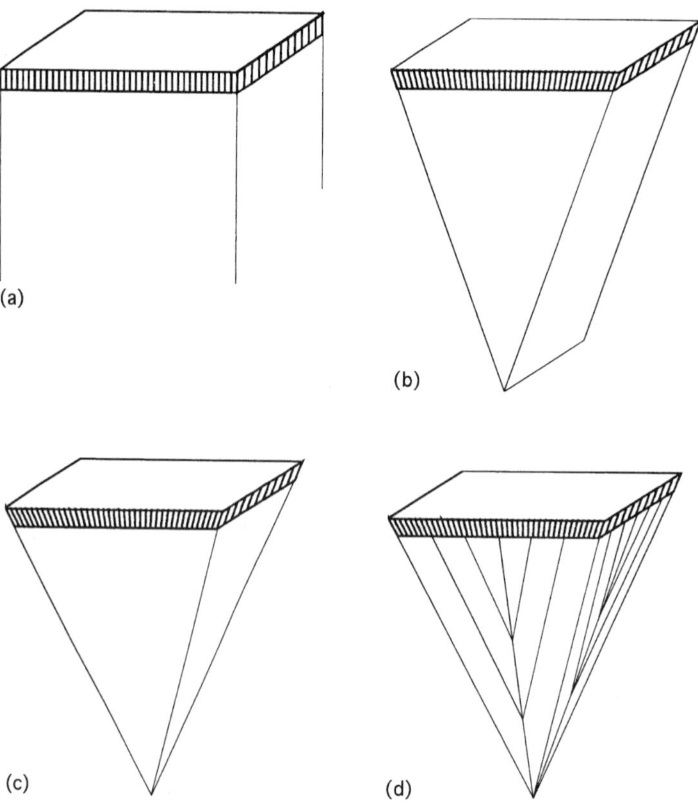

FIGURE 11.10 Collimator designs used in camera-based SPECT systems. (a) The commonly used parallel-hole collimator. (b) The fan-beam collimator, where the collimator holes are converged to a line that is parallel to the axis of rotation. (c) The cone-beam collimator, where the collimator holes are converged to a point. (d) A varifocal collimator, where the collimator holes are converged to various focal points.

spatial resolution of parallel-hole collimator is a limitating factor for SPECT. A means to improve SPECT system performance is to improve the trade-off imposed by the parallel-hole collimation.

To achieve this goal, converging-hole collimator designs that increase the angle of acceptance of incoming photons without sacrificing spatial resolution have been developed. Examples are fan-beam [Jaszczak et al., 1979b; Tsui et al., 1986], cone-beam [Jaszczak et al., 1987], astigmatic [Hawman and Hsieh, 1986], and more recently varifocal collimators. As shown in Fig. 11.10b–d, the collimator holes converge to a line that is oriented parallel to the axis of rotation for a fan-beam collimator, to a point for a cone-beam collimator, and to various points for a varifocal collimator, respectively. The gain in detection efficiency of a typical fan-beam and cone-beam collimator is about 1.5 and 2 times of that of a parallel-hole collimator with the same spatial resolution. The anticipated gain in detection efficiency and corresponding decrease in image noise are the main reasons for the interest in applying converging-hole collimators in SPECT.

Despite the advantage of increased detection efficiency, the use of converging-hole collimators in SPECT poses special problems. The trade-off for increase in detection efficiency as compared with parallel-hole collimators is a decrease in field of view (see Fig. 11.10). Consequently, converging-hole collimators are restricted to imaging small organs or body parts such as the head [Jaszczak et al., 1979b; Tsui et al., 1986] and heart [Gullberg et al., 1991]. In addition, the use of converging-hole collimators requires special data-acquisition strategies and image reconstruction algorithms. For example, for cone-beam tomography using a conventional single planar orbit, the acquired projection data become increasingly insufficient for reconstructing transaxial image sections that are further away from the central plane of the cone-beam geometry. Active research is under way to study special rotational orbits for sufficient projection data acquisition and 3D image reconstruction methods specific for cone-beam SPECT.

Reconstruction Methods

As discussed earlier, SPECT combines conventional nuclear medicine image techniques and methods for image reconstruction from projections. Aside from radiopharmaceuticals and instrumentation, image reconstruction methods are another important engineering and technological aspect of the SPECT imaging technique.

In x-ray CT, accurate transaxial images can be obtained through the use of standard algorithms for image reconstruction from projections. The results are images of attenuation coefficient distribution of various organs within the patient's body. In SPECT, the goal of image reconstruction is to determine the distribution of administered radiopharmaceutical in the patient. However, the presence of photon attenuation affects the measured projection data. If conventional reconstruction algorithms are used without proper compensation for the attenuation effects, inaccurate reconstructed images will be obtained. Effects of scatter and the finite collimator-detector response impose additional difficulties on image reconstruction in SPECT.

In order to achieve quantitatively accurate images, special reconstruction methods are required for SPECT. Quantitatively accurate image reconstruction methods for SPECT consist of two major components. They are the standard algorithms for image reconstruction from projections and methods that compensate for the image-degrading effects described earlier. Often, image reconstruction algorithms are inseparable from the compensation methods, resulting in a new breed of reconstruction method not found in other tomographic medical imaging modalities. The following subsections will present the reconstruction problem and a brief review of conventional algorithms for image reconstruction from projections. Then quantitative SPECT reconstruction methods that include additional compensation methods will be described.

Image Reconstruction Problem

Figure 11.11 shows a schematic diagram of the two-dimensional (2D) image reconstruction problem. Let $f(x, y)$ represent a 2D object distribution that is to be determined. A one-dimensional (1D) detector array is oriented at an angle θ with respect to the x axis of the laboratory coordinates system (x, y). The

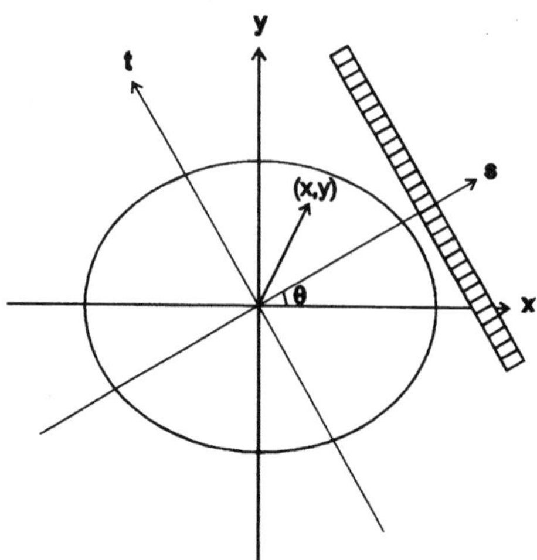

FIGURE 11.11 Schematic diagram of the two-dimensional image reconstruction problem. The projection data are line integrals of the object distribution along rays that are perpendicular to the detector. A source point (x, y) is projected onto a point $p\ (t, \theta)$, where t is a position along the projection and θ is the projection angle.

data collected into each detector element at location t, called the *projection data* $p(t, \theta)$, is equal to the sum of $f(x, y)$ along a ray that is perpendicular to the detector array and intersects the detector at position t; that is,

$$p(t, \theta) = c \int_{-\alpha}^{\alpha} f(x, y)\, ds \tag{11.1}$$

where (s, t) represents a coordinate system with s along the direction of the ray sum and t parallel to the 1D detector array, and c is the gain factor of the detection system. The angle between the s and x axes is θ. The relationship between the source position (x, y), the projection angle θ, and the position of detection on the 1D detector array is given by

$$t = y \cos\theta - x \sin\theta \tag{11.2}$$

In 2D tomographic imaging, the 1D detector array rotates around the object distribution $f(x, y)$ and collects projection data from various projection data from various projection angles θ. The integral transform of the object distribution to its projections given by Eq. (11.1) is called the *Radon transform* [Radon, 1917]. The goal of image reconstruction is to solve the inverse Radon transform. The solution is the reconstructed image estimate $\hat{f}(x, y)$ of the object distribution $f(x, y)$.

In x-ray CT, the measured projection data is given by

$$p'(t, \theta) = c_t I_o \exp\left[-\int_{-\alpha}^{+\alpha} \mu(x, y)\, ds\right] \tag{11.3}$$

where I_o is the intensity of the incident x-ray, $\mu(x, y)$ is the 2D attenuation coefficient, and c_t is the gain factor which transforms x-ray intensity to detected signals. The reconstruction problem can be rewritten as

$$p(t, \theta) = \ln\left[\frac{I_o}{p'(t, \theta)}\right] = \int_{-\alpha}^{+\alpha} \mu(x, y)\, ds \tag{11.4}$$

with the goal to solve for the attenuation coefficient distribution $\mu(x, y)$. Also, in x-ray CT, if parallel rays are used, the projection data at opposing views are the same, i.e., $p(t, \theta) = p(\theta + \pi)$, and projection data acquired over 180° will be sufficient for reconstruction. The number of linear samples along the 1D projection array and angular samples, i.e., the number of projection views, over 180° must be chosen carefully to avoid aliasing error and resolution loss in the reconstructed images.

In SPECT, if the effects of attenuation, scatter, and collimator-detector response are ignored, the measured projection data can be written as the integral of radioactivity along the projection rays; that is,

$$p(t, \theta) = c_e \int_{-\alpha}^{+\alpha} \rho(x, y)\, ds \tag{11.5}$$

where $\rho(x, y)$ is the radioactivity concentration distribution of the object, and c_e is the gain factor which transforms radioactivity concentration to detected signals. Equation (11.5) fits in the form of the Radon transform, and similar to x-ray CT, the radioactivity distribution can be obtained by solving the inverse Radon transform problem.

If attenuation is taken into consideration, the attenuated Radon transform [Gullberg, 1979] can be written as

$$p(t, \theta_i) = c_e \int_{-\alpha}^{+\alpha} \rho(x, y) \exp\left[-\int_{(x,y)}^{+\alpha} \mu(u, v)\, ds'\right] ds \tag{11.6}$$

where $\mu(u, v)$ is the 2D attenuation coefficient distribution, and $\int_{(x,y)}^{\alpha} \mu(u, v)\, ds$ is the attenuation factor for photons that originate from (x, y), travel along the direction perpendicular to the detector array, and are detected by the collimator-detector. A major difficulty in SPECT image reconstruction lies in the attenuation factor, which makes the inverse problem given by Eq. (11.6) difficult to solve analytically. However, the solution is important in cardiac SPECT, where the widely different attenuation coefficients are found in various organs within the thorax. Also, due to the attenuation factor, the projection views at opposing angles are different. Hence full 360° projection data are usually necessary for image reconstruction in SPECT.

Different from x-ray CT, small differences in attenuation coefficient are not as important in SPECT. When the attenuation coefficient in the body region can be considered constant, the attenuated Radon transform given by Eq. (11.6) can be written as [Tretiak and Metz, 1980]

$$p(t, \theta) = c_e \int_{-\alpha}^{+\alpha} \rho(x, y) \exp\left[-\mu l(x, y)\right] ds \tag{11.7}$$

where μ is the constant attenuation coefficient in the body region, and $l(x, y)$ is the path length between the point (x, y) and the edge of the attenuator (or patient's body) along the direction of the projection ray. The solution of the inverse problem with constant attenuator has been a subject of several investigations. It forms the basis for analytical methods for compensation of uniform attenuation described later in this chapter.

When scatter and collimator-detector response are taken into consideration, the assumption that the projection data can be represented by line integrals given by Eqs. (11.1) to (11.7) will no longer be exactly correct. Instead, the integration will have to include a wider region covering the field of view of the collimator-detector (or the collimator-detector response function). The image reconstruction problem is further complicated by the nonstationary properties of the collimator-detector and scatter response functions and their dependence on the size and composition of the patient's body.

Algorithms for Image Reconstruction from Projections

The application of methods for image reconstruction from projections was a major component in the development of x-ray CT in the 1970s. The goal was to solve for the inverse Radon transform problem given in Eq. (11.1). There is an extensive literature on these reconstruction algorithms. Reviews of the applications of these algorithms to SPECT can be found in several articles [Barrett, 1986; Brooks and Di Chiro, 1975, 1976; Budinger and Gullberg, 1974].

Simple Backprojection. An intuitive image reconstruction method is *simple backprojection.* Here, the reconstructed image is formed simply by spreading the values of the measured projection data uniformly along the projection ray into the reconstructed image array. By backprojecting the measured projection data from all projection views, an estimate of the object distribution can be obtained. Mathematically, the simple backproject operation is given by

$$\hat{f}(x, y) = \sum_{j=1}^{m} p(y \cos \theta_j - x \sin \theta_j, \theta_j) \Delta\theta \tag{11.8}$$

where θ_j is the jth projection angle, m is the number of projection views, and $\Delta\theta$ is the angular spacing between adjacent projections. The simple backprojected image $\hat{f}(x, y)$ is a poor approximation of the true object distribution $f(x, y)$. It is equivalent to the true object distribution blurred by a blurring function in the form of $1/r$.

There are two approaches for accurate image reconstruction, and both have been applied to SPECT. The first approach is based on direct analytical methods and is widely used in commercial SPECT systems. The second approach is based on statistical criteria and iterative algorithms. They have been found useful in reconstruction methods that include compensation for the image-degrading effects.

Analytical Reconstruction Algorithms: Filtered Backprojection. The most widely used analytical image-reconstruction algorithm is the *filtered backprojection* (FBP) method, which involves backprojecting the filtered projections [Bracewell and Riddle, 1967; Ramachandran and Lakshminarayanan, 1971]. The algorithm consists of two major steps:

1. Filter the measured projection data at different projection angles with a special function.
2. Backproject the filtered projection data to form the reconstructed image.

The first step of the filtered backprojection method can be implemented in two different ways. In the spatial domain, the filter operation is equivalent to convolving the measured projection data using a special convolving function $h(t)$; that is,

$$p'(t, \theta) = p(t, \theta) \circledast h(t) \tag{11.8a}$$

where $\circledast$ is the convolution operation. With the advance of fast Fourier transform (FFT) methods, the convolution operation can be replaced by a more efficient multiplication in the spatial frequency domain. The equivalent operation consists of three steps:

1. Fourier-transform the measured projection data into spatial frequency domain using the FFT method, i.e., $P(\nu, \theta) = \mathrm{FT}\{p(t, \theta)\}$, where FT is the Fourier transform operation.
2. Multiply the Fourier-transformed projection data with a special function that is equal to the Fourier transform of the special function used in the convolution operation described above, i.e., $P'(\nu, \theta) = P(\nu, \theta) \cdot H(\nu)$, where $H(\nu) = \mathrm{FT}\{h(x)\}$ is the Fourier transform of $h(x)$.
3. Inverse Fourier transform the product $P'(\nu, \theta)$ into spatial domain.

Again, the filtered projections from different projection angles are backprojected to form the reconstructed images.

The solution of the inverse Radon transform given in Eq. (11.1) specifies the form of the special function. In the spatial domain, the special function $h(x)$ used in the convolution operation in Eq. (11.8) is given by

$$h(x) = \frac{1}{2(\Delta x)^2}\left\{\text{sinc}\left[\frac{x}{(\Delta x)}\right]\right\} - \frac{1}{4(\Delta x)^2}\left\{\text{sinc}^2\left[\frac{x}{2(\Delta x)}\right]\right\} \tag{11.9}$$

where Δx is the linear sampling interval, and $\text{sinc}(z) = [\sin(z)]/z$. The function $h(x)$ consists of a narrow central peak with high magnitude and small negative side lobes. It removes the blurring from the $1/r$ function found in the simple backprojected images.

In the frequency domain, the special function $H(v)$ is equivalent to the Fourier transform of $h(x)$ and is a truncated ramp function given by

$$H(v) = |v| \cdot \text{rect}(v) \tag{11.10}$$

where $|v|$ is the ramp function, and

$$\text{rect}(v) = \begin{cases} 1 & |v| \le 0.5 \\ 0 & |v| < 0.5 \end{cases} \tag{11.11}$$

that is, the rectangular function $\text{rect}(v)$ has a value of 1 when the absolute value of v is less than the Nyquist frequency at 0.5 cycles per pixel.

For noisy projection data, the ramp function tends to amplify the high-frequency noise. In these situations, an additional smoothing filter is often applied to smoothly roll off the high-frequency response of the ramp function. Examples are Hann and Butterworth filters [Huesman et al., 1977]. Also, deconvolution filters have been used to provide partial compensation of spatial resolution loss due to the collimator-detection response and noise smoothing. Examples are the Metz and Wiener filters (see below).

Iterative Reconstruction Algorithms. Another approach to image reconstruction is based on statistical criteria and iterative algorithms. They were investigated for application in SPECT before the development of analytical image reconstruction methods [Gilbert, 1972; Goitein, 1972; Gordon et al., 1970; Kuhl and Edwards, 1968]. The major drawbacks of iterative reconstruction algorithms are the extensive computations and long processing time required. For these reasons, the analytical reconstruction methods have gained widespread acceptance in clinical SPECT systems. In recent years, there has been renewed interest in the use of iterative reconstruction algorithms in SPECT to achieve accurate quantitation by compensating for the image-degrading effects.

A typical iterative reconstruction algorithm starts with an initial estimate of the object source distribution. A set of projection data is estimated from the initial estimate using a projector that models the imaging process. The estimated projection data are compared with the measured projection data at the same projection angles, and their differences are calculated. Using an algorithm derived from specific statistical criteria, the differences are used to update the initial image estimate. The updated image estimate is then used to recalculate a new set of estimated projection data that are again compared with the measured projection data. The procedure is repeated until the difference between the estimated and measured projection data are smaller than a preselected small value. Statistical criteria that have been used in formulating iterative reconstruction algorithms include the minimum mean squares error (MMSE) [Budinger and Gullberg, 1977], weighted least squares (WLS) [Huesman et al., 1977], maximum entropy (ME) [Minerbo, 1979], maximum likelihood (ML) [Shepp and Vardi, 1982], and maximum a posteriori approaches [Barrett, 1986; Geman and McClure, 1985; Johnson et al., 1991; Levitan and Herman, 1987; Liang and Hart, 1987]. Iterative algorithms that have been used in estimating the reconstructed images include the conjugate gradient (CG) [Huesman et al., 1977] and expectation maximization (EM) [Lange and Carson, 1984].

Recently, interest in the application of iterative reconstruction algorithms in SPECT has been revitalized. The interest is sparked by the need to compensate for the spatially variant and/or nonstationary image-degrading factors in the SPECT imaging process. The compensation can be achieved by modeling the imaging process that includes the image-degrading factors in the projection and backprojection operations of the iterative steps. The development is aided by advances made in computer technology and custom-dedicated processors. The drawback of long processing time in using these algorithms is substantially reduced. Discussion of the application of iterative reconstruction algorithms in SPECT will be presented in a later subsection.

Compensation Methods

For a typical SPECT system, the measured projection data are severely affected by attenuation, scatter, and collimator-detector response. Direct reconstruction of the measured projection data without compensation of these effects produces images with artifacts, distortions, and inaccurate quantitation. In recent years, substantial efforts have been made to develop compensation methods for these image-degrading effects. This development has produced much improved quality and quantitatively accurate reconstructed images. The following subsections will present a brief review of some of these compensation methods.

Compensation for Attenuation. Methods for attenuation compensation can be grouped into two categories: (1) methods that assume the attenuation coefficient is uniform over the body region, and (2) methods that address situations of nonuniform attenuation coefficient distribution. The assumption of uniform attenuation can be applied to SPECT imaging of the head and abdomen regions. The compensation methods seek to solve for the inverse of the attenuated Radon transform given in Eq. (11.7). For cardiac and lung SPECT imaging, nonuniform attenuation compensation methods must be used due to the very different attenuation coefficient values in various organs in the thorax. Here, the goal is to solve the more complicated problem of the inverse of the attenuated Radon transform in Eq. (11.6).

There are several approximate methods for compensating uniform attenuation. They include methods that preprocess the projection data or postprocess the reconstructed image. The typical preprocess methods are those which use the geometric or arithmetic mean [Sorenson, 1974] of projections from opposing views. These compensation methods are easy to implement and work well with a single, isolated source. However, they are relatively inaccurate for more complicated source configurations. Another method achieves uniform attenuation compensation by processing the Fourier transform of the sinogram [Bellini et al., 1979]. The method provides accurate compensation even for complicated source configurations.

A popular compensation method for uniform attenuation is that proposed by Chang [1978]. The method requires knowledge of the body contour. The information is used in calculating the average attenuation factor at each image point from all projection views. The array of attenuation factors is used to multiply the reconstructed image obtained without attenuation compensation. The result is the attenuation-compensated image. An iterative scheme also can be implemented for improved accuracy. In general, the Chang method performs well for uniform attenuation situations. However, the noise level in the reconstructed images increases with iteration number. Also, certain image features tend to fluctuate as a function of iteration. For these reasons, no more than one or two iterations are recommended.

Another class of methods for uniform attenuation compensation is based on analytical solution of the inverse of the attenuation Radon transform given in Eq. (11.7) for a convex-shaped medium [Gullberg and Budinger, 1981; Tretiak and Metz, 1980]. The resultant compensation method involves multiplying the projection data by an exponential function. Then the FBP algorithm is used in the image reconstruction except that the ramp filter is modified such that its value is zero in the frequency range between 0 and $\mu/2\pi$, where μ is the constant attenuation coefficient. The compensation method is easy to implement and provides good quantitative accuracy. However, it tends to amplify noise in the resulting image, and smoothing is required to obtain acceptable image quality [Gullberg and Budinger, 1981].

An analytical solution for the more complicated inverse attenuated Radon transform with nonuniform attenuation distribution [Eq. (11.6)] has been found difficult [Gullberg, 1979]. Instead, iterative approaches have been used to estimate a solution of the problem. The application is especially important in cardiac and lung SPECT studies. The iterative methods model the attenuation distribution in the projection and backprojection operations [Manglos et al., 1987; Tsui et al., 1989]. The ML criterion with the EM algorithm [Lange and Carson, 1984] has been used with success [Tsui et al., 1989]. The compensation method requires information about the attenuation distribution of the region to be imaged. Recently, transmission CT methods are being developed using existing SPECT systems to obtain attenuation distribution from the patient. The accurate attenuation compensation of cardiac SPECT promises to provide much improved quality and quantitative accuracy in cardiac SPECT images [Tsui et al., 1989, 1994a].

Compensation for Scatter. As described earlier in this chapter, scattered photons carry misplaced positional information about the source distribution resulting in lower image contrast and inaccurate quantitation in SPECT images. Compensation for scatter will improve image contrast for better image quality and images that will more accurately represent the true object distribution. Much research has been devoted to develop scatter compensation methods that can be grouped into two general approaches. In the first approach, various methods have been developed to estimate the scatter contribution in the measured data. The scatter component is then subtracted from the measured data or from the reconstructed images to obtain scatter-free reconstructed images. The compensation method based on this approach tends to increase noise level in the compensated images.

One method estimates the scatter contribution as a convolution of the measured projection data with an empirically derived function [Axelsson et al., 1984]. Another method models the scatter component as the convolution of the primary (or unscattered) component of the projection data with an exponential function [Floyd et al., 1985]. The convolution method is extended to 3D by estimating the 2D scatter component [Yanch et al., 1988]. These convolution methods assume that the scatter response function is stationary, which is only an approximation.

The scatter component also has been estimated using two energy windows acquisition methods. One method estimates the scatter component in the primary energy window from the measured data obtained from a lower and adjacent energy window [Jaszczak et al., 1984, 1985b]. In a dual photopeak window (DPW) method, two nonoverlapping windows spanning the primary photopeak window are used [King et al., 1992]. This method provides more accurate estimation of the scatter response function.

Multiple energy windows also have been used to estimate the scatter component. One method uses two satellite energy windows that are placed directly above and below the photopeak window to estimate the scatter component in the center window [Ogawa et al., 1991]. In another method, the energy spectrum detected at each image pixel is used to predict the scatter contribution [Koral et al., 1988]. An energy-weighted acquisition (EWA) technique acquires data from multiple energy windows. The images reconstructed from these data are weighted with energy-dependent factors to minimize scatter contribution to the weighted image [DeVito et al., 1989; DeVito and Hamill, 1991]. Finally, the holospectral imaging method [Gagnon et al., 1989] estimates the scatter contribution from a series of eigenimages derived from images reconstructed from data obtained from a series of multiple energy windows.

In the second approach, the scatter photons are utilized in estimating the true object distribution. Without subtracting the scatter component, the compensated images are less noisy than those obtained from the first approach. In one method, an average scatter response function can be combined with the geometric response of the collimator-detector to form the total response of the imaging system [Gilland et al., 1988; Tsui et al., 1994a]. The total response function is then used to generate a restoration filter for an approximate geometric and scatter response compensation (see below).

Another class of methods characterizes the exact scatter response function and incorporates it into iterative reconstruction algorithms for accurate compensation for scatter [Floyd et al., 1985; Frey and Tsui, 1992]. Since the exact scatter response functions are nonstationary and are asymmetric in shape, implementation of the methods requires extensive computations. However, efforts are being made to parameterize the scatter response function and to optimize the algorithm for substantial reduction in processing time [Frey et al., 1993; Frey and Tsui, 1991].

Compensation for Collimator-Detector Response. As described earlier, for a typical collimator-detector, the response function broadens as the distance from the collimator face increases. The effect of the collimator-detector response is loss of spatial resolution and blurring of fine detail in SPECT images.

Also, the spatially variant detector response function will cause nonisotropic point response in SPECT images [Knesaurek et al., 1989; Maniawski et al., 1991]. The spatially variant collimator-detector response is a major difficulty in its exact compensation.

By assuming an average and stationary collimator-detector response function, restoration filters can be used to provide partial and approximate compensation for the effects of the collimator-detector. Examples are the Metz [King et al., 1984, 1986] and Wiener [Penney et al., 1990] filters, where the inverse of the average collimator-detector response function is used in the design of the restoration filters. Two-dimensional (2D) compensation is achieved by applying the 1D restoration filters to the 1D projection data, and 3D compensation by applying the 2D filters to the 2D projection images [Tsui et al., 1994b].

Analytical methods have been developed for compensation of the spatially variant detector response. A spatially variant filtering method has been proposed which is based on the frequency distance principle (FDP) [Edholm et al., 1986; Lewitt et al., 1989]. The method has been shown to provide an isotropic point response function in phantom SPECT images [Glick et al., 1993].

Iterative reconstruction methods also have been used to accurately compensate for both nonuniform attenuation and collimator-detector response by modeling the attenuation distribution and spatially variant detector response function in the projection and backprojection steps. The compensation methods have been applied in 2D reconstruction [Formiconi et al., 1990; Tsui et al., 1988], and more recently in 3D reconstruction [Tsui et al., 1994b; Zeng et al., 1991]. It has been found that the iterative reconstruction methods provide better image quality and more accurate quantitation when compared with the conventional restoration filtering techniques. Furthermore, 3D compensation outperforms 2D compensation at the expense of more extensive computations [Tsui et al., 1994b].

Sample SPECT Images

This subsection presents sample SPECT images to demonstrate the performance of various reconstruction and compensation methods. Two data sets were used. The first set was acquired from a 3D physical phantom that mimics a human brain perfusion study. The phantom study provided knowledge of the true radioactivity distribution for evaluation purposes. The second data set was obtained from a patient myocardial SPECT study using thallium-201.

Figure 11.12a shows the radioactivity distribution from a selected slice of a 3D brain phantom manufactured by the Data Spectrum Corporation. The phantom design was based on PET images from a normal patient to simulate cerebral blood flow [Hoffman et al., 1990]. The phantom was filled with water containing 74 mBq of Tc-99m. A single-camera-based GE 400AC/T SPECT system fitted with a high-resolution collimator was used for data collection. The projection data were acquired into 128×128 matrices at 128 views over 360°. Figure 11.12b shows the reconstructed image obtained from the FBP algorithm without any compensation. The poor image quality is due to statistical noise fluctuations, effects of attenuation (especially at the central portion of the image), loss of spatial resolution due to the collimator-detector response, and loss of contrast due to scatter.

Figure 11.12c shows the reconstructed image obtained with the application of a noise-smoothing filter and compensation for the uniform attenuation and scatter. The resulting image has lower noise level, reduced attenuation effect, and higher contrast as compared with the image shown in Fig. 11.12b. Figure 11.12d is similar to Fig. 11.12c except for an additional application of a Metz filter to partially compensate for the collimator-detector blurring. Figure 11.12e shows the reconstructed image obtained from the iterative ML-EM algorithm that accurately modeled the attenuation and spatially variant detector response. The much superior image quality is apparent.

Figure 11.13a shows a selected FBP reconstructed transaxial image slice from a typical patient myocardial SPECT study using thallium-201. Figure 11.13b shows the reconstructed image obtained from the Chang algorithm for approximate nonuniform attenuation compensation and 2D processing using a Metz filter for approximate compensation for collimator-detector response. Figure 11.13c shows the reconstructed image obtained from the iterative ML-EM algorithm using a measured transmission CT image for accurate attenuation compensation and a 2D model of the collimator-detector response for accurate collimator-detector response compensation. The reconstructed image in Fig. 11.13d is similar to that in

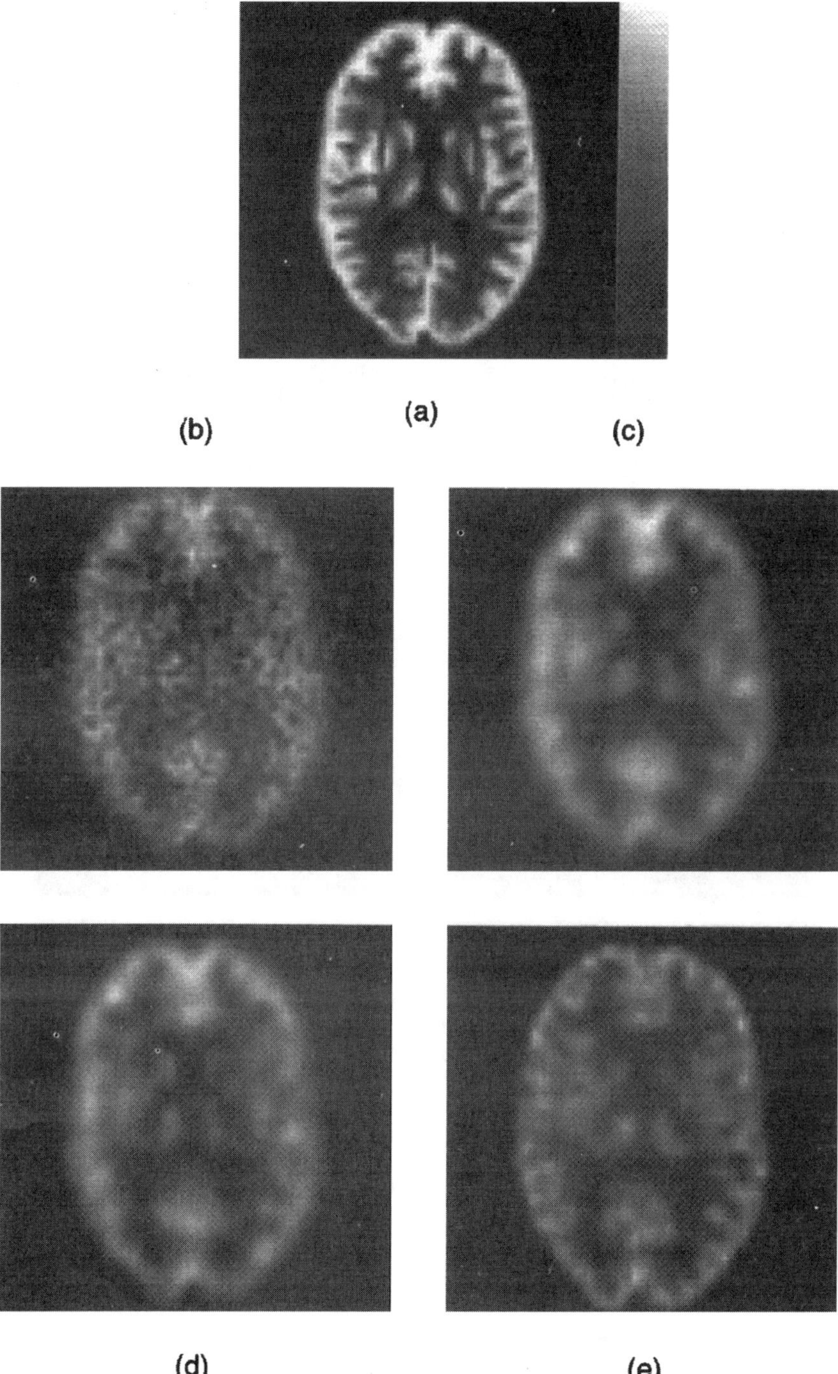

FIGURE 11.12 Sample images from a phantom SPECT study. (a) Radioactivity distribution from a selected slice of a 3D brain phantom. (b) Reconstructed image obtained from the FBP algorithm without any compensation. (c) Reconstructed image obtained with the application of noise-smoothing filter and compensation for uniform attenuation and scatter. (d) Similar to (c) except for an additional application of a Metz filter to partially compensate for the collimator-detector blurring. (e) Reconstructed image similar to that obtained from the iterative ML-EM algorithm that accurately models the attenuation and spatially variant detector response. (From Tsui BMW, Frey EC, Zhao X-D, et al. 1994. Reprinted with permission.)

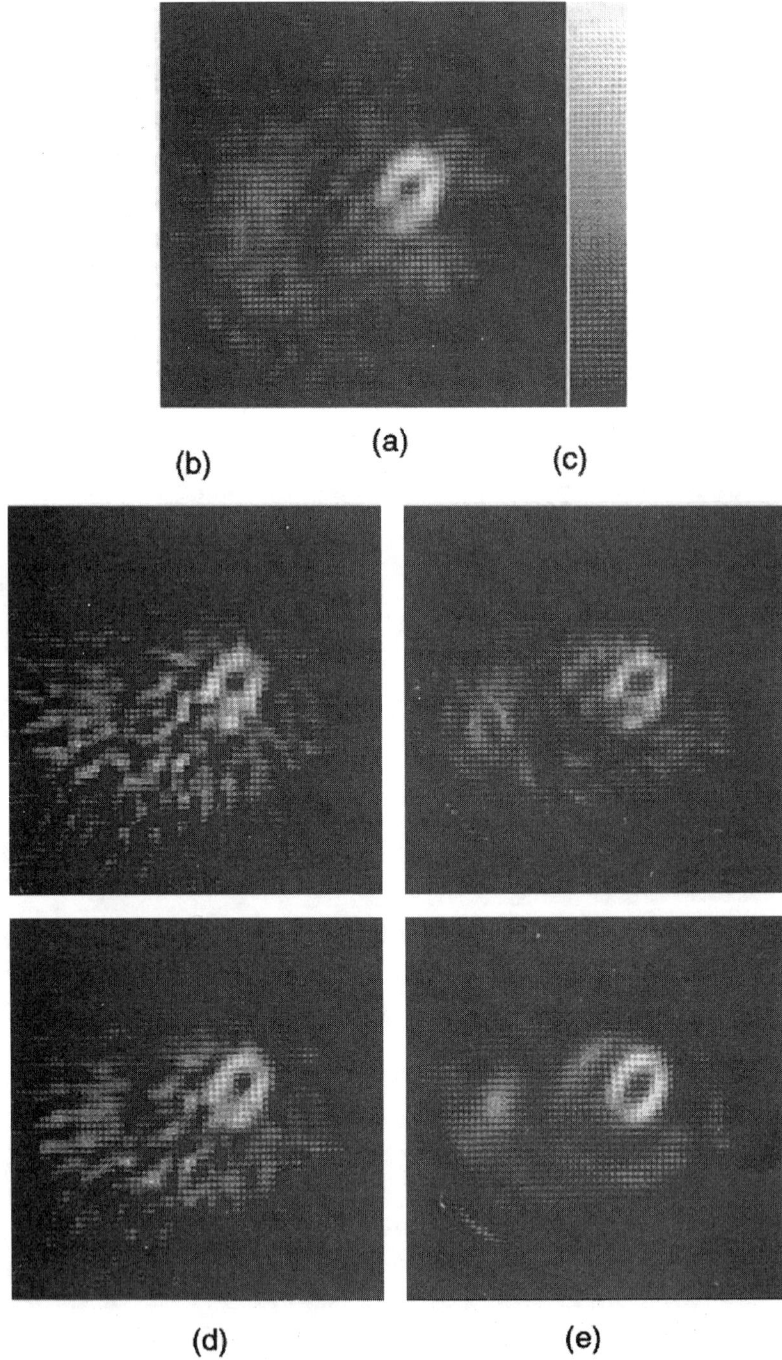

FIGURE 11.13 Sample images from a patient myocardial SPECT study using TI-201. (a) A selected transaxial image slice from a typical patient myocardial SPECT study using TI-201. The reconstructed image was obtained with the FBP algorithm without any compensation. (b) Reconstructed image obtained from the Chang algorithm for approximate nonuniform attenuation compensation and 2D processing using a Metz filter for approximate compensation for collimator-detector response. (c) Reconstructed image obtained from the iterative ML-EM algorithm using a measured transmission CT image for accurate attenuation compensation and 2D model of the collimator-detector response for accurate collimator-detector response compensation. (d) Similar to (b) except that the Metz filter was implemented in 3D. (e) Similar to (c) except that a 3D model of the collimator-detector response is used.

Fig. 11.13b except that the Metz filter was implemented in 3D. Finally, the reconstructed image in Fig. 11.13e is similar to that in Fig. 11.13c except that a 3D model of the collimator-detector response is used. The superior image quality obtained from using an accurate 3D model of the imaging process is evident.

Discussion

The development of SPECT has been a combination of advances in radiopharmaceuticals, instrumentation, image processing and reconstruction methods, and clinical applications. Although substantial progress has been made during the last decade, there are many opportunities for contributions from biomedical engineering in the future.

The future SPECT instrumentation will consist of more detector area to fully surround the patient for high detection efficiency and multiple contiguous transaxial slice capability. Multicamera SPECT systems will continue to dominate the commercial market. The use of new radiation detector materials and detector systems with high spatial resolution will receive increased attention. Continued research is needed to investigate special converging-hole collimator design geometries, fully 3D reconstruction algorithms, and their clinical applications.

To improve image quality and to achieve quantitatively accurate SPECT images will continue to be the goals of image processing and image reconstruction methods for SPECT. An important direction of research in analytical reconstruction methods will involve solving the inverse Radon transform, which includes the effects of attenuation, the spatially variant collimator-detector response function, and scatter. The development of iterative reconstruction methods will require more accurate models of the complex SPECT imaging process, faster and more stable iterative algorithms, and more powerful computers and special computational hardware.

These improvements in SPECT instrumentation and image reconstruction methods, combined with newly developed radiopharmaceuticals, will bring SPECT images with increasingly higher quality and more accurate quantitation to nuclear medicine clinics for improved diagnosis and patient care.

References

Anger HO. 1958. Scintillation camera. Rev Sci Instrum 29:27.

Anger HO. 1964. Scintillation camera with multichannel collimators. J Nucl Med 5:515.

Axelsson B, Msaki P, Israelsson A. 1984. Subtraction of Compton-scattered photons in single-photon emission computed tomography. J Nucl Med 25:490.

Barrett HH. 1986. Perspectives on SPECT. SPIE 671:178.

Bellini S, Piacentini M, Cafforio C, et al. 1979. Compensation of tissue absorption in emission tomography. IEEE Trans Acoust Speech Signal Processing ASSP-27:213.

Bracewell RN, Riddle AC. 1967. Inversion of fan-beam scans in radio astronomy. Astrophys J 150:427.

Brooks RA, Di Chiro G. 1975. Theory of image reconstruction in computed tomography. Radiology 117:561.

Brooks RA, Di Chiro G. 1976. Principles of computer assisted tomography (CAT) in radiographic and radioisotopic imaging. Phys Med Biol 21:689.

Budinger TF, Gullberg GT. 1974. Three-dimensional reconstruction in nuclear medicine emission imaging. IEEE Trans Nucl Sci NS-21:2.

Budinger TF, Gullberg GT. 1977. Transverse section reconstruction of gamma-ray emitting radionuclides in patients. In MM Ter-Pogossian, ME Phelps, GL Brownell, et al. (eds), Reconstruction Tomography in Diagnostic Radiology and Nuclear Medicine. Baltimore, University Park Press.

Chang LT. 1978. A method for attenuation correction in radionuclide computed tomography. IEEE Trans Nucl Sci NS-25:638.

Chang W, Huang G, Wang L. 1990. A multi-detector cylindrical SPECT system for phantom imaging. In Conference Record of the 1990 Nuclear Science Symposium, vol 2, pp 1208–1211. Piscataway, NJ, IEEE.

Cho ZH, Yi W, Jung KJ, et al. 1982. Performance of single photon tomography system-Gamma-tom-1. IEEE Trans Nucl Sci NS-29:484.

DeVito RP, Hamill JJ. 1991. Determination of weighting functions for energy-weighted acquisition. J Nucl Med 32:343.

DeVito RP, Hamill JJ, Treffert JD, Stoub EW. 1989. Energy-weighted acquisition of scintigraphic images using finite spatial filters. J Nucl Med 30:2029.

Edholm PR, Lewitt RM, Lindholm B. 1986. Novel properties of the Fourier decomposition of the sinogram. Proc SPIE 671:8.

Evans RD. 1955. The Atomic Nucleus. Malabar, FL, Robert E. Krieger.

Floyd CE, Jaszczak RJ, Greer KL, Coleman RE. 1985. Deconvolution of Compton scatter in SPECT. J Nucl Med 26:403.

Formiconi AR, Pupi A, Passeri A. 1990. Compensation of spatial system response in SPECT with conjugate gradient reconstruction technique. Phys Med Biol 34:69.

Frey EC, Ju Z-W, Tsui BMW. 1993. A fast projector-backprojector pair modeling the asymmetric, spatially varying scatter response function for scatter compensation in SPECT imaging. IEEE Trans Nucl Sci NS-40(4):1192.

Frey EC, Tsui BMW. 1991. Spatial properties of the scatter response function in SPECT. IEEE Trans Nucl Sci NS-38:789.

Frey EC, Tsui BMW. 1992. A comparison of scatter compensation methods in SPECT: Subtraction-based techniques versus iterative reconstruction with an accurate scatter model. In Conference Record of the 1992 Nuclear Science Symposium and the Medical Imaging Conference, October 27–31, Orlando, FL, pp 1035–1037.

Gagnon D, Todd-Pokropek A, Arsenault A, Dupros G. 1989. Introduction to holospectral imaging in nuclear medicine for scatter subtraction. IEEE Trans Med Imaging 8:245.

Geman S, McClure DE. 1985. Bayesian image analysis: An application to single photon emission tomography. In Proceedings of the Statistical Computing Section. Washington, American Statistical Association.

Genna S, Smith A. 1988. The development of ASPECT, an annular single crystal brain camera for high efficiency SPECT. IEEE Trans Nucl Sci NS-35:654.

Gilland DR, Tsui BMW, Perry JR, et al. 1988. Optimum filter function for SPECT imaging. J Nucl Med 29:643.

Gilbert P. 1972. Iterative methods for the three-dimensional reconstruction of an object from projections. J Theor Biol 36:105.

Glick SJ, Penney BC, King MA, Byrne CL. 1993. Non-iterative compensation for the distance-dependent detector response and photon attenuation in SPECT imaging. IEEE Trans Med Imaging 13(2):363.

Goitein M. 1972. Three-dimensional density reconstruction from a series of two-dimensional projections. Nucl Instrum Methods 101:509.

Gordon R. 1974. A tutorial on ART (Algebraic reconstruction techniques). IEEE Trans Nucl Sci 21:78.

Gordon R, Bender R, Herman GT. 1970. Algebraic reconstruction techniques (ART) for three-dimensional electron microscopy and x-ray photography. J Theor Biol 29:471.

Gullberg GT. 1979. The attenuated Radon transform: Theory and application in medicine and biology. Ph.D. dissertation, University of California at Berkeley.

Gullberg GT, Budinger TF. 1981. The use of filtering methods to compensate for constant attenuation in single-photon emission computed tomography. IEEE Trans Biomed Eng BME-28:142.

Gullberg GT, Christian PE, Zeng GL, et al. 1991. Cone beam tomography of the heart using single-photon emission-computed tomography. Invest Radiol 26:681.

Hawman EG, Hsieh J. 1986. An astigmatic collimator for high sensitivity SPECT of the brain. J Nucl Med 27:930.

Hirose Y, Ikeda Y, Higashi Y, et al. 1982. A hybrid emission CT-HEADTOME II. IEEE Trans Nucl Sci NS-29:520.

Hoffman EJ, Cutler PD, Kigby WM, Mazziotta JC. 1990. 3-D phantom to simulate cerebral blood flow and metabolic images for PET. IEEE Trans Nucl Sci NS-37:616.

Huesman RH, Gullberg GT, Greenberg WL, Budinger TF. 1977. RECLBL Library Users Manual, Donner Algorithms for Reconstruction Tomography. Lawrence Berkeley Laboratory, University of California.

Jaszczak RJ, Chang LT, Murphy PH. 1979. Single photon emission computed tomography using multi-slice fan beam collimators. IEEE Trans Nucl Sci NS-26:610.

Jaszczak RJ, Chang LT, Stein NA, Moore FE. 1979. Whole-body single-photon emission computed tomography using dual, large-field-of-view scintillation cameras. Phys Med Biol 24:1123.

Jaszczak RJ, Coleman RE. 1985. Single photon emission computed tomography (SPECT) principles and instrumentation. Invest Radiol 20:897.

Jaszczak RJ, Coleman RE, Lim CB. 1980. SPECT: Single photon emission computed tomography. IEEE Trans Nucl Sci NS-27:1137.

Jaszczak RJ, Coleman RE, Whitehead FR. 1981. Physical factors affecting quantitative measurements using camera-based single photon emission computed tomography (SPECT). IEEE Trans Nucl Sci NS-28:69.

Jaszczak RJ, Floyd CE, Coleman RE. 1985. Scatter compensation techniques for SPECT. IEEE Trans Nucl Sci NS-32:786.

Jaszczak RJ, Floyd CE, Manglos SM, et al. 1987. Cone beam collimation for single photon emission computed tomography: Analysis, simulation, and image reconstruction using filtered backprojection. Med Phys 13:484.

Jaszczak RJ, Greer KL, Floyd CE, et al. 1984. Improved SPECT quantification using compensation for scattered photons. J Nucl Med 25:893.

Jaszczak RJ, Murphy PH, Huard D, Burdine JA. 1977. Radionuclide emission computed tomography of the head with ^{99m}Tc and a scintillation camera. J Nucl Med 18:373.

Jaszczak RJ, Tsui BMW. 1994. Single photon emission computed tomography. In HN Wagner and Z Szabo (eds), Principles of Nuclear Medicine, 2nd ed. Philadelphia, Saunders.

Johnson VE, Wong WH, Hu X, Chen CT. 1991. Image restoration using Gibbs priors: Boundary modeling, treatment of blurring and selection of hyperparameters. IEEE Trans Pat 13:413.

Keller EL. 1968. Optimum dimensions of parallel-hole, multiaperture collimators for gamma-ray camera. J Nucl Med 9:233.

Keyes JW Jr, Orlandea N, Heetderks WJ, et al. 1977. The humogotron—A scintillation-camera transaxial tomography. J Nucl Med 18:381.

King MA, Hademenos G, Glick SJ. 1992. A dual photopeak window method for scatter correction. J Nucl Med 33:605.

King MA, Schwinger RB, Doherty PW, Penney BC. 1984. Two-dimensional filtering of SPECT images using the Metz and Wiener filters. J Nucl Med 25:1234.

King MA, Schwinger RB, Penney BC. 1986. Variation of the count-dependent Metz filter with imaging system modulation transfer function. Med Phys 25:139.

Knesaurek K, King MA, Glick SJ, et al. 1989. Investigation of causes of geometric distortion in 180 degree and 360 degree angular sampling in SPECT. J Nucl Med 30:1666.

Koral KF, Wang X, Rogers WL, Clinthorne NH. 1988. SPECT Compton-scattering correction by analysis of energy spectra. J Nucl Med 29:195.

Kuhl DE, Edwards RQ. 1963. Image separation radioisotope scanning. Radiology 80:653.

Kuhl DE, Edwards RQ. 1964. Cylindrical and section radioisotope scanning of the liver and brain. Radiology 83:926.

Kuhl DE, Edwards RQ. 1968. Reorganizing data from transverse section scans of the brain using digital processing. Radiology 91:975.

Lange K, Carson R. 1984. EM reconstruction algorithms for emission and transmission tomography. J Comput Assist Tomogr 8:306.

Levitan E, Herman GT. 1987. A maximum a posteriori probability expectation maximization algorithm for image reconstruction in emission tomography. IEEE Trans Med Imaging MI-6:185.

Liang Z, Hart H. 1987. Bayesian image processing of data from constrained source distribution: I. Nonvalued, uncorrelated and correlated constraints. Bull Math Biol 49:51.

Larsson SA, Hohm C, Carnebrink T, et al. 1991. A new cylindrical SPECT Anger camera with a decentralized transputer based data acquisition system. IEEE Trans Nucl Sci NS-38:654.

Lassen NA, Sveinsdottir E, Kanno I, et al. 1978. A fast moving single photon emission tomograph for regional cerebral blood flow studies in man. J Comput Assist Tomog 2:661.

Lewitt RM, Edholm PR, Xia W. 1989. Fourier method for correction of depth dependent collimator blurring. SPIE Proc 1092:232.

Lim CB, Chang JT, Jaszczak RJ. 1980. Performance analysis of three camera configurations for single photon emission computed tomography. IEEE Trans Nucl Sci NS-27:559.

Lim CB, Gottschalk S, Walker R, et al. 1985. Tri-angular SPECT system for 3-D total organ volume imaging: Design concept and preliminary imaging results. IEEE Trans Nucl Sci NS-32:741.

Manglos SH, Jaszczak RJ, Floyd CE, et al. 1987. Nonisotropic attenuation in SPECT: Phantom test of quantitative effects and compensation techniques. J Nucl Med 28:1584.

Maniawski PJ, Morgan HT, Wackers FJT. 1991. Orbit-related variations in spatial resolution as a source of artifactual defects in thallium-201 SPECT. J Nucl Med 32:871.

Milster TD, Aarsvold JN, Barrett HH, et al. 1990. A full-field modular gamma camera. J Nucl Med 31:632.

Minerbo G. 1979. Maximum entropy reconstruction from cone-beam projection data. Comput Biol Med 9:29.

Moore SC, Doherty MD, Zimmerman RE, Holman BL. 1984. Improved performance from modifications to the multidetector SPECT brain scanner. J Nucl Med 25:688.

Ogawa K, Harata Y, Ichihara T, et al. 1991. A practical method for position-dependent Compton scatter correction in SPECT. IEEE Trans Med Imaging 10:408.

Penney BC, Glick SJ, King MA. 1990. Relative importance of the errors sources in Wiener restoration of scintigrams. IEEE Trans Med Imaging 9:60.

Radon J. 1917. Uber die Bestimmung von Funktionen durch ihre integral-werte langs gewisser Mannigfaltigkeiten. Ber Verh Sachs Akad Wiss 67:26.

Ramachandran GN, Lakshminarayanan AV. 1971. Three-dimensional reconstruction from radiographs and electron micrographs: Application of convolutions instead of Fourier transforms. Proc Natl Acad Sci USA 68:2236.

Roger WL, Ackermann RJ. 1992. SPECT Instrumentation. Am J Physiol Imaging 314:105.

Rogers WL, Clinthorne NH, Shao L, et al. 1988. SPRINT II: A second-generation single photon ring tomograph. IEEE Trans Med Imaging 7:291.

Rowe RK, Aarsvold JN, Barrett HH, et al. 1992. A stationary, hemispherical SPECT imager for 3D brain imaging. J Nucl Med 34:474.

Sorenson JA. 1974. Quantitative measurement of radiation in vivo by whole body counting. In GH Hine and JA Sorenson (eds), Instrumentation in Nuclear Medicine, vol 2, pp 311–348. New York, Academic Press.

Shepp LA, Vardi Y. 1982. Maximum likelihood reconstruction for emission tomography. IEEE Trans Med Imaging MI-1:113.

Stoddart HF, Stoddart HA. 1979. A new development in single gamma transaxial tomography Union Carbide focused collimator scanner. IEEE Trans Nucl Sci NS-26:2710.

Stokely EM, Sveinsdottir E, Lassen NA, Rommer P. 1980. A single photon dynamic computer assisted tomography (DCAT) for imaging brain function in multiple cross-sections. J Comput Assist Tomogr 4:230.

Tretiak OJ, Metz CE. 1980. The exponential Radon transform. SIAM J Appl Math 39:341.

Tsui BMW. 1988. Collimator design, properties and characteristics. Chapter 2. In GH Simmons (ed), The Scintillation Camera, pp 17–45. New York, Society of Nuclear Medicine.

Tsui BMW, Frey EC, Zhao X-D, et al. 1994. The importance and implementation of accurate 3D compensation methods for quantitative SPECT. Phys Med Biol 39:509.

Tsui BMW, Gullberg GT, Edgerton ER, et al. 1986. The design and clinical utility of a fan beam collimator for a SPECT system. J Nucl Med 247:810.

Tsui BMW, Gullberg GT, Edgerton ER, et al. 1989. Correction of nonuniform attenuation in cardiac SPECT imaging. J Nucl Med 30:497.

Tsui BMW, Hu HB, Gilland DR, Gullberg GT. 1988. Implementation of simultaneous attenuation and detector response correction in SPECT. IEEE Trans Nucl Sci NS-35:778.

Tsui BMW, Zhao X-D, Frey EC, McCartney WH. 1994. Quantitative single-photon emission computed tomography: Basics and clinical considerations. Semin Nucl Med 24(1):38.

Yanch JC, Flower MA, Webb S. 1988. Comparison of deconvolution and windowed subtraction techniques for scatter compensation in SPECT. IEEE Trans Med Imaging 7:13.

Zeng GL, Gullberg GT, Tsui BMW, Terry JA. 1991. Three-dimensional iterative reconstruction algorithms with attenuation and geometric point response correction. IEEE Trans Nucl Sci NS-38:693.

12

Ultrasound

Richard L. Goldberg
University of North Carolina

Stephen W. Smith
Duke University

Jack G. Mottley
University of Rochester

K. Whittaker Ferrara
Riverside Research Institute

12.1 Transducers

Richard L. Goldberg and Stephen W. Smith

An ultrasound transducer generates acoustic waves by converting magnetic, thermal, and electrical energy into mechanical energy. The most efficient technique for medical ultrasound uses the piezoelectric effect, which was first demonstrated in 1880 by Jacques and Pierre Curie [Curie and Curie, 1880]. They applied a stress to a quartz crystal and detected an electrical potential across opposite faces of the material. The Curies also discovered the inverse piezoelectric effect by applying an electric field across the crystal to induce a mechanical deformation. In this manner, a piezoelectric transducer converts an oscillating electric signal into an acoustic wave, and vice versa.

Many significant advances in ultrasound imaging have resulted from innovation in transducer technology. One such instance was the development of linear-array transducers. Previously, ultrasound systems had made an image by manually moving the transducer across the region of interest. Even the faster scanners had required several seconds to generate an ultrasound image, and as a result, only static targets could be scanned. On the other hand, if the acoustic beam could be scanned rapidly, clinicians could visualize moving targets such as a beating heart. In addition, real-time imaging would provide instantaneous feedback to the clinician of the transducer position and system settings.

To implement real-time imaging, researchers developed new types of transducers that rapidly steer the acoustic beam. Piston-shaped transducers were designed to wobble or rotate about a fixed axis to *mechanically* steer the beam through a sector-shaped region. Linear sequential arrays were designed to *electronically* focus the beam in a rectangular image region. Linear phased-array transducers were designed to *electronically* steer and focus the beam at high speed in a sector image format.

This section describes the application of piezoelectric ceramics to transducer arrays for medical ultrasound. Background is presented on transducer materials and beam steering with phased arrays. Array performance is described, and the design of an idealized array is presented.

0-8493-1810-6/03/$0.00+$1.50

TABLE 12.1 Maerial Properties of Linear-Array Elements Made of PZT-5H

Parameter	Symbol	Value	Units
Density	ρ	7500	kg/m^3
Speed of sound	c	3970	m/s
Acoustic impedance	Z	29.75	MRayls
Relative dielectric constant	$\varepsilon/\varepsilon_0$	1475	None
Electromechanical coupling coefficient	k	0.698	None
Mechanical loss tangent	$\tan \delta_m$	0.015	None
Electrical loss tangent	$\tan \delta_e$	0.02	None

Transducer Materials

Ferroelectric materials strongly exhibit the piezoelectric effect, and they are ideal materials for medical ultrasound. For many years, the ferroelectric ceramic lead-zirconate-titanate (PZT) has been the standard transducer material for medical ultrasound, in part because of its high electromechanical conversion efficiency and low intrinsic losses. The properties of PZT can be adjusted by modifying the ratio of zirconium to titanium and introducing small amounts of other substances, such as lanthanum [Berlincourt, 1971]. Table 12.1 shows the material properties of linear-array elements made from PZT-5H.

PZT has a high dielectric constant compared with many piezoelectric materials, resulting in favorable electrical characteristics. The ceramic is mechanically strong, and it can be machined to various shapes and sizes. PZT can operate at temperatures up to 100°C or higher, and it is stable over long periods of time.

The disadvantages of PZT include its high acoustic impedance ($Z = 30$ MRayls) compared with body tissue ($Z = 1.5$ MRayls) and the presence of lateral modes in array elements. One or more acoustic matching layers can largely compensate for the acoustic impedance mismatch. The effect of lateral modes can be diminished by choosing the appropriate element dimensions or by subdicing the elements.

Other piezoelectric materials are used for various applications. Composites are made from PZT interspersed in an epoxy matrix [Smith, 1992]. Lateral modes are reduced in a composite because of its inhomogeneous structure. By combining the PZT and epoxy in different ratios and spatial distributions, one can tailor the composite's properties for different applications. Polyvinylidene difluoride (PVDF) is a ferroelectric polymer that has been used effectively in high-frequency transducers [Sherar and Foster, 1989]. The copolymer of PVDF with trifluoroethylene has an improved electromechanical conversion efficiency. Relaxor ferroelectric materials, such as lead-magnesium-niobate (PMN), become piezoelectric when a large direct-current (dc) bias voltage is applied [Takeuchi et al., 1990]. They have a very large dielectric constant ($\varepsilon > 20{,}000\varepsilon_0$), resulting in higher transducer capacitance and a lower electrical impedance.

Scanning with Array Transducers

Array transducers use the same principles as acoustic lenses to focus an acoustic beam. In both cases, variable delays are applied across the transducer aperture. With a sequential or phased array, however, the delays are electronically controlled and can be changed instantaneously to focus the beam in different regions. Linear arrays were first developed for radar, sonar, and radio astronomy [Allen, 1964; Bobber, 1970], and they were implemented in a medical ultrasound system by Somer in 1968 [Somer, 1968].

Linear-array transducers have increased versatility over piston transducers. Electronic scanning involves no moving parts, and the focal point can be changed dynamically to any location in the scanning plane. The system can generate a wide variety of scan formats, and it can process the received echoes for other applications, such as dynamic receive focusing [von Ramm and Thurstone, 1976], correction for phase aberrations [Flax and O'Donnell, 1988; Trahey et al., 1990], and synthetic aperture imaging [Nock and Trahey, 1992].

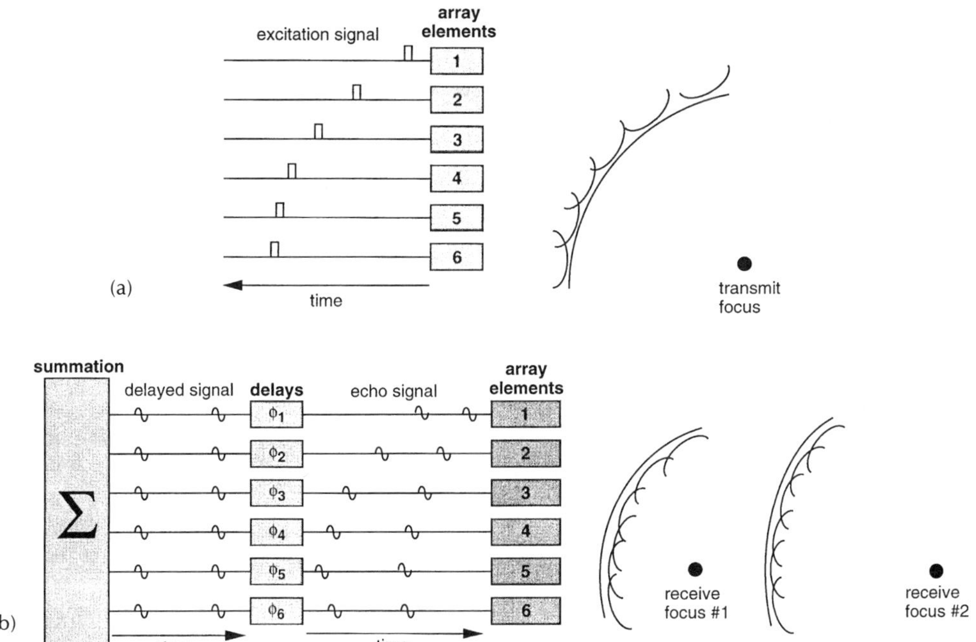

FIGURE 12.1 Focusing and steering an acoustic beam using a phased array. A six-element linear array is shown (a) in the transmit mode and (b) in the receive mode. Dynamic focusing in receive allows the scanner focus to track the range of returning echoes.

The disadvantages of linear arrays are due to the increased complexity and higher cost of the transducers and scanners. For high-quality ultrasound images, many identical array elements are required (currently 128 and rising). The array elements are typically less than a millimeter on one side, and each has a separate connection to its own transmitter and receiver electronics.

The widespread use of array transducers for many applications indicates that the advantages often outweigh the disadvantages. In addition, improvement in transducer fabrication techniques and integrated circuit technology have led to more advanced array transducers and scanners.

Focusing and Steering with Phased Arrays

This subsection describes how a phased-array transducer can focus and steer an acoustic beam along a specific direction. An ultrasound image is formed by repeating this process over 100 times to interrogate a two- (2D) or three-dimensional (3D) region of the medium.

Figure 12.1a illustrates a simple example of a six-element linear array focusing the transmitted beam. One can assume that each array element is a point source that radiates a spherically shaped wavefront into the medium. Since the top element is farthest from the focus in this example, it is excited first. The remaining elements are excited at the appropriate time intervals so that the acoustic signals from all the elements reach the focal point at the same time. According to Huygens' principle, the net acoustic signal is the sum of the signals that have arrived from each source. At the focal point, the contributions from every element add in phase to produce a peak in the acoustic signal. Elsewhere, at least some of the contributions add out of phase, reducing the signal relative to the peak.

For receiving an ultrasound echo, the phased array works in reverse. Fig. 12.1b shows an echo originating from focus 1. The echo is incident on each array element at a different time interval. The received signals are electronically delayed so that the delayed signals add in phase for an echo originating at the focal point. For echoes originating elsewhere, at least some of the delayed signals will add out of phase, reducing the receive signal relative to the peak at the focus.

In the receive mode, the focal point can be dynamically adjusted so that it coincides with the range of returning echoes. After transmission of an acoustic pulse, the initial echoes return from targets near the transducer. Therefore, the scanner focuses the phased array on these targets, located at focus 1 in Fig. 12.1b. As echoes return from more distant targets, the scanner focuses at a greater depth (focus 2 in the figure). Focal zones are established with adequate depth of field so that the targets are always in focus in receive. This process is called *dynamic receive focusing* and was first implemented by von Ramm and Thurstone in 1976 [von Ramm and Thurstone, 1976].

Array-Element Configurations

An ultrasound image is formed by repeating the preceding process many times to scan a 2D or 3D region of tissue. For a 2D image, the scanning plane is the **azimuth dimension;** the **elevation dimension** is perpendicular to the azimuth scanning plane. The shape of the region scanned is determined by the array-element configuration, described in the paragraphs below.

Linear Sequential Arrays. Sequential liner arrays have as many as 512 elements in current commercial scanners. A subaperture of up to 128 elements is selected to operate at a given time. As shown in Fig. 12.2a, the scanning lines are directed perpendicular to the face of the transducer; the acoustic beam is focused but not steered. The advantage of this scheme is that the array elements have high sensitivity when the beam is directed straight ahead. The disadvantage is that the field of view is limited to the rectangular region directly in front of the transducer. Linear-array transducers have a large footprint to obtain an adequate field of view.

Curvilinear Arrays. Curvilinear or convex arrays have a different shape than sequential linear arrays, but they operate in the same manner. In both cases, the scan lines are directed perpendicular to the transducer face. A curvilinear array, however, scans a wider field of view because of its convex shape, as shown in Fig. 12.2b.

Linear Phased Arrays. The more advanced linear phased arrays have 128 elements. All the elements are used to transmit and receive each line of data. As shown in Fig. 12.2c, the scanner steers the ultrasound beam through a sector-shaped region in the azimuth plane. Phased arrays scan a region that is significantly wider than the footprint of the transducer, making them suitable for scanning through restricted acoustic windows. As a result, these transducers are ideal for cardiac imaging, where the transducer must scan through a small window to avoid the obstructions of the ribs (bone) and lungs (air).

1.5D Arrays. The so-called 1.5D array is similar to a 2D array in construction but a 1D array in operation. The 1.5D array contains elements along both the azimuth and elevation dimensions. Features such as dynamic focusing and phase correction can be implemented in both dimensions to improve image quality. Since a 1.5D array contains a limited number of elements in elevation (e.g., three to nine elements), steering is not possible in that direction. Figure 12.2d illustrates a B-scan made with a 1.5D phased array. Linear sequential scanning is also possible with 1.5D arrays.

2D Phased Arrays. A 2D phased-array has a large number of elements in both the azimuth and elevation dimensions. Therefore, 2D arrays can focus and steer the acoustic beam in both dimensions. Using parallel receive processing [Shattuck et al., 1984], a 2D array can scan a pyramidal region in real time to produce a volumetric image, as shown in Fig. 12.2e [von Ramm and Smith, 1990].

Linear-Array Transducer Performance

Designing an ultrasound transducer array involves many compromises. Ideally, a transducer has high sensitivity or SNR, good spatial resolution, and no artifacts. The individual array elements should have wide angular response in the steering dimensions, low cross-coupling, and an electrical impedance matched to the transmitter.

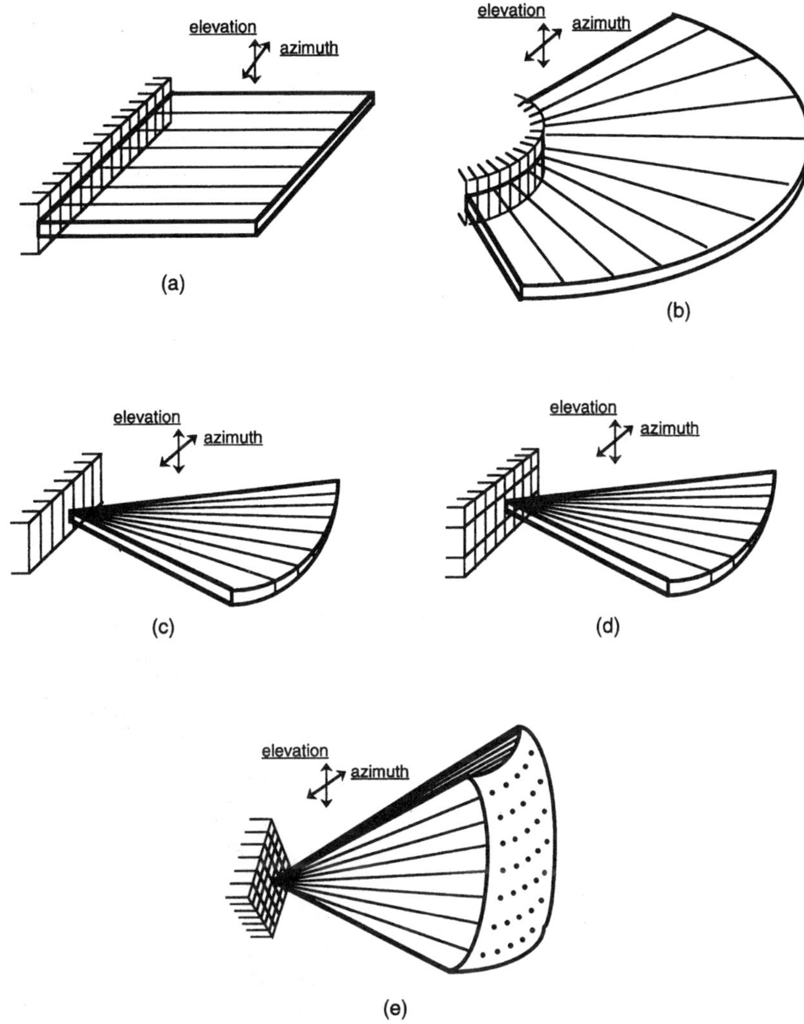

FIGURE 12.2 Array-element configurations and the region scanned by the acoustic beam. (a) A sequential linear array scans a rectangular region; (b) a curvilinear array scans a sector-shaped region; (c) a linear phased array scans a sector-shaped region; (d) a 1.5D array scans a sector-shaped region; (e) a 2D array scans a pyramidal-shaped region.

Figure 12.3a illustrates the connections to the transducer assembly. The transmitter and receiver circuits are located in the ultrasound scanner and are connected to the array elements through 1 to 2 m of coaxial cable. Electrical matching networks can be added to tune out the capacitance of the coaxial cable and/or the transducer element and increase the signal-to-noise ratio (SNR).

A more detailed picture of six-transducer elements is shown in Fig. 12.3b. Electrical leads connect to the ground and signal electrodes of the piezoelectric material. Acoustically, the array elements are loaded on the front side by one or two quarter-wave matching layers and the tissue medium. The matching layers may be made from glass or epoxy. A backing material, such as epoxy, loads the back side of the array elements. The faceplate protects the transducer assembly and also may act as an acoustic lens. Faceplates are often made from silicone or polyurethane.

The following subsections describe several important characteristics of an array transducer. Figure 12.3c shows a six-element array and its dimensions. The element thickness, width, and length are labeled as t, a, and b, respectively. The interelement spacing is d, and the total aperture size is D in

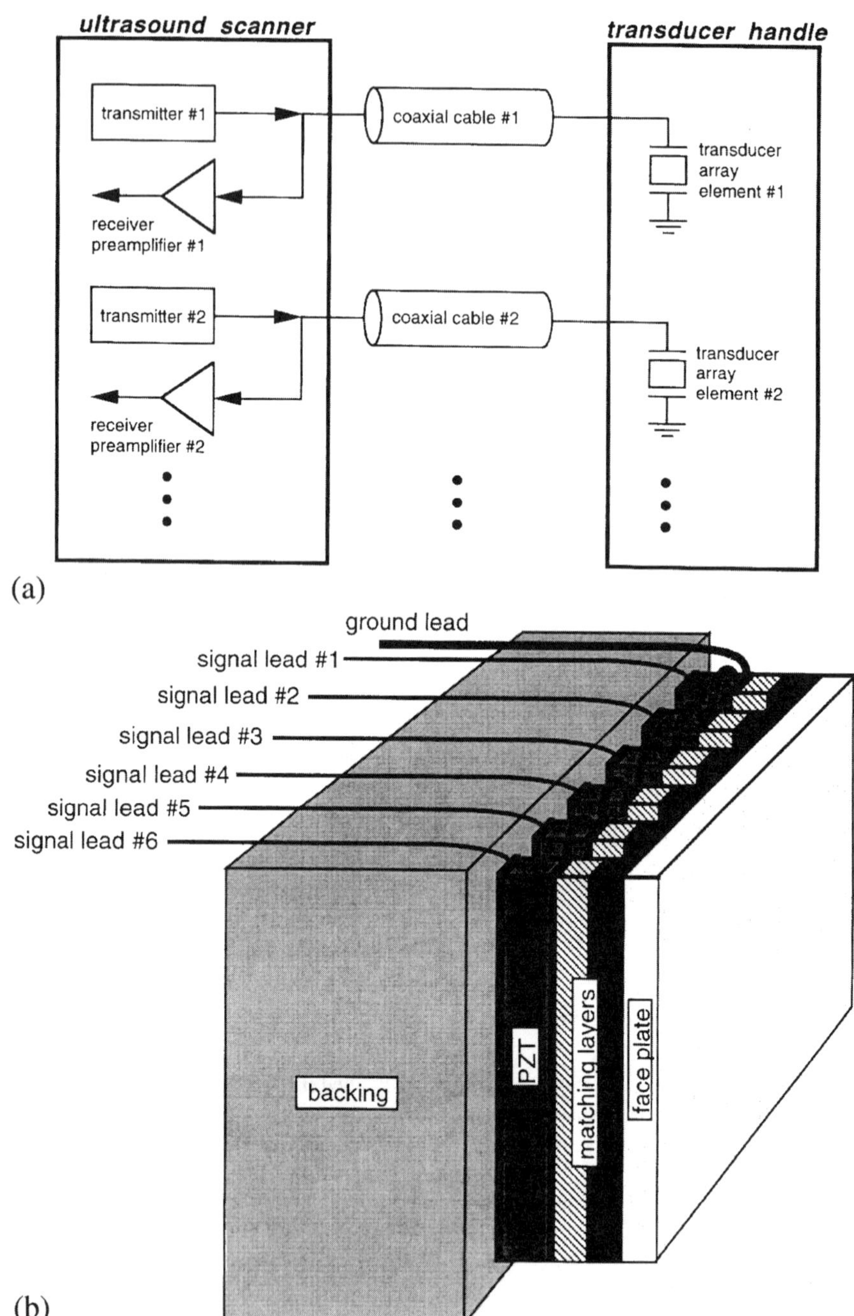

FIGURE 12.3 (a) The connections between the ultrasound scanner and the transducer assembly for two elements of an array. (b) A more detailed picture of the transducer assembly for six elements of an array. (c) Coordinate system and labeling used to describe an array transducer.

azimuth. The acoustic wavelength in the load medium, usually human tissue, is designated as λ, while the wavelength in the transducer material is λ_t.

Examples are given below for a 128-element linear array operating at 5 MHz. The array is made of PZT-5H with element dimensions of $0.1 \times 5 \times 0.3$ mm. The interelement spacing is $d = 0.15$ mm in

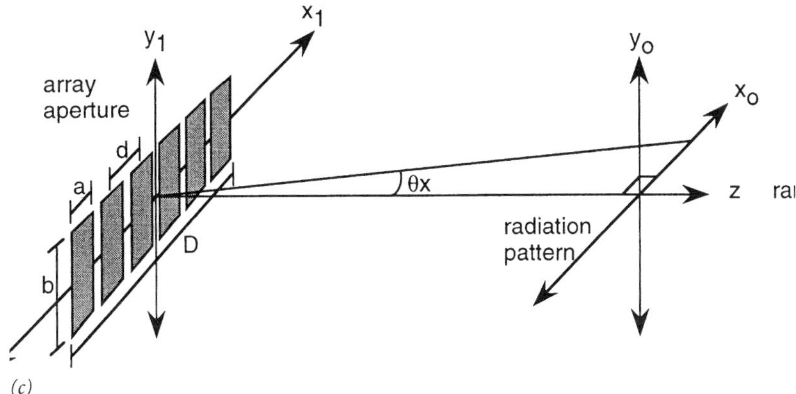

(c)

FIGURE 12.3 (continued)

azimuth, and the total aperture is $D = 128 \cdot 0.15$ mm $= 19.3$ mm. See Table 12.1 for the piezoelectric material characteristics. The elements have an epoxy backing of $Z = 3.25$ MRayls. For simplicity, the example array does not contain a $\lambda/4$ matching layer.

Axial Resolution

Axial resolution determines the ability to distinguish between targets aligned in the axial direction (the direction of acoustic propagation). In pulse-echo imaging, the echoes off of two targets separated by $r/2$ have a path length difference of r. If the acoustic pulse length is r, then echoes off the two targets are just distinguishable. As a result, the axial resolution is often defined as one-half the pulse length [Christensen, 1988]. A transducer with a high resonant frequency and a broad bandwidth has a short acoustic pulse and good axial resolution.

Radiation Pattern

The radiation pattern of a transducer determines the insonified region of tissue. For good lateral resolution and sensitivity, the acoustic energy should be concentrated in a small region. The radiation pattern for a narrow-band or continuous-wave (CW) transducer is described by the Rayleigh-Sommerfeld diffraction formula [Goodman, 1986]. For a pulse-echo imaging system, this diffraction formula is not exact due to the broadband acoustic waves used. Nevertheless, the Rayleigh-Sommerfeld formula is a reasonable first-order approximation to the actual radiation pattern.

The following analysis considers only the azimuth scanning dimension. Near the focal point or in the far field, the Fraunhofer approximation reduces the diffraction formula to a Fourier transform formula. For a circular or rectangular aperture, the far field is at a range of

$$z > \frac{D^2}{4\lambda} \tag{12.1}$$

Figure 12.3c shows the coordinate system used to label the array aperture and its radiation pattern. The array aperture is described by

$$\text{Array}\left(x_1\right) = \text{rect}\left(\frac{x_1}{a}\right) * \text{comb}\left(\frac{x_1}{d}\right) \cdot \text{rect}\left(\frac{x_1}{D}\right) \tag{12.2}$$

where the rect(x) function is a rectangular pulse of width x, and the comb(x) function is a delta function repeated at intervals of x. The diffraction pattern is evaluated in the x_0 plane at a distance z from the

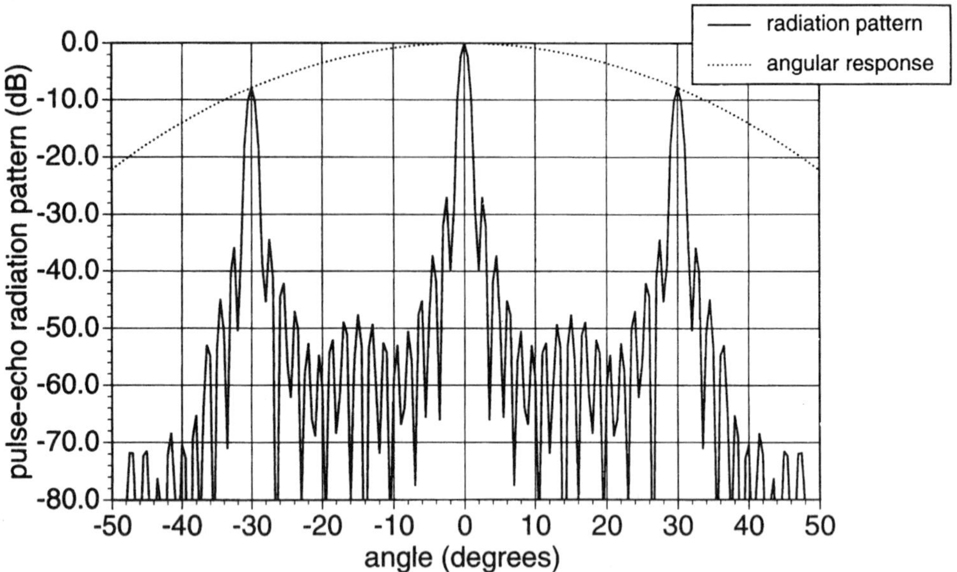

FIGURE 12.4 Radiation pattern of Eq. (12.3) for a 16-element array with $a = \lambda$, $d = 2\lambda$, and $D = 32\lambda$. The angular response, the first term of Eq. (12.3), is also shown as a dashed line.

transducer, and θ_x is the angle of the point x_0 from the normal axis. With the Fraunhofer approximation, the normalized diffraction pattern is given by

$$P_x(\theta_x) = \text{sinc}\left(\frac{a \sin \theta_x}{\lambda}\right) \cdot \text{comb}\left(\frac{d \sin \theta_x}{\lambda}\right) * \text{sinc}\left(\frac{D \sin \theta_x}{\lambda}\right) \tag{12.3}$$

in azimuth, where the Fourier transform of Eq. (12.2) has been evaluated at the spatial frequency

$$f_x = \frac{x_0}{\lambda z} = \frac{\sin \theta_x}{\lambda} \tag{12.4}$$

Figure 12.4 shows a graph of Eq. (12.3) for a 16-element array with $a = \lambda$, $d = 2\lambda$, and $D = 32\lambda$. In the graph, the significance of each term is easily distinguished. The first term determines the angular response weighting, the second term determines the location of grating lobes off-axis, and the third term determines the shape of the main lobe and the grating lobes. The significance of **lateral resolution, angular response,** and **grating lobes** is seen from the CW diffraction pattern.

Lateral resolution determines the ability to distinguish between targets in the azimuth and elevation dimensions. According to the Rayleigh criterion [Goodman, 1986], the *lateral resolution* can be defined by the first null in the main lobe, which is determined from the third term of Eq. (12.3).

$$\theta_x = \sin^{-1} \frac{\lambda}{D} \tag{12.5}$$

in the azimuth dimension. A larger aperture results in a more narrow main lobe and better resolution.

A broad angular response is desired to maintain sensitivity while steering off-axis. The first term of Eq. (12.3) determines the one-way angular response. The element is usually surrounded by a soft baffle, such as air, resulting in an additional cosine factor in the radiation pattern [Selfridge et al., 1980]. Assuming transmit/receive reciprocity, the pulse-echo angular response for a single element is

$$P_x(\theta_x) = \frac{\sin^2(\pi a/\lambda \cdot \sin\theta_x)}{(\pi a/\lambda \cdot \sin\theta_x)^2} \cdot \cos^2\theta_x \tag{12.6}$$

in the azimuth dimension. As the aperture size becomes smaller, the element more closely resembles a point source, and the angular response becomes broader. Another useful indicator is the –6-dB angular response, defined as the full-width half-maximum of the angular response graph.

Grating lobes are produced at a location where the path length difference to adjacent array elements is a multiple of a wavelength (the main lobe is located where the path length difference is zero). The acoustic contributions from the elements constructively interfere, producing off-axis peaks. The term *grating lobe* was originally used to describe the optical peaks produced by a diffraction grating. In ultrasound, grating lobes are undesirable because they represent acoustic energy steered away from the main lobe. From the Comb function in Eq. (12.3), the grating lobes are located at

$$\theta_x = \sin^{-1}\frac{i\lambda}{d} \qquad i = 1, 2, 3, \ldots \tag{12.7}$$

in azimuth.

If d is a wavelength, then grating lobes are centered at ±90° from the steering direction in that dimension. Grating lobes at such large angles are less significant because the array elements have poor angular response in those regions. If the main lobe is steered at a large angle, however, the grating lobes are brought toward the front of the array. In this case, the angular response weighting produces a relatively weak main lobe and a relatively strong grating lobe. To eliminate grating lobes at all steering angles, the interelement spacing is set to $\lambda/2$ or less [Steinberg, 1967].

Figure 12.5 shows the theoretical radiation pattern of the 128-element example. For this graph, the angular response weighting of Eq. (12.6) was substituted into Eq. (12.3). The lateral resolution, as defined by Eq. (12.7), $\theta_x = 0.9$ degrees at the focal point. The –6-dB angular response is ±40° from Eq. (12.6).

Electrical Impedance

The electric impedance of an element relative to the electrical loads has a significant impact on transducer signal-to-noise ratio (SNR). At frequencies away from resonance, the transducer has electrical characteristics of a capacitor. The construction of the transducer is a parallel-plate capacitor with clamped capacitance of

$$C_0 = \varepsilon^s \frac{ab}{t} \tag{12.8}$$

where ε^S is the clamped dielectric constant.

Near resonance, equivalent circuits help to explain the impedance behavior of a transducer. The simplified circuit of Fig. 12.6a is valid for transducers operating at series resonance without losses and with low acoustic impedance loads [Kino, 1987]. The mechanical resistance R_m represents the acoustic loads as seen from the electrical terminals:

$$R_m = \frac{\pi}{4k^2\omega C_0} \cdot \frac{Z_1 + Z_2}{Z_C} \tag{12.9}$$

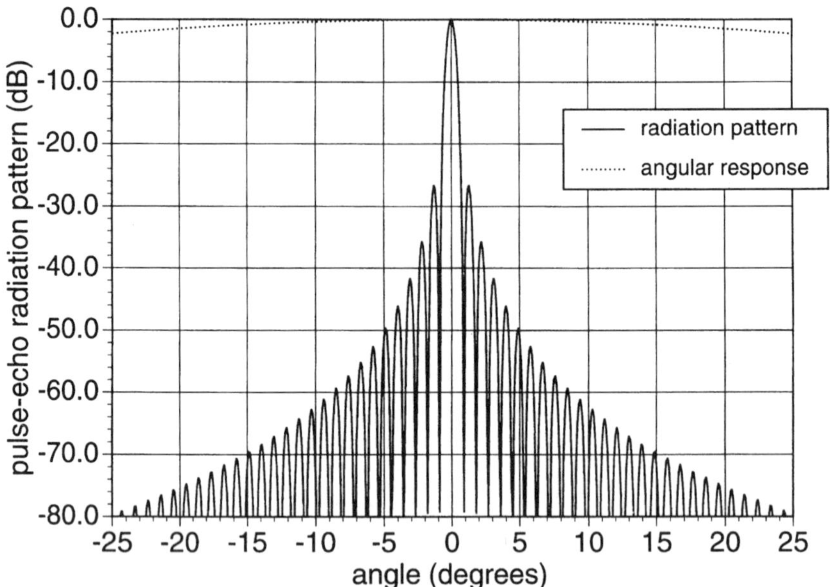

FIGURE 12.5 Radiation pattern of the example array element with $a = 0.1$ mm, $d = 0.15$ mm, $D = 19.2$ mm, and $\lambda = 0.3$ mm. The angular response of Eq. (12.6) was substituted into Eq. (12.3) for this graph.

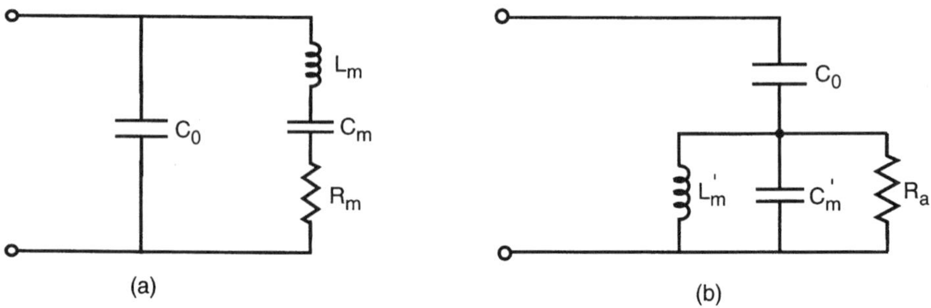

FIGURE 12.6 Simplified equivalent circuits for a piezoelectric transducer: (a) near-series resonance and (b) near-parallel resonance.

where k is the electromechanical coupling coefficient of the piezoelectric material, Z_C is the acoustic impedance of the piezoelectric material, Z_1 is the acoustic impedance of the transducer backing, and Z_2 is the acoustic impedance of the load medium (body tissue). The power dissipated through R_m corresponds to the acoustic output power from the transducer.

The mechanical inductance L_m and mechanical capacitance C_m are analogous to the inductance and capacitance of a mass-spring system. At the series resonant frequency of

$$f_s = \frac{1}{2\pi\sqrt{L_m C_m}} \tag{12.10}$$

the impedances of these components add to zero, resulting in a local impedance minimum.

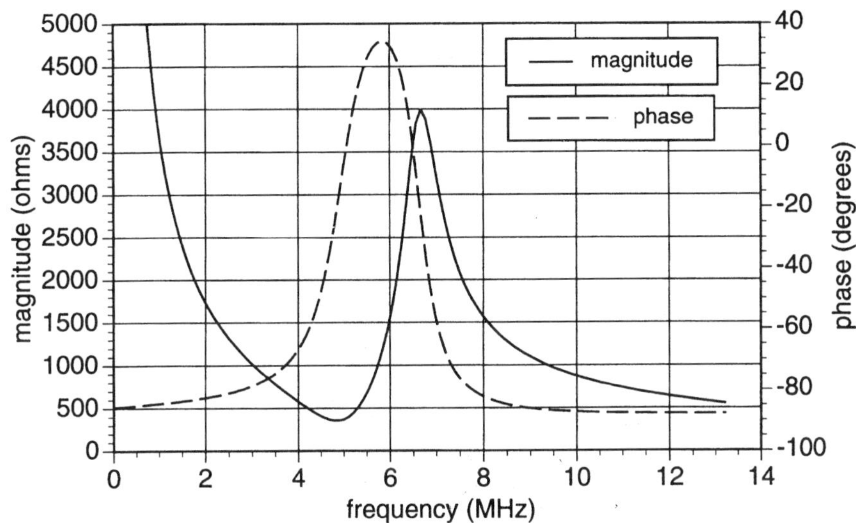

FIGURE 12.7 Complex electrical impedance of the example array element. Series resonance is located at 5.0 MHz, and parallel resonance is located at 6.7 MHz.

The equivalent circuit of Fig. 12.6a can be redrawn in the form shown in Fig. 12.6b. In this circuit, C_0 is the same as before, but the mechanical impedances have values of L_m', C_m', and R_a. The resistive component R_a is

$$R_a = \frac{4k^2}{\pi\omega C_0} \cdot \frac{Z_C}{Z_1 + Z_2} \tag{12.11}$$

The inductor and capacitor combine to form an open circuit at the parallel resonant frequency of

$$f_p = \frac{1}{2\pi\sqrt{L_m' C_m'}} \tag{12.12}$$

The parallel resonance, which is at a slightly higher frequency than the series resonance, is indicated by a local impedance maximum.

Figure 12.7 shows a simulated plot of magnitude and phase versus frequency for the example array element described at the beginning of this subsection. The series resonance frequency is immediately identified at 5.0 MHz with an impedance minimum of $|Z| = 350\ \Omega$. Parallel resonance occurs at 6.7 MHz with an impedance maximum of $|Z| = 4000\ \Omega$. Note the capacitive behavior (approximately –90° phase) at frequencies far from resonance.

Designing a Phased-Array Transducer

In this subsection the design of an idealized phased-array transducer is considered in terms of the performance characteristics described above. Criteria are described for selecting array dimensions, acoustic backing and matching layers, and electrical matching networks.

Choosing Array Dimensions

The array element thickness is determined by the parallel resonant frequency. For $\lambda/2$ resonance, the thickness is

$$t = \frac{\lambda_t}{2} = \frac{c_t}{2f_p} \tag{12.13}$$

where c_t is the longitudinal speed of sound in the transducer material.

There are three constraints for choosing the element width and length: (1) a nearly square cross-section should be avoided so that lateral vibrations are not coupled to the thickness vibration; as a rule of thumb [Kino and DeSilets, 1979],

$$a/t \le 0.6 \quad \text{or} \quad a/t \ge 10 \tag{12.14}$$

(2) a small width and length are also desirable for a wide angular response weighting function; and (3) an interelement spacing of $\lambda/2$ or less is necessary to eliminate grating lobes.

Fortunately, these requirements are consistent for PZT array elements. For all forms of PZT, $c_t > 2c$, where c is the speed of sound in body tissue (an average of 1540 m/s). At a given frequency, then $\lambda_t > 2\lambda$. Also, Eq. (12.13) states that $\lambda_t = 2t$ at a frequency of f_p. By combining these equations, $t > \lambda$ for PZT array elements operating at a frequency of f_p. If $d = \lambda/2$, then $a < \lambda/2$ because of the finite kerf width that separates the elements. Given this observation, then $a < t/2$. This is consistent with Eq. (12.14) to reduce lateral modes.

An element having $d = \lambda/2$ also has adequate angular response. For illustrative purposes, one can assume a zero kerf width so that $a = \lambda/2$. In this case, the –6-dB angular response is $\theta_x = \pm 35°$ according to Eq. (12.6).

The array dimensions determine the transducer's lateral resolution. In the azimuth dimension, if $d = \lambda/2$, then the transducer aperture is $D = n\lambda/2$, where n is the number of elements in a fully sampled array. From Eq. (12.5), the lateral resolution in azimuth is

$$\theta_x = \sin^{-1}\frac{2}{n} \tag{12.15}$$

Therefore, the lateral resolution is independent of frequency in a fully sampled array with $d = \lambda/2$. For this configuration, the lateral resolution is improved by increasing the number of elements.

Acoustic Backing and Matching Layers

The backing and matching layers affect the transducer bandwidth and sensitivity. While a lossy, matched backing improves bandwidth, it also dissipates acoustic energy that could otherwise be transmitted into the tissue medium. Therefore, a low-impedance acoustic backing is preferred because it reflects the acoustic pulses toward the front side of the transducer. In this case, adequate bandwidth is maintained by acoustically matching the transducer to the tissue medium using matching layers.

Matching layers are designed with a thickness of $\lambda/4$ at the center frequency and an acoustic impedance between those of the transducer Z_T and the load medium Z_L. The ideal acoustic impedances can be determined from several different models [Hunt et al., 1983]. Using the KLM equivalent circuit model [Desilets et al., 1978], the ideal acoustic impedance is

$$Z_1 = \sqrt[3]{Z_T Z_L^2} \tag{12.16}$$

for a single matching layer. For matching PZT-5H array elements ($Z_T = 30$ MRayls) to a water load ($Z_L = 1.5$ MRayls), a matching layer of $Z_1 = 4.1$ MRayls should be chosen. If two matching layers are used, they should have acoustic impedances of

$$Z_1 = \sqrt[7]{Z_T^4 Z_L^3} \tag{12.17a}$$

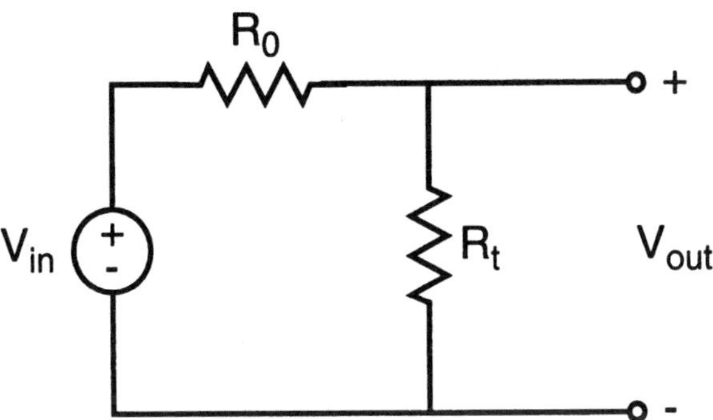

FIGURE 12.8 A transducer of real impedance R_t being excited by a transmitter with source impedance R_0 and source voltage V_{in}.

$$Z_2 = \sqrt[7]{Z_T Z_L^6} \tag{12.17b}$$

In this case, Z_1 = 8.3 MRayls and Z_2 = 2.3 MRayls for matching PZT-5H to a water load.

When constructing a transducer, a practical matching layer material is not always available, with the ideal acoustic impedance [Eq. (12.16) or (12.17)]. Adequate bandwidth is obtained by using materials that have an impedance close to the ideal value. With a single matching layer, for example, conductive epoxy can be used with Z = 5.1 MRayls.

Electrical Impedance Matching

Signal-to-noise ratio and bandwidth are also improved when electrical impedance of an array element is matched to that of the transmit circuitry. Consider the simplified circuit in Fig. 12.8 with a transmitter of impedance R_0 and a transducer of real impedance R_t. The power output is proportional to the power dissipated in R_t, as expressed as

$$P_{out} = \frac{V_{out}^2}{R_t} \quad \text{where } V_{out} = \frac{R_t}{R_0 + R_t} V_{in} \tag{12.18}$$

The power available from the transmitter is

$$P_{in} = \frac{\left(V_{in}/2\right)^2}{R_0} \tag{12.19}$$

into a matched load. From the two previous equations, the power efficiency is

$$\frac{P_{out}}{P_{in}} = \frac{4R_0 R_t}{\left(R_0 + R_t\right)^2} \tag{12.20}$$

For a fixed-source impedance, the maximum efficiency is obtained by taking the derivative of Eq. (12.20) with respect to R_t and setting it to zero. Maximum efficiency occurs when the source impedance is matched to the transducer impedance, $R_0 = R_t$.

In practice, the transducer has a complex impedance of R_m in parallel with C_0 (see Fig. 12.6), which is excited by a transmitter with a real impedance of 50 Ω. The transducer has a maximum efficiency

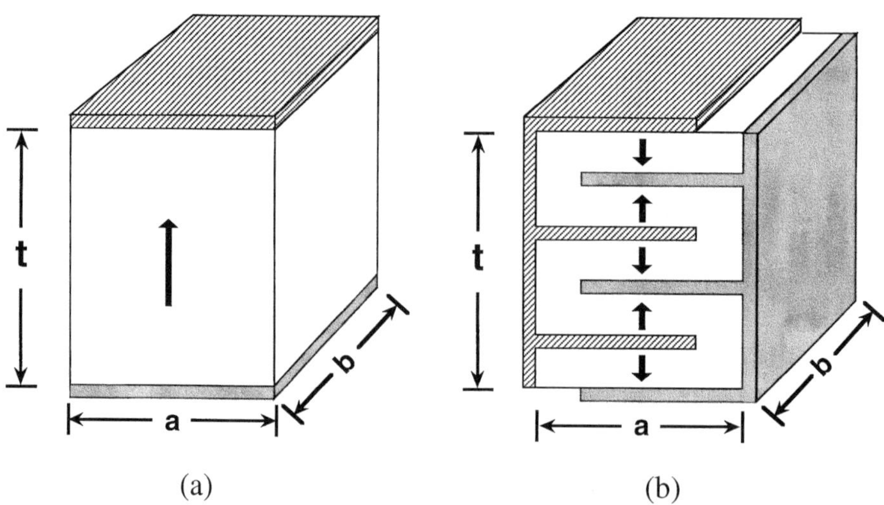

FIGURE 12.9 (a) Conventional single-layer ceramic; (b) five-layer ceramic of the same overall dimensions. The layers are electrically in parallel and acoustically in series. The arrows indicate the piezoelectric poling directions of each layer.

when the imaginary component is tuned out and the real component is 50 Ω. This can be accomplished with electrical matching networks.

The capacitance C_0 is tuned out in the frequency range near ω_0 using an inductor of

$$L_0 = \frac{1}{\omega_0^2 C_0} \tag{12.21}$$

for an inductor in shunt, or

$$L_1 = \frac{1}{\omega_0^2 C_0 + 1/R_m^2 C_0} \tag{12.22}$$

for an inductor in series. The example array elements described in the preceding subsection have C_0 = 22 pF and R_m = 340 Ω at series resonance of 5.0 MHz. Therefore, tuning inductors of L_0 = 46 μH or L_1 = 2.4 μH should be used.

A shunt inductor also raises the impedance of the transducer, as seen from the scanner, while a series inductor lowers the terminal impedance [Hunt et al., 1983]. For more significant changes in terminal impedance, transformers are used.

A transformer of turns ratio 1:N multiplies the terminal impedance by $1/N^2$. In the transmit mode, N can be adjusted so that the terminal impedance matches the transmitter impedance. In the receive mode, the open-circuit sensitivity varies as $1/N$ because of the step-down transformer. The lower terminal impedance of the array element, however, provides increased ability to drive an electrical load.

More complicated circuits can be used for better electrical matching across a wide bandwidth [Hunt et al., 1983]. These circuits can be either passive, as above, or active. Inductors also can be used in the scanner to tune out the capacitance of the coaxial cable that loads the transducer on receive.

Another alternative for electrical matching is to use multilayer piezoelectric ceramics [Goldberg and Smith, 1994]. Figure 12.9 shows an example of a single layer and a five-layer array element with the same overall dimensions of a, b, and t. Since the layers are connected electrically in parallel, the clamped capacitance of a multilayer ceramic (MLC) element is

$$C_0 = N \cdot \varepsilon^S \cdot \frac{ab}{t/N} = N^2 \cdot C_{\text{single}} \tag{12.23}$$

where C_{single} is the capacitance of the single-layer element (Eq. 12.8). As a result, the MLC impedance is reduced by a factor of N^2. Acoustically, the layers of the MLC are in series so the $\lambda/2$ resonant thickness is t, the stack thickness.

To a first order, an N-layer ceramic has identical performance compared with a 1:N transformer, but the impedance is transformed within the ceramic. MLCs also can be fabricated in large quantities more easily than hand-wound transformers. While MLCs do not tune out the reactive impedance, they make it easier to tune a low capacitance array element. By lowering the terminal impedance of an array element, MLCs significantly improve transducer SNR.

Summary

The piezoelectric transducer is an important component in the ultrasound imaging system. The transducer often consists of a liner array that can electronically focus an acoustic beam. Depending on the configuration of array elements, the region scanned may be sector shaped or rectangular in two dimensions or pyramidal shaped in three dimensions.

The transducer performance large determines the resolution and the signal-to-noise ratio of the resulting ultrasound image. The design of an array involves many compromises in choosing operating frequency and array-element dimensions. Electrical matching networks and quarter-wave matching layers may be added to improve transducer performance.

Further improvements in transducer performance may result from several areas of research. Newer materials, such as composites, are gaining widespread use in medical ultrasound. In addition, 1.5D arrays or 2D arrays may be employed to control the acoustic beam in both azimuth and elevation. Problems in fabrication and electrical impedance matching must be overcome to implement these arrays in an ultrasound system.

Defining Terms

Acoustic impedance: In an analogy to transmission line impedance, the acoustic impedance is the ratio of pressure to particle velocity in a medium; more commonly, it is defined as $Z = \rho c$, where ρ = density and c = speed of sound in a medium [the units are kg/(m^2·s) or Rayls].

Angular response: The radiation pattern versus angle for a single element of an array.

Axial resolution: The ability to distinguish between targets aligned in the axial direction (the direction of acoustic propagation).

Azimuth dimension: The lateral dimension that is along the scanning plane for an array transducer.

Electrical matching networks: Active or passive networks designed to tune out reactive components of the transducer and/or match the transducer impedance to the source and receiver impedance.

Elevation dimension: The lateral dimension that is perpendicular to the scanning plane for an array transducer.

Grating lobes: Undesirable artifacts in the radiation pattern of a transducer; they are produced at a location where the path length difference to adjacent array elements is a multiple of a wavelength.

Lateral modes: Transducer vibrations that occur in the lateral dimensions when the transducer is excited in the thickness dimension.

Lateral resolution: The ability to distinguish between targets in the azimuth and elevation dimensions (perpendicular to the axial dimension).

Quarter-wave matching layers: One or more layers of material placed between the transducer and the load medium (water or human tissue); they effectively match the acoustic impedance of the transducer to the load medium to improve the transducer bandwidth and signal-to-noise ratio.

References

Allen JL. 1964. Array antennas: New applications for an old technique. IEEE Spect 1:115.

Berlincourt D. 1971. Piezoelectric crystals and ceramics. In OE Mattiat (ed), Ultrasonic Transducer Materials. New York, Plenum Press.

Bobber RJ. 1970. Underwater Electroacoustic Measurements. Washington, Naval Research Laboratory.

Christensen DA. 1988. Ultrasonic Bioinstrumentation. New York, Wiley.

Curie P, Curie J. 1980. Development par pression de l'electricite polaire dans les cristaux hemiedres a faces enclinees. Comp Rend 91:383.

Desilets CS, Fraser JD, Kino GS. 1978. The design of efficient broad-band piezoelectric transducers. IEEE Trans Son Ultrason SU-25:115.

Flax SW, O'Donnell M. 1988. Phase aberration correction using signals from point reflectors and diffuse scatters: Basic principles. IEEE Trans Ultrason Ferroelec Freq Contr 35:758.

Goldberg RL, Smith SW. 1994. Multi-layer piezoelectric ceramics for two-dimensional array transducers. IEEE Trans Ultrason Ferroelec Freq Contr.

Goodman W. 1986. Introduction to Fourier Optics. New York, McGraw-Hill.

Hunt JW, Arditi M, Foster FS. 1983. Ultrasound transducers for pulse-echo medical imaging. IEEE Trans Biomed Eng 30:453.

Kino GS. 1987. Acoustic Waves. Englewood Cliffs, NJ, Prentice-Hall.

Kino GS, DeSilets CS. 1979. Design of slotted transducer arrays with matched backings. Ultrason Imag 1:189.

Nock LF, Trahey GE. 1992. Synthetic receive aperture imaging with phase correction for motion and for tissue inhomogeneities: I. Basic principles. IEEE Trans Ultrason Ferroelec Freq Contr 39:489.

Selfridge AR, Kino GS, Khuri-Yahub BT. 1980. A theory for the radiation pattern of a narrow strip acoustic transducer. Appl Phys Lett 37:35.

Shattuck DP, Weinshenker MD, Smith SW, von Ramm OT. 1984. Explososcan: A parallel processing technique for high speed ultrasound imaging with linear phased arrays. J Acoust Soc Am 75:1273.

Sherar MD, Foster FS. 1989. The design and fabrication of high frequency poly(vinylidene fluoride) transducers. Ultrason Imag 11:75.

Smith WA. 1992. New opportunities in ultrasonic transducers emerging from innovations in piezoelectric materials. In FL Lizzi (ed), New Developments in Ultrasonic Transducers and Transducer Systems, pp 3–26. New York, SPIE.

Somer JC. 1968. Electronic sector scanning for ultrasonic diagnosis. Ultrasonics 153.

Steinberg BD. 1976. Principles of Aperture and Array System Design. New York, Wiley.

Takeuchi H, Masuzawa H, Nakaya C, Ito Y. 1990. Relaxor ferroelectric transducers. Proc IEEE Ultrasonics Symposium, IEEE cat no 90CH2938-9, pp 697–705.

Trahey GE, Zhao D, Miglin JA, Smith SW. 1990. Experimental results with a real-time adaptive ultrasonic imaging system for viewing through distorting media. IEEE Trans Ultrason Ferroelec Freq Contr 37:418.

von Ramm OT, Smith SW. 1990. Real time volumetric ultrasound imaging system. In SPIE Medical Imaging IV: Image Formation, vol 1231, pp 15–22. New York, SPIE.

von Ramm OT, Thurstone FL. 1976. Cardiac imaging using a phased array ultrasound system: I. System design. Circulation 53:258.

Further Information

A good overview of linear array design and performance is contained in von O.T. Ramm and S.W. Smith (1983), Beam steering with linear arrays, *IEEE Trans Biomed Eng* 30:438. The same issue contains a more general article on transducer design and performance: J.W. Hunt, M. Arditi, and F.S. Foster (1983), Ultrasound transducers for pulse-echo medical imaging, *IEEE Trans Biomed Eng* 30:453.

The journal *IEEE Transactions on Ultrasonics, Ferroelectrics, and Frequency Control* frequently contains articles on medical ultrasound transducers. For subscription information, contact IEEE Service Center, 445 Hoes Lane, P.O. Box 1331, Piscataway, NJ 08855-1331, phone (800) 678-IEEE.

Another good source is the proceedings of the IEEE Ultrasonics Symposium, published each year. Also, the proceedings from *New Developments in Ultrasonics Transducers and Transducer Systems*, edited by F.L. Lizzi, was published by SPIE, Vol. 1733, in 1992.

12.2 Ultrasonic Imaging

Jack G. Mottley

It was recognized long ago that the tissues of the body are inhomogeneous and that signals sent into them, like pulses of high-frequency sound, are reflected and scattered by those tissues. Scattering, or redirection of some of an incident energy signal to other directions by small particles, is why we see the beam of a spotlight in fog or smoke. That part of the scattered energy that returns to the transmitter is called the backscatter.

Ultrasonic imaging of the soft tissues of the body really began in the early 1970s. At that time, the technologies began to become available to capture and display the echoes backscattered by structures within the body as images, at first as static compound images and later as real-time moving images. The development followed much the same sequence (and borrowed much of the terminology) as did radar and sonar, from initial crude single-line-of-sight displays (A-mode) to recording these side by side to build up recordings over time to show motion (M-mode), to finally sweeping the transducer either mechanically or electronically over many directions and building up two-dimensional views (B-mode or 2D).

Since this technology was intended for civilian use, applications had to wait for the development of inexpensive data handling, storage, and display technologies. A-mode was usually shown on oscilloscopes, M-modes were printed onto specially treated light-sensitive thermal paper, and B-mode was initially built up as a static image in analog scan converters and shown on television monitors. Now all modes are produced in real time in proprietary scan converters, shown on television monitors, and recorded either on commercially available videotape recorders (for organs or studies in which motion is a part of the diagnostic information) or as still frames on photographic film (for those cases in which organ dimensions and appearance are useful, but motion is not important).

Using commercial videotape reduces expenses and greatly simplifies the review of cases for quality control and training, since review stations can be set up in offices or conference rooms with commonly available monitors and videocassette recorders, and tapes from any imaging system can be played back. Also, the tapes are immediately available and do not have to be chemically processed.

Since the earliest systems were mostly capable of showing motion, the first applications were in studying the heart, which must move to carry out its function. A-mode and M-mode displays (see Figs. 12.10 through 12.12) were able to demonstrate the motion of valves, thickening of heart chamber walls, relationships between heart motion and pressure, and other parameters that enabled diagnoses of heart problems that had been difficult or impossible before. For some valvular diseases, the preferred display format for diagnosis is still the M-mode, on which the speed of valve motions can be measured and the relations of valve motions to the electrocardiogram (ECG) are easily seen.

Later, as 2D displays became available, ultrasound was applied more and more to imaging of the soft abdominal organs and in obstetrics (Fig. 12.13). In this format, organ dimensions and structural relations are seen more easily, and since the images are now made in real time, motions of organs such as the heart are still well appreciated. These images are used in a wide variety of areas from obstetrics and gynecology to ophthalmology to measure the dimensions of organs or tissue masses and have been widely accepted as a safe and convenient imaging modality.

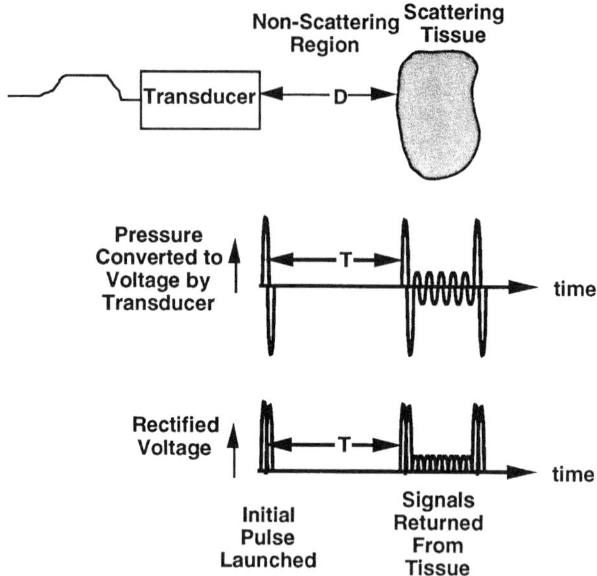

FIGURE 12.10 Schematic representation of the signal received from along a single line of sight in a tissue. The rectified voltage signals are displayed for A-mode.

Fundamentals

Strictly speaking, ultrasound is simply any sound wave whose frequency is above the limit of human hearing, which is usually taken to be 20 kHz. In the context of imaging of the human body, since frequency and wavelength (and therefore resolution) are inversely related, the lowest frequency of sound commonly used is around 1 MHz, with a constant trend toward higher frequencies in order to obtain better resolution. Axial resolution is approximately one wavelength, and at 1 MHz, the wavelength is 1.5 mm in most soft tissues, so one must go to 1.5 MHz to achieve 1-mm resolution.

Attenuation of ultrasonic signals increases with frequency in soft tissues, and so a trade-off must be made between the depth of penetration that must be achieved for a particular application and the highest frequency that can be used. Applications that require deep penetration (e.g., cardiology, abdominal, obstetrics) typically use frequencies in the 2- to 5-MHz range, while those applications which only require shallow penetration but high resolution (e.g., ophthalmology, peripheral vascular, testicular) use frequencies up to around 20 MHz. Intra-arterial imaging systems, requiring submillimeter resolution, use even higher frequencies of 20 to 50 MHz, and laboratory applications of ultrasonic microscopy use frequencies up to 100 or even 200 MHz to examine structures within individual cells.

There are two basic equations used in ultrasonic imaging. One relates the (one-way) distance d of an object that caused an echo from the transducer to the (round-trip) time delay t and speed of sound in the medium c:

$$d = \frac{1}{2} tc \tag{12.24}$$

The speed of sound in soft body tissues lies in a fairly narrow range from 1450 to 1520 m/s. For rough estimates of time of flight, one often uses 1500 m/s, which can be converted to 1.5 mm/μs, a more convenient set of units. This leads to delay times for the longest-range measurements (20 cm) of 270 μs. To allow echoes and reverberations to die out, one needs to wait several of these periods before launching the next interrogating pulse, so pulse repetition frequencies of about a kilohertz are possible.

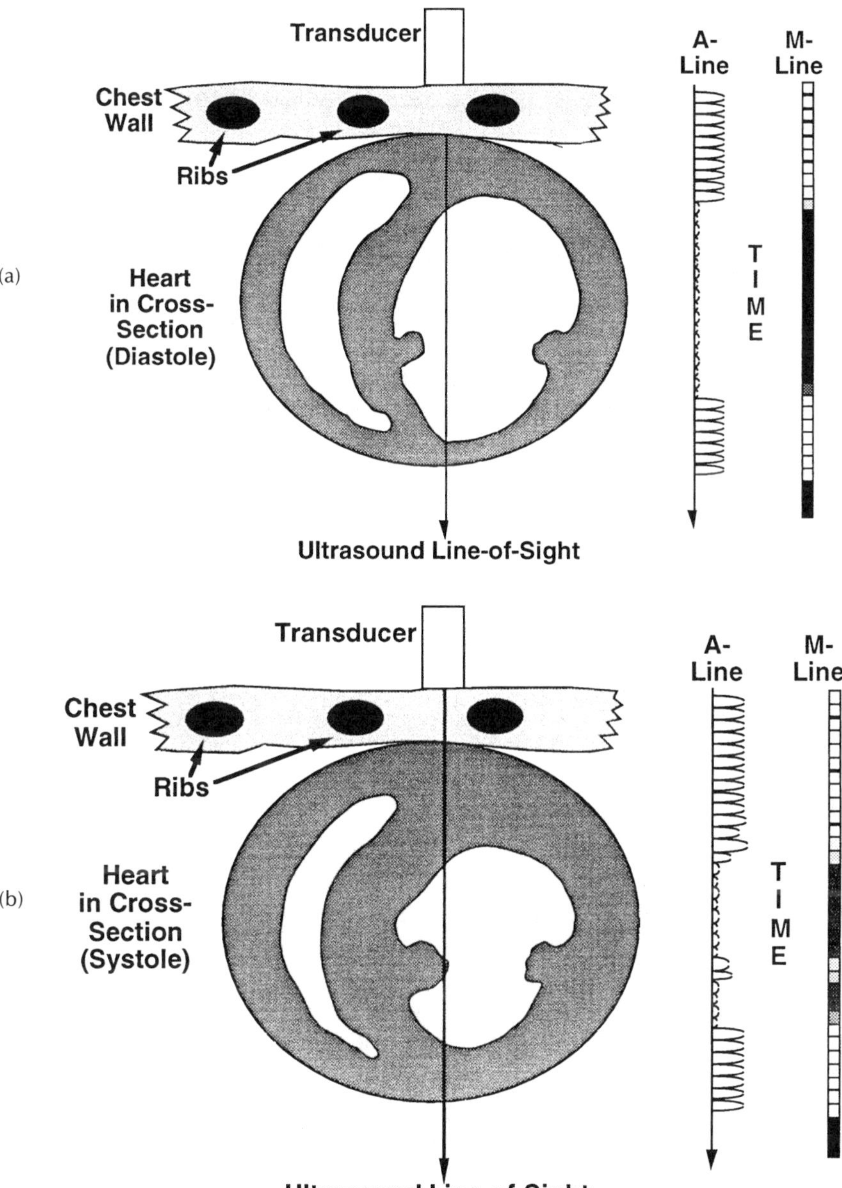

FIGURE 12.11 Example of M-mode imaging of a heart at two points during the cardiac cycle. (a) Upper panel shows heart during diastole (relaxation) with a line of sight through it and the corresponding A-line converted to an M-line. (b) The lower panel shows the same heart during systole (contraction) and the A- and M-lines. Note the thicker walls and smaller ventricular cross-section during systole.

The other equation relates the received signal strength $S(t)$ to the transmitted signal $T(t)$, the transducer's properties $B(t)$, the attenuation of the signal path to and from the scatterer $A(t)$, and the strength of the scatterer $\eta(t)$:

$$S(t) = T(t) \otimes B(t) \otimes A(t) \otimes \eta(t) \tag{12.25}$$

where $\otimes$ denotes time-domain convolution. Using the property of Fourier transforms that a convolution in the time domain is a multiplication in the frequency domain, this is more often written in the frequency domain as

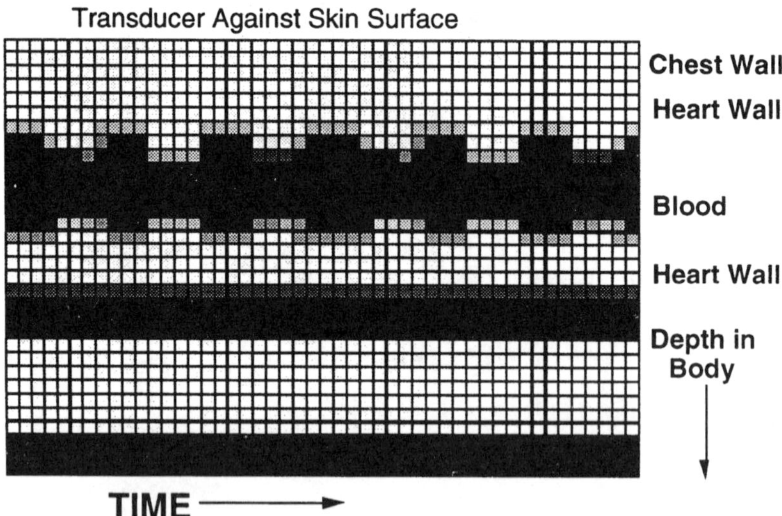

FIGURE 12.12 Completed M-mode display obtained by showing the M-lines of Fig. 12.11 side by side. The motion of the heart walls and their thickening and thinning are well appreciated. Often the ECG or heart sounds are also shown in order to coordinate the motions of the heart with other physiologic markers.

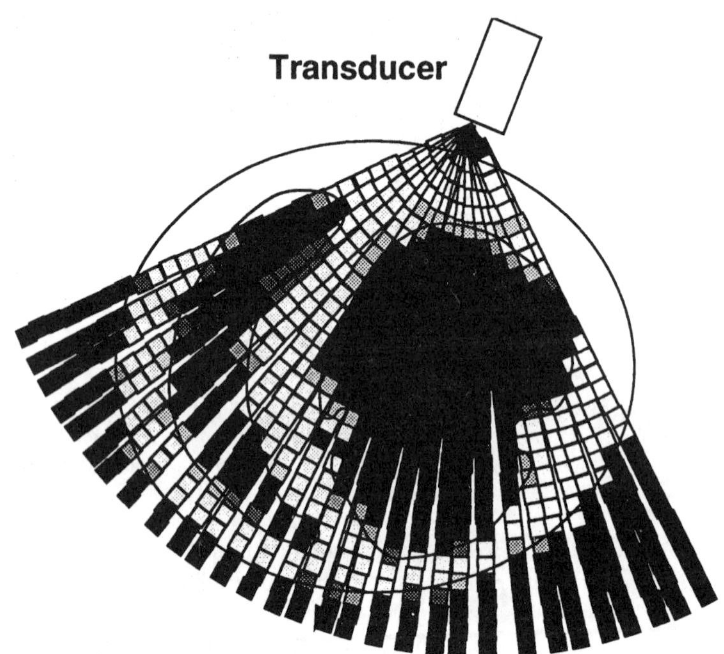

FIGURE 12.13 Schematic representation of a heart and how a 2D image is constructed by scanning the transducer.

$$S(f) = T(f)B(f)A(f)\eta(f) \tag{12.26}$$

where each term is the Fourier transform of the corresponding term in the time-domain expression (12.25) and is written as a function of frequency *f*.

The goal of most imaging applications is to measure and produce an image based on the local values of the scattering strength, which requires some assumptions to be made concerning each of the other terms. The amplitude of the transmitted signal *T*(*f*) is a user-adjustable parameter that simply adds a scale factor to the image values, unless it increases the returned signal to the point of saturating the receiver amplifier. Increasing the transmit power increases the strength of return from distant or faint echoes simply by increasing the power that illuminates them, like using a more powerful flashlight lets you see farther at night. Some care must be taken to not turn the transmit power up too high, since very high power levels are capable of causing acoustic cavitation or local heating of tissues, both of which can cause cellular damage. Advances in both electronics and transducers make it possible to transmit more and more power. For this reason, new ultrasonic imaging systems are required to display an index value that indicates the transmitted power. If the index exceeds established thresholds, it is possible that damage may occur, and the examiner should limit the time of exposure.

Most imaging systems are fairly narrow band, so the transducer properties *B*(*f*) are constant and produce only a scale factor to the image values. On phased-array systems it is possible to change the depth of focus on both transmit and receive. This improves image quality and detection of lesions by matching the focusing characteristics of the transducer to best image the object in question, like focusing a pair of binoculars on a particular object.

As the ultrasonic energy travels along the path from transmitter to scatterer and back, attenuation causes the signal to decrease with distance. This builds up as a line integral from time 0 to time *t* as

$$A(f,t) = e^{-\int_0^t \alpha(f)cdt'}$$

An average value of attenuation can be corrected for electronically by increasing the gain of the imaging system as a function of time [variously called time gain compensation (TGC) or depth gain compensation (DGC)]. In addition, some systems allow for lateral portions of the image region to have different attenuation by adding a lateral gain compensation in which the gain is increased to either side of the center region of the image.

Time gain compensation is usually set to give a uniform gray level to the scattering along the center of the image. Most operators develop a "usual" setting on each machine, and if it becomes necessary to change those settings to obtain acceptable images on a patient, then that indicates that the patient has a higher attenuation or that there is a problem with the electronics, transducer, or acoustic coupling.

Applications and Example Calculations

As an example of calculating the time of flight of an ultrasonic image, consider the following.

Example 1. A tissue has a speed of sound c = 1460 m/s, and a given feature is 10 cm deep within. Calculate the time it will take an ultrasonic signal to travel from the surface to the feature and back.

Answer: $t = 2 \times (10 \text{ cm})/(1460 \text{ m/s}) = 137\ \mu\text{s}$, where the factor of 2 is to account for the round trip the signal has to make (i.e., go in and back out).

Example 2. Typical soft tissues attenuate ultrasonic signals at a rate of 0.5 dB/cm/MHz. How much attenuation would be suffered by a 3-MHz signal going through 5 cm of tissue and returning?

Answer: a = 3 MHz × (0.5 dB/cm/MHz) / (8.686 dB/neper) = 0.173 neper/cm, A(3 MHz, 5 cm) = $e^{(-0.173 \text{ neper/cm})\times(5 \text{ cm})\times 2} = 0.177$.

Economics

Ultrasonic imaging has many economic advantages over other imaging modalities. The imaging systems are typically much less expensive than those used for other modalities and do not require special preparations of facilities such as shielding for x-rays or uniformity of magnetic field for MRI. Most ultrasonic imaging systems can be rolled easily from one location to another, so one system can be shared among technicians or examining rooms or even taken to patients' rooms for critically ill patients.

There are minimal expendables used in ultrasonic examinations, mostly the coupling gel used to couple the transducer to the skin and videotape or film for recording. Transducers are reusable and amortized over many examinations. These low costs make ultrasonic imaging one of the least expensive modalities, far preferred over others when indicated. The low cost also means these systems can be a part of private practices and used only occasionally.

As an indication of the interest in ultrasonic imaging as an alternative to other modalities, in 1993, the *Wall Street Journal* reported that spending in the United States on MRI units was approximately \$520 million, on CT units \$800 million, and on ultrasonic imaging systems \$1000 million, and that sales of ultrasound systems was growing at 15% annually [1].

Defining Terms

A-mode: The original display of ultrasound measurements, in which the amplitude of the returned echoes along a single line is displayed on an oscilloscope.

Attenuation: The reduction is signal amplitude that occurs per unit distance traveled. Some attenuation occurs in homogeneous media such as water due to viscous heating and other phenomena, but that is very small and is usually taken to be negligible over the 10- to 20-cm distances typical of imaging systems. In inhomogeneous media such as soft tissues, the attenuation is much higher and increases with frequency. The values reported for most soft tissues lie around 0.5 dB/cm/MHz.

Backscatter: That part of a scattered signal that goes back toward the transmitter of the energy.

B-mode or 2D: The current display mode of choice. This is produced by sweeping the transducer from side to side and displaying the strength of the returned echoes as bright spots in their geometrically correct direction and distance.

Compound images: Images built up by adding, or compounding, data obtained from a single transducer or multiple transducers swept through arcs. Often these transducers were not fixed to a single point of rotation but could be swept over a surface of the body like the abdomen in order to build up a picture of the underlying organs such as the liver. This required an elaborate position-sensing apparatus attached to the patient's bed or the scanner and that the organ in question be held very still throughout the scanning process, or else the image was blurred.

M-mode: Followed A-mode by recording the strength of the echoes as dark spots on moving light-sensitive paper. Objects that move, such as the heart, caused standard patterns of motion to be displayed, and a lot of diagnostic information such as valve closure rates, whether valves opened or closed completely, and wall thickness could be obtained from M-mode recordings.

Real-time images: Images currently made on ultrasound imaging systems by rapidly sweeping the transducer through an arc either mechanically or electronically. Typical images might have 120 scan lines in each image, each 20 cm long. Since each line has a time of flight of 267 μs, a single frame takes $120 \times 267\ \mu s = 32$ ms. It is therefore possible to produce images at standard video frame rates (30 frames/s, or 33.3 ms/frame).

Reflection: Occurs at interfaces between large regions (much larger than a wavelength) of media with differing acoustic properties such as density or compressibility. This is similar to the reflection of light at interfaces and can be either *total,* like a mirror, or *partial,* like a half-silvered mirror or the ghostlike reflection seen in a sheet of glass.

Scattering: Occurs when there are irregularities or inhomogeneities in the acoustic properties of a medium over distances comparable with or smaller than the wavelength of the sound. Scattering from objects much smaller than a wavelength typically increases with frequency (the blue-sky law in optics), while that from an object comparable to a wavelength is constant with frequency (why clouds appear white).

Reference

1. Naj AK. 1993. Industry focus: Big medical equipment makers try ultrasound market; cost-cutting pressures prompt shift away from more expensive devices. Wall Street Journal, November 30, B-4.

Further Information

There are many textbooks that contain good introductions to ultrasonic imaging. *Physical Principles of Ultrasonic Diagnosis,* by P. N. Wells, is a classic, and there is a new edition of another classic, *Diagnostic Ultrasound: Principles, Instruments and Exercises,* 4th ed., by Frederick Kremkau. Books on medical imaging that contain introductions to ultrasonic imaging include *Medical Imaging Systems,* by Albert Macovski; *Principles of Medical Imaging,* by Kirk Shung, Michael Smith, and Benjamin Tsui; and *Foundations of Medical Imaging,* by Zang-Hee Cho, Joie P. Jones, and Manbir Singh.

The monthly journals *IEEE Transactions on Ultrasonics, Ferroelectrics, and Frequency Control* and *IEEE Transactions on Biomedical Engineering* often contain information and research reports on ultrasonic imaging. For subscription information, contact IEEE Service Center, 445 Hoes Lane, P.O. Box 1331, Piscataway, NJ 08855-1331, phone (800) 678-4333. Another journal that often contains articles on ultrasonic imaging is the *Journal of the Acoustical Society of America.* For subscription information, contact AIP Circulation and Fulfillment Division, 500 Sunnyside Blvd., Woodbury, NY 11797-2999, phone (800) 344-6908; e-mail: elecprod\@pinet.aip.org.

There are many journals that deal with medical ultrasonic imaging exclusively. These include *Ultrasonic Imaging,* the *Journal of Ultrasound in Medicine,* American Institute of Ultrasound of Medicine (AIUM), 14750 Sweitzer Lane, Suite 100, Laurel, MD 20707-5906, and the *Journal of Ultrasound in Medicine and Biology,* Elsevier Science, Inc., 660 White Plains Road, Tarrytown, NY 10591-5153, e-mail: esuk.usa@elsevier.com.

There are also specialty journals for particular medical areas, e.g., the *Journal of the American Society of Echocardiography,* that are available through medical libraries and are indexed in Index Medicus, Current Contents, Science Citation Index, and other databases.

12.3 Blood Flow Measurement Using Ultrasound

K. Whittaker Ferrara

In order to introduce the fundamental challenges of blood velocity estimation, a brief description of the unique operating environment produced by the ultrasonic system, intervening tissue, and the scattering of ultrasound by blood is provided. In providing an overview of the parameters that differentiate this problem from radar and sonar target estimation problems, an introduction to the fluid dynamics of the cardiovascular system is presented, and the requirements of specific clinical applications are summarized. An overview of blood flow estimation systems and their performance limitations is then presented. Next, an overview of the theory of moving target estimation, with its roots in radar and sonar signal processing, is provided. The application of this theory to blood velocity estimation is then reviewed, and a number of signal processing strategies that have been applied to this problem are considered. Areas of new research including three-dimensional (3D) velocity estimation and the use of ultrasonic contrast agents are described in the final section.

Fundamental Concepts

In blood velocity estimation, the goal is not simply to estimate the mean target position and mean target velocity. The goal instead is to measure the velocity profile over the smallest region possible and to repeat this measurement quickly and accurately over the entire target. Therefore, the joint optimization of spatial, velocity, and temporal resolution is critical. In addition to the mean velocity, diagnostically useful information is contained in the volume of blood flowing through various vessels, spatial variations in the velocity profile, and the presence of turbulence. While current methods have proven extremely valuable in the assessment of the velocity profile over an entire vessel, improved *spatial resolution* is required in several diagnostic situations. Improved *velocity resolution* is also desirable for a number of clinical applications. Blood velocity estimation algorithms implemented in current systems also suffer from a velocity ambiguity due to aliasing.

Unique Features of the Operating Environment

A number of features make blood flow estimation distinct from typical radar and sonar target estimation situations. The combination of factors associated with the beam formation system, properties of the intervening medium, and properties of the target medium lead to a difficult and unique operating environment. Figure 12.14 summarizes the operating environment of an ultrasonic blood velocity estimation system, and Table 12.2 summarizes the key parameters.

Beam Formation–Data Acquisition System. *The transducer bandwidth is limited.* Most current transducers are limited to a 50% to 75% fractional bandwidth due to their finite dimensions and a variety of electrical and mechanical properties. This limits the form of the transmitted signal. The transmitted pulse is typically a short pulse with a carrier frequency, which is the center frequency in the spectrum of the transmitted signal.

Federal agencies monitor four distinct intensity levels. The levels are *TASA, TASP, TPSA,* and *TPSP,* where *T* represents temporal, *S* represents spatial, *A* represents average, and *P* represents peak. Therefore, the

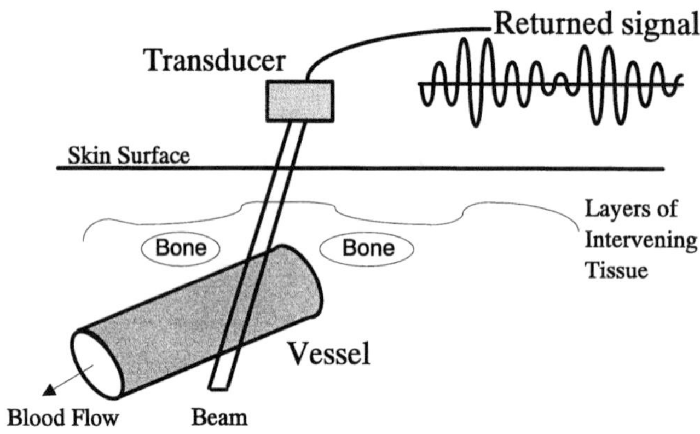

FIGURE 12.14 Operating environment for the estimation of blood velocity.

TABLE 12.2 Important Parameters

Typical transducer center frequency	2–10 MHz
Maximum transducer fractional bandwidth	50–75%
Speed of sound *c*	1500–1600 m/s
Acoustic wavelength (c = 1540)	0.154–1.54 mm
Phased-array size	>32·wavelength
Sample volume size	mm^3
Blood velocity	Normal; up to 1 m/s Pathological: up to 8 m/s
Vessel wall echo/blood echo	20–40 dB
Diameter of a red blood cell	8.5 μm
Thickness of a red blood cell	2.4 μm
Volume of a red blood cell	87 ± 6 μm^3
Volume concentration of cells (hematocrit)	45%
Maximum concentration without cell deformation	58%

use of long bursts requires a proportionate reduction in the transmitted peak power. This may limit the signal-to-noise ratio (SNR) obtained with a long transmitted burst due to the weak reflections from the complex set of targets within the body.

Intervening Medium. Acoustic windows, which are locations for placement of a transducer to successfully interrogate particular organs, are limited in number and size. Due to the presence of bone and air, the number of usable acoustic windows is extremely limited. The reflection of acoustic energy from bone is only 3 dB below that of a perfect reflector [Wells, 1977]. Therefore, transducers cannot typically surround a desired imaging site. In many cases, it is difficult to find a single small access window. This limits the use of inverse techniques.

Intervening tissue produces acoustic refraction and reflection. Energy is reflected at unpredictable angles.

The clutter-to-signal ratio is very high. Clutter is the returned signal from stationary or slowly moving tissue, which can be 40 dB above the returned signal from blood. Movement of the vessel walls and valves during the cardiac cycle introduces a high-amplitude, low-frequency signal. This is typically considered to be unwanted noise, and a high-pass filter is used to eliminate the estimated wall frequencies.

The sampling rate is restricted. The speed of sound in tissue is low (approximately 1540 m/s), and each transmitted pulse must reach the target and return before the returned signal is recorded. Thus the sampling rate is restricted, and the aliasing limit is often exceeded.

The total observation time is limited (due to low acoustic velocity). In order to estimate the velocity of blood in all locations in a 2D field in real time, the estimate for each region must be based on the return from a limited number of pulses because of the low speed of sound.

Frequency-dependent attenuation affects the signal. Tissue acts as a low-pass transmission filter; the scattering functions as a high-pass filter. The received signal is therefore a distorted version of the transmitted signal. In order to estimate the effective filter function, the type and extent of each tissue type encountered by the wave must be known. Also, extension of the bandwidth of the transmitted signal to higher frequencies increases absorption, requiring higher power levels that can increase health concerns.

Target Scattering Medium (Red Blood Cells). Multiple groups of scatterers are present. The target medium consists of multiple volumes of diffuse moving scatterers with velocity vectors that vary in magnitude and direction. The target medium is spread in space and velocity. The goal is to estimate the velocity over the smallest region possible.

There is a limited period of statistical stationarity. The underlying cardiac process can only be considered to be stationary for a limited time. This time was estimated to be 10 ms for the arterial system by Hatle and Angelsen [1985]. If an observation interval greater than this period is used, the average scatterer velocity cannot be considered to be constant.

Overview of Ultrasonic Flow Estimation Systems

Current ultrasonic imaging systems operate in a pulse-echo (PE) or continuous-wave (CW) intensity mapping mode. In pulse-echo mode, a very short pulse is transmitted, and the reflected signal is analyzed. For a continuous-wave system, a lower-intensity signal is continuously transmitted into the body, and the reflected energy is analyzed. In both types of systems, an acoustic wave is launched along a specific path into the body, and the return from this wave is processed as a function of time. The return is due to reflected waves from structures along the line of sight, combined with unwanted noise. Spatial selectivity is provided by beam formation performed on burst transmission and reception. Steering of the beam to a particular angle and creating a narrow beam width at the depth of interest are accomplished by an effective lens applied to the ultrasonic transducer. This lens may be produced by a contoured material, or it may be simulated by phased pulses applied to a transducer array. The spatial weighting pattern will ultimately be the product of the effective lens on transmission and reception. The returned signal from the formed beam can be used to map the backscattered intensity into a two-dimensional gray-scale image, or to estimate target velocity. *We shall focus on the use of this information to estimate the velocity of red blood cells moving through the body.*

Single Sample Volume Doppler Instruments. One type of system uses the Doppler effect to estimate velocity in a single volume of blood, known as the sample volume, which is designated by the system operator. The Doppler shift frequency from a moving target can be shown to equal $2f_c v/c$, where f_c is the transducer center frequency in hertz, c is the speed of sound within tissue, and v is the velocity component of the blood cells toward or away from the transducer. These "Doppler" systems transmit a train of long pulses with a well-defined carrier frequency and measure the Doppler shift in the returned signal. The spectrum of Doppler frequencies is proportional to the distribution of velocities present in the sample volume. The sample volume is on a cubic millimeter scale for typical pulse-echo systems operating in the frequency range of 2 to 10 MHz. Therefore, a thorough cardiac or peripheral vascular examination requires a long period. In these systems, 64 to 128 temporal samples are acquired for each estimate. The spectrum of these samples is typically computed using a fast Fourier transform (FFT) technique [Kay and Marple, 1981]. The range of velocities present within the sample volume can then be estimated. The spectrum is scaled to represent velocity and plotted on the vertical axis. Subsequent spectral estimates are then calculated and plotted vertically adjacent to the first estimate.

Color Flow Mapping. In color flow mapping, a pseudo-color velocity display is overlaid on a 2D gray-scale image. Simultaneous amplitude and velocity information is thus available for a 2D sector area of the body. The clinical advantage is a reduction in the examination time and the ability to visualize the velocity profile as a 2D map. Figure 12.15 shows a typical color flow map of ovarian blood flow combined with the Doppler spectrum of the region indicated by the small graphic sample volume. The color flow map shows color-encoded velocities superimposed on the gray-scale image with the velocity magnitude indicated by the color bar on the side of the image. Motion toward the transducer is shown in yellow and red, and motion away from the transducer is shown in blue and green, with the range of colors representing a range of velocities to a maximum of 6 cm/s in each direction. Velocities above this limit would produce aliasing for the parameters used in optimizing the instrument for the display of ovarian flow. A velocity of 0 m/s would be indicated by black, as shown at the center of the color bar. Early discussions of the implementation of color flow mapping systems can be found in Curry and White [1978] and Nowicki and Reid [1981].

The lower portion of the image presents an intensity-modulated display of instantaneous Doppler components along the vertical axis. As time progresses, the display is translated along the horizontal axis to generate a Doppler time history for the selected region of interest [provided by Acuson Corporation, Mountain View, California].

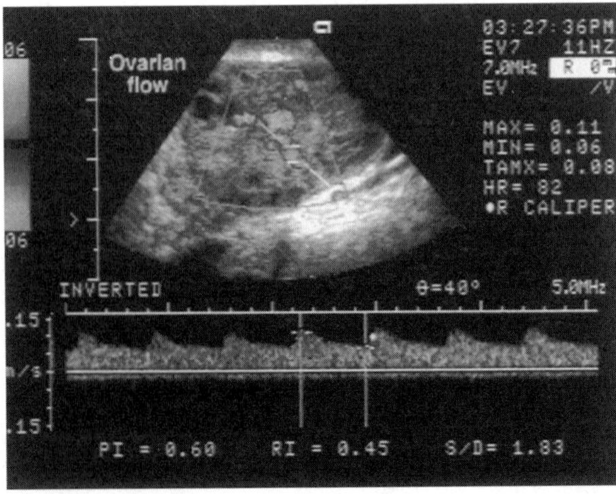

FIGURE 12.15 Flow map and Doppler spectrum for ovarian blood flow.

Limitations of color flow instruments result in part from the transmission of a narrowband (long) pulse that is needed for velocity estimation but degrades spatial resolution and prevents mapping of the spatial-velocity profile. Due to the velocity gradient in each blood vessel, the transmission of a long pulse also degrades the velocity resolution. This is caused by the simultaneous examination of blood cells moving at different velocities and the resulting mixing of regions of the scattering medium, which can be distinctly resolved on a conventional B-mode image. Since the limited speed of acoustic propagation velocity limits the sampling rate, a second problem is aliasing of the Doppler frequency. Third, information regarding the presence of velocity gradients and turbulence is desired and is not currently available. Finally, estimation of blood velocity based on the Doppler shift provides only an estimate of the axial velocity, which is the movement toward or away from the transducer, and cannot be used to estimate movement across the transducer beam. It is the 3D velocity magnitude that is of clinical interest.

For a color flow map, the velocity estimation technique is based on estimation of the mean Doppler shift using signal-processing techniques optimized for rapid (real-time) estimation of velocity in each region of the image. The transmitted pulse is typically a burst of 4 to 8 cycles of the carrier frequency. Data acquisition for use in velocity estimation is interleaved with the acquisition of information for the gray-scale image. Each frame of acquired data samples is used to generate one update of the image display. An azimuthal line is a line that describes the direction of the beam from the transducer to the target. A typical 2D ultrasound scanner uses 128 azimuthal lines per frame and 30 frames per second to generate a gray-scale image. Data acquisition for the velocity estimator used in color flow imaging requires an additional 4 to 18 transducer firings per azimuthal line and therefore reduces both the number of azimuthal lines and the number of frames per second. If the number of lines per frame is decreased, spatial undersampling or a reduced examination area results. If the number of frames per second is decreased, temporal undersampling results, and the display becomes difficult to interpret.

The number of data samples available for each color flow velocity estimate is reduced to 4 to 18 in comparison with the 64 to 128 data samples available to estimate velocity in a single sample volume Doppler mode. This reduction, required to estimate velocity over the 2D image, produces a large increase in the estimator variance.

Fluid Dynamics and the Cardiovascular System

In order to predict and adequately assess blood flow profiles within the body, the fluid dynamics of the cardiovascular system will be briefly reviewed. The idealized case known as *Poiseuille flow* will be considered first, allowed by a summary of the factors that disturb Poiseuille flow.

A Poiseuille flow model is appropriate in a long rigid circular pipe at a large distance from the entrance. The velocity in this case is described by the equation $v/v_0 = 1 - (r/a)^2$, where v represents the velocity parallel to the wall, v_0 represents the center-line velocity, r is the radial distance variable, and a is the radius of the tube. In this case, the mean velocity is half the center-line velocity, and the volume flow rate is given by the mean velocity multiplied by the cross-sectional area of the vessel.

For the actual conditions within the arterial system, Poiseuille flow is only an approximation. The actual arterial geometry is tortuous and individualistic, and the resulting flow is perturbed by entrance effects and reflections. Reflections are produced by vascular branches and the geometric taper of the arterial diameter. In addition, spatial variations in vessel elasticity influence the amplitude and wave velocity of the arterial pulse. Several parameters can be used to characterize the velocity profile, including the Reynolds number, the Womersly number, the pulsatility index, and the resistive index. The pulsatility and resistive indices are frequently estimated during a clinical examination.

The Reynolds number is denoted Re and measures the ratio of fluid inertia to the viscous forces acting on the fluid. The Reynolds number is defined by $\mathrm{Re} = Dv'/\mu_k$, where v' is the average cross-sectional velocity μ_k is the kinematic viscosity, and D is the vessel diameter. *Kinematic viscosity* is defined as the fluid viscosity divided by the fluid density. When the Reynolds number is high, fluid inertia dominates. This is true in the aorta and larger arteries, and bursts of turbulence are possible. When the number is low, viscous effects dominate.

The Womersly number is used to describe the effect introduced by the unsteady, pulsatile nature of the flow. This parameter, defined by $a(\omega/\mu_k)^{1/2}$, where ω represents radian frequency of the wave, governs propagation along an elastic, fluid-filled tube. When the Womersly number is small, the instantaneous profile will be parabolic in shape, the flow is viscous dominated, and the profile is oscillatory and Poiseuille in nature. When the Womersly number is large, the flow will be blunt, inviscid, and have thin wall layers [Nicholas and O'Rourke, 1990].

The pulsatility index represents the ratio of the unsteady and steady velocity components of the flow. This shows the magnitude of the velocity changes that occur during acceleration and deceleration of blood constituents. Since the arterial pulse decreases in magnitude as it travels, this index is maximum in the aorta. The pulsatility index is given by the difference between the peak systolic and minimum diastolic values divided by the average value over one cardiac cycle. The Pourcelot, or resistance, index is the peak-to-peak swing in velocity from systole to diastole divided by the peak systolic value [Nichols and O'Rourke, 1990].

Blood Velocity Profiles. Specific factors that influence the blood velocity profile include the entrance effect, vessel curvature, skewing, stenosis, acceleration, secondary flows, and turbulence. These effects are briefly introduced in this subsection.

The entrance effect is a result of fluid flow passing from a large tube or chamber into a smaller tube. The velocity distribution at the entrance becomes blunt. At a distance known as the *entry length,* the fully developed parabolic profile is restored, where the entry length is given by $0.06\mathrm{Re}\cdot(2a)$ [Nerem, 1985]. Distal to this point the profile is independent of distance.

If the vessel is curved, there will also be an entrance effect. The blunt profile in this case is skewed, with the peak velocity closer to the inner wall of curvature. When the fully developed profile occurs downstream, the distribution will again be skewed, with the maximal velocity toward the outer wall of curvature. Skewing also occurs at a bifurcation where proximal flow divides into daughter vessels. The higher-velocity components, which occurred at the center of the parent vessel, are then closer to the flow divider, and the velocity distribution in the daughter vessels is skewed toward the divider.

Stenosis, a localized narrowing of the vessel diameter, dampens the pulsatility of the flow and pressure waveforms. The downstream flow profile depends on the shape and degree of stenosis. Acceleration adds a flat component to the velocity profile. It is responsible for the flat profile during systole, as well as the negative flat component near the walls in the deceleration phase.

Secondary flows are swirling components which are superimposed on the main velocity profile. These occur at bends and branches, although regions of secondary flow can break away from the vessel wall and are then known as *separated flow.* These regions reattach to the wall at a point downstream.

One definition of turbulent flow is flow that demonstrates a random fluctuation in the magnitude and direction of velocity as a function of space and time. The intensity of turbulence is calculated using the magnitude of the fluctuating velocities. The relative intensity of turbulence is given by $I_t = u_{\mathrm{rms}}/u_{\mathrm{mean}}$, where u_{rms} represents the root-mean-square value of the fluctuating portion of the velocity, and u_{mean} represents the nonfluctuating mean velocity [Hinze, 1975].

Clinical Applications and Their Requirements

Blood flow measurement with ultrasound is used in estimating the velocity and volume of flow within the heart and peripheral arteries and veins. Normal blood vessels vary in diameter up to a maximum of 2 cm, although most vessels examined with ultrasound have a diameter of 1 to 10 mm. Motion of the vessel wall results in a diameter change of 5% to 10% during a cardiac cycle.

Carotid Arteries (Common, Internal, External). The evaluation of flow in the carotid arteries is of great clinical interest due to their importance in supplying blood to the brain, their proximity to the skin, and the wealth of experience that has been developed in characterizing vascular pathology through an evaluation of flow. The size of the carotid arteries is moderate; they narrow quickly from a maximum diameter of 0.8 cm. The shape of carotid flow waveforms over the cardiac cycle can be related to the pathophysiology of the circulation. Numerous attempts have been made to characterize the parameters of carotid waveforms and to compare these parameters in normal and stenotic cases. A number of indices have been used to summarize the information contained in these waveforms. The normal range of the Pourcelot index is 0.55 to 0.75. Many researchers have shown that accurate detection of a minor stenosis requires accurate quantitation of the entire Doppler spectrum and remains very difficult with current technology. The presence of a stenosis causes spectral broadening with the introduction of lower frequency or velocity components.

Cardiology. Blood velocity measurement in cardiology requires analysis of information at depths up to 18 cm. A relatively low center frequency (e.g., 2.5 to 3.5 MHz) typically is used in order to reduce attenuation. Areas commonly studied and the maximum rate of flow include the following [Hatle, 1985]:

Normal Adult Maximal Velocity (m/s)	
Mitral flow	0.9
Tricuspid flow	0.5
Pulmonary artery	0.75
Left ventricle	0.9

Aorta. Aortic flow exhibits a blunt profile with entrance region characteristics. The entrance length is approximately 30 cm. The vessel diameter is approximately 2 cm. The mean Reynolds number is 2500 [Nerem, 1985], although the peak Reynolds number in the ascending aorta can range from 4300 to 8900, and the peak Reynolds number in the abdominal aorta is in the range of 400 to 1100 [Nichols and O'Rourke, 1990]. The maximal velocity is on the order of 1.35 m/s. The flow is skewed in the aortic arch with a higher velocity at the inner wall. The flow is unsteady and laminar with possible turbulent bursts at peak systole.

Peripheral Arteries [Hatsukami et al., 1992]. The peak systolic velocity in centimeters per second and standard deviation of the velocity measurement technique are provided below for selected arteries.

Artery	Peak Systolic Velocity (cm/s)	Standard Deviation
Proximal external iliac	99	22
Distal external iliac	96	13
Proximal common femoral	89	16
Distal common femoral	71	15
Proximal popliteal	53	9
Distal popliteal	53	24
Proximal peroneal	46	14
Distal peroneal	44	12

Nearly all the vessels above normally show some flow reversal during early diastole. A value of the pulsatility index of 5 or more in a limb artery is considered to be normal.

Velocity Estimation Techniques

Prior to the basic overview of theoretical approaches to target velocity estimation, it is necessary to understand a few basic features of the received signal from blood scatterers. It is the statistical correlation of the received signal in space and time that provides the opportunity to use a variety of velocity estimation strategies. Velocity estimation based on analysis of the frequency shift or the temporal correlation can be justified by these statistical properties.

Blood velocity mapping has unique features due to the substantial viscosity of blood and the spatial limitations imposed by the vessel walls. Because of these properties, groups of red blood cells can be tracked over a significant distance. Blood consists of a viscous incompressible fluid containing an average

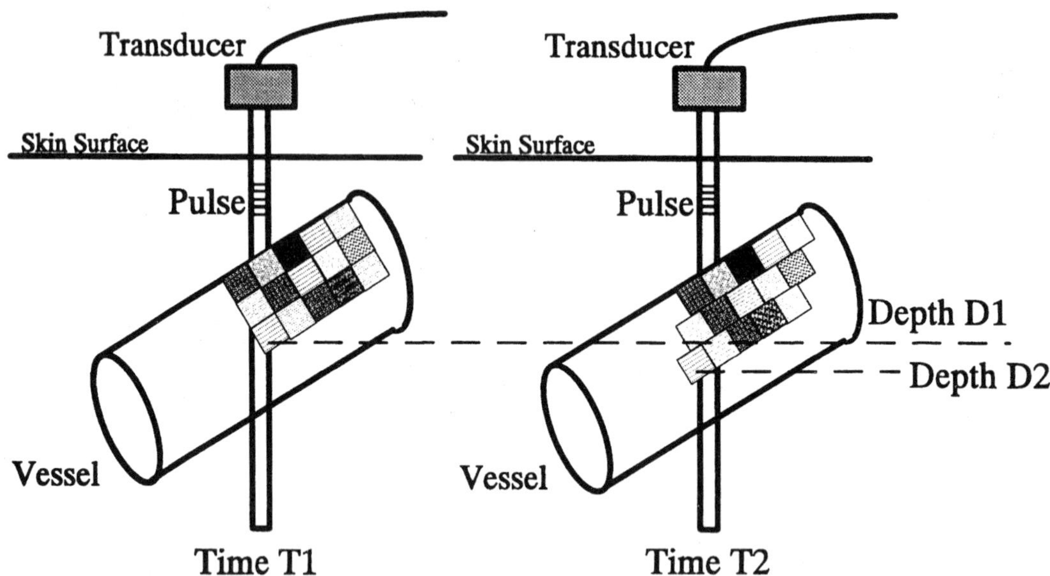

FIGURE 12.16 Random concentration of red blood cells within a vessel at times T_1 and T_2, where the change in depth from D_1 to D_2 would be used to estimate velocity.

volume concentration of red blood cells of 45%, although this concentration varies randomly through the blood medium. The red blood cells are primarily responsible for producing the scattered wave, due to the difference in their acoustic properties in comparison with plasma. Recent research into the characteristics of blood has led to stochastic models for its properties as a function of time and space [Angelson, 1980; Atkinson and Berry, 1974; Mo and Cobbold, 1986; Shung et al., 1976, 1992]. The scattered signal from an insonified spatial volume is a random process that varies with the fluctuations in the density of scatterers in the insonified area, the shear rate within the vessel, and the hematocrit [Atkinson and Berry, 1974; Ferrara and Algazi, 1994a, 1994b; Mo and Cobbold, 1986].

Since the concentration of cells varies randomly through the vessel, the magnitude of the returned signal varies when the group of scatterers being insonified changes. The returned amplitude from one spatial region is independent of the amplitude of the signal from adjacent spatial areas. As blood flows through a vessel, it transports cells whose backscattered signals can be tracked to estimate flow velocities.

Between the transmission of one pulse and the next, the scatterers move a small distance within the vessel. As shown in Fig. 12.16, a group of cells with a particular concentration which are originally located at depth D_1 at time T_1 move to depth D_2 at time T_2. The resulting change in axial depth produces a change in the delay of the signal returning to the transducer from each group of scatterers. This change in delay of the radiofrequency (RF) signal can be estimated in several ways. As shown in Fig. 12.17, the returned signal from a set of sequential pulses then shows a random amplitude that can be used to estimate the velocity. Motion is detected using signal-processing techniques that estimate the shift of the signal between pulses.

Clutter. In addition to the desired signal from the blood scatterers, the received signal contains clutter echoes returned from the surrounding tissue. An important component of this clutter signal arises from slowly moving vessel walls. The wall motion produces Doppler frequency shifts typically below 1 kHz, while the desired information from the blood cells exists in frequencies up to 15 kHz. Due to the smooth structure of the walls, energy is scattered coherently, and the clutter signal can be 40 dB above the scattered signal from blood. High-pass filters have been developed to remove the unwanted signal from the surrounding vessel walls.

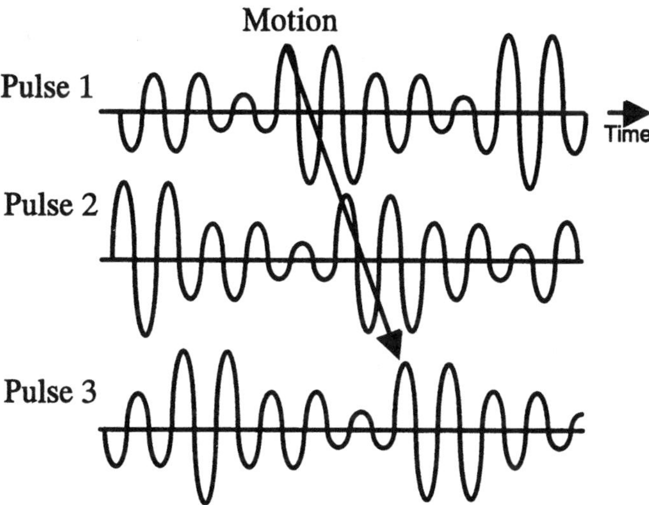

FIGURE 12.17 Received RF signal from three transmitted pulses, with a random amplitude which can be used to estimate the axial movement of blood between pulses. Motion is shown by the shift in the signal with a recognizable amplitude.

Classic Theory of Velocity Estimation. Most current commercial ultrasound systems transmit a train of long pulses with a carrier frequency of 2 to 10 MHz and estimate velocity using the Doppler shift of the reflected signal. The transmission of a train of short pulses and new signal-processing strategies may improve the spatial resolution and quality of the resulting velocity estimate. In order to provide a basis for discussion and comparison of these techniques, the problem of blood velocity estimation is considered in this subsection from the view of classic velocity estimation theory typically applied to radar and sonar problems.

Important differences exist between classic detection and estimation for radar and sonar and the application of such techniques to medical ultrasound. The Van Trees [1971] approach is based on joint estimation of the Doppler shift and position over the entire target. In medical ultrasound, the velocity is estimated in small regions of a large target, where the target position is assumed to be known. While classic theories have been developed for estimation of all velocities within a large target by Van Trees and others, such techniques require a model for the velocity in each spatial region of interest. For the case of blood velocity estimation, the spatial variation in the velocity profile is complex, and it is difficult to postulate a model that can be used to derive a high-quality estimate. The theory of velocity estimation in the presence of spread targets is also discussed by Kennedy [1969] and Price [1968] as it applies to radar astronomy and dispersive communication channels.

It is the desire to improve the spatial and velocity resolution of the estimate of blood velocity that has motivated the evaluation of alternative wideband estimation techniques. Narrowband velocity estimation techniques use the Doppler frequency shift produced by the moving cells with a sample volume that is fixed in space. Wideband estimation techniques incorporate the change in delay of the returned pulse due to the motion of the moving cells. Within the classification of narrowband techniques are a number of estimation strategies to be detailed below. These include the fast Fourier transform (FFT), finite derivative estimation, the autocorrelator, and modern spectral estimation techniques, including autoregressive strategies. Within the classification of wideband techniques are cross-correlation strategies and the wideband maximum likelihood estimator (WMLE).

For improving the spatial mapping of blood velocity within the body, the transmission of short pulses is desirable. Therefore, it is of interest to assess the quality of velocity estimates made using narrowband and wideband estimators with transmitted signals of varying lengths. If $(2v/c)BT << 1$, where v represents the axial velocity of the target, c represents the speed of the wave in tissue, B represents the transmitted

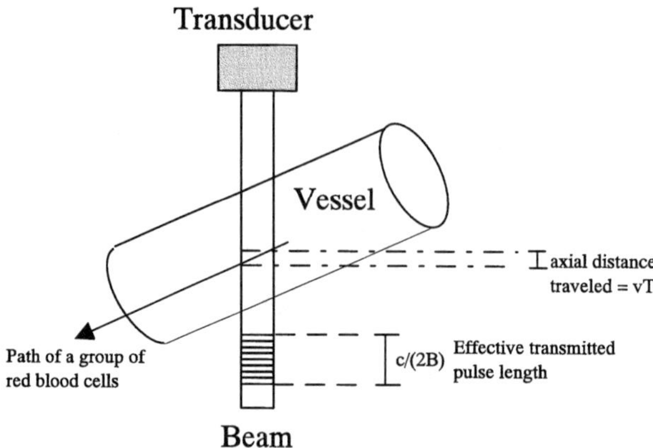

FIGURE 12.18 Comparison of the axial distance traveled and the effective length of the transmitted pulse.

signal bandwidth, and T represents the total time interval used in estimating velocity within an individual region, then the change in delay produced by the motion of the red blood cells can be ignored [Van Trees, 1971].

This inequality is interpreted for the physical conditions of medical ultrasound in Fig. 12.18. As shown in Fig. 12.18, the value vT represents the axial distance traveled by the target while it is observed by the transducer beam, and $c/(2B)$ represents the effective length of the signal that is used to observe the moving cells. If $vT << c/(2B)$, the shift in the position of a group of red blood cells during their travel though the ultrasonic beam is not a detectable fraction of the signal length. This leads to two important restrictions on estimation techniques. First, under the "narrowband" condition of transmission of a long (narrowband) pulse, motion of a group of cells through the beam can only be estimated using the Doppler frequency shift. Second, if the inequality is not satisfied and therefore the transmitted signal is short (wideband), faster-moving red blood cells leave the region of interest, and the use of a narrowband estimation technique produces a biased velocity estimate. Thus two strategies can be used to estimate velocity. A long (narrowband) pulse can transmitted, and the signal from a fixed depth then can be used to estimate velocity. Alternatively, a short (wideband) signal can be transmitted in order to improve spatial resolution, and the estimator used to determine the velocity must move along with the red blood cells.

The inequality is now evaluated for typical parameters. When the angle between the axis of the beam and the axis of the vessel is 45°, the axial distance traveled by the red blood cells while they cross the beam is equivalent to the lateral beam width. Using an axial distance vT of 0.75 mm, which is a reasonable lateral beam width, and an acoustic velocity of 1540 m/s, the bandwidth of the transmitted pulse must be much less than 1.026 MHz for the narrowband approximation to be valid.

Due to practical advantages in the implementation of the smaller bandwidth required by baseband signals, the center frequency of the signal is often removed before velocity estimation. The processing required for the extraction of the baseband signal is shown in Fig. 12.19. The returned signal from the transducer is amplified and coherently demodulated, through multiplication by the carrier frequency, and then a low-pass filter is applied to remove the signal sideband frequencies and noise. The remaining signal is the complex envelope. A high-pass filter is then applied to the signal from each fixed depth to remove the unwanted echoes from stationary tissue. The output of this processing is denoted as $I_k(t)$ for the in-phase signal from the kth pulse as a function of time and $Q_k(t)$ for the quadrature signal from the kth pulse.

Narrowband Estimation

Narrowband estimation techniques that estimate velocity for blood at a fixed depth are described in this subsection. Both the classic Doppler technique, which frequently is used in single-sample volume systems,

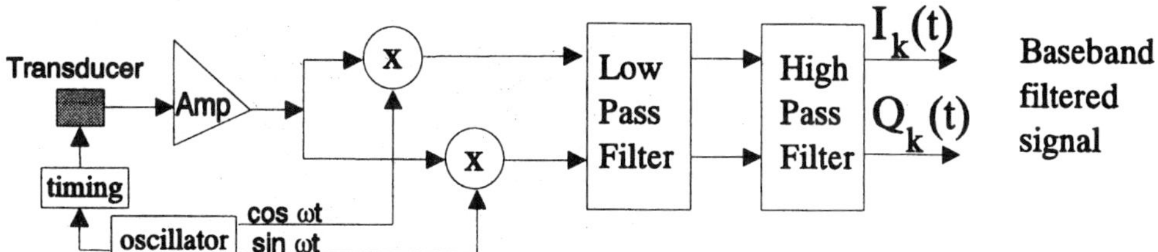

FIGURE 12.19 Block diagram of the system architecture required to generate the baseband signal used by several estimation techniques.

and the autocorrelator, which frequently is used in color flow mapping systems, are included, as well as a finite derivative estimator and an autoregressive estimator, which have been the subject of previous research. The autocorrelator is used in real-time color flow mapping systems due to the ease of implementation and the relatively small bias and variance.

Classic Doppler Estimation. If the carrier frequency is removed by coherently demodulating the signal, the change in delay of the RF signal becomes a change in the phase of the baseband signal. The Doppler shift frequency from a moving target equals $2f_c v/c$. With a center frequency of 5 MHz, sound velocity of 1540 m/s, and blood velocity of 1 m/s, the resulting frequency shift is 6493.5 Hz. For the estimation of blood velocity, the Doppler shift is not detectable using a single short pulse, and therefore, the signal from a fixed depth and a train of pulses is acquired.

A pulse-echo Doppler processing block diagram is shown in Fig. 12.20. The baseband signal, from Figure 12.19, is shown as the input to this processing block. The received signal from each pulse is multiplied by a time window that is typically equal to the length of the transmitted pulse and integrated to produce a single data sample from each pulse. The set of data samples from a train of pulses is then Fourier-transformed, with the resulting frequency spectrum related to the axial velocity using the Doppler relationship.

Estimation of velocity using the Fourier transform of the signal from a fixed depth suffers from the limitations of all narrowband estimators, in that the variance of the estimate increases when a short pulse is transmitted. In addition, the velocity resolution produced using the Fourier transform is inversely proportional to the length of the data window. Therefore, if 64 pulses with a pulse repetition frequency of 5 kHz are used in the spectral estimate, the frequency resolution is on the order of 78.125 Hz (5000/64). The velocity resolution for a carrier frequency of 5 MHz and speed of sound of 1540 m/s is then on the order of 1.2 cm/s, determined from the Doppler relationship. Increasing the data window only improves the velocity resolution if the majority of the red blood cells have not left the sample volume and the flow conditions have not produced a decorrelation of the signal. It is this relationship between the data window and velocity resolution, a fundamental feature of Fourier transform techniques, that has motivated the use of autoregressive estimators. The frequency and velocity resolution are not fundamentally constrained by the data window using these modern spectral estimators introduced below.

Autoregressive Estimation (AR). In addition to the classic techniques discussed previously, higher-order modern spectral estimation techniques have been used in an attempt to improve the velocity

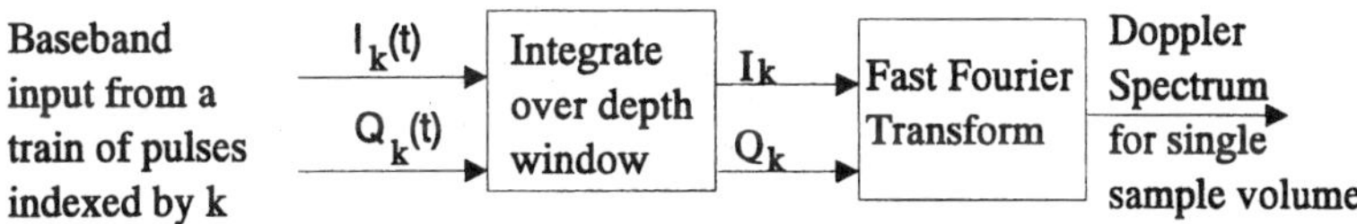

FIGURE 12.20 Block diagram of the system architecture required to estimate the Doppler spectrum from a set of baseband samples from a fixed depth.

resolution of the estimate. These techniques are again narrowband estimation techniques, since the data samples used in computing the estimate are obtained from a fixed depth. The challenges encountered in applying such techniques to blood velocity estimation include the selection of an appropriate order which adequately models the data sequence while providing the opportunity for real-time velocity estimation and determination of the length of the data sequence to be used in the estimation process.

The goal in autoregressive velocity estimation is to model the frequency content of the received signal by a set of coefficients which could be used to reconstruct the signal spectrum. The coefficients $a(m)$ represent the AR parameters of the AR(p) process, where p is the number of poles in the model for the signal. Estimation of the AR parameters has been accomplished using the Burg and Levinson-Durban recursion methods. The spectrum $P(f)$ is then estimated using the following equation:

$$P(f) = k\left|1 + \sum_{m=1}^{p} a(m)\exp\left[-i2\pi mf\right]\right|^{-2}$$

The poles of the AR transfer function which lie within the unit circle can then be determined based on these parameters, and the velocity associated with each pole is determined by the Doppler equation.

Both autoregressive and autoregressive moving-average estimation techniques have been applied to single-sample-volume Doppler estimation. Order selection for single-sample-volume AR estimators is discussed in Kaluzinski [1989]. Second-order autoregressive estimation has been applied to color flow mapping by Loupas and McDicken [1990] and Ahn and Park [1991]. Although two poles are not sufficient to model the data sequence, the parameters of a higher-order process cannot be estimated in real time. In addition, the estimation of parameters of a higher-order process using the limited number of data points available in color flow mapping produces a large variance. Loupas and McDicken have used the two poles to model the signal returned from blood. Ahn and Park have used one pole to model the received signal from blood and the second pole to model the stationary signal from the surrounding tissue.

While AR techniques are useful in modeling the stationary tissue and blood and in providing a high-resolution estimate of multiple velocity components, several problems have been encountered in the practical application to blood velocity estimation. First, the order required to adequately model any region of the vessel can change when stationary tissue is present in the sample volume or when the range of velocity components in the sample volume increases. In addition, the performance of an AR estimate degrades rapidly in the presence of white noise, particularly with a small number of data samples.

Autocorrelator. Kasai et al. [1985] and Barber et al. [1985] discussed a narrowband *mean* velocity estimation structure for use in color flow mapping. The phase of the signal correlation at a lag of one transmitted period is estimated and used in an inverse tangent calculation of the estimated mean Doppler shift f_{mean} of the returned signal. A block diagram of the autocorrelator is shown in Fig. 12.21. The baseband signal is first integrated over a short depth window. The phase of the correlation at a lag of one pulse period is then estimated as the inverse tangent of the imaginary part of the correlation divided by the real part of the correlation. The estimated mean velocity v_{mean} of the scattering medium is then

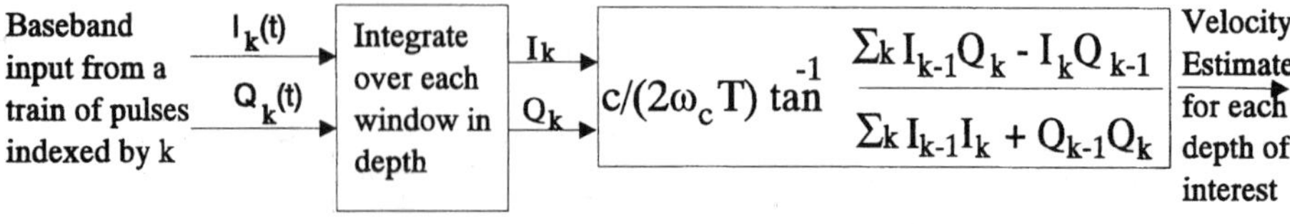

FIGURE 12.21 Block diagram of the system architecture required to estimate the mean Doppler shift for each depth location using the autocorrelator.

determined by scaling the estimated Doppler shift by several factors, including the expected center frequency of the returned signal.

The autocorrelator structure can be derived from the definition of instantaneous frequency, from the phase of the correlation at a lag of one period, or as the first-order autoregressive estimate of the mean frequency of a baseband signal. The contributions of uncorrelated noise should average to zero in both the numerator and denominator of the autocorrelator. This is an advantage because the autocorrelation estimate is unbiased when the input signal includes the desired flow signal and noise. Alternatively, in the absence of a moving target, the input to the autocorrelator may consist only of white noise. Under these conditions, both the numerator and denominator can average to values near zero, and the resulting output of the autocorrelator has a very large variance. This estimation structure must therefore be used with a power threshold that can determine the presence or absence of a signal from blood flow and set the output of the estimator to zero when this motion is absent.

The variance of the autocorrelation estimate increases with the transmitted bandwidth, and therefore, the performance is degraded by transmitting a short pulse.

Finite Derivative Estimator (FDE). A second approach to mean velocity or frequency estimation is based on a finite implementation of a derivative operator. The *finite derivative* estimator is derived based on the first and second moments of the spectrum. The basis for this estimator comes from the definition of the spectral centroid:

$$v_{\text{mean}} = \frac{\int \omega S(\omega)\, d\omega}{\int S(\omega)\, d\omega} \tag{12.27}$$

The mean velocity is given by v_{mean}, which is a scaled version of the mean frequency, where the scaling constant is given by k' and $S(\omega)$ represents the power spectral density. Letting $R_r(\cdot)$ represent the complex signal correlation and τ represent the difference between the two times used in the correlation estimate, Eq. (12.27) is equivalent to

$$v_{\text{mean}} = k' \frac{\left[\frac{\partial}{\partial \tau} R_r(\tau)\Big|_{\tau=0}\right]}{R_r(0)} \tag{12.28}$$

Writing the baseband signal as the sum $I(t) + jQ(t)$ and letting E indicate the statistical expectation, Brody and Meindl [1974] have shown that the mean velocity estimate can be rewritten as

$$v_{\text{mean}} = \frac{k'\, E\left\{\frac{\partial}{\partial t}[I(t)]Q(t) - \frac{\partial}{\partial t}[Q(t)]I(t)\right\}}{E\left[I^2(t) + Q^2(t)\right]} \tag{12.29}$$

The estimate of this quantity requires estimation of the derivative of the in-phase portion $I(t)$ and quadrature portion $Q(t)$ of the signal. For an analog, continuous-time implementation, the bias and variance were evaluated by Brody and Meindl [1974]. The discrete case has been studied by Kristoffersen [1986]. The differentiation has been implemented in the discrete case as a finite difference or as a finite impulse response differentiation filter. The estimator is biased by noise, since the denominator represents power in the returned signal. Therefore, for nonzero noise power, the averaged noise power in the denominator will not be zero mean and will constitute a bias. The variance of the finite derivative estimator depends on the shape and bandwidth of the Doppler spectrum, as well as on the observation interval.

Wideband Estimation Techniques

It is desirable to transmit a short ultrasonic pulse in order to examine blood flow in small regions individually. For these short pulses, the narrowband approximation is not valid, and the estimation techniques used should track the motion of the red blood cells as they move to a new position over time. Estimation techniques that track the motion of the red blood cells are known as *wideband estimation techniques* and include cross-correlation techniques, the wideband maximum likelihood estimator and high time bandwidth estimation techniques. A thorough review of time-domain estimation techniques to estimate tissue motion is presented in Hein and O'Brien [1993].

Cross-Correlation Estimator. The use of time shift to estimate signal parameters has been studied extensively in radar. If the transmitted signal is known, a maximum likelihood (ML) solution for the estimation of delay has been discussed by Van Trees [1971] and others. If the signal shape is not known, the use of cross-correlation for delay estimation has been discussed by Helstrom [1968] and Knapp and Carter [1976]. If information regarding the statistics of the signal and noise are available, an MLE based on cross-correlation has been proposed by Knapp and Carter [1976] known as the *generalized correlation method for the estimation of time delay.*

Several researchers have applied cross-correlation analysis to medical ultrasound. Bonnefous and Pesque [1986], Embree and O'Brien [1986], Foster et al. [1990], and Trahey et al. [1987] have studied the estimation of mean velocity based on the change in delay due to target movement. This analysis has assumed the shape of the transmitted signal to be unknown, and a cross-correlation technique has been used to estimate the difference in delay between successive pulses. This differential delay has then been used to estimate target velocity, where the velocity estimate is now based on the change in delay of the signal over an axial window, by maximizing the cross-correlation of the returned signal over all possible target velocities. Cross-correlation processing is typically performed on the radiofrequency (RF) signal, and a typical cross-correlation block diagram is shown in Fig. 12.22. A high-pass filter is first applied to the signal from a fixed depth to remove the unwanted return from stationary tissue. One advantage of this strategy is that the variance is now inversely proportional to bandwidth of the transmitted signal rather than proportional.

Wideband Maximum Likelihood Estimator (WMLE). Wideband maximum likelihood estimation is a baseband strategy with performance properties that are similar to cross-correlation. The estimate of the velocity of the blood cells is jointly based on the shift in the signal envelope and the shift in the carrier frequency of the returned signal. This estimator can be derived using a model for the signal that is expected to be reflected from the moving blood medium after the signal passes through intervening tissue. The processing of the signal can be interpreted as a filter matched to the expected signal. A diagram of the processing required for the wideband maximum likelihood estimator is shown in Fig. 12.23 [Ferrara and Algazi, 1991]. Assume that P pulses were transmitted. Required processing involves the delay of the signal from the $(P - k)$th pulse by an amount equal to $2v/ckT$, which corresponds to the movement of the cells between pulses for a specific v, followed by multiplication by a frequency which corresponds to the expected Doppler shift frequency of the baseband returned signal. The result of this multiplication

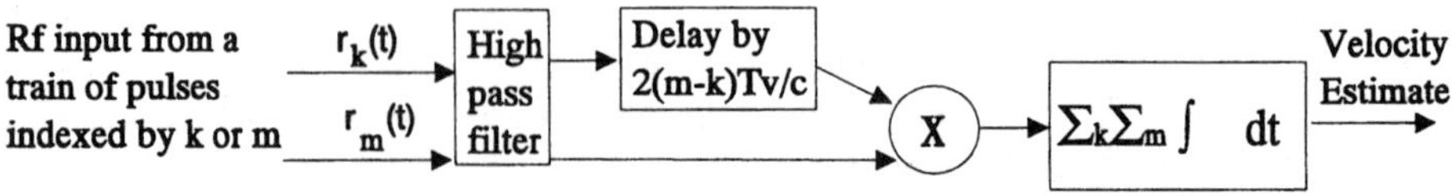

FIGURE 12.22 Block diagram of the system architecture required to estimate the velocity at each depth using a cross-correlation estimator.

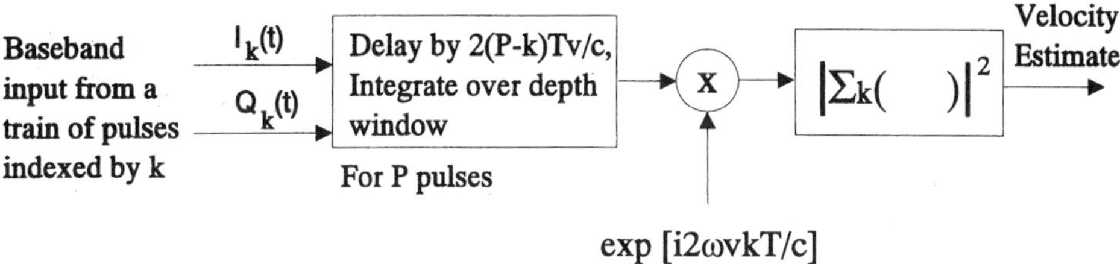

FIGURE 12.23 Block diagram of the system architecture required to estimate the velocity at each depth using the wideband MLE.

is summed for all pulses, and the maximum likelihood velocity is then the velocity which produces the largest output from this estimator structure.

Estimation Using High-Time-Bandwidth Signals. Several researchers have also investigated the use of long wideband signals including "chirp" modulated signals and pseduo-random noise for the estimation of blood velocity. These signals are transmitted continuously (or with a short "flyback" time). Since these signals require continual transmission, the instantaneous power level must be reduced in order to achieve safe average power levels.

Bertram [1979] concluded that transmission of a "chirp" appears to give inferior precision for range measurement and inferior resolution of closely spaced multiple targets than a conventional pulse-echo system applied to a similar transducer. Multiple targets confuse the analysis. Using a simple sawtooth waveform, it is not possible to differentiate a stationary target at one range from a moving target at a different range. This problem could possibly be overcome with increasing and decreasing frequency intervals. Axial resolution is independent of the modulation rate, dependent only on the spectral frequency range (which is limited).

The limitations of systems that have transmitted a long pulse of random noise and correlated the return with the transmitted signal include reverberations from outside the sample volume which degrade the signal-to-noise ratio (the federally required reduction in peak transmitted power also reduces SNR), limited signal bandwidth due to frequency-dependent attenuation in tissue, and the finite transducer bandwidth [Bendick and Newhouse, 1974; Cooper and McGillem, 1972].

New Directions

Areas of research interest, including estimation of the 3D velocity magnitude, volume flow estimation, the use of high-frequency catheter-based transducers, mapping blood flow within malignant tumors, a new display mode known as *color Doppler energy,* and the use of contrast agents, are summarized in this subsection.

Estimation of the 3D Velocity Magnitude and Beam Vessel Angle. Continued research designed to provide an estimate of the 3D magnitude of the flow velocity includes the use of crossed-beam Doppler systems [Overbeck et al., 1992; Wang and Yao, 1982] and tracking of speckle in two and three dimensions [Trahey et al., 1987]. Mapping of the velocity estimate in two and three dimensions, resulting in a 3D color flow map has been described by Carson et al. [1992], Picot et al. [1993], and Cosgrove et al. [1990].

Volume Flow Estimation. Along with the peak velocity, instantaneous velocity profile, and velocity indices, a parameter of clinical interest is the volume of flow through vessels as a function of time. Estimation strategies for the determination of the volume of flow through a vessel have been described by Embree and O'Brien [1990], Gill [1979], Hottinger and Meindl [1979], and Uematsu [1981].

Intravascular Ultrasound. It has been shown that intravascular ultrasonic imaging can provide information about the composition of healthy tissue and atheroma as well as anatomic data. A number of researchers have now shown that using frequencies of 30 MHz or above, individual layers and tissue types can be differentiated [de Kroon et al., 1991a, 1991b; Lockwood et al., 1991]. Although obvious changes in the vessel wall, such as dense fibrosis and calcification, have been identified with lower-frequency transducers, more subtle changes have been difficult to detect. Recent research has indicated that the character of plaque may be a more reliable predictor of subsequent cerebrovascular symptoms than the degree of vessel narrowing or the presence of ulceration [Merritt et al., 1992]. Therefore, the recognition of subtle differences in tissue type may be extremely valuable. One signal-processing challenge in imaging the vascular wall at frequencies of 30 MHz or above is the removal of the unwanted echo from red blood cells, which is a strong interfering signal at high frequencies.

Vascular Changes Associated with Tumors. Three-dimensional color flow mapping of the vascular structure is proposed to provide new information for the differentiation of benign and malignant masses. Judah Folkman and associates first recognized the importance of tumor vascularity in 1971 [Folkman et al., 1971]. They hypothesized that the increased cell population required for the growth of a malignant tumor must be preceded by the production of new vessels. Subsequent work has shown that the walls of these vessels are deficient in muscular elements, and this deficiency results in a low impedance to flow [Gammill et al., 1976]. This change can be detected by an increase in diastolic flow and a change in the resistive index.

More recently, Less et al. [1991] have shown that the vascular architecture of solid mammary tumors has several distinct differences from normal tissues, at least in the microvasculature. A type of network exists that exhibits fluctuations in both the diameter and length of the vessel with increasing branch order. Current color flow mapping systems with a center frequency of 5 MHz or above have been able to detect abnormal flow with varying degrees of clinical sensitivity from 40% to 82% [Balu-Maestro et al., 1991; Belcaro et al., 1988; Luska et al., 1992]. Researchers using traditional Doppler systems have also reported a range of clinical sensitivity, with a general reporting of high sensitivity but moderate to low specificity. Burns et al. [1982] studied the signal from benign and malignant masses with 10-MHz CW Doppler. They hypothesized, and confirmed through angiography, that the tumors under study were fed by multiple small arteries, with a mean flow velocity below 10 cm/s. Carson et al. [1992] compared 10-MHz CW Doppler to 5- and 7.5-MHz color flow mapping and concluded that while 3D reconstruction of the vasculature could provide significant additional information, color flow mapping systems must increase their ability to detect slow flow in small vessels in order to effectively map the vasculature.

Ultrasound Contrast Agents. The introduction of substances that enhance the ultrasonic echo signal from blood primarily through the production of microbubbles is of growing interest in ultrasonic flow measurement. The increased echo power may have a significant impact in contrast echocardiography, where acquisition of the signal from the coronary arteries has been difficult. In addition, such agents have been used to increase the backscattered signal from small vessels in masses that are suspected to be malignant. Contrast agents have been developed using sonicated albumen, saccharide microbubbles, and gelatin-encapsulated microbubbles.

Research to improve the sensitivity of flow measurement systems to low-velocity flow and small volumes of flow, with the goal of mapping the vasculature architecture, includes the use of ultrasonic contrast agents with conventional Doppler signal processing [Hartley et al., 1993], as well as the detection of the second harmonic of the transducer center frequency [Shrope and Newhouse, 1993].

Color Doppler Energy. During 1993, a new format for the presentation of the returned signal from the blood scattering medium was introduced and termed *color Doppler energy* (CDE) or *color power imaging* (CPI). In this format, the backscattered signal is filtered to remove the signal from stationary tissue, and the remaining energy in the backscattered signal is color encoded and displayed as an overlay on the gray-scale image. The advantage of this signal-processing technique is the sensitivity to very low flow velocities.

Defining Terms

Baseband signal: The received signal after the center frequency component (carrier frequency) has been removed by demodulation.

Carrier frequency: The center frequency in the spectrum of the transmitted signal.

Clutter: An unwanted fixed signal component generated by stationary targets typically outside the region of interest (such as vessel walls).

Complex envelope: A signal expressed by the product of the carrier, a high-frequency component, and other lower-frequency components that comprise the envelope. The envelope is usually expressed in complex form.

Maximum likelihood: A statistical estimation technique that maximizes the probability of the occurrence of an event to estimate a parameter. ML estimate is the minimum variance, unbiased estimate.

References

Ahn Y, Park S. 1991. Estimation of mean frequency and variance of ultrasonic Doppler signal by using second-order autoregressive model. IEEE Trans Ultrason Ferroelec Freq Cont 38(3):172.

Angelson B. 1980. Theoretical study of the scattering of ultrasound from blood. IEEE Trans Biomed Eng 27(2):61.

Atkinson P, Berry MV. 1974. Random noise in ultrasonic echoes diffracted by blood. J Phys A Math Nucl Gen 7(11):1293.

Balu-Maestro C, Bruneton JN, Giudicelli T, et al. 1991. Color Doppler in breast tumor pathology. J Radiol 72(11):579.

Barber W, Eberhard JW, Karr S. 1985. A new time domain technique for velocity measurements using Doppler ultrasound. IEEE Trans Biomed Eng 32(3):213.

Belcaro G, Laurora G, Ricci A, et al. 1988. Evaluation of flow in nodular tumors of the breast by Doppler and duplex scanning. Acta Chir Belg 88(5):323.

Bertram CD. 1979. Distance resolution with the FM-CW ultrasonic echo-ranging system. Ultrasound Med Biol (5):61.

Bonnefous O, Pesque P. 1986. Time domain formulation of pulse-Doppler ultrasound and blood velocity estimators by cross correlation. Ultrasonic Imaging 8:73.

Brody W, Meindl J. 1974. Theoretical analysis of the CW Doppler ultrasonic flowmeter. IEEE Trans Biomed Eng 21(3):183.

Burns PN, Halliwell M, Wells PNT, Webb AJ. 1982. Ultrasonic Doppler studies of the breast. Ultrasound Med Biol 8(2):127.

Carson PL, Adler DD, Fowlkes JB, et al. 1992. Enhanced color flow imaging of breast cancer vasculature: Continuous wave Doppler and three-dimensional display. J Ultrasound Med 11(8):77.

Cosgrove DO, Bamber JC, Davey JB, et al. 1990. Color Doppler signals from breast tumors: Work in progress. Radiology 176(1):175.

Curry GR, White DN. 1978. Color coded ultrasonic differential velocity arterial scanner. Ultrasound Med Biol 4:27.

de Kroon MGM, Slager CJ, Gussenhoven WJ, et al. 1991. Cyclic changes of blood echogenicity in high-frequency ultrasound. Ultrasound Med Biol 17(7):723.

de Kroon MGM, van der Wal LF, Gussenhoven WJ, et al. 1991. Backscatter directivity and integrated backscatter power of arterial tissue. Int J Cardiac Imaging 6:265.

Embree PM, O'Brien WD Jr. 1990. Volumetric blood flow via time-domain correlation: Experimental verification. IEEE Trans Ultrason Ferroelec Freq Cont 37(3):176.

Ferrara KW, Algazi VR. 1994a. A statistical analysis of the received signal from blood during laminar flow. IEEE Trans Ultrason Ferroelec Freq Cont 41(2):185.

Ferrara KW, Algazi VR. 1994b. A theoretical and experimental analysis of the received signal from disturbed blood flow. IEEE Trans Ultrason Ferroelec Freq Cont 41(2):172.

Ferrara KW, Algazi VR. 1991. A new wideband spread target maximum likelihood estimator for blood velocity estimation: I. Theory. IEEE Trans Ultrason Ferroelec Freq Cont 38(1):1.

Folkman J, Nerler E, Abernathy C, Williams G. 1971. Isolation of a tumor factor responsible for angiogenesis. J Exp Med 33:275.

Foster SG, Embree PM, O'Brien WD Jr. 1990. Flow velocity profile via time-domain correlation: Error analysis and computer simulation. IEEE Trans Ultrason Ferroelec Freq Cont 37(3):164.

Gammill SL, Stapkey KB, Himmellarb EH. 1976. Roenigenology—Pathology correlative study of neovascular ray. AJR 126:376.

Gill RW. 1979. Pulsed Doppler with B-mode imaging for quantitative blood flow measurement. Ultrasound Med Biol 5:223.

Hartley CJ, Cheirif J, Collier KR, Bravenec JS. 1993. Doppler quantification of echo-contrast injections in vivo. Ultrasound Med Biol 19(4):269.

Hatle L, Angelsen B. 1985. Doppler Ultrasound in Cardiology, 3d ed. Philadelphia, Lea & Febiger.

Hatsukami TS, Primozich J, Zierler RE, Strandness DE. 1992. Color Doppler characteristics in normal lower extremity arteries. Ultrasound Med Biol 18(2):167.

Hein I, O'Brien W. 1993. Current time domain methods for assessing tissue motion. IEEE Trans Ultrason Ferroelec Freq Cont 40(2):84.

Helstrom CW. 1968. Statistical Theory of Signal Detection. London, Pergamon Press.

Hinze JO. 1975. Turbulence. New York, McGraw-Hill.

Hottinger CF, Meindl JD. 1979. Blood flow measurement using the attenuation compensated volume flowmeter. Ultrasonic Imaging (1)1:1.

Kaluzinski K. 1989. Order selection in Doppler blood flow signal spectral analysis using autoregressive modelling. Med Biol Eng Com 27:89.

Kasai C, Namekawa K, Koyano A, Omoto R. 1985. Real-time two-dimensional blood flow imaging using an autocorrelation technique. IEEE Trans Sonics Ultrason 32(3).

Kay S, Marple SL. 1981. Spectrum analysis. A modern perspective. Proc IEEE 69(11):1380.

Kennedy RS. 1969. Fading Dispersive Channel Theory. New York, Wiley Interscience.

Knapp CH, Carter GC. 1976. The generalized correlation method for estimation of time delay. IEEE Trans Acoust Speech Signal Proc 24(4):320.

Kristoffersen K, Angelsen BJ. 1985. A comparison between mean frequency estimators for multigated Doppler systems with serial signal processing. IEEE Trans Biomed Eng 32(9):645.

Less JR, Skalak TC, Sevick EM, Jain RK. 1991. Microvascular architecture in a mammary carcinoma: Branching patterns and vessel dimensions. Cancer Res 51(1):265.

Lockwood GR, Ryan LK, Hunt JW, Foster FS. 1991. Measurement of the ultrasonic properties of vascular tissues and blood from 35–65 MHz. Ultrasound Med Biol 17(7):653.

Loupas T, McDicken WN. 1990. Low-order AR models for mean and maximum frequency estimation in the context of Doppler color flow mapping. IEEE Trans Ultrason Ferroelec Freq Cont 37(6):590.

Luska G, Lott D, Risch U, von Boetticher H. 1992. The findings of color Doppler sonography in breast tumors. Rofo Forts Gebiete Rontgens Neuen Bildg Verf 156(2):142.

Merritt C, Bluth E. 1992. The future of carotid sonography. AJR 158:37.

Mo L, Cobbold R. 1986. A stochastic model of the backscattered Doppler ultrasound from blood. IEEE Trans Biomed Eng 33(1):20.

Nerem RM. 1985. Fluid dynamic considerations in the application of ultrasound flowmetry. In SA Altobelli, WF Voyles, ER Greene (eds), Cardiovascular Ultrasonic Flowmetry. New York, Elsevier.

Nichols WW, O'Rourke MF. 1990. McDonald's Blood Flow in Arteries: Theoretic, Experimental and Clinical Principles. Philadelphia, Lea & Febiger.

Nowicki A, Reid JM. 1981. An infinite gate pulse Doppler. Ultrasound Med Biol 7:1.

Overbeck JR, Beach KW, Strandness DE Jr. 1992. Vector Doppler: Accurate measurement of blood velocity in two dimensions. Ultrasound Med Biol 18(1):19.

Picot PA, Rickey DW, Mitchell R, et al. 1993. Three dimensional color Doppler mapping. Ultrasound Med Biol 19(2):95.
Price R. 1968. Detectors for radar astronomy. In J Evans, T Hagfors (eds), Radar Astronomy. New York, McGraw-Hill.
Schrope BA, Newhouse VL. 1993. Second harmonic ultrasound blood perfusion measurement. Ultrasound Med Biol 19(7):567.
Shung KK, Sigelman RA, Reid JM. 1976. Scattering of ultrasound by blood. IEEE Trans Biomed Eng 23(6):460.
Shung KK, Cloutier G, Lim CC. 1992. The effects of hematocrit, shear rate, and turbulence on ultrasonic Doppler spectrum from blood. IEEE Trans Biomed Eng 39(5):462.
Trahey GE, Allison JW, Von Ramm OT. 1987. Angle independent ultrasonic detection of blood flow. IEEE Trans Biomed Eng 34(12):964.
Uematsu S. 1981. Determination of volume of arterial blood flow by an ultrasonic device. J Clin Ultrason 9:209.
Van Trees HL. 1971. Detection, Estimation and Modulation Theory, Part III. New York, Wiley.
Wang W, Yao L. 1982. A double beam Doppler ultrasound method for quantitative blood flow velocity measurement. Ultrasound Med Biol (8):421.
Wells PNT. 1977. Biomedical Ultrasonics. London, Academic Press.

Further Information

The bimonthly journal *IEEE Transactions on Ultrasonics Ferroelectrics and Frequency Control* reports engineering advances in the area of ultrasonic flow measurement. For subscription information, contact IEEE Service Center, 445 Hoes Lane, P.O. Box 1331, Piscataway, NJ 08855-1331. Phone (800) 678-IEEE. The journal and the yearly conference proceedings of the IEEE Ultrasonic Symposium are published by the IEEE Ultrasonic Ferroelectrics and Frequency Control Society. Membership information can be obtained from the IEEE address above or from K. Ferrara, Riverside Research Institute, 330 West 42nd Street, New York, NY 10036.

The journal *Ultrasound in Medicine and Biology,* published 10 times per year, includes new developments in ultrasound signal processing and the clinical application of these developments. For subscription information, contact Pergamon Press, Inc., 660 White Plains Road, Tarrytown, NY 10591-5153. The American Institute of Ultrasound Medicine sponsors a yearly meeting which reviews new developments in ultrasound instrumentation and the clinical applications. For information, contact American Institute of Ultrasound in Medicine, 11200 Rockville Pike, Suite 205, Rockville, MD 20852-3139; phone: (800) 638-5352.

13

Magnetic Resonance Microscopy

Xiaohong Zhou
Duke University Medical Center

G. Allan Johnson
Duke University Medical Center

Visualization of internal structures of opaque biologic objects is essential in many biomedical studies. Limited by the penetration depth of the probing sources (photons and electrons) and the lack of endogenous contrast, conventional forms of microscopy such as optical microscopy and electron microscopy require tissues to be sectioned into thin slices and stained with organic chemicals or heavy-metal compounds prior to examination. These invasive and destructive procedures, as well as the harmful radiation in the case of electron microscopy, make it difficult to obtain three-dimensional information and virtually impossible to study biologic tissues *in vivo*.

Magnetic resonance (MR) microscopy is a new form of microscopy that overcomes the aforementioned limitations. Operating in the radiofrequency (RF) range, MR microscopy allows biologic samples to be examined in the living state without bleaching or damage by ionizing radiation and in fresh and fixed specimens after minimal preparation. It also can use a number of endogenous contrast mechanisms that are directly related to tissue biochemistry, physiology, and pathology. Additionally, MR microscopy is digital and three dimensional; internal structures of opaque tissues can be quantitatively mapped out in three dimensions to accurately reveal their histopathologic status. These unique properties provide new opportunities for biomedical scientists to attack problems that have been difficult to investigate using conventional techniques.

Conceptually, MR microscopy is an extension of magnetic resonance imaging (MRI) to the microscopic domain, generating images with spatial resolution better than 100 μm [Lauterbur, 1984]. As such, MR microscopy is challenged by a new set of theoretical and technical problems [Johnson et al., 1992]. For example, to improve isotropic resolution from 1 mm to 10 μm, signal-to-noise ratio (SNR) per voxel must be increased by a million times to maintain the same image quality. In order to do so, almost every component of hardware must be optimized to the fullest extent, pulse sequences have to be carefully designed to minimize any potential signal loss, and special software and dedicated computation facilities must be involved to handle large image arrays (e.g., 256^3). Over the past decade, development of MR microscopy has focused mainly on these issues. Persistent efforts by many researchers have recently led to images with isotropic resolution of the order of ~10 μm [Cho et al., 1992; Jacobs and Fraser, 1994; Johnson et al., 1992; Zhou and Lauterbur, 1992]. The significant resolution improvement opens up a

0-8493-1810-6/03/$0.00+$1.50

broad range of applications, from histology to cancer biology and from toxicology to plant biology [Johnson et al., 1992]. In this chapter we will first discuss the basic principles of MR microscopy, with special attention to such issues as resolution limits and sensitivity improvements. Then we will give an overview of the instrumentation. Finally, we will provide some examples to demonstrate the applications.

13.1 Basic Principles

Spatial Encoding and Decoding

Any digital imaging system involves two processes. First, spatially resolved information must be encoded into a measurable signal, and second, the spatially encoded signal must be decoded to produce an image. In MR microscopy, the spatial encoding process is accomplished by acquiring nuclear magnetic resonance (NMR) signals under the influence of three orthogonal magnetic field gradients. There are many ways that a gradient can interact with a spin system. If the gradient is applied during a frequency-selective RF pulse, then the NMR signal arises only from a thin slab along the gradient direction. Thus a slice is selected from a three-dimensional (3D) object. If the gradient is applied during the acquisition of an NMR signal, the signal will consist of a range of spatially dependent frequencies given by

$$\omega(\vec{r}) = \gamma B_0 + \gamma \vec{G} \cdot \vec{r} \tag{13.1}$$

where γ is gyromagnetic ratio, B_0 is the static magnetic field, $\vec{G}$ is the magnetic field gradient, and $\vec{r}$ is the spatial variable. In this way, the spatial information along $\vec{G}$ direction is encoded into the signal as frequency variations. This method of encoding is called *frequency encoding,* and the gradient is referred to as a *frequency-encoding gradient* (or *read-out gradient*). If the gradient is applied for a fixed amount of time t_{pe} before the signal acquisition, then the phase of the signal, instead of the frequency, becomes spatially dependent, as given by

$$\phi(\vec{r}) = \int_0^{t_{pe}} \omega(\vec{r})\,dt = \phi_0 + \int_0^{t_{pe}} \gamma \vec{G} \cdot \vec{r}\,dt \tag{13.2}$$

where ϕ_0 is the phase originated from the static magnetic field. This encoding method is known as *phase encoding,* and the gradient is called a *phase-encoding gradient.*

Based on the three basic spatial encoding approaches, many imaging schemes can be synthesized. For two-dimensional (2D) imaging, a slice-selection gradient is first applied to confine the NMR signal in a slice. Spatial encoding within the slice is then accomplished by frequency encoding and/or by phase encoding. For 3D imaging, the slice-selection gradient is replaced by either a frequency-encoding or a phase-encoding gradient. If all spatial directions are frequency-encoded, the encoding scheme is called *projection acquisition,* and the corresponding decoding method is called *projection reconstruction* [Lai and Lauterbur, 1981; Lauterbur, 1973]. If one of the spatial dimensions is frequency encoded while the rest are phase encoded, the method is known as *Fourier imaging,* and the image can be reconstructed simply by a multidimensional Fourier transform [Edelstein et al., 1980; Kumar et al., 1975]. Although other methods do exist, projection reconstruction and Fourier imaging are the two most popular in MR microscopy.

Projection reconstruction is particularly useful for spin systems with short apparent T_2 values, such as protons in lung and liver. Since the T_2 of most tissues decreases as static magnetic field increases, the advantage of projection reconstruction is more obvious at high magnetic fields. Another advantage of projection reconstruction is its superior SNR to Fourier imaging. This advantage has been theoretically analyzed and experimentally demonstrated in a number of independent studies [Callaghan and Eccles, 1987; Gewalt et al., 1993; Zhou and Lauterbur, 1992]. Recently, it also has been shown that projection reconstruction is less sensitive to motion and motion artifacts can be effectively reduced using sinograms [Glover and Noll, 1993; Glover and Pauly, 1992; Gmitro and Alexander, 1993]. Unlike projection reconstruction, data acquisition in

TABLE 13.1 Choice of Acquisition Parameters for Different Image Contrasts

Contrast	TR#	TE#	Pulse Sequences§
ρ	3–5 $T_{1,max}$	<< $T_{2,min}$	SE, GE
T_1	–$T_{1,avg}$	<< $T_{2,min}$	SE, GE
T_2	3–5 $T_{1,max}$	~$T_{2,avg}$	SE, FSE
T_2^*	3–5 $T_{1,max}$	~$T_{s,avg}^*$	GE
D†	3–5 $T_{1,max}$	<< $T_{2,min}$	Diffusion-weighted SE, GE, or FSE

#Subscripts *min*, *max*, and *avg* stand for minimum, maximum, and average values, respectively.

§SE: spin-echo; GE: gradient echo; FSE: fast spin echo.

†A pair of diffusion weighting gradients must be used.

Fourier imaging generates Fourier coefficients of the image in a Cartesian coordinate. Since multidimensional fast Fourier transform algorithms can be applied directly to the raw data, Fourier imaging is computationally more efficient than projection reconstruction. This advantage is most evident when reconstructing 3D images with large arrays (e.g., 256^3). In addition, Fourier transform imaging is less prone to image artifacts arising from various off-resonance effects and is more robust in applications such as chemical shift imaging [Brown et al., 1982] and flow imaging [Moran, 1982].

Image Contrast

A variety of contrast mechanisms can be exploited in MR microscopy, including spin density (ρ), spin-spin relaxation time (T_1), spin-lattice relaxation time (T_2), apparent T_2 relaxation time (T_2^*), diffusion coefficient (D), flow and chemical shift (δ). One of the contrasts can be highlighted by varying data-acquisition parameters or by choosing different pulse sequences. Table 13.1 summarizes the pulse sequences and data-acquisition parameters to obtain each of the preceding contrasts.

In high-field MR microscopy (>1.5 T), T_2 and diffusion contrast are strongly coupled together. An increasing number of evidences indicate that the apparent T_2 contrast observed in high-field MR microscopy is largely due to microscopic magnetic susceptibility variations [Majumdar and Gore, 1988; Zhong and Gore, 1991]. The magnetic susceptibility difference produces strong local magnetic field gradients. Molecular diffusion through the induced gradients causes significant signal loss. In addition, the large external magnetic field gradients required for spatial encoding further increase the diffusion-induced signal loss. Since the signal loss has similar dependence on echo time (TE) to T_2-related loss, the diffusion contrast mechanism is involved in virtually all T_2-weighted images. This unique contrast mechanism provides a direct means to probe the microscopic tissue heterogeneities and forms the basis for many histopathologic studies [Benveniste et al., 1992; Zhou et al., 1994].

Chemical shift is another unique contrast mechanism. Changes in chemical shift can directly reveal tissue metabolic and histopathologic stages. This mechanism exists in many spin systems such as ^1H, ^{31}P, and ^{13}C. Recently, Lean et al. [1993] showed that based on proton chemical shifts, MR microscopy can detect tissue pathologic changes with superior sensitivity to optical microscopy in a number of tumor models. A major limitation for chemical-shift MR microscopy is the rather poor spatial resolution, since most spin species other than water protons are of considerably low concentration and/or sensitivity. In addition, the long data-acquisition time required to resolve both spatial and spectral information also appears as an obstacle.

13.2 Resolution Limits

Intrinsic Resolution Limit

Intrinsic resolution is defined as the width of the point-spread function originated from physics laws. In MR microscopy, the intrinsic resolution arises from two sources: natural linewidth broadening and diffusion [Callaghan and Eccles, 1988; Cho et al., 1988; House, 1984].

In most conventional pulse sequences, natural linewidth broadening affects the resolution limit only in the frequency-encoding direction. In some special cases, such as fast spin echo [Hennig et al., 1986] and echo planar imaging [Mansfield and Maudsley, 1977], natural linewidth broadening also imposes resolution limits in the phase-encoding direction [Zhou et al., 1993]. The natural linewidth resolution limit, defined by

$$\Delta r_{\text{n.l.w.}} = \frac{2}{\gamma G T_2} \tag{13.3}$$

is determined by the T_2 relaxation time and can be improved using a stronger gradient G. To obtain 1-μm resolution from a specimen with T_2 = 50 ms, the gradient should be at least 14.9 G/cm. This gradient requirement is well within the range of most MR microscopes.

Molecular diffusion affects the spatial resolution in a number of ways. The bounded diffusion is responsible for many interesting phenomena known as *edge enhancements* [Callaghan et al., 1993; Hills et al., 1990; Hyslop and Lauterbur, 1991; Putz et al., 1991]. They are observable only at the microscopic resolution and are potentially useful to detect microscopic boundaries. The unbounded diffusion, on the other hand, causes signal attenuation, line broadening, and phase misregistration. All these effects originate from an incoherent and irreversible phase-dispersion. The root-mean-square value of the phase dispersion is

$$\sigma = \gamma \left\{ 2D \int_0^t \left[\int_{t'}^t G(t'')\,dt'' \right]^2 dt' \right\}^{1/2} \tag{13.4}$$

where t' and t are pulse-sequence-dependent time variables defined by Ahn and Cho [1989]. Because of the phase uncertainty, an intrinsic resolution limit along the phase encoding direction arises:

$$\Delta r_{pe} = \frac{\sigma}{\gamma \int_0^t G_{pe}(t')\,dt'} \tag{13.5}$$

For a rectangularly shaped phase-encoding gradient, the preceding equation can be reduced to a very simple form:

$$\Delta r_{pe} = \sqrt{\frac{2}{3} D t_{pe}} \tag{13.6}$$

This simple result indicates that the diffusion resolution limit in the phase-encoded direction is determined only by the phase-encoding time t_{pe} (D is a constant for a chosen sample). This is so because the phase uncertainty is introduced only during the phase-encoding period. Once the spins are phase encoded, they always carry the same spatial information no matter where they diffuse to. In the frequency-encoding direction, diffusion imposes resolution limits by broadening the point-spread function. Unlike natural linewidth broadening, broadening caused by diffusion is pulse sequence dependent. For the simplest pulse sequence, a 3D projection acquisition using free induction decays, the full width at half maximum [Callaghan and Eccles, 1988; McFarland, 1992; Zhou, 1992] is

$$\Delta r_{fr} = 8 \left[\frac{D (\ln 2)^2}{3 \gamma G_{fr}} \right]^{1/3} \tag{13.7}$$

Compared with the case of the natural linewidth broadening (Eq. 13.3), the resolution limit caused by diffusion varies slowly with the frequency-encoding gradient G_{fr}. Therefore, to improve resolution by the same factor, a much larger gradient is required. With the currently achievable gradient strength, the diffusion resolution limit is estimated to be 5 to 10 μm.

Digital Resolution Limit

When the requirements imposed by intrinsic resolution limits are satisfied, image resolution is largely determined by the voxel size, provided that SNR is sufficient and the amplitude of physiologic motion is limited to a voxel. The voxel size, also known as *digital resolution*, can be calculated from the following equations:

Frequency-encoding direction:
$$\Delta x \equiv \frac{L_x}{N_x} = \frac{\Delta v}{2\pi\gamma G_x N_x} \tag{13.8}$$

Phase-encoding direction:
$$\Delta y \equiv \frac{L_y}{N_y} = \frac{\Delta\phi}{\gamma G_y t_{pe}} \tag{13.9}$$

where L is the field of view, N is the number of data points or the linear matrix size, G is the gradient strength, Δv is the receiver bandwidth, $\Delta\phi$ is the phase range of the phase-encoding data (e.g., if the data cover a phase range from $-\pi$ to $+\pi$, then $\Delta\phi = 2\pi$), and the subscripts x and y represent frequency- and phase-encoding directions, respectively. To obtain a high digital resolution, L should be kept minimal, while N maximal. In practice, the minimal field of view and the maximal data points are constrained by other experimental parameters. In the frequency-encoding direction, decreasing field of view results in an increase in gradient amplitude at a constant receiver bandwidth or a decrease in the bandwidth for a constant gradient (Eq. 13.8). Since the receiver bandwidth must be large enough to keep the acquisition of NMR signals within a certain time window, the largest available gradient strength thus imposes the digital resolution limit. In the phase-encoding direction, $\Delta\phi$ is fixed at 2π in most experiments, and the maximum t_{pe} value is refrained by the echo time. Thus digital resolution is also determined by the maximum available gradient, as indicated by Eq. (13.9). It has been estimated that in order to achieve 1-μm resolution with a phase-encoding time of 4 ms, the required gradient strength is as high as 587 G/cm. This gradient requirement is beyond the range of current MR microscopes. Fortunately, the requirement is fully relaxed in projection acquisition where no phase encoding is involved.

Practical Resolution Limit

The intrinsic resolution limits predict that MR microscopy can theoretically reach the micron regime. To realize the resolution, one must overcome several technical obstacles. These obstacles, or practical resolution limits, include insufficient SNR, long data-acquisition times, and physiologic motion. At the current stage of development, these practical limitations are considerably more important than other resolution limits discussed earlier and actually determine the true image resolution.

SNR is of paramount importance in MR microscopy. As resolution improves, the total number of spins per voxel decreases drastically, resulting in a cubic decrease in signal intensity. When the voxel signal intensity becomes comparable with noise level, structures become unresolvable even if the digital resolution and intrinsic resolution are adequate.

SNR in a voxel depends on many factors. The relationship between SNR and common experimental variables is given by

$$\text{SNR} \propto \frac{B_1 B_0^2 \sqrt{n}}{\sqrt{4kT\Delta v\left(R_{\text{coil}} + R_{\text{sample}}\right)}} \tag{13.10}$$

where B_1 is the RF magnetic field, B_0 is the static magnetic field, n is the number of average, T is the temperature, Δv is the bandwidth, k is the Boltzmann constant, and R_{coil} and R_{sample} are the coil and sample resistance, respectively. When small RF coils are used, R_{sample} is negligible. Since R_{coil} is proportional to $\sqrt{B_0}$ due to skin effects, the overall SNR increases as $B_0^{7/4}$. This result strongly suggests that MR microscopy be performed at high magnetic field. Another way to improve SNR is to increase the B_1 field. This is accomplished by reducing the size of RF coils [McFarland and Mortara, 1992; Peck et al., 1990; Schoeniger et al., 1991; Zhou and Lauterbur, 1992]. Although increasing B_0 and B_1 is the most common approach to attacking the SNR problem, other methods such as signal averaging, pulse-sequence optimization, and post data processing are also useful in MR microscopy. For example, diffusion-induced signal loss can be effectively minimized using diffusion-reduced-gradient (DRG) echo pulse sequences [Cho et al., 1992]. Various forms of projection acquisition techniques [Gewalt et al., 1993; Hedges, 1984; McFarland and Mortara, 1992; Zhou and Lauterbur, 1992], as well as new k-space sampling schemes [Zhou et al., 1993], also have proved useful in SNR improvements. Recently, Black et al. used high-temperature superconducting materials for coil fabrication to simultaneously reduce coil resistance R_{coil} and coil temperature T [Black et al., 1993]. This novel approach can provide up to 70-fold SNR increase, equivalent to the SNR gain by increasing the magnetic field strength 11 times.

Long data-acquisition time is another practical limitation. Large image arrays, long repetition times (TR), and signal averaging all contribute to the overall acquisition time. For instance, a T_2-weighted image with a 256^3 image array requires a total acquisition time of more than 18 h (assuming $TR = 500$ ms and $n = 2$). Such a long acquisition time is unacceptable for most applications. To reduce the acquisition time while still maintaining the desired contrast, fast-imaging pulse sequences such as echo-planar imaging (EPI) [Mansfield and Maudsley, 1977], driven equilibrium Fourier transform (DEFT) [Maki et al., 1988], fast low angle shot (FLASH) [Haase et al., 1986], gradient refocused acquisition at steady state (GRASS) [Karis et al., 1987], and rapid acquisition with relaxation enhancement (RARE) [Hennig et al., 1986] have been developed and applied to MR microscopy. The RARE pulse sequence, or fast spin-echo (FSE) [Mulkern et al., 1990], is particularly useful in high-field MR microscopy because of its insensitivity to magnetic susceptibility effects as well as the reduced diffusion loss [Zhou et al., 1993]. Using fast spin-echo techniques, a 256^3 image has been acquired in less than 2 h [Zhou et al., 1993].

For *in vivo* studies, the true image resolution is also limited by physiologic motion [Hedges, 1984; Wood and Henkelman, 1985]. Techniques to minimize the motion effects have been largely focused on pulse sequences and post data processing algorithms, including navigator echoes [Ehman and Felmlee, 1989], motion compensation using even echo or moment nulling gradients, projection acquisition [Glover and Noll, 1993], and various kinds of ghost-image decomposition techniques [Xiang and Henkelman, 1991]. It should be noted, however, that by refining animal handling techniques and using synchronized data acquisition, physiologic motion effects can be effectively avoided and very high quality images can be obtained [Hedlund et al., 1986; Johnson et al., 1992].

13.3 Instrumentation

An MR microscope consists of a high-field magnet (>1.5 T), a set of gradient coils, an RF coil (or RF coils), and the associated RF systems, gradient power supplies, and computers. Among these components, RF coils and gradient coils are often customized for specific applications in order to achieve optimal performance. Some general guidelines to design customized RF coils and gradient coils are presented below.

Radiofrequency Coils

Many types of RF coils can be used in MR microscopy (Fig. 13.1). The choice of a particular coil configuration is determined by specific task and specimen size. If possible, the smallest coil size should always be chosen in order to obtain the highest SNR. For *ex vivo* studies of tissue specimens, solenoid coils are a common choice because of their superior B_1 field homogeneity, high sensitivity, as well as

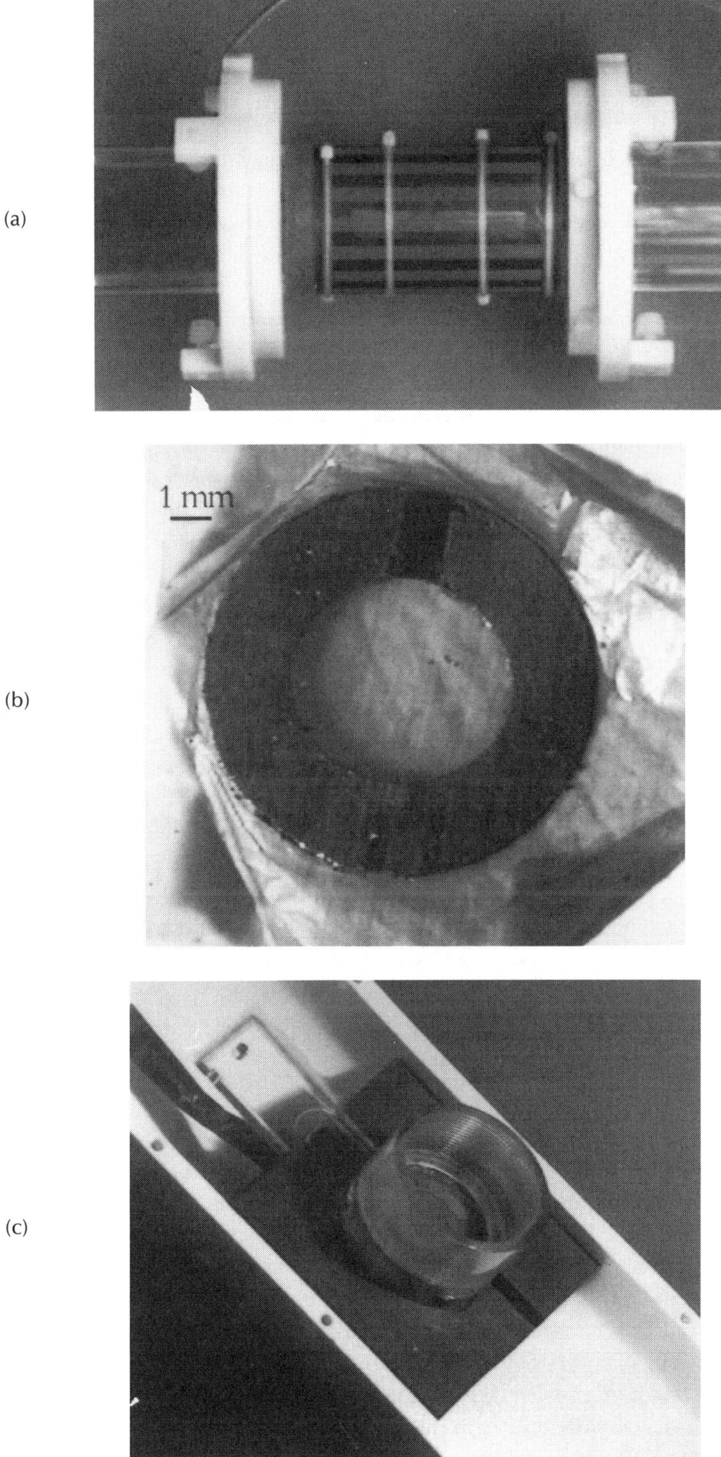

FIGURE 13.1 A range of radiofrequency coils are used in MR microscopy. (a) A quadrature birdcage coil scaled to the appropriate diameter for rats (6 cm) is used for whole-body imaging. (b) Resonant coils have been constructed on microwave substrate that can be surgically implanted to provide both localization and improved SNR. (c) MR microscopy of specimens is accomplished with a modified Helmholz coil providing good filling factors, high *B* homogeneity, and ease of access.

simplicity in fabrication. Using a 2.9-mm solenoid coil (5 turn), Zhou and Lauterbur [1992] have achieved the highest ever reported spatial resolution at 6.4 μm^3. Solenoid coil configurations are also used by others to obtain images with similar resolution (~10 μm) [Cho et al., 1988; Hedges, 1984; McFarland and Mortara, 1992; Schoeniger et al., 1991]. Recently, several researchers began to develop microscopic solenoid coils with a size of a few hundred microns [McFarland and Mortara, 1992; Peck et al., 1990]. Fabrication of these microcoils often requires special techniques, such as light lithography and electron-beam lithography.

The direction of the B_1 field generated by a solenoid coil prevents the coil from being coaxially placed in the magnet. Thus accessing and positioning samples are difficult. To solve this problem, Banson et al. [1992] devised a unique Helmholtz coil that consists of two separate loops. Each loop is made from a microwave laminate with a dielectric material sandwiched between two copper foils. By making use of the distributed capacitance, the coil can be tuned to a desired frequency. Since the two loops of the coil are mechanically separated, samples can be easily slid into the gap between the loops without any obstruction. Under certain circumstances, the Helmholtz coil can outperform an optimally designed solenoid coil with similar dimensions.

For *in vivo* studies, although volume coils such as solenoid coils and birdcage coils can be employed, most high-resolution experiments are carried out using local RF coils, including surface coils [Banson et al., 1992; Rudin, 1987] and implanted coils [Farmer et al., 1989; Hollett et al., 1987; Zhou et al., 1994]. Surface coils can effectively reduce coil size and simultaneously limit the field of view to a small region of interest. They can be easily adaptable to the shape of samples and provide high sensitivity in the surface region. The problem of inhomogeneous B_1 fields can be minimized using composite pulses [Hetherington et al., 1986] or adiabatic pulses [Ugurbil et al., 1987]. To obtain high-resolution images from regions distant from the surface, surgically implantable coils become the method of choice. These coils not only give better SNR than optimized surface coils [Zhou et al., 1992] but also provide accurate and consistent localization. The latter advantage is particularly useful for time-course studies on dynamic processes such as the development of pathology and monitoring the effects of therapeutic drugs.

The recent advent of high-temperature superconducting (HTS) RF coils has brought new excitement to MR microscopy [Black et al., 1993]. The substantial improvement, as discussed earlier, makes signal averaging unnecessary. Using these coils, the total imaging time will be solely determined by the efficiency to traverse the *k*-space. Although much research is yet to be done in this new area, combination of the HTS coils with fast-imaging algorithms will most likely provide a unique way to fully realize the potential of MR microscopy and eventually bring the technique into routine use.

Magnetic Field Gradient Coils

As discussed previously, high spatial resolution requires magnetic field gradients. The gradient strength increases proportional to the coil current and inversely proportional to the coil size. Since increasing current generates many undesirable effects (overheating, mechanical vibrations, eddy current, etc.), strong magnetic field gradient is almost exclusively achieved by reducing the coil diameter.

Design of magnetic field gradient coils for MR microscopy is a classic problem. Based on Maxwell equations, ideal surface current density can be calculated for a chosen geometry of the conducting surface. Two conducting surfaces are mostly used: a cylindrical surface parallel to the axis of the magnet and a cylindrical surface perpendicular to the axis. The ideal surface current density distributions for these two geometries are illustrated in Fig. 13.2 [Suits and Wilken, 1989]. After the ideal surface current density distribution is obtained, design of gradient coils is reduced to a problem of using discrete conductors with a finite length to approximate the continuous current distribution function. The error in the approximation determines the gradient linearity. Recent advancements in computer-based fabrication and etching techniques have made it feasible to produce complicated current density distributions. Using these techniques, nonlinear terms up to the 11th order can be eliminated over a predefined cylindrical volume.

Another issue in gradient coil design involves minimizing the gradient rise time so that fast-imaging techniques can be implemented successfully and short echo times can be achieved to minimize signal

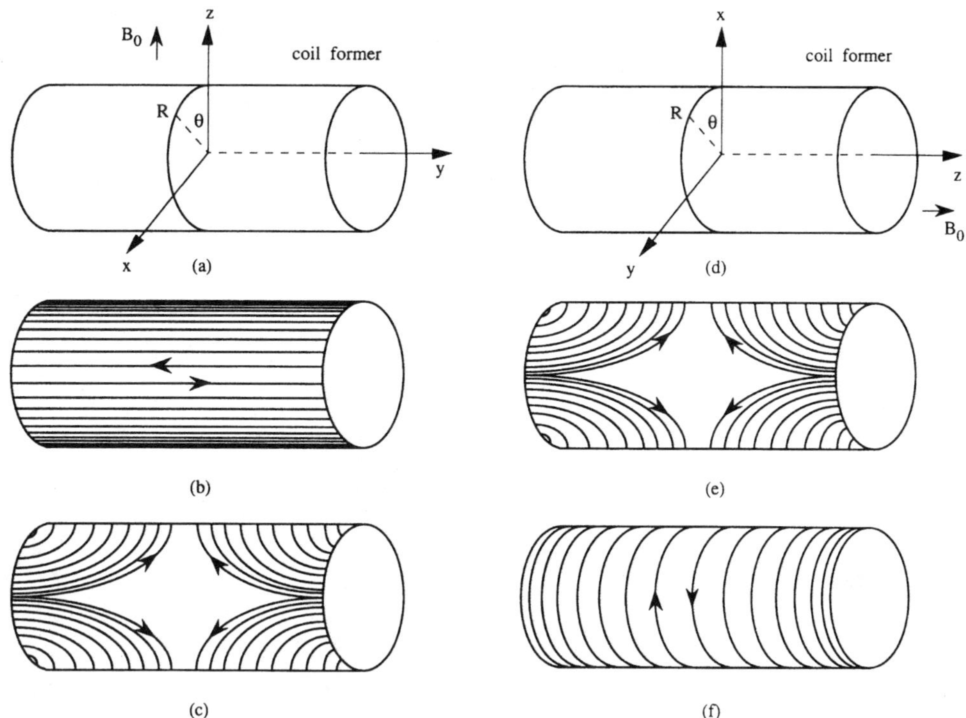

FIGURE 13.2 (*Left*) Ideal surface current distributions to generate linear magnetic field gradients when the gradient coil former is parallel to the magnet bore: (b) for x gradient and (c) for z gradient. The analytical expressions for the current density distribution functions are $J_x = KG_x[R \cos \theta(\sin \theta i - \cos \theta j) - z \sin \theta k]$ and $J_z = KG_z Z[\sin \theta i - \cos \theta j]$. The y gradient can be obtained by rotating J_x 90°. (*Right*) Ideal surface current distributions to generate linear magnetic field gradients when the gradient coil former is perpendicular to the magnet bore: (e for x gradient and (f) for y gradient. The analytical expressions for the current density distribution functions are: $J_x = KG_x R(\sin 2\theta j)$ and $J_y = KG_y(-R \cos^2 \theta i + y \sin j + 0.5R \sin 2\theta k)$. The z gradient can be obtained by rotating J_x 45°. (The graphs are adapted based on Suits and Wilken [1989]).

loss for short T_2 specimens. The gradient rise time relies on three factors: the inductance over resistance ratio of the gradient coil, the time constant of the feedback circuit of the gradient power supply, and the decay rate of eddy current triggered by gradient switching. The time constant attributed to inductive resistance (L/R) is relatively short (<100 μs) for most microscopy gradient coils, and the inductive resistance from the power supply can be easily adjusted to match the time constant of the coil. However, considering the high magnetic field gradient strength used in MR microscopy, eddy currents can be a serious problem. This problem is even worse when the gradient coils are closely placed in a narrow magnet bore. To minimize the eddy currents, modern design of gradient coils uses an extra set of coils so that the eddy currents can be actively canceled [Mansfield and Chapman, 1986]. Under close to optimal conditions, a rise time of <150 μs can be achieved with a maximum gradient of 82 G/cm in a set of 8-cm coils [Johnson et al., 1992].

Although the majority of microscopic MR images are obtained using cylindrical gradient coils, surface gradient coils have been used recently in several studies [Cho et al., 1992]. Similar to surface RF coils, surface gradient coils can be easily adapted to the shape of samples and are capable of producing strong magnetic field gradient in limited areas. The surface gradient coils also provide more free space in the magnet, allowing easy access to samples. A major problem with surface gradient coils is the gradient nonlinearity. But when the region of interest is small, high-quality images can still be obtained with negligible distortions.

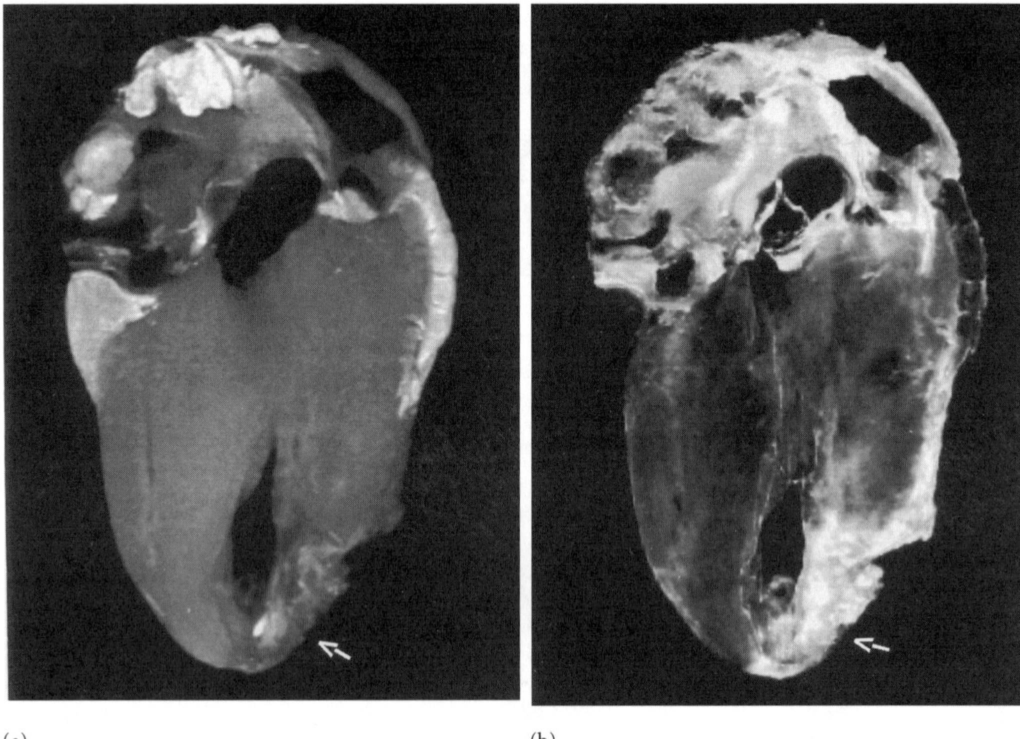

(a) (b)

FIGURE 13.3 Selected sections of 3D isotropic images of a sheep heart with experimentally induced infarct show the utility of MRM in pathology studies. A 3D FSE sequence has been designed to allow rapid acquisition of either (a) T_1-weighted or (b) T_2-weighted images giving two separate "stains" for the pathology. Arrows indicate areas of necrosis.

13.4 Applications

MR microscopy has a broad range of applications. We include here several examples. Figure 13.3 illustrates an application of MR microscopy in *ex vivo* histology. In this study, a fixed sheep heart with experimentally induced infarct is imaged at 2 T using 3D fast-spin-echo techniques with T_1 (Fig. 13.3a) and T_2 (Fig. 13.3b) contrasts. The infarct region is clearly detected in both images. The region of infarct can be segmented from the rest of the tissue and its volume can be accurately measured. Since the image is three dimensional, the tissue pathology can be examined in any arbitrary orientation. The nondestructive nature of MR microscopy also allows the same specimen to be restudied using other techniques as well as using other contrast mechanisms of MR microscopy. Obtaining this dimension of information from conventional histologic studies would be virtually impossible.

The *in vivo* capability of MR microscopy for toxicologic studies is illustrated in Fig. 13.4. In this study [Farmer et al., 1989], the effect of mercuric chloride in rat kidney is monitored in a single animal. Therefore, development of tissue pathology over a time period is directly observed without the unnecessary interference arising from interanimal variabilities. Since the kidney was the only region of interest in this study, a surgically implanted coil was chosen to optimize SNR and to obtain consistent localization. Figure 13.4 shows four images obtained from the same animal at different time points to show the progression and regression of the $HgCl_2$-induced renal pathology. Tissue damage is first observed 24 h after the animal was treated by the chemical, as evident by the blurring between the cortex and the outer medulla. The degree of damage is greater in the image obtained at 48 h. Finally, at 360 h, the blurred boundary between the two tissue regions completely disappeared, indicating full recovery of the organ.

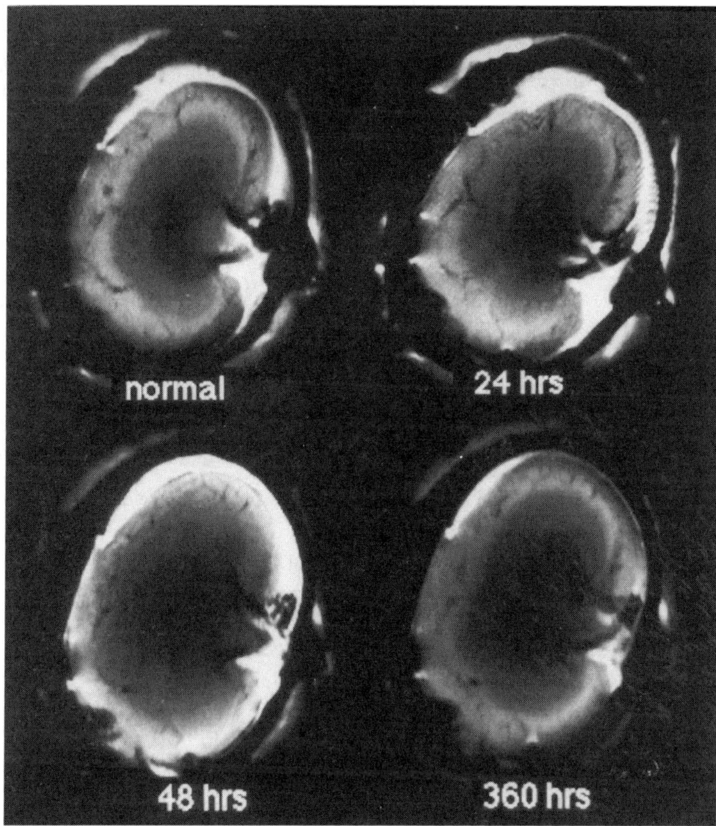

FIGURE 13.4 Implanted RF coils allow *in vivo* studies of deep structures with much higher spatial resolution by limiting the field of view during excitation and by increasing the SNR over volume coils. An added benefit is the ability to accurately localize the same region during a time course study. Shown here is the same region of a kidney at four different time points following exposure to mercuric chloride. Note the description of boundaries between the several zones of the kidney in the early part of the study followed by regeneration of the boundaries upon repair.

The capability to monitor tissue pathologic changes *in vivo*, as illustrated in this example, bodes well for a broad range of applications in pharmacology, toxicology, and pathology.

Development biology is another area where MR microscopy has found an increasing number of applications, Jacobs and Fraser [1994] used MR microscopy to follow cell movements and lineages in developing frog embryos. In their study, 3D images of the developing embryo were obtained on a time scale faster than the cell division time and analyzed forward and backward in time to reconstruct full cell divisions and cell movements. By labeling a 16-cell embryo with an exogenous contrast agent (Gd-DTPA), they successfully followed the progression from early cleavage and blastula stage through gastrulation, neurulation, and finally to tail bud stage. More important, they found that external ectodermal and internal mesodermal tissues extend at different rates during amphibian gastrulation and neurulation. This and many other key events in vertebrate embryogenesis would be very difficult to observe with optical microscopy. Another example in developmental biology is given in Fig. 13.5. Using 3D high-field (9.4-T) MR microscopy with large image arrays (256^3), Smith et al. [1993] studied the early development of the circulatory system of mouse embryos. With the aid of a T_1 contrast agent made from bovine serum albumin and Gd-DTPA, vasculature such as ventricles, atria, aorta, cardinal sinuses, basilar arteries, and thoracic arteries are clearly identified in mouse embryos at between 9.5 and 12.5 days of gestation. The ability to study embryonic development in a noninvasive fashion provided great opportunities to explore many problems in transgenic studies, gene targeting, and *in situ* hybridization.

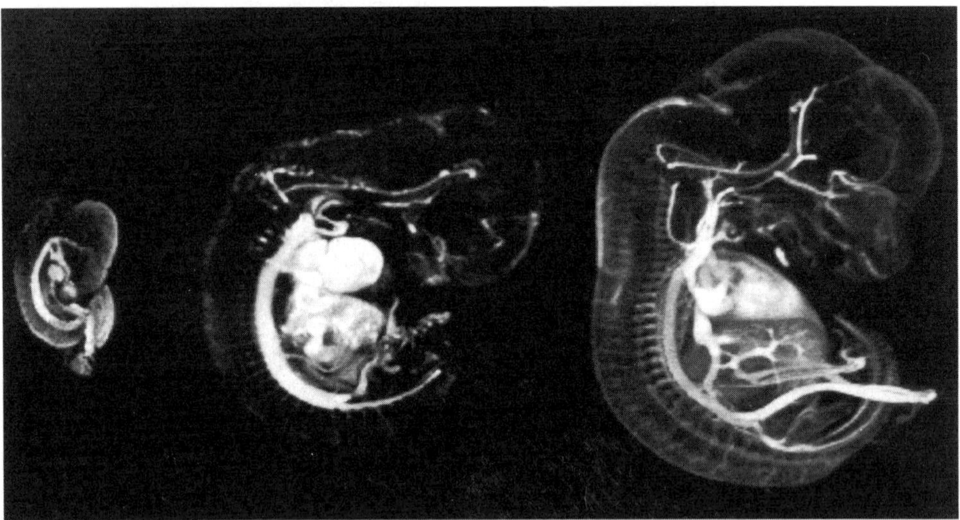

FIGURE 13.5 Isotropic 3D images of fixed mouse embryos at three stages of development have been volume rendered to allow visualization of the developing vascular anatomy.

In less than 10 years, MR microscopy has grown from a scientific curiosity to a tool with a wide range of applications. Although many theoretical and experimental problems still exist at the present time, there is no doubt that MR microscopy will soon make a significant impact in many areas of basic research and clinical diagnosis.

References

Ahn CB, Cho ZH. 1989. A generalized formulation of diffusion effects in μm resolution nuclear magnetic resonance imaging. Med Phys 16:22.

Banson MB, Cofer GP, Black RD, Johnson GA. 1992. A probe for specimen magnetic resonance microscopy. Invest Radiol 27:157.

Banson ML, Cofer GP, Hedlund LW, Johnson GA. 1992. Surface coil imaging of rat spine at 7.0 T. Magn Reson Imaging 10:929.

Benveniste H, Hedlund LW, Johnson GA. 1992. Mechanism of detection of acute cerebral ischemia in rats by diffusion-weighted magnetic resonance microscopy. Stroke 23:746.

Black RD, Early TA, Roemer PB, et al. 1993. A high-temperature superconducting receiver for NMR microscopy. Science 259:793.

Brown TR, Kincaid BM, Ugurbil K. 1982. NMR chemical shift imaging in three dimensions. Proc Natl Acad Sci USA 79:3523.

Callaghan PT, Coy A, Forde LC, Rofe CJ. 1993. Diffusive relaxation and edge enhancement in NMR microscopy. J Magn Reson Series A 101:347.

Callaghan PT, Eccles CD. 1987. Sensitivity and resolution in NMR imaging. J Magn Reson 71:426.

Callaghan PT, Eccles CD. 1988. Diffusion-limited resolution in nuclear magnetic resonance microscopy. J Magn Reson 78:1.

Cho ZH, Ahn CB, Juh SC, et al. 1988. Nuclear magnetic resonance microscopy with 4 μm resolution: Theoretical study and experimental results. Med Phys 15(6):815.

Cho ZH, Yi JH, Friedenberg RM. 1992. NMR microscopy and ultra-high resolution NMR imaging. Rev Magn Reson Med 4:221.

Edelstein WA, Hutchison JMS, Johnson G, Redpath T. 1980. Spin warp NMR imaging and applications to human whole-body imaging. Phys Med Biol 25:751.

Ehman RL, Felmlee JP. 1989. Adaptive technique for high-definition MR imaging of moving structures. Radiology 173:255.

Farmer THR, Johnson GA, Cofer GP, et al. 1989. Implanted coil MR microscopy of renal pathology. Magn Reson Med 10:310.

Gewalt SL, Glover GH, MacFall JR, et al. 1993. MR microscopy of the rat lung using projection reconstruction. Magn Reson Med 29:99.

Glover GH, Noll DC. 1993. Consistent projection reconstruction techniques for MRI. Magn Reson Med 29:345.

Glover GH, Pauly JM. 1992. Projection reconstruction techniques for suppression of motion artifacts. Magn Reson Med 28:275.

Gmitro A, Alexander AL. 1993. Use of a projection reconstruction method to decrease motion sensitivity in diffusion-weighted MRI. Magn Reson Med 29:835.

Haase A, Frahm J, Matthaei D, et al. 1986. FLASH imaging: Rapid NMR imaging using low flip angle pulses. J Magn Reson 67:258.

Hedges HK. 1984. Nuclear magnetic resonance microscopy. Ph.D. dissertation, State University of New York at Stony Brook.

Hedlund LW, Dietz J, Nassar R, et al. 1986. A ventilator for magnetic resonance imaging. Invest Radiol 21:18.

Hennig J, Nauerth A, Friedburg H. 1986. RARE imaging: A fast imaging method for clinical MR. Magn Reson Med 3:823.

Hetherington HP, Wishart D, Fitzpatrick SM, et al. 1986. The application of composite pulses to surface coil NMR. J Magn Reson 66:313.

Hills BP, Wright KM, Belton PS. 1990. The effects of restricted diffusion in nuclear magnetic resonance microscopy. Magn Reson Imaging 8:755.

Hollett MD, Cofer GP, Johnson GA. 1987. In situ magnetic resonance microscopy. Invest Radiol 22:965.

House WV. 1984. NMR microscopy. IEEE Trans Nucl Sci NS-31:570.

Hyslop WB, Lauterbur PC. 1991. Effects of restricted diffusion on microscopic NMR imaging. J Magn Reson 94:501.

Jacobs RE, Fraser SE. 1994. Magnetic resonance microscopy of embryonic cell lineages and movements. Science 263:681.

Johnson GA, Hedlund LW, Cofer GP, Suddarth SA. 1992. Magnetic resonance microscopy in the life sciences. Rev Magn Reson Med 4:187.

Karis JP, Johnson GA, Glover GH. 1987. Signal to noise improvements in three dimensional NMR microscopy using limited angle excitation. J Magn Reson 71:24.

Kumar A, Welti D, Ernst RR. 1975. NMR Fourier zeugmatography. J Magn Reson 18:69.

Lai CM, Lauterbur PC. 1981. True three-dimensional image reconstruction by nuclear magnetic resonance zeugmatography. Phys Med Biol 26:851.

Lauterbur PC. 1984. New direction in NMR imaging. IEEE Trans Nucl Sci NS-31:1010.

Lauterbur PC. 1973. Image formation by induced local interactions: Examples employing nuclear magnetic resonance. Nature 242:190.

Lean CL, Russell P, Delbridge L, et al. 1993. Metastatic follicular thyroid diagnosed by ^{1}H MRS. Proc Soc Magn Reson Med 1:71.

Majumdar S, Gore JC. 1988. Studies of diffusion in random fields produced by variations in susceptibility. J Magn Reson 78:41.

Maki JH, Johnson GA, Cofer GP, MacFall JR. 1988. SNR improvement in NMR microscopy using DEFT. J Magn Reson 80:482.

Mansfield P, Chapman B. 1986. Active magnetic screening of gradient coils in NMR imaging. J Magn Reson 66:573.

Mansfield P, Maudsley AA. 1977. Planar spin imaging by NMR. J Magn Reson 27:129.

McFarland EW. 1992. Time independent point-spread function for MR microscopy. Magn Reson Imaging 10:269.

McFarland EW, Mortara A. 1992. Three-dimensional NMR microscopy: Improving SNR with temperature and microcoils. Magn Reson Imaging 10:279.

Moran PR. 1982. A flow velocity zeugmatographic interface for NMR imaging in humans. Magn Reson Imaging 1:197.

Mulkern RV, Wong STS, Winalski C, Jolesz FA. 1990. Contrast manipulation and artifact assessment of 2D and 3D RARE sequences. Magn Reson Imaging 8:557.

Peck TL, Magin RL, Lauterbur PC. 1990. Microdomain magnetic resonance imaging. Proc Soc Magn Reson Med 1:207.

Putz B, Barsky D, Schulten K. 1991. Edge enhancement by diffusion: Microscopic magnetic resonance imaging of an ultrathin glass capillary. Chem Phys 183:391.

Rudin M. 1987. MR microscopy on rats in vivo at 4.7 T using surface coils. Magn Reson Med 5:443.

Schoeniger JS, Aiken NR, Blackband SJ. 1991. NMR microscopy of single neurons. Proc Soc Magn Reson Med 2:880.

Smith BR, Johnson GA, Groman EV, Linney E. 1993. Contrast enhancement of normal and abnormal mouse embryo vasculature. Proc Soc Magn Reson Med 1:303.

Suits BH, Wilken DE. 1989. Improving magnetic field gradient coils for NMR imaging. J Phys E: Sci Instrum 22:565.

Ugurbil K, Garwood M, Bendall R. 1987. Amplitude- and frequency-modulated pulses to achieve 90° plane rotation with inhomogeneous B_1 fields. J Magn Reson 72:177.

Wood ML, Henkelman RM. 1985. NMR image artifacts from periodic motion. Med Phys 12:143.

Xiang Q-S, Henkelman RM. 1991. Motion artifact reduction with three-point ghost phase cancellation. J Magn Reson Imaging 1:633.

Zhong J, Gore JC. 1991. Studies of restricted diffusion in heterogeneous media containing variations in susceptibility. Magn Reson Med 19:276.

Zhou Z. 1992. Nuclear magnetic resonance microscopy: New theoretical and technical developments. Ph.D. dissertation, University of Illinois at Urbana-Champaign.

Zhou X, Cofer GP, Mills GI, Johnson GA. 1992. An inductively coupled probe for MR microscopy at 7 T. Proc Soc Magn Reson Med 1:971.

Zhou X, Cofer GP, Suddarth SA, Johnson GA. 1993. High-field MR microscopy using fast spin-echoes. Magn Reson Med 31:60.

Zhou X, Lauterbur PC. 1992. NMR microscopy using projection reconstruction. In B Blümich, W Kuhn (eds), Magnetic Resonance Microscopy, pp 1–27. Weinheim, Germany, VCH.

Zhou X, Liang Z-P, Cofer GP, et al. 1993. An FSE pulse sequence with circular sampling for MR microscopy. Proc Soc Magn Reson Med 1:297.

Zhou X, Maronpot RR, Mills GI, et al. 1994. Studies on bromobenzene-induced hepatotoxicity using in vivo MR microscopy. Magn Reson Med 31:619.

Further Information

A detailed description of the physics of NMR and MRI can be found in *Principles of Magnetic Resonance*, by C. S. Slichter (3rd edition, Springer-Verlag, 1989), in *NMR Imaging in Biology and Medicine*, by P. Morris (Clarendon Press, 1986), and in *Principles of Magnetic Resonance Microscopy*, by P. T. Callaghan (Oxford Press, 1991). The latter two books also contain detailed discussions on instrumentation, data acquisition, and image reconstruction for conventional and microscopic magnetic resonance imaging.

Magnetic Resonance Microscopy, edited by Blümich and Kuhn (VCH, 1992), is particularly helpful to understand various aspects of MR microscopy, both methodology and applications. Each chapter of the book covers a specific topic and is written by experts in the field.

Proceedings of the Society of Magnetic Resonance (formerly Society of Magnetic Resonance in Medicine, Berkeley, California), published annually, documents the most recent developments in the field of MR microscopy. *Magnetic Resonance in Medicine*, *Journal of Magnetic Resonance Imaging*, and *Magnetic Resonance Imaging*, all monthly journals, contain original research articles and are good sources for up-to-date developments.

14

Positron-Emission Tomography (PET)

Thomas F. Budinger
University of California at Berkeley

Henry F. VanBrocklin
University of California at Berkeley

14.1 Radiopharmaceuticals

Thomas F. Budinger and Henry F. VanBrocklin

Since the discovery of artificial radioactivity a half century ago, radiotracers, radionuclides, and radionuclide compounds have played a vital role in biology and medicine. Common to all is radionuclide (radioactive isotope) production. This section describes the basic ideas involved in radionuclide production and gives examples of the applications of radionuclides. The field of radiopharmaceutical chemistry has fallen into subspecialties of positron-emission tomography (PET) chemistry and general radiopharmaceutical chemistry, including specialists in technetium chemistry, taking advantage of the imaging attributes of technetium-99m.

The two general methods of radionuclide production are neutron addition (activation) from neutron reactors to make neutron-rich radionuclides which decay to give off electrons and gamma rays and charged-particle accelerators (linacs and cyclotrons) which usually produce neutron-deficient isotopes that decay by electron capture and emission of x-rays, gamma rays, and positrons. The production of artificial radionuclides is governed by the number of neutrons or charged particles hitting an appropriate target per time, the cross section for the particular reaction, the number of atoms in the target, and the half-life of the artificial radionuclide:

$$A(t) = \frac{N\sigma\phi}{3.7 \times 10^{10}} \left(1 - e \frac{0.693t}{T_{1/2}} \right) \tag{14.1}$$

where $A(t)$ is the produced activity in number of atoms per second, N is the number of target nuclei, σ is the cross section (probability that the neutron or charged particles will interact with the nucleus to form the artificial radioisotope) for the reaction, ϕ is the flux of charged particles, and $T_{1/2}$ is the half-life of the product. Note that N is the target mass divided by the atomic weight and multiplied by

0-8493-1810-6/03/$0.00+$1.50

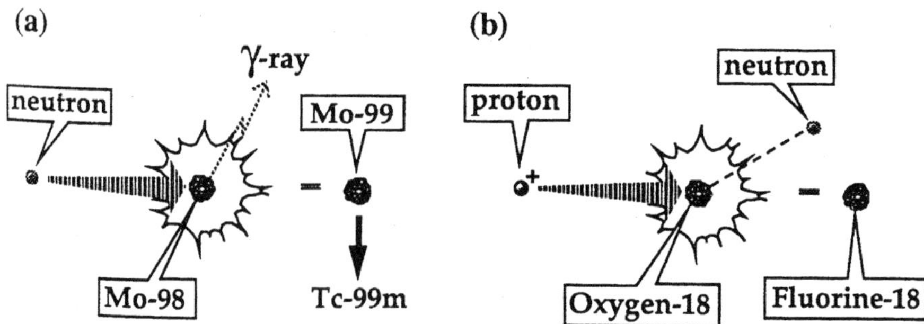

FIGURE 14.1 (a) High specific activity neutron-excess radionuclides are produced usually through the (n, γ), (n, p), or (n, α) reactions. The product nuclides usually decay β^- followed by γ. Most of the reactor produced radionuclides are produced by the (n, γ) reaction. (b) Cyclotrons and linear accelerators (linacs) are sources of beams of protons, deuterons, or helium ions which bombard targets to produce neutron-deficient radionuclides.

Avogadro's number (60.24×10^{23}) and σ is measured in cm^2. The usual flux is about 10^{14} neutrons per second or, for charged particles, 10 to 100 μA, which is equivalent to 6.25×10^{13} to 6.25×10^{14} charged particles per second.

Nuclear Reactor–Produced Radionuclides

Thermal neutrons of the order of 10^{14} neutrons/s/cm^2 are produced in a nuclear reactor usually during a controlled nuclear fission of uranium, though thorium or plutonium are also used. High specific activity neutron-rich radionuclides are produced usually through the (n, γ), (n, p), or (n, α) reactions (Fig. 14.1a). The product nuclides usually decay by β^- followed by γ. Most of the reactor-produced radionuclides are produced by the (n, γ) reaction. The final step in the production of a radionuclide consists of the separation of the product nuclide from the target container by chemical or physical means.

An alternative method for producing isotopes from a reactor is to separate the fission fragments from the spent fuel rods. This is the leading source of ^{99}Mo for medical applications. The following two methods of ^{99}Mo production are examples of carrier-added and no-carrier-added radionuclide synthesis, respectively. In Fig. 14.1a, the ^{99}Mo is production from ^{98}Mo. Only a small fraction of the ^{98}Mo nuclei will be converted to ^{99}Mo. Therefore, at the end of neutron bombardment, there is a mixture of both isotopes. These are inseparable by conventional chemical separation techniques, and both isotopes would participate equally well in chemical reactions. The ^{99}Mo from fission of ^{238}U would not contain any other isotopes of Mo and is considered carrier-free. Thus radioisotopes produced by any means having the same atomic number as the target material would be considered carrier-added. Medical tracer techniques obviate the need for carrier-free isotopes.

Accelerator-Produced Radionuclides

Cyclotrons and linear accelerators (linacs) are sources of beams of protons, deuterons, or helium ions that bombarded targets to produce neutron-deficient (proton-rich) radionuclides (Fig. 14.1b). The neutron-deficient radionuclides produced through these reactions are shown in Table 14.1. These product nuclides (usually carrier-free) decay either by electron capture or by positron emission tomography or both, followed by γ emission. In Table 14.2, most of the useful charged-particle reactions are listed.

The heat produced by the beam current on the target material can interfere with isotope production and requires efficient heat-removal strategies using extremely stable heat-conducting target materials such as metal foils, electroplate metals, metal powders, metal oxides, and salts melted on duralmin plate. All the modern targets use circulating cold deionized water and/or chilled helium gas to aid in cooling the target body and window foils. Cyclotrons used in medical studies have ^{11}C, ^{13}N, ^{15}O, and ^{18}F production capabilities that deliver the product nuclides on demand through computer-executed commands. The

TABLE 14.1 Radionuclides Used in Biomedicine

Radionuclide	Half-Life	Application(s)
Arsenic-74*	17.9 d	A positron-emitting chemical analogue of phosphorus
Barium-128*	2.4 d	Parent in the generator system for producing the positron emitting ^{128}Cs, a potassium analogue
Berylium-7*	53.37 d	Berylliosis studies
Bromine-77	57 h	Radioimmunotherapy
Bromine-82	35.3 h	Used in metabolic studies and studies of estrogen receptor content
*Carbon-11**	20.3 min	*Positron emitter for metabolism imaging*
Cobalt-57*	270 d	Calibration of imaging instruments
Copper-62	9.8 min	Heart perfusion
Copper-64	12.8 h	Used as a clinical diagnostic agent for cancer and metabolic disorders
Copper-67	58.5 h	Radioimmunotherapy
Chromium-51	27.8 d	Used to assess red blood cell survival
Fluorine-18	109.7 min	*Positron emitter used in glucose analogue uptake and neuroreceptor imaging*
Gallium-68	68 min	Required in calibrating PET tomographs. Potential antibody level
Germanium-68*	287 d	Parent in the generator system for producing the positron emitting ^{68}Ga
Indium-111*	2.8 d	Radioimmunotherapy
Iodine-122	3.76 min	*Positron emitter for blood flow studies*
Iodine-123*	13.3 h	SPECT brain imaging agent
Iodine-124*	4.2 d	Radioimmunotherapy, *positron emitter*
Iodine-125	60.2 d	Used as a potential cancer therapeutic agent
Iodine-131	8.1 d	Used to diagnose and treat thyroid disorders including cancer
*Iron-52**	8.2 h	*Used as an iron tracer, positron emitter for bone-marrow imaging*
Magnesium-28*	21.2 h	Magnesium tracer which decays to 2.3 in aluminum-28
Manganese-52m	5.6 d	Flow tracer for heart muscle
Mercury-195m*	40 h	Parent in the generator system for producing ^{195m}Au, which is used in cardiac blood pool studies
Molybdenum-99	67 h	Used to produce technetium-99m, the most commonly used radioisotope in clinical nuclear medicine
*Nitrogen-13**	9.9 min	*Positron emitter used as ^{13}NH for heart perfusion studies*
Osmium-191	15 d	Decays to iridium-191 used for cardiac studies
*Oxygen-15**	123 s	*Positron emitter used for blood flow studies as $H_2^{15}O$*
Palladium-103	17 d	Used in the treatment of prostate cancer
Phosphorus-32	14.3 d	Used in cancer treatment, cell metabolism and kinetics, molecular biology, genetics research, biochemistry, microbiology, enzymology, and as a starter to make many basic chemicals and research products
Rhenium-188	17 h	Used for treatment of medullary thyroid carcinoma and alleviation of pain in bone metastases
*Rubidium-82**	1.2 min	*Positron emitter used for heart perfusion studies*
Ruthenium-97*	2.9 d	Hepatobiliary function, tumor and inflammation localization
Samarium-145	340 d	Treatment of ocular cancer
Samarium-153	46.8 h	Used to radiolabel various molecules as cancer therapeutic agents and to alleviate bone cancer pain
Scandium-47	3.4 d	Radioimmunotherapy
Scandium-47*	3.4 d	Used in the therapy of cancer
Strontium-82*	64.0 d	Parent in the generator system for producing the positron emitting ^{82}Rb, a potassium analogue
Strontium-85	64 d	Used to study bone formation metabolism
Strontium-89	52 d	Used to alleviate metastatic bone pain
Sulfur-35	87.9 d	Used in studies of cell metabolism and kinetics, molecular biology, genetics research, biochemistry, microbiology, enzymology, and as a start to make many basic chemicals and research products
Technetium-99m	6 h	The most widely used radiopharmaceutical in nuclear medicine and produced from molybdenum-99
Thalium-201*	74 h	Cardiac imaging agent
Tin-117m	14.0 d	Palliative treatment of bone cancer pain
Tritium (hydrogen-3)	12.3 yr	Used to make tritiated water which is used as a starter for thousands of different research products and basic chemicals; used for life science and drug metabolism studies to ensure the safety of potential new drugs

TABLE 14.1 (continued) Radionuclides Used in Biomedicine

Radionuclide	Half-Life	Application(s)
Tungsten-178*	21.5 d	Parent in generator system for producing ^{178}Ta, short lived scanning agent
Tungsten-188	69 d	Decays to rhenium-188 for treatment of cancer and rheumatoid arthritis
Vanadium-48*	16.0 d	Nutrition and environmental studies
Xenon-122*	20 h	Parent in the generator system for producing the positron emitting ^{122}I
Xenon-127*	36.4 d	Used in lung ventilation studies
Xenon-133	5.3 d	Used in lung ventilation and perfusion studies
Yttrium-88*	106.6 d	Radioimmunotherapy
Yttrium-90	64 h	Used to radiolabel various molecules as cancer therapeutic agents
Zinc-62*	9.13 h	Parent in the generator system for producing the positron emitting ^{62}Cu
Zirconium-89*	78.4 h	Radioimmunotherapy, positron emitter

* Produced by accelerated charged particles. Others are produced by neutron reactors.

radionuclide is remotely transferred into a lead-shielded hot cell for processing. The resulting radionuclides are manipulated using microscale radiochemical techniques: small-scale synthetic methodology, ion-exchange chromatography, solvent extraction, electrochemical synthesis, distillation, simple filtration, paper chromatography, and isotopic carrier precipitation. Various relevant radiochemical techniques have been published in standard texts.

TABLE 14.2 Important Reactions for Cyclotron-Produced Radioisotopes

1.	*p*, *n*	7.	*p*, *pn*
2.	*p*, 2*n*	8.	*p*, 2*p*
3.	*d*, *n*	9.	*d*, *p*
4.	*d*, 2*n*	10.	*d*, ^{4}He
5.	*p*, ^{4}He	11.	*p*, *d*
6.	*p*, ^{4}He*n*	12.	^{4}He, *n*
		13.	^{3}He, *p*

Generator-Produced Radionuclides

If the reactor, cyclotron, or natural product radionuclide of long half-life decays to a daughter with nuclear characteristics appropriate for medical application, the system is called a *medical radionuclide generator.* There are several advantages afforded by generator-produced isotopes. These generators represent a convenient source of short-lived medical isotopes without the need for an on-site reactor or particle accelerator. Generators provide delivery of the radionuclide on demand at a site remote from the production facility. They are a source of both gamma- and positron-emitting isotopes.

The most common medical radionuclide generator is the ^{99}Mo $\rightarrow$ ^{99m}Tc system, the source of ^{99m}Tc, a gamma-emitting isotope currently used in 70% of the clinical nuclear medicine studies. The ^{99}Mo has a 67-h half-life, giving this generator a useful life of about a week. Another common generator is the ^{68}Ge $\rightarrow$ ^{68}Ga system. Germanium (half-life is 287 days) is accelerator-produced in high-energy accelerators (e.g., BLIP, LAMPF, TRIUMF) through the alpha-particle bombardment of ^{66}Zn. The ^{68}Ge decays to ^{68}Ga, a positron emitter, which has a 68-min half-life. Gallium generators can last for several months.

The generator operation is fairly straightforward. In general, the parent isotope is bound to a solid chemical matrix (e.g., alumina column, anionic resin, Donux resin). As the parent decays, the daughter nuclide grows in. The column is then flushed ("milked") with a suitable solution (e.g., saline, hydrochloric acid) that elutes the daughter and leaves the remaining parent absorbed on the column. The eluent may be injected directly or processed into a radiopharmaceutical.

Radiopharmaceuticals

^{99m}Tc is removed from the generator in the form of TcO_4^- (pertechnetate). This species can be injected directly for imaging or incorporated into a variety of useful radiopharmaceuticals. The labeling of ^{99m}Tc usually involves reduction complexation/chelation. ^{99m}Tc-Sestamibi (Fig. 14.2) is a radiopharmaceutical used to evaluate myocardial perfusion or in the diagnosis of cancer. There are several reduction methods employed, including Sn(II) reduction in $NaHCO_3$ at pH of 8 and other reduction and complexation reactions such as S_2O_3 + HCl, $FeCl_3$ + ascorbic acid, $LiBH_4$, Zn + HCl, HCl, Fe(II), Sn(II)F_2, Sn(II) citrate, and Sn(II) tartrate reduction and complexation, electrolytic reduction, and *in vivo* labeling of red cells following Sn(II) pyrophosphate or Sn(II) DTPA administration. ^{131}I, ^{125}I, and ^{123}I labeling requires special reagents or conditions such as chloramine-T, widely used for protein labeling at 7.5 pH; peroxidase + H_2O_2 widely used for radioassay tracers; isotopic exchange for imaging tracers; excitation labeling as in ^{123}Xe → ^{123}I diazotization plus iodination for primary amines; conjugation labeling with Bolton Hunter agent (*N*-succinimidyl 3-[4-hydroxy 5-(^{131,125,123}I)iodophenyl] propionate); hydroboration plus iodination; electrophilic destannylation; microdiffusion with fresh iodine vapor; and other methods. Radiopharmaceuticals in common use for brain perfusion studies are *N*-isopropyl-*p* [^{123}I] iodoamphetamine and ^{99m}Tc-labeled hexamethylpropyleneamine.

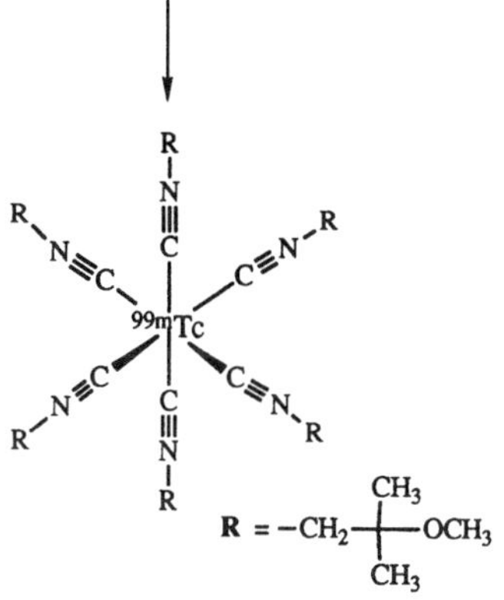

FIGURE 14.2 ^{99m}Tc-Sestamibi is a radiopharmaceutical used to evaluate myocardial perfusion or in the diagnosis of cancer using both computed tomography and scintigraphy techniques.

PET Radionuclides

For ^{11}C, ^{13}N, ^{15}O, and ^{18}F, the modes of production of short-lived positron emitters can dictate the chemical form of the product, as shown in Table 14.3. Online chemistry is used to make various PET agents and precursors. For example, ^{11}C cyanide, an important precursor for synthesis of other labeled compounds, is produced in the cyclotron target by first bombarding N_2 + 5% H_2 gas target with 20-MeV protons. The product is carbon-labeled methane, $^{11}CH_4$, which when combined with ammonia and passed over a platinum wool catalyst at 1000°C becomes $^{11}CN^-$, which is subsequently trapped in NaOH.

Molecular oxygen is produced by bombarding a gas target of $^{14}N_2$ + 2% O_2 with deuterons (6 to 8 MeV). A number of products (e.g., $^{15}O_2$, $C^{15}O_2$, $N^{15}O_2$, $^{15}O_3$, and $H_2{}^{15}O$) are trapped by soda lime followed by charcoal to give $^{15}O_2$ as the product. However, if an activated charcoal trap at 900°C is used before the soda lime trap, the $^{15}O_2$ will be converted to $C^{15}O$. The specific strategies for other online PET agents is given in Rayudu [1990].

Fluorine-18 (^{18}F) is a very versatile positron emitting isotope. With a 2-h half-life and two forms (F^+ and F^-), one can develop several synthetic methods for incorporating ^{18}F into medically useful compounds [Kilbourn, 1990]. Additionally, fluorine forms strong bonds with carbon and is roughly the same size as a hydrogen atom, imparting metabolic and chemical stability of the molecules without drastically altering biologic activity. The most commonly produced ^{18}F radiopharmaceutical is 2-deoxy-2-[^{18}F]fluoroglucose (FDG). This radiotracer mimics part of the glucose metabolic pathway and has shown both hypo- and hypermetabolic abnormalities in cardiology, oncology, and neurology. The synthetic pathway for the production of FDG is shown in Fig. 14.3.

TABLE 14.3 Major Positron-Emitting Radionuclides Produced by Accelerated Protons

Radionuclide	Half-Life	Reaction
Carbon-11	20 min	^{12}C (*p*, *pn*) ^{11}C
		^{14}N (*p*, α) ^{11}C
Nitrogen-13	10 min	^{16}O (*p*, α) ^{13}N
		^{13}C (*p*, *n*) ^{13}N
Oxygen-15	2 min	^{15}N (*p*, *n*) ^{15}O
		^{14}N (*d*, *n*) ^{15}O
Fluorine-18	110 min	^{18}O (*p*, *n*) ^{18}F
		^{20}Ne (*d*, α) ^{18}F

Note: A(*x*, *y*)*B*: *A* is target, *x* is the bombarding particle, *y* is the radiation product, and *B* is the isotope produced.

The production of positron radiopharmaceuticals requires the rapid incorporation of the isotope into the desired molecule. Chemical techniques and synthetic strategies have been developed to facilitate these reactions. Many of these synthetic manipulations require hands-on operations by a highly trained chemist. Additionally, since positrons give off 2- to 511-keV gamma rays upon annihilation, proximity to

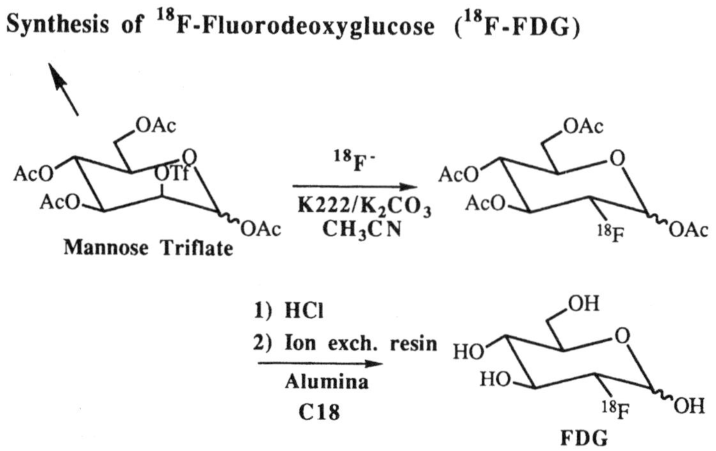

Synthesis of ^{18}F-Fluorodeoxyglucose (^{18}F-FDG)

Mannose Triflate

$^{18}F^-$

K222/K_2CO_3

CH_3CN

1) HCl

2) Ion exch. resin

Alumina

C18

FDG

FIGURE 14.3 Schematic for the chemical production of deoxyglucose labeled with fluorine-18. Here K222 refers to Kryptofix and C18 denotes a reverse-phase high-pressure liquid chromatography column.

the source can increase one's personal dose. The demand for the routine production of positron radiopharmaceuticals such as FDG has led to the development of remote synthetic devices. These devices can be human-controlled (i.e., flipping switches to open air-actuated valves), computer-controlled, or robotic. A sophisticated computer-controlled chemistry synthesis unit has been assembled for the fully automated production of ^{18}FDG [Padgett, 1989]. A computer-controlled robot has been programmed to produce 6α-[^{18}F]fluoroestradiol for breast cancer imaging [Brodack, 1986; Mathias, 1987]. Both these types of units increase the availability and reduce the cost of short-lived radiopharmaceutical production through greater reliability and reduced need for a highly trained staff. Additionally, these automated devices reduce personnel radiation exposure. These and other devices are being designed with greater versatility in mind to allow a variety of radiopharmaceuticals to be produced just by changing the programming and the required reagents.

These PET radionuclides have been incorporated into a wide variety of medically useful radiopharmaceuticals through a number of synthetic techniques. The development of PET scanner technology has added a new dimension to synthetic chemistry by challenging radiochemists to devise labeling and purification strategies that proceed on the order of minutes rather than hours or days as in conventional synthetic chemistry. To meet this challenge, radiochemists are developing new target systems to improve isotope production and sophisticated synthetic units to streamline routine production of commonly desired radiotracers as well as preparing short-lived radiopharmaceuticals for many applications.

Acknowledgment

This work was supported in part by the Director, Office of Energy Research, Office of Health and Environmental Research, Medical Applications and Biophysical Research Division of the U.S. Department of Energy, under Contract No. DE-AC03-SF00098, and in part by NIH Grant HL25840.

References

Brodack JW, Dence CS, Kilbourn MR, Welch MJ. 1988. Robotic production of 2-deoxy-2-[18F]fluoro-D-glucose: A routine method of synthesis using tetrabutylammonium [18F]fluoride. Int J Radiat Appl Instrum Part A: Appl Radiat Isotopes 39(7):699.

Brodack JW, Kilbourn MR, Welch MJ, Katzenellenbogen JA. 1986. Application of robotics to radiopharmaceutical preparation: Controlled synthesis of fluorine-18 16 alpha-fluoroestradiol-17 beta. J Nucl Med 27(5):714.

Hupf HB. 1976. Production and purification of radionuclides. In Radiopharmacy. New York, Wiley.

Kilbourn MR. 1990. Fluorine-18 Labeling of Radiopharmaceuticals. Washington, National Academy Press.

Lamb J, Kramer HH. 1983. Commercial production of radioisotopes for nuclear medicine. In Radiotracers for Medical Applications, pp 17–62. Boca Raton, FL, CRC Press.

Mathias CJ, Welch MJ, Katzenellenbogen JA, et al. 1987. Characterization of the uptake of 16 alpha-([18F]fluoro)-17 beta-estradiol in DMBA-induced mammary tumors. Int J Radiat Appl Instrum Part B: Nucl Med Biol 14(1):15.

Padgett HC, Schmidt DG, Luxen A, et al. 1989. Computed-controlled radiochemical synthesis: A chemistry process control unit for the automated production of radiochemicals. Int J Radiat Appl Instrum Part A: Appl Radiat Isotopes 40(5):433.

Rayudu GV. 1990. Production of radionuclides for medicine. Semin Nucl Med 20(2):100.

Sorenson JA, Phelps ME. 1987. Physics in Nuclear Medicine. New York, Grune & Stratton.

Steigman J, Eckerman WC. 1992. The Chemistry of Technetium in Medicine. Washington, National Academy Press.

Stocklin G. 1992. Tracers for metabolic imaging of brain and heart: Radiochemistry and radiopharmacology. Eur J Nucl Med 19(7):527.

14.2 Instrumentation

Thomas F. Budinger

Background

The history of positron-emission tomography (PET) can be traced to the early 1950s, when workers in Boston first realized the medical imaging possibilities of a particular class of radioactive substances. It was recognized then that the high-energy photons produced by annihilation of the positron from positron-emitting isotopes could be used to describe, in three dimensions, the physiologic distribution of "tagged" chemical compounds. After two decades of moderate technological developments by a few research centers, widespread interest and broadly based research activity began in earnest following the development of sophisticated reconstruction algorithms and improvements in detector technology. By the mid-1980s, PET had become a tool for medical diagnosis and for dynamic studies of human metabolism.

Today, because of its million-fold sensitivity advantage over magnetic resonance imaging (MRI) in tracer studies and its chemical specificity, PET is used to study neuroreceptors in the brain and other body tissues. In contrast, MRI has exquisite resolution for anatomic (Fig. 14.4) and flow studies as well as unique attributes of evaluating chemical composition of tissue but in the millimolar range rather than the nanomolar range of much of the receptor proteins in the body. Clinical studies include tumors of the brain, breast, lungs, lower gastrointestinal tract, and other sites. Additional clinical uses include Alzheimer's disease, Parkinson's disease, epilepsy, and coronary artery disease affecting heart muscle metabolism and flow. Its use has added immeasurably to our current understanding of flow, oxygen utilization, and the metabolic changes that accompany disease and that change during brain stimulation and cognitive activation.

PET Theory

PET imaging begins with the injection of a metabolically active tracer—a biologic molecule that carries with it a positron-emitting isotope (e.g., ^{11}C, ^{13}N, ^{15}O, or ^{18}F). Over a few minutes, the isotope accumulates in an area of the body for which the molecule has an affinity. As an example, glucose labeled with ^{11}C, or a glucose analogue labeled with ^{18}F, accumulates in the brain or tumors, where glucose is used as the primary source of energy. The radioactive nuclei then decay by positron emission. In positron (positive electron) emission, a nuclear proton changes into a positive electron and a neutron. The atom maintains

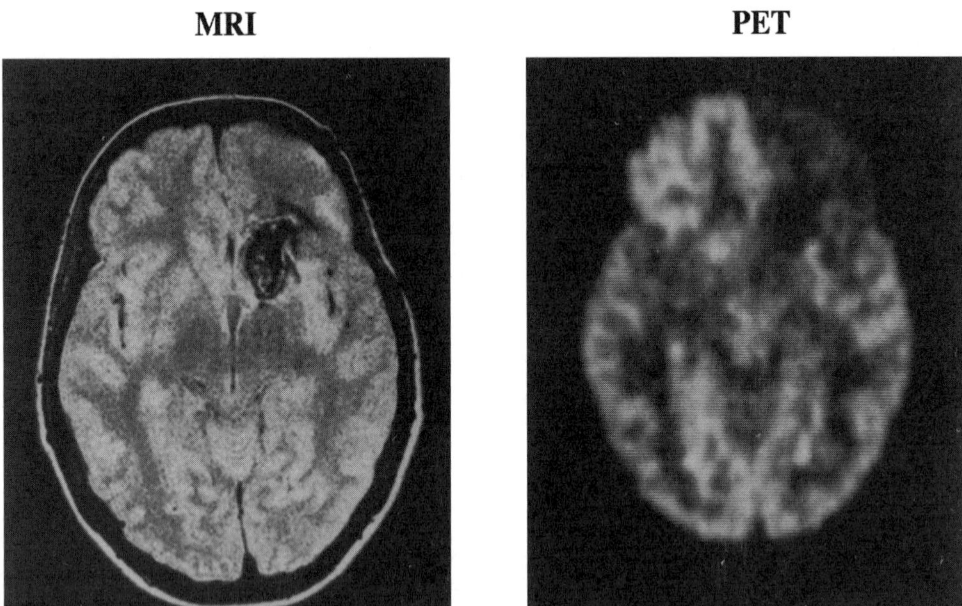

FIGURE 14.4 The MRI image shows the arteriovenous malformation (AVM) as an area of signal loss due to blood flow. The PET image shows the AVM as a region devoid of glucose metabolism and also shows decreased metabolism in the adjacent frontal cortex. This is a metabolic effect of the AVM on the brain and may explain some of the patient's symptoms.

its atomic mass but decreases its atomic number by 1. The ejected positron combines with an electron almost instantaneously, and these two particles undergo the process of annihilation. The energy associated with the masses of the positron and electron particles is 1.022 MeV in accordance with the energy E to mass m equivalence $E = mc^2$, where c is the velocity of light. This energy is divided equally between two photons that fly away from one another at a 180° angle. Each photon has an energy of 511 keV. These high-energy gamma rays emerge from the body in opposite directions, to be detected by an array of detectors that surround the patient (Fig. 14.5). When two photons are recorded simultaneously by a pair of detectors, the annihilation event that gave rise to them must have occurred somewhere along the line connecting the detectors. Of course, if one of the photons is scattered, then the line of coincidence will be incorrect. After 100,000 or more annihilation events are detected, the distribution of the positron-emitting tracer is calculated by tomographic reconstruction procedures. PET reconstructs a two-dimensional (2D) image from the one-dimensional projections seen at different angles. Three-dimensional (3D) reconstructions also can be done using 2D projections from multiple angles.

PET Detectors

Efficient detection of the annihilation photons from positron emitters is usually provided by the combination of a crystal, which converts the high-energy photons to visible-light photons, and a photomultiplier tube that produces an amplified electric current pulse proportional to the amount of light photons interacting with the photocathode. The fact that imaging system sensitivity is proportional to the square of the detector efficiency leads to a very important requirement that the detector be nearly 100% efficient. Thus other detector systems such as plastic scintillators or gas-filled wire chambers, with typical individual efficiencies of 20% or less, would result in a coincident efficiency of only 4% or less.

Most modern PET cameras are multilayered with 15 to 47 levels or transaxial layers to be reconstructed (Fig. 14.6). The lead shields prevent activity from the patient from causing spurious counts in the tomograph ring, while the tungsten septa reject some of the events in which one (or both) of the 511-keV

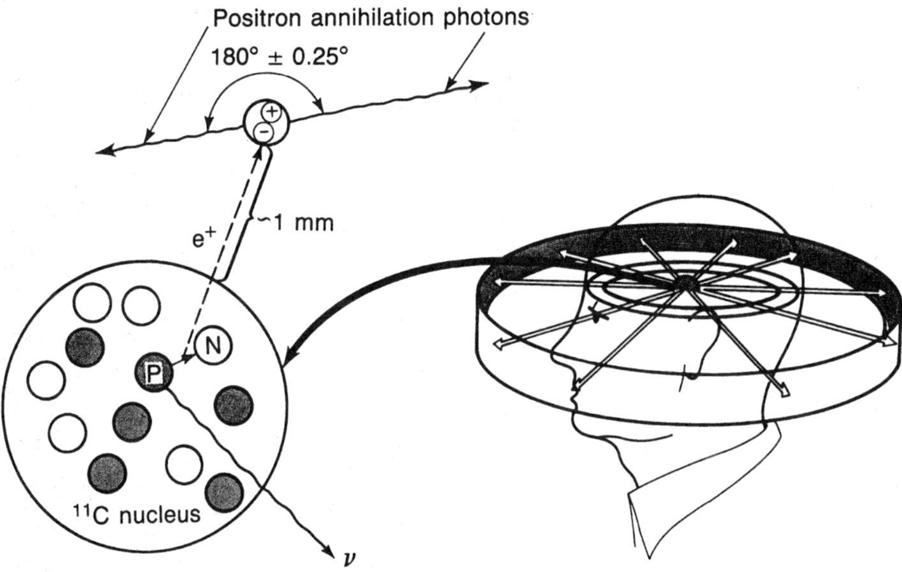

FIGURE 14.5 The physical basis of positron-emission tomography. Positrons emitted by "tagged" metabolically active molecules annihilate nearby electrons and give rise to a pair of high-energy photons. The photons fly off in nearly opposite directions and thus serve to pinpoint their source. The biologic activity of the tagged molecule can be used to investigate a number of physiologic functions, both normal and pathologic.

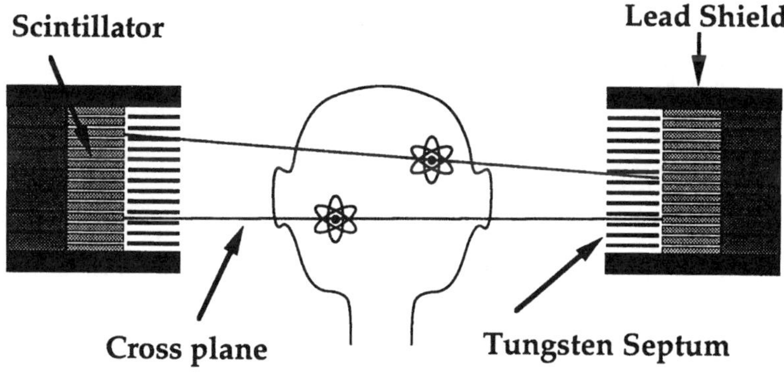

FIGURE 14.6 Most modern PET cameras are multilayered with 15 to 47 levels or transaxial layers to be reconstructed. The lead shields prevent activity from the patient from causing spurious counts in the tomograph ring, while the tungsten septa reject some of the events in which one (or both) of the 511-keV photons suffer a Compton scatter in the patient. The sensitivity of this design is improved by collection of data from cross-planes.

photons suffer a Compton scatter in the patient. The sensitivity of this design is improved by collection of data from cross-planes (Fig. 14.6). The arrangement of scintillators and phototubes is shown in Fig. 14.7.

The "individually coupled" design is capable of very high resolution, and because the design is very parallel (all the photomultiplier tubes and scintillator crystals operate independently), it is capable of very high data throughput. The disadvantages of this type of design are the requirement for many expensive photomultiplier tubes and, additionally, that connecting round photomultiplier tubes to rectangular

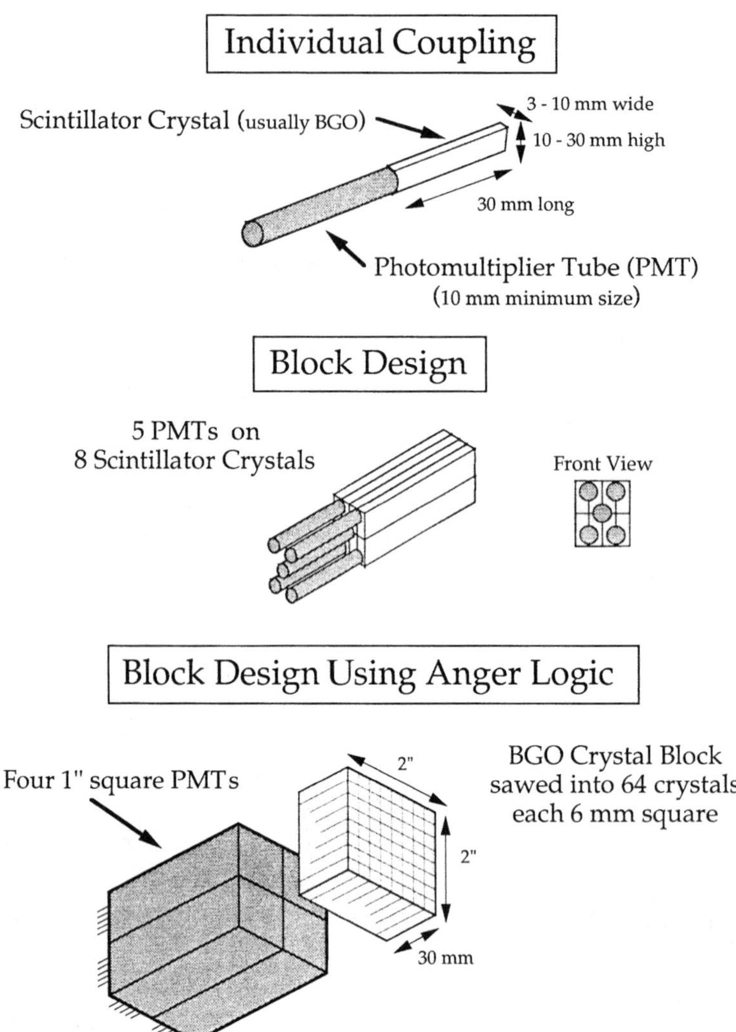

FIGURE 14.7 The arrangement of scintillators and phototubes is shown. The "individually coupled" design is capable of very high resolution, and because the design is very parallel (all the photomultiplier tubes and scintillator crystals operate independently), it is capable of very high data throughput. A block detector couples several photomultiplier tubes to a bank of scintillator crystals and uses a coding scheme to determine the crystal of interaction. In the two-layer block, five photomultiplier tubes are coupled to eight scintillator crystals.

scintillation crystals leads to problems of packing rectangular crystals and circular phototubes of sufficiently small diameter to form a solid ring.

The contemporary method of packing many scintillators for 511 keV around the patient is to use what is called a *block detector design.* A block detector couples several photomultiplier tubes to a bank of scintillator crystals and uses a coding scheme to determine the crystal of interaction. In the two-layer block (Fig. 14.7), five photomultiplier tubes are coupled to eight scintillator crystals. Whenever one of the outside four photomultiplier tubes fires, a 511-keV photon has interacted in one of the two crystals attached to that photomultiplier tube, and the center photomultiplier tube is then used to determine whether it was the inner or outer crystal. This is known as a *digital* coding scheme, since each photomultiplier tube is either "hit" or "not hit" and the crystal of interaction is determined by a "digital" mapping of the hit pattern. Block detector designs are much less expensive and practical to form into a multilayer camera. However, errors in the decoding scheme reduce the spatial resolution, and since the entire block is "dead" whenever one of its member crystals is struck by a photon, the dead time is worse than with individual coupling. The electronics necessary to decode the output of the block are straightforward but more complex than that needed for the individually coupled design.

Most block detector coding schemes use an *analog* coding scheme, where the ratio of light output is used to determine the crystal of interaction. In the example above, four photomultiplier tubes are coupled to a block of BGO that has been partially sawed through to form 64 "individual" crystals. The depth of the cuts are critical; that is, deep cuts tend to focus the scintillation light onto the face of a single photomultiplier tube, while shallow cuts tend to spread the light over all four photomultiplier tubes. This type of coding scheme is more difficult to implement than digital coding, since analog light ratios place more stringent requirements on the photomultiplier tube linearity and uniformity as well as scintillator crystal uniformity. However, most commercial PET cameras use an analog coding scheme because it is much less expensive due to the lower number of photomultiplier tubes required.

Physical Factors Affecting Resolution

The factors that affect the spatial resolution of PET tomographs are shown in Fig. 14.8. The size of the detector is critical in determining the system's geometric resolution. If the block design is used, there is a degradation in this geometric resolution by 2.2 mm for BGO. The degradation is probably due to the limited light output of BGO and the ratio of crystals (cuts) per phototube.

The angle between the paths of the annihilation photons can deviated from 180° as a result of some residual kinetic motion (Fermi motion) at the time of annihilation. The effect on resolution of this deviation increases as the detector ring diameter increases so that eventually this factor can have a significant effect.

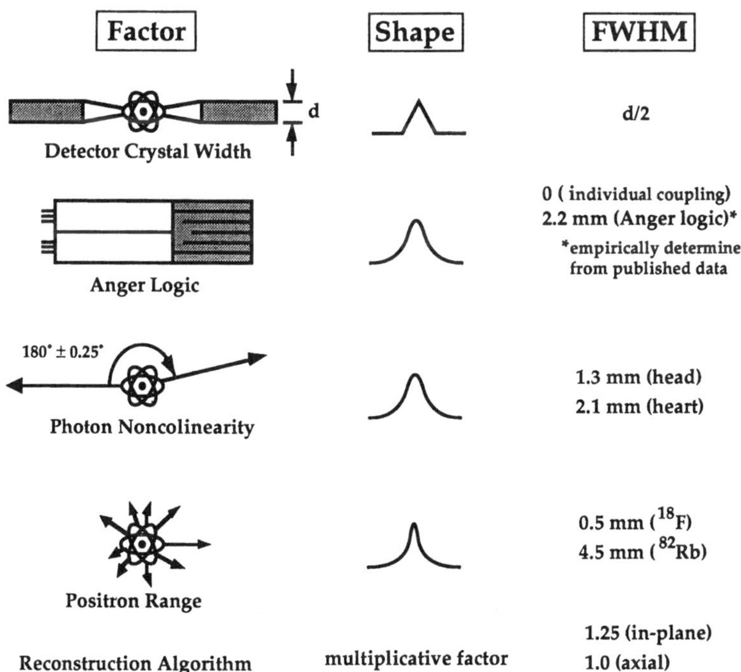

FIGURE 14.8 Factors contributing to the resolution of the PET tomograph. The contribution most accessible to further reduction is the size of the detector crystals.

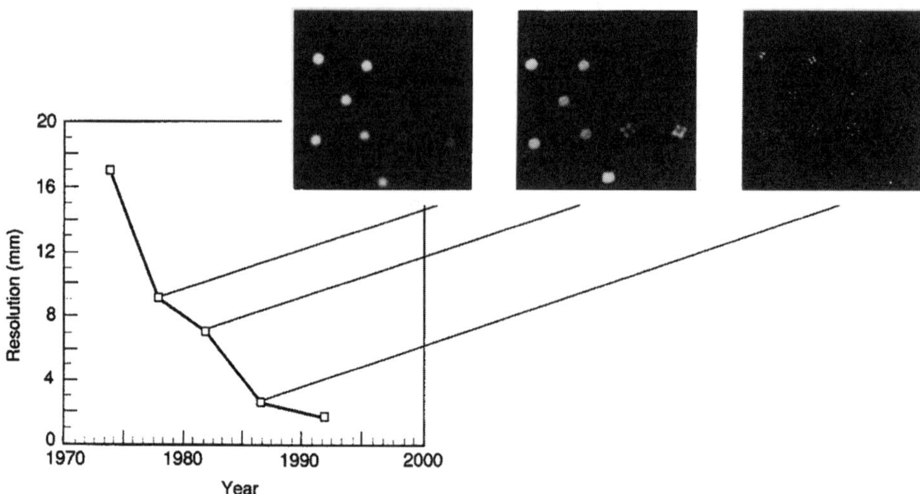

FIGURE 14.9 The evolution of resolution. Over the past decade, the resolving power of PET has improved from about 9 to 2.6 mm. This improvement is graphically illustrated by the increasing success with which one is able to resolve "hot spots" of an artificial sample that are detected and imaged by the tomographs.

The distance the positron travels after being emitted from the nucleus and before annihilation causes a deterioration in spatial resolution. This distance depends on the particular nuclide. For example, the range of blurring for ^{18}F, the isotope used for many of the current PET studies, is quite small compared with that of the other isotopes. Combining values for these factors for the PET-600 tomograph, we can estimate a detector-pair spatial resolution of 2.0 mm and a reconstructed image resolution of 2.6 mm. The measured resolution of this system is 2.6 mm, but most commercially available tomographs use a block detector design (Fig. 14.7), and the resolution of these systems is above 5 mm. The evolution of resolution improvement is shown in Fig. 14.9.

The resolution evolutions discussed above pertain to results for the center or axis of the tomograph. The resolution at the edge of the object (e.g., patient) will be less by a significant amount due to two factors. First, the path of the photon from an "off-center" annihilation event typically traverses more than one detector crystal, as shown in Fig. 14.10. This results in an elongation of the resolution spread function along the radius of the transaxial plane. The loss of resolution is dependent on the crystal density and the diameter of the tomograph detector ring. For a 60-cm-diameter system, the resolution can deteriorate by a factor of 2 from the axis to 10 cm.

The coincidence circuitry must be able to determine coincident events with 10- to 20-ns resolution for each crystal-crystal combination (i.e., chord). The timing requirement is set jointly by the time of flight across the detector ring (4 ns) and the crystal-to-crystal resolving time (typically 3 ns). The most stringent requirement, however, is the vast number of chords in which coincidences must be determined (over 1.5 million in a 24-layer camera with septa in place and 18 million with the septa removed).

It is obviously impractical to have an individual coincidence circuit for each chord, so tomograph builders use parallel organization to solve this problem. A typical method is to use a high-speed clock (typically 200 MHz) to mark the arrival time of each 511-keV photon and a digital coincidence processor to search for coincident pairs of detected photons based on this time marker. This search can be done extremely quickly by having multiple sorters working in parallel.

The maximum event rate is also quite important, especially in septaless systems. The maximum rate in a single detector crystals is limited by the dead time due to the scintillator fluorescent lifetime (typically 1 μs per event), but as the remainder of the scintillator crystals are available, the instrument has much higher event rates (e.g., number of crystals × 1 μs). Combining crystals together to form contiguous blocks reduces the maximum event rate because the fluorescent lifetime applies to the entire block and a fraction of the tomograph is dead after each event.

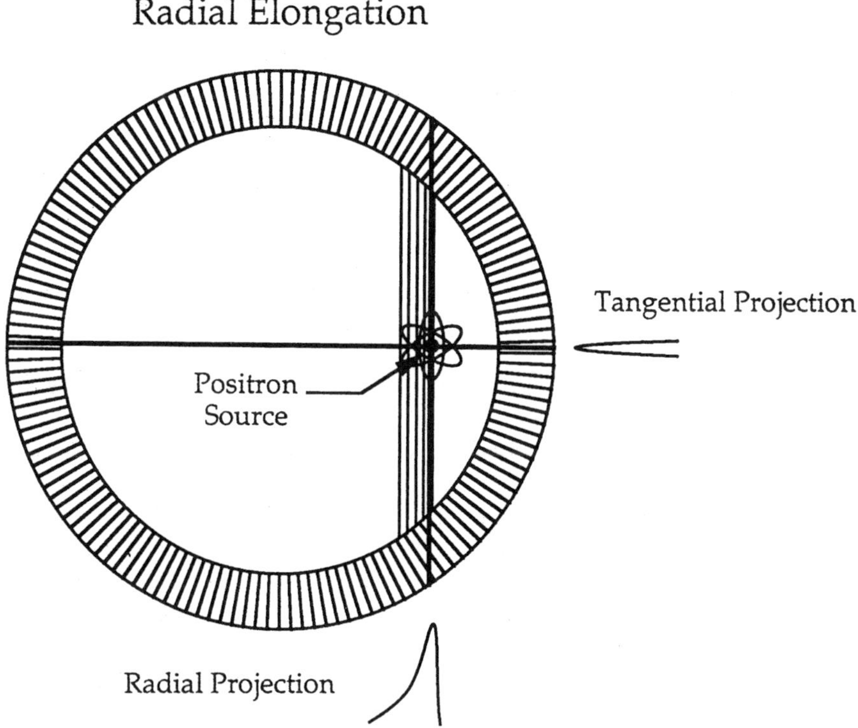

FIGURE 14.10 Resolution astigmatism in detecting off-center events. Because annihilation photons can penetrate crystals to different depths, the resolution is not equal in all directions, particularly at the edge of the imaging field. This problem of astigmatism will be taken into account in future PET instrumentation.

Random Coincidences

If two annihilation events occur within the time resolution of the tomograph (e.g., 10 ns), then random coincident "events" add erroneous background activity to the tomograph and are significant at high event rates. These can be corrected for on a chord-by-chord basis. The noncoincidence event rate of each crystal pair is measured by observing the rate of events beyond the coincident timing window. The random rate for the particular chord R_{ij} corresponding to a crystal pair is

$$R_{ij} = r_i \times r_j \times 2\tau \quad R_{ij} = R_{ij} \tag{14.2}$$

where r_i and r_j are the event rates of crystal i and crystal j, and τ is the coincidence window width. As the activity in the subject increases, the event rate in each detector increases. Thus the random event rate will increase as the square of the activity.

Tomographic Reconstruction

Before reconstruction, each projection ray or chord receives three corrections: crystal efficiency, attenuation, and random efficiency. The efficiency for each chord is computed by dividing the observed count rate for that chord by the average court rate for chords with a similar geometry (i.e., length). This is typically done daily using a transmission source without the patient or object in place. Once the patient is in position in the camera, a transmission scan is taken, and the attenuation factor for each chord is computed by dividing its transmission count rate by its efficiency count rate. The patient is then injected with the isotope, and an emission scan is taken, during which time the random count rate is also measured.

For each chord, the random event rate is subtracted from the emission rate, and the difference is divided by the attenuation factor and the chord efficiency. (The detector efficiency is divided twice because two separate detection measurements are made—transmission and emission). The resulting value is reconstructed, usually with the filtered backprojection algorithm. This is the same algorithm used in x-ray computed tomography (CT) and in projection MRI. The corrected projection data are formatted onto parallel- or fan-beam data sets for each angle. These are modified by a high-pass filter and backprojected.

The process of PET reconstruction is linear and shown by operators successively operating on the projection P:

$$A = \sum_{\theta} BPF^{-1}\ RF\left(P\right) \tag{14.3}$$

where A is the image, F is the Fourier transform, R is the ramp-shaped high-pass filter, F^{-1} is the inverse Fourier transform, BP is the backprojection operation, and ϵ denotes the superposition operation.

The alternative class of reconstruction algorithms involves iterative solutions to the classic inverse problem:

$$P = FA \tag{14.4}$$

where P is the projection matrix, A is the matrix of true data being sought, and F is the projection operation. The inverse is

$$A = F^{-1}P$$

which is computed by iteratively estimating the data A' and modifying the estimate by comparison of the calculated projection set P' with the true observed projections P. The expectation-maximization algorithm solves the inverse problem by updating each pixel value a_i in accord with

$$a_1^{k+1} = \sum p_j \frac{a_i^k f_{ij}}{\sum_i a_l^k f_{ij}} \tag{14.5}$$

where P is the measured projection, f_{ij} is the probability a source at pixel i will be detected in projection detector j, and k is the iteration.

Sensitivity

The sensitivity is a measure of how efficiently the tomograph detects coincident events and has units of count rate per unit activity concentration. It is measured by placing a known concentration of radionuclide in a water-filled 20-cm-diameter cylinder in the field of view. This cylinder, known as a *phantom*, is placed in the tomograph, and the coincidence event rate is measured. High sensitivity is important because emission imaging involves counting each event, and the resulting data are as much as 1000 times less than experienced in x-ray CT. Most tomographs have high individual detection efficiency for 511-keV photons impinging on the detector (>90%), so the sensitivity is mostly determined by geometric factors, i.e., the solid angle subtended by the tomograph:

$$S = \frac{A\varepsilon^2\gamma \times 3.7 \times 10^4}{4\pi r^2}\left(\text{events}/\text{s}\right)/\left(\text{mCi}/\text{cc}\right) \tag{14.6}$$

where: r = radius of tomograph
A = area of detector material seen by each point in the object ($2\pi r \times$ axial aperture)
ε = efficiency of scintillator
γ = attenuation factor

For a single layer, the sensitivity of a tomograph of 90 cm diameter (2-cm axial crystals) will be 15,000 events/s/μCi/ml for a disk of activity 20 cm in diameter and 1 cm thick. For a 20-cm-diameter cylinder, the sensitivity will be the same for a single layer with shields or septa that limit the off-slice activity from entering the collimators. However, modern multislice instruments use septa that allow activity from adjacent planes to be detected, thus increasing the solid angle and therefore the sensitivity. This increase comes at some cost due to increase in scatter. The improvement in sensitivity is by a factor of 7, but after correction for the noise, the improvement is 4. The noise equivalent sensitivity S_{NE} is given by

$$S_{NE} = \frac{(\text{true events})^2}{\text{true} \times \text{scatter} \times \text{random}} \tag{14.7}$$

Statistical Properties of PET

The ability to map quantitatively the spatial distribution of a positron-emitting isotope depends on adequate spatial resolution to avoid blurring. In addition, sufficient data must be acquired to allow a statistically reliable estimation of the tracer concentration. The amount of available data depends on the biomedical accumulation, the imaging system sensitivity, and the dose of injected radioactivity. The propagation of errors due to the reconstruction process results in an increase in the noise over that expected for an independent signal (e.g., $\sqrt{\text{signal}}$) by a factor proportional to the square root of the number of resolution elements (true pixels) across the image. The formula that deals with the general case of emission reconstruction (PET or SPECT) is

$$\%\ \text{uncertainty} = \frac{1.2 \times 100\,(\text{total no. of events})^{3/4}}{(\text{total no. of events})^{1/2}} \tag{14.8}$$

The statistical requirements are closely related to the spatial resolution, as shown in Fig. 14.11.

For a given accuracy or a signal-to-noise ratio for a uniform distribution, the ratio of the number of events needed in a high-resolution system to that needed in a low-resolution system is proportional to the 3/2 power of the ratio of the number of effective resolution elements in the two systems. Equation (14.8) and Fig. 14.11 should be used not with the total pixels in the image but with the effective resolution cells. The number of effective resolution cells is the sum of the occupied resolution elements weighted by the activity within each element. Suppose, however, that the activity is mainly in a few resolution cells (e.g., 100 events per cell) and the remainder of the 10,000 cells have a background of 1 event per cell. The curves of Fig. 14.11 would suggest unacceptable statistics; however, in this case, the effective number of resolution cells is below 100. The relevant equation for this situation is

$$\%\ \text{uncertainty} = \frac{1.2 \times 100\,(\text{no. of resolution cells})^{3/4}}{(\text{avg no. of events per resolution cell in target})^{3/4}} \tag{14.9}$$

The better resolution gives improved results without the requirement for a drastic increase in the number of detected events in that the improved resolution increases contrast. (It is well known that the number of events needed to detect an object is inversely related to the square of the contrast.)

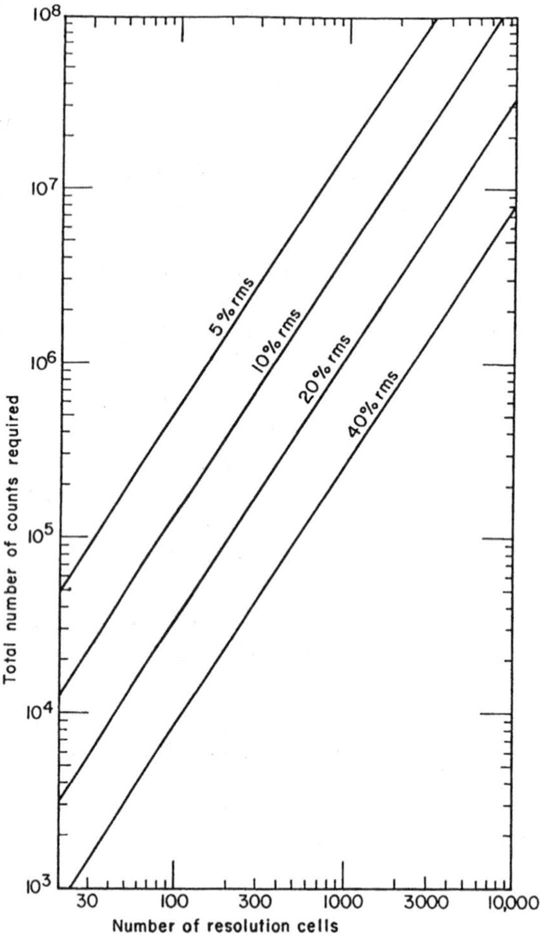

FIGURE 14.11 Statistical requirements and spatial resolution. The general relationship between the detected number of events and the number of resolution elements in an image is graphed for various levels of precision. These are relations for planes of constant thickness.

Acknowledgments

This work was supported in part by the Director, Office of Energy Research, Office of Health and Environmental Research, Medical Applications and Biophysical Research Division of the U.S. Department of Energy under Contract No. DE-AC03-SF00098 and in part by NIH Grant HL25840. I wish to thank Drs. Stephen Derenzo and William Moses, who contributed material to this presentation.

References

1. Anger HO. 1963. Gamma-ray and positron scintillator camera. Nucleonics 21:56.
2. Bailey DL. 1992. 3D acquisition and reconstruction in positron emission tomography. Ann Nucl Med 6:123.
3. Brownell GL, Sweet WH. 1953. Localization of brain tumors with positron emitters. Nucleonics 11:40.
4. Budinger TF, Greenberg WL, Derenzo SE, et al. 1978. Quantitative potentials of dynamic emission computed tomography. J Nucl Med 19:309.

5. Budinger TF, Gullberg GT, Huesman RH. 1979. Emission computed tomography. In GT Herman (ed), Topics in Applied Physics: Image Reconstruction from Projections: Implementation and Applications, pp 147–246. Berlin, Springer-Verlag.
6. Cherry SR, Dahlbom M, Hoffman EJ. 1991. 3D PET using a conventional multislice tomograph without septa. J Comput Assist Tomogr 15:655.
7. Daube-Witherspoon ME, Muehllehner G. 1987. Treatment of axial data in three-dimensional PET. J Nucl Med 28:1717.
8. Derenzo SE, Huesman RH, Cahoon JL, et al. 1988. A positron tomograph with 600 BGO crystals and 2.6 mm resolution. IEEE Trans Nucl Sci 35:659.
9. Kinahan PE, Rogers JG. 1989. Analytic 3D image reconstruction using all detected events. IEEE Trans Nucl Sci 36:964–968.
10. Shepp LA, Vardi Y. 1982. Maximum likelihood reconstruction for emission tomography. IEEE Trans Med Imaging 1:113.
11. Ter-Pogossian MM, Phelps ME, Hoffman EJ, et al. 1975. A positron-emission transaxial tomograph for nuclear imaging (PETT). Radiology 114:89.

15

Electrical Impedance Tomography

D.C. Barber
University of Sheffield

15.1 The Electrical Impedance of Tissue

The specific conductance (conductivity) of human tissues varies from 15.4 mS/cm for cerebrospinal fluid to 0.06 mS/cm for bone. The difference in the value of conductivity is large between different tissues (Table 15.1). Cross-sectional images of the distribution of conductivity, or alternatively specific resistance (resistivity), should show good contrast. The aim of electrical impedance tomography (EIT) is to produce such images. It has been shown [Kohn and Vogelius, 1984a, 1984b; Sylvester and Uhlmann, 1986] that for reasonable isotropic distributions of conductivity it is possible in principle to reconstruct conductivity images from electrical measurements made on the surface of an object. Electrical impedance tomography (EIT) is the technique of producing these images. In fact, human tissue is not simply conductive. There is evidence that many tissues also demonstrate a capacitive component of current flow and, therefore, it is appropriate to speak of the specific admittance (admittivity) or specific impedance (impedivity) of tissue rather than the conductivity; hence the word *impedance* is used in electrical impedance tomography.

15.2 Conduction in Human Tissues

Tissue consists of cells with conducting contents surrounded by insulating membranes embedded in a conducting medium. Inside and outside the cell wall is conducting fluid. At low frequencies of applied current, the current cannot pass through the membranes, and conduction is through the extracellular space. At high frequencies, current can flow through the membranes, which act as capacitors. A simple model of bulk tissue impedance based on this structure, which was proposed by Cole and Cole [1941], is shown by Fig. 15.1.

Clearly, this model as it stands is too simple, since an actual tissue sample would be better represented as a large network of interconnected modules of this form. However, it has been shown that this model fits experimental data if the values of the components, especially the capacitance, are made a power

0-8493-1810-6/03/$0.00+$1.50

function of the applied frequency ω. An equation which describes the behavior of tissue impedance as a function of frequency reasonably well is

$$\mathbf{Z} = \mathbf{Z}_\infty + \frac{\mathbf{Z}_0 - \mathbf{Z}_\infty}{1 + \left(j\dfrac{f}{f_c} \right)^\alpha} \tag{15.1}$$

where $\mathbf{Z}_0$ and $\mathbf{Z}_\infty$ are the (complex) limiting values of tissue impedance low and high frequency and f_c is a characteristic frequency. The value of α allows for the frequency dependency of the components of the model and is tissue dependent. Numerical values for *in vivo* human tissues are not well established.

TABLE 15.1 Values of Specific Conductance for Human Tissues

Tissue	Conductivity, mS/cm
Cerebrospinal fluid	15.4
Blood	6.7
Liver	2.8
Skeletal muscle	8.0 (longitudinal)
	0.6 (transverse)
Cardiac muscle	6.3 (longitudinal
	2.3 (transverse)
Neural tissue	1.7
Gray matter	3.5
White matter	1.5
Lung	1.0 (expiration)
	0.4 (inspiration)
Fat	0.36
Bone	0.06

Making measurements of the real and imaginary components of tissue impedivity over a range of frequencies will allow the components in this model to be extracted. Since it is known that tissue structure alters in disease and that *R, S, C* are dependent on structure, it should be possible to use such measurements to distinguish different types of tissue and different disease conditions. It is worth noting that although maximum accuracy in the determination of the model components can be obtained if both real and imaginary components are available, in principle, knowledge of the resistive component alone should enable the values to be determined, provided an adequate range of frequencies is used. This can have practical consequences for data collection, since accurate measurement of the capacitive component can prove difficult.

Although on a microscopic scale tissue is almost certainly electrically isotropic, on a macroscopic scale this is not so for some tissues because of their anisotropic physical structure. Muscle tissue is a prime example (see Table 15.1), where the bulk conductivity along the direction of the fibers is significantly higher than across the fibers. Although unique solutions for conductivity are possible for isotropic conductors, it can be shown that for anisotropic conductors unique solutions for conductivity do not exist. There are sets of different anisotropic conductivity distributions that give the same surface voltage distributions and which therefore cannot be distinguished by these measurements. It is not yet clear how limiting anisotropy is to electrical impedance tomography. Clearly, if sufficient data could be obtained to resolve down to the microscopic level (this is not possible practically), then tissue becomes isotropic. Moreover, the tissue distribution of conductivity, including anisotropy, often can be modeled as a network of conductors, and it is known that a unique solution will always exist for such a network. In practice, use of some prior knowledge about the anisotropy of tissue may remove the ambiguities of conductivity distribution associated with anisotropy. The degree to which anisotropy might inhibit useful image reconstruction is still an open question.

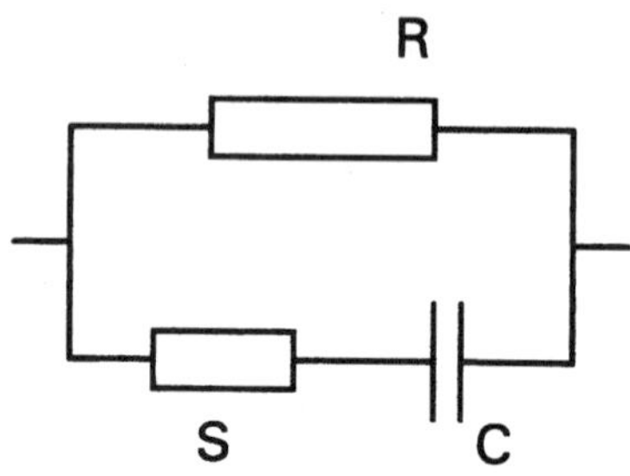

FIGURE 15.1 The Cole-Cole model of tissue impedance.

15.3 Determination of the Impedance Distribution

The distribution of electrical potential within an isotropic conducting object through which a low-frequency current is flowing is given by

$$\nabla(\sigma \nabla \phi) = 0 \tag{15.2}$$

where ϕ is the potential distribution within the object and σ is the distribution of conductivity (generally admittivity) within the object. If the conductivity is uniform, this reduces to Laplace's equation. Strictly speaking, this equation is only correct for direct current, but for the frequencies of alternating current used in EIT (up to 1 MHz) and the sizes of objects being imaged, it can be assumed that this equation continues to describe the instantaneous distribution of potential within the conducting object. If this equation is solved for a given conductivity distribution and current distribution through the surface of the object, the potential distribution developed on the surface of the object may be determined. The distribution of potential will depend on several things. It will depend on the pattern of current applied and the shape of the object. It will also depend on the internal conductivity of the object, and it is this that needs to be determined. In theory, the current may be applied in a continuous and nonuniform pattern at every point across the surface. In practice, current is applied to an object through electrodes attached to the surface of the object. Theoretically, potential may be measured at every point on the surface of the object. Again, voltage on the surface of the object is measured in practice using electrodes (possibly different from those used to apply current) attached to the surface of the object. There will be a relationship, the forward solution, between an applied current pattern j_i, the conductivity distribution σ, and the surface potential distribution ϕ_i which can be formally represented as

$$\phi_i = R(j_i, \sigma) \tag{15.3}$$

If σ and j_i are known, ϕ_i can be computed. For one current pattern j_i, knowledge of ϕ_i is not in general sufficient to uniquely determine σ. However, by applying a complete set of independent current patterns, it becomes possible to obtain sufficient information to determine σ, at least in the isotropic case. This is the **inverse solution.** In practice, measurements of surface potential or voltage can only be made at a finite number of positions, corresponding to electrodes placed on the surface of the object. This also means that only a finite number of independent current patterns can be applied. For N electrodes, $N - 1$ independent current patterns can be defined and $N(N - 1)/2$ independent measurements made. This latter number determines the limit of image resolution achievable with N electrodes. In practice, it may not be possible to collect all possible independent measurements. Since only a finite number of current patterns and measurements is available, the set of equations represented by Eq. (15.3) can be rewritten as

$$\mathbf{v} = \mathbf{A}_c \mathbf{c} \tag{15.4}$$

where $\mathbf{v}$ is now a concatenated vector of *all* voltage values for *all* current patterns, $\mathbf{c}$ is a vector of conductivity values, representing the conductivity distribution divided into uniform image pixels, and $\mathbf{A}_c$ a matrix representing the transformation of this conductivity vector into the voltage vector. Since $\mathbf{A}_c$ depends on the conductivity distribution, this equation is nonlinear. Although formally the preceding equation can be solved for $\mathbf{c}$ by inverting $\mathbf{A}_c$, the nonlinear nature of this equation means that this cannot be done in a single step. An iterative procedure will therefore be needed to obtain $\mathbf{c}$.

Examination of the physics of current flow shows that current tends to take the easiest path possible in its passage through the object. If the conductivity at some point is changed, the current path redistributes in such a way that the effects of this change are minimized. The practical effect of this is that it is possible to have fairly large changes in conductivity within the object which only produce relatively small changes in voltage at the surface of the object. The converse of this is that when reconstructing the conductivity distribution, small errors on the measured voltage data, both random and systematic, can translate into large errors in the estimate of the conductivity distribution. This effect forms, and will continue to form, a limit to the quality of reconstructed conductivity images in terms of resolution, accuracy, and sensitivity.

Any measurement of voltage must always be referred to a reference point. Usually this is one of the electrodes, which is given the nominal value of 0 V. The voltage on all other electrodes is determined by measuring the voltage difference between each electrode and the reference electrode. Alternatively, voltage

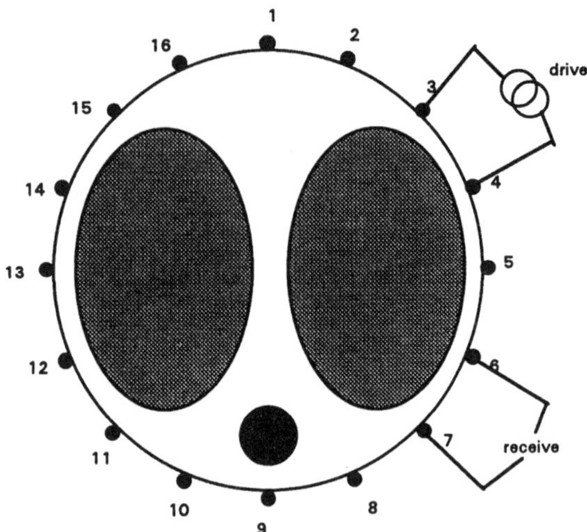

FIGURE 15.2 Idealized electrode positions around a conducting object with typical drive and measurement electrode pairs indicated.

differences may be measured between pairs of electrodes. A common approach is to measure the voltage between adjacent pairs of electrodes (Fig. 15.2). Clearly, the measurement scheme affects the form of $\mathbf{A}_c$. Choice of the pattern of applied currents and the voltage measurement scheme used can affect the accuracy with which images of conductivity can be reconstructed.

Electrical impedance tomography (EIT) is not a mature technology. However, it has been the subject of intensive research over the past few years, and this work is still continuing. Nearly all the research effort has been devoted to exploring the different possible ways of collecting data and producing images of tissue resistivity, with the aim of optimizing image reconstruction in terms of image accuracy, spatial resolution, and sensitivity.

Very few areas of medical application have been explored in any great depth, although in a number of cases preliminary work has been carried out. Although most current interest is in the use of EIT for medical imaging, there is also some interest in its use in geophysical measurements and some industrial uses. A recent detailed review of the state of electrical impedance tomography is given in Boone et al. [1997].

Data Collection

Basic Requirements

Data are collected by applying a current to the object through electrodes connected to the surface of the object and then making measurements of the voltage on the object surface through the same or other electrodes. Although conceptually simple, technically this can be difficult. Great attention must be paid to the reduction of noise and the elimination of any voltage offsets on the measurements. The currents applied are alternating currents usually in the range 10 kHz to 1 MHz. Since tissue has a complex impedance, the voltage signals will contain in-phase and out-of-phase components. In principle, both of these can be measured. In practice, measurement of the out-of-phase (the capacitive) component is significantly more difficult because of the presence of unwanted (stray) capacitances between various parts of the voltage measurement system, including the leads from the data-collection apparatus to the electrodes. These stray capacitances can lead to appreciable leakage currents, especially at the higher frequencies, which translate into systematic errors on the voltage measurements. The signal measured on an electrode, or between a pair of electrodes, oscillates at the same frequency as the applied current. The magnitude of this signal (usually separated into real and imaginary components) is determined, typically by demodulation and integration. The frequency of the demodulated signal is much less than the frequency of the applied signal, and the effects of stray capacitances on this signal are generally negligible. This realization has led some workers to propose that the signal demodulation and detection system be mounted as close to the electrodes as possible, ideally at the electrode site itself, and some systems have been developed that use this approach, although none with sufficient miniaturization of the electronics to be practical in a clinical setting. This solution is not in itself free of problems, but this approach is likely to be of increasing importance if the frequency range of applied currents is to be extended beyond 1 MHz, necessary if the value of the complex impedance is to be adequately explored as a function of frequency.

Various data-collection schemes have been proposed. Most data are collected from a two-dimensional (2D) configuration of electrodes, either from 2D objects or around the border of a plane normal to the principal axis of a cylindrical (in the general sense) object where that plane intersects the object surface. The simplest data-collection protocol is to apply a current between a pair of electrodes (often an adjacent pair) and measure the voltage difference between other adjacent pairs (see Fig. 15.2). Although in principle voltage could be measured on electrodes though which current is simultaneously flowing, the presence of an electrode impedance, generally unknown, between the electrode and the body surface means that the voltage measured is not actually that on the body surface. Various means have been suggested for either measuring the electrode impedance in some way or including it as an unknown in the image-reconstruction process. However, in many systems, measurements from electrodes through which current is flowing are simply ignored. Electrode impedance is generally not considered to be a problem when making voltage measurements on electrodes through which current is not flowing, provided a voltmeter with sufficiently high input impedance is used, although, since the input impedance is always finite, every attempt should be made to keep the electrode impedance as low as possible. Using the same electrode for driving current and making voltage measurements, even at different times in the data collection cycle, means that at some point in the data-collection apparatus wires carrying current and wires carrying voltage signals will be brought close together in a switching system, leading to the possibility of leakage currents. There is a good argument for using separate sets of electrodes for driving and measuring to reduce this problem. Paulson et al. [1992] have also proposed this approach and also have noted that it can aid in the modeling of the forward solution (see Image Reconstruction). Brown et al. [1994] have used this approach in making multifrequency measurements.

Clearly, the magnitude of the voltage measured will depend on the magnitude of the current applied. If a constant-current drive is used, this must be able to deliver a known current to a variety of input impedances with a stability of better than 0.1%. This is technically demanding. The best approach to this problem is to measure the current being applied, which can easily be done to this accuracy. These measurements are then used to normalize the voltage data.

The current application and data-collection regime will depend on the reconstruction algorithm used. Several EIT systems apply current in a distributed manner, with currents of various magnitudes being applied to several or all of the electrodes. These optimal currents (see Image Reconstruction) must be specified accurately, and again, it is technically difficult to ensure that the correct current is applied at each electrode. Although there are significant theoretical advantages to using distributed current patterns, the increased technical problems associated with this approach, and the higher noise levels associated with the increase in electronic complexity, may outweigh these advantages.

Although most EIT at present is 2D in the sense given above, it is intrinsically a three-dimensional (3D) imaging procedure, since current cannot be constrained to flow in a plane through a 3D object. 3D data collection does not pose any further problems apart from increased complexity due to the need for more electrodes. Whereas most data-collection systems to date have been based on 16 or 32 electrodes, 3D systems will require four times or more electrodes distributed over the surface of the object if adequate resolution is to be maintained. Technically, this will require "belts" or "vests" of electrodes that can be rapidly applied [McAdams et al., 1994]. Some of these are already available, and the application of an adequate number of electrodes should not prove insuperable provided electrode-mounted electronics are not required. Metherell et al. [1996] describe a 3D data collection system and reconstruction algorithm and note the improved accuracy of 3D images compared to 2D images constructed using data collected from 3D objects.

Performance of Existing Systems

Several research groups have produced EIT systems for laboratory use [Brown and Seagar, 1987; Smith et al., 1990; Rigaud et al., 1990; Jossinet and Trillaud, 1992; Lidgey et al., 1992; Riu et al., 1992; Gisser et al., 1991; Cook et al., 1994; Brown et al., 1994; Zhu et al., 1994; Cusick et al., 1994] and some clinical trials. The complexity of the systems largely depends on whether current is applied via a pair of electrodes (usually adjacent) or whether through many electrodes simultaneously. The former systems are much simpler in design and construction and can deliver higher signal-to-noise ratios. The Sheffield Mark II system (Smith et al., 1990) used 16 electrodes and was capable of providing signal-to-noise ratios of up to 68 dB at 25 data sets per second. The average image resolution achievable across the image was 15% of the image diameter. In general, multifrequency systems have not yet delivered similar performance, but are being continuously improved.

Spatial resolution and noise levels are the most important constraints on possible clinical applications of EIT. As images are formed through a reconstruction process the values of these parameters will depend critically on the quality of the data collected and the reconstruction process used. However, practical limitations to the number of electrodes which can be used and the ill-posed nature of the reconstruction problem make it unlikely that high-quality images, comparable to other medical imaging modalities, can be produced. The impact of this on diagnostic performance still needs to be evaluated.

Image Reconstruction

Basics of Reconstruction

Although several different approaches to image reconstruction have been tried [Wexler, 1985; Yorkey et al., 1986; Barber and Seagar, 1987; Kim et al., 1987; Hua et al., 1988; Cheny et al., 1990; Breckon, 1990; Zadecoochak et al., 1991; Kotre et al., 1992; Bayford et al., 1994; Morucci et al., 1994], the most accurate approaches are based broadly on the following algorithm. For a given set of current patterns, a forward transform is set up for determining the voltages **v** produced form the conductivity distribution **c** (Eq. 15.4). $\mathbf{A}_c$ is dependent on **c**, so it is necessary to assume an initial starting conductivity distribution $\mathbf{c}_0$. This is usually taken to be uniform. Using $\mathbf{A}_c$, the expected voltages $\mathbf{v}_0$ are calculated and compared with the actual measured voltages $\mathbf{v}_m$. Unless $\mathbf{c}_0$ is correct (which it will not be initially), $\mathbf{v}_0$ and $\mathbf{v}_m$ will differ. It can be shown that an improved estimate of **c** is given by

$$\Delta \mathbf{c} = \left(\mathbf{S}_c^t \mathbf{S}_c\right)^{-1} \mathbf{S}_c^t \left(\mathbf{v}_0 - \mathbf{v}_m\right) \tag{15.5}$$

$$\mathbf{c}_1 = \mathbf{c}_0 + \Delta \mathbf{c} \tag{15.6}$$

where $\mathbf{S}_c$ is the differential of $\mathbf{A}_c$ with respect to **c**, the sensitivity matrix and $\mathbf{S}_c^t$ is the transpose of $\mathbf{S}_c$. The improved value of **c** is then used in the next iteration to compute an improved estimate of $\mathbf{v}_m$, i.e., $\mathbf{v}_1$. This iterative process is continued until some appropriate endpoint is reached. Although convergence is not guaranteed, in practice, convergence to the correct **c** in the absence of noise can be expected, provided a good starting value is chosen. Uniform conductivity seems to be a reasonable choice. In the presence of noise on the measurements, iteration is stopped when the difference between **v** and $\mathbf{v}_m$ is within the margin of error set by the known noise on the data.

There are some practical difficulties associated with this approach. One is that large changes in **c** may only produce small changes in **v**, and this will be reflected in the structure of $\mathbf{S}_c$, making $\mathbf{S}_c^t\mathbf{S}_c$ very difficult to invert reliably. Various methods of regularization have been used, with varying degrees of success, to achieve stable inversion of this matrix although the greater the regularization applied, the poorer the resolution that can be achieved. A more difficult practical problem is that for convergence to be possible the computed voltages **v** must be equal to the measured voltages $\mathbf{v}_m$ when the correct conductivity values are used in the forward calculation. Although in a few idealized cases analytical solutions of the forward problem are possible, in general, numerical solutions must be used. Techniques such as the finite-element method (FEM) have been developed to solve problems of this type numerically. However, the accuracy of these methods has to be carefully examined [Paulson et al., 1992] and, while they are adequate for many applications, they may not be adequate for the EIT reconstruction problem, especially in the case of 3D objects. Accuracies of rather better than 1% appear to be required if image artifacts are to be minimized. Consider a situation in which the actual distortion of conductivity is uniform. Then the initial $\mathbf{v}$ should be equal to the $\mathbf{v}_m$ to an accuracy less than the magnitude of the noise. If this is not the case, then the algorithm will alter the conductivity distribution from uniform, which will clearly result in error. While the required accuracies have been approached under ideal conditions, there is only a limited amount of evidence at present to suggest that they can be achieved with data taken from human subjects.

Optimal Current Patterns

So far little has been said about the form of the current patterns applied to the object except that a set of independent patterns is needed. The simplest current patterns to use are those given by passing current into the object through one electrode and extracting current through a second electrode (a bipolar pattern). This pattern has the virtue of simplicity and ease of application. However, other current patterns are possible. Current can be passed simultaneously through many electrodes, with different amounts passing through each electrode. Indeed, an infinite number of patterns are possible, the only limiting condition being that the magnitude of the current flowing into the conducting object equals the magnitude of the current flowing out of the object. Isaacson [1986] has shown that for any conducting object there is a set of optimal current patterns and has provided an algorithm to compute them even if the conductivity distribution is initially unknown. Isaacson showed that by using optimal patterns, significant improvements in sensitivity could be obtained compared with simpler two-electrode current patterns. However, the additional computation and hardware required to use optimal current patterns compared with fixed, nonoptimal patterns are considerable.

Use of suboptimal patterns close to optimum also will produce significant gains. In general, the optimal patterns are very different from the patterns produced in the simple two-electrode case. The optimal patterns are often cosine-like patterns of current amplitude distributed around the object boundary rather than being localized at a pair of points, as in the two-electrode case. Since the currents are passed simultaneously through many electrodes, it is tempting to try and use the same electrodes for voltage measurements. This produces two problems. As noted above, measurement of voltage on an electrode through which an electric current is passing is compromised by the presence of electrode resistance, which causes a generally unknown voltage drop across the electrode, whereas voltage can be accurately measured on an electrode through which current is not flowing using a voltmeter of high input impedance. In addition, it has proved difficult to model current flow around an electrode through which current is flowing with sufficient accuracy to allow the reliable calculation of voltage on that electrode, which is needed for accurate reconstruction. It seems that separate electrodes should be used for voltage measurements with distributed current systems.

Theoretically, distributed (near-) optimal current systems have some advantages. As each of the optimal current patterns is applied, it is possible to determine if the voltage patterns produced contain any useful information or if they are simply noise. Since the patterns can be generated and applied in order of decreasing significance, it is possible to terminate application of further current patterns when no further information can be obtained. A consequence of this is that SNRs can be maximized for a given total data-collection time. With bipolar current patterns this option is not available. All patterns must be applied. Provided the SNR in the data is sufficiently good and only a limited number of electrodes are used, this may not be too important, and the extra effort involved in generating the optimal or near-optimal patterns may not be justified. However, as the number of electrodes is increased, the use of optimal patterns becomes more significant. It also has been suggested that the distributed nature of the optimal patterns makes the forward problem less sensitive to modeling errors. Although there is currently no firm evidence for this, this seems a reasonable assertion.

Three-Dimensional Imaging

Most published work so far on image reconstruction has concentrated on solving the 2D problem. However, real medical objects, i.e., patients, are three dimensional. Theoretically, as the dimensionality of the object increases, reconstruction should become better conditioned. However, unlike 3D x-ray images, which can be constructed from a set of independent 2D images, EIT data from 3D objects cannot be so decomposed and data from over the whole surface of the object is required for 3D reconstruction. The principles of reconstruction in 3D are identical to the 2D situation although practically the problem is quite formidable, principally because of the need to solve the forward problem in three dimensions. Some early work on 3D imaging was presented by Goble and Isaacson [1990]. More recently Metherall et al. [1996] have shown images using data collected from human subjects.

Single-Step Reconstruction

The complete reconstruction problem is nonlinear and requires iteration. However, each step in the iterative process is linear. Images reconstructed using only the first step of iteration effectively treat image formation as a linear process, an assumption approximately justified for small changes in conductivity from uniform. In the case the functions $\mathbf{A}_c$ and $\mathbf{S}_c$ often can be precomputed with reasonable accuracy because they usually are computed for the case of uniform conductivity. Although the solution cannot be correct, since the nonlinearity is not taken into account, it may be useful, and first-step linear approximations have gained some popularity. Cheney et al. [1990] have published some results from a first-step process using optimal currents. Most, if not all, of the clinical images produced to date have used a single-step reconstruction algorithm [Barber and Seagar, 1987; Barber and Brown, 1990]. Although this algorithm uses very nonoptimal current patterns, this has not so far been a limitation because of the high quality of data collected and the limited number of electrodes used (16). With larger numbers of electrodes, this conclusion may need to be revised.

Differential Imaging

Ideally, the aim of EIT is to reconstruct images of the absolute distribution of conductivity (or admittivity). These images are known as absolute (or static) images. However, this requires that the forward problem can be solved to an high degree of accuracy, and this can be difficult. The magnitude of the voltage signal measured on an electrode or between electrodes will depend on the body shape, the electrode shape and position, and the internal conductivity distribution. The signal magnitude is in fact dominated by the first two effects rather than by conductivity. However, if a *change* in conductivity occurs within the object, then it can often be assumed that the *change* in surface voltage is dominated by this conductivity change. In differential (or dynamic) imaging, the aim is to image changes in conductivity rather than absolute values. If the voltage difference between a pair of (usually adjacent) electrodes before a conductivity change occurs is $\mathbf{g}_1$ and the value after change occurs is $\mathbf{g}_2$, then a normalized data value is defined as

$$\Delta\mathbf{g}_n = 2\frac{\mathbf{g}_1 - \mathbf{g}_2}{\mathbf{g}_1 + \mathbf{g}_2} = \frac{\Delta\mathbf{g}}{\mathbf{g}_{\text{mean}}} \tag{15.7}$$

Many of the effects of body shape (including interpreting the data as coming from a 2D object when in fact it is from a 3D object) and electrode placing at least partially cancel out in this definition. The values of the normalized data are determined largely by the conductivity changes. It can be argued that the relationship between the (normalized) changes in conductivity $\Delta\mathbf{c}_n$ and the normalized changes in boundary data $\Delta\mathbf{g}_n$ is given by

$$\Delta\mathbf{g}_n = \mathbf{F}\Delta\mathbf{c}_n \tag{15.8}$$

where $\mathbf{F}$ is a sensitivity matrix which it can be shown is much less sensitive to object shape end electrode positions than the sensitivity matrix of Eq. 15.5. Although images produced using this algorithm are not

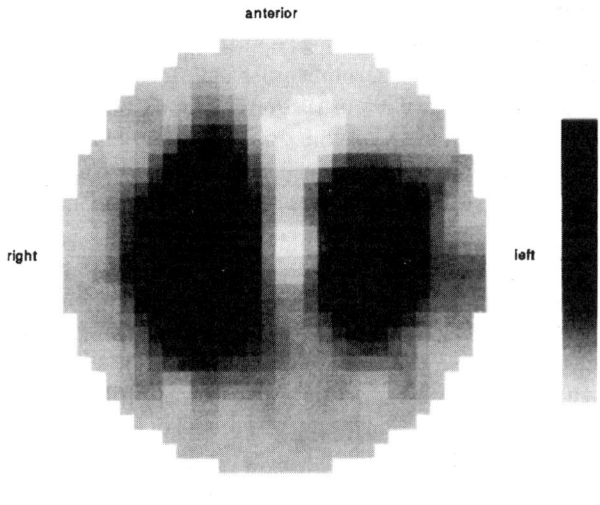

FIGURE 15.3 A differential conductivity image representing the changes in conductivity in going from maximum inspiration (breathing in) to maximum expiration (breathing out). Increasing blackness represents increasing conductivity.

completely free of artifact that is the only algorithm which has reliably produced images using data taken from human subjects. Metherall et al. [1996] used a version of this algorithm for 3D imaging and Brown et al. [1994] for multifrequency imaging, in this case imaging changes in conductivity with frequency.

The principal disadvantage of this algorithm is that it can only image changes in conductivity, which must be either natural or induced. Figure 15.3 shows a typical differential image. This represents the changes in the conductivity of the lungs between expiration and inspiration.

Multifrequency Measurements

Differential algorithms can only image changes in conductivity. Absolute distributions of conductivity cannot be produced using these methods. In addition, any gross movement of the electrodes, either because they have to be removed and replaced or even because of significant patient movement, make the use of this technique difficult for long-term measurements of changes. As an alternative to changes in time, differential algorithms can image changes in conductivity with frequency. Brown et al. [1994] have shown that if measurements are made over a range of frequencies and differential images produced using data from the lowest frequency and the other frequencies in turn, these images can be used to compute parametric images representing the distribution of combinations of the circuit values in Fig. 15.1. For example, images representing the ratio of S to R, a measure of the ratio of intracellular to extracellular volume, can be produced, as well as images of $f_o = 1/2\pi(RC + SC)$, the tissue characteristic frequency. Although not images of the absolute distribution of conductivity, they are images of absolute tissue properties. Since these properties are related to tissue structure, they should produce images with useful contrast. Data sufficient to reconstruct an image can be collected in a time short enough to preclude significant patient movement, which means these images are robust against movement artifacts. Changes of these parameters with time can still be observed.

15.4 Areas of Clinical Application

There is no doubt that the clinical strengths of EIT relate to its ability to be considered as a functional imaging modality that carries no hazard and can therefore be used for monitoring purposes. The best spatial resolution that might become available will still be much worse than anatomic imaging methods such as magnetic resonance imaging and x-ray computed tomography. However, EIT is able to image small changes in tissue conductivity such as those associated with blood perfusion, lung ventilation, and fluid shifts. Clinical applications seek to take advantage of the ability of EIT to follow rapid changes in physiologic function.

There are several areas in clinical medicine where EIT might provide advantages over existing techniques. These have been received elsewhere [Brown et al., 1985; Dawids, 1987; Holder and Brown, 1990; Boone et al., 1997].

Possible Biomedical Applications

Gastrointestinal System

A priori, it seems likely that EIT could be applied usefully to measurement of motor activity in the gut. Electrodes can be applied with ease around the abdomen, and there are no large bony structures likely to seriously violate the assumption of constant initial conductivity. During motor activity, such as gastric emptying or peristalsis, there are relatively large movements of the conducting fluids within the bowel. The quantity of interest is the timing of activity, e.g., the rate at which the stomach empties, and the absolute impedance change and its exact location in space area of secondary importance. The principal limitations of EIT of poor spatial resolution and amplitude measurement are largely circumvented in this application [Avill et al., 1987]. There has also been some interest in the measurement of other aspects of gastrointestinal function such as esophageal activity [Erol et al., 1995].

Respiratory System

Lung pathology can be imaged by conventional radiography, x-ray computed tomography, or magnetic resonance imaging, but there are clinical situations where it would be desirable to have a portable means of imaging regional lung ventilation which could, if necessary, generate repeated images over time. Validation studies have shown that overall ventilation can be measured with good accuracy [Harris et al., 1988]. More recent work [Hampshire et al., 1995] suggests that multifrequency measurements may be useful in the diagnosis of some lung disorders.

EIT Imaging of Changes in Blood Volume

The conductivity of blood is about 6.7 mS/cm, which is approximately three times that of most intrathoracic tissues. It therefore seems possible that EIT images related to blood flow could be accomplished. The imaged quantity will be the change in conductivity due to replacement of tissue by blood (or vice versa) as a result of the pulsatile flow through the thorax. This may be relatively large in the cardiac ventricles but will be smaller in the peripheral lung fields.

The most interesting possibility is that of detecting pulmonary embolus (PE). If a blood clot is present in the lung, the lung beyond the clot will not be perfused, and under favorable circumstances, this may be visualized using a gated blood volume image of the lung. In combination with a ventilation image, which should show normal ventilation in this region, pulmonary embolism could be diagnosed. Some data [Leathard et al., 1994] indicate that PE can be visualized in human subjects. Although more sensitive methods already exist for detecting PE, the noninvasiveness and bedside availability of EIT mean that treatment of the patient could be monitored over the period following the occurrence of the embolism, an important aim, since the use of anticoagulants, the principal treatment for PE, needs to be minimized in postoperative patients, a common class of patients presenting with this complication.

15.5 Summary and Future Developments

EIT is still an emerging technology. In its development, several novel and difficult measurement and image-reconstruction problems have had to be addressed. Most of these have been satisfactorily solved. The current generation of EIT imaging systems are multifrequency, with some capable of 3D imaging. These should be capable of greater quantitative accuracy and be less prone to image artifact and are likely to find a practical role in clinical diagnosis. Although there are still many technical problems to be answered and many clinical applications to be addressed, the technology may be close to coming of age.

Defining Terms

Absolute imaging: Imaging the actual distribution of conductivity.

Admittivity: The specific admittance of an electrically conducting material. For simple biomedical materials such as saline with no reactive component of resistance, this is the same as conductivity.

Anisotropic conductor: A material in which the conductivity is dependent on the direction in which it is measured through the material.

Applied current pattern: In EIT, the electric current is applied to the surface of the conducting object via electrodes placed on the surface of the object. The spatial distribution of current flow through the surface of the object is the applied current pattern.

Bipolar current pattern: A current pattern applied between a single pair of electrodes.

Conductivity: The specific conductance of an electrically conducting material. The inverse of resistivity.

Differential imaging: An EIT imaging technique that specifically images changes in conductivity.

Distributed current: A current pattern applied through more than two electrodes.

Dynamic imaging: The same as differential imaging.

EIT: Electrical impedance tomography.

Forward transform or problem or solution: The operation, real or computational, that maps or transforms the conductivity distribution to surface voltages.

Impedivity: The specific impedance of an electrically conducting material. The inverse of admittivity. For simple biomedical materials such as saline with no reactive component of resistance, this is the same as resistivity.

Inverse transform or problem or solution: The computational operation that maps voltage measurements on the surface of the object to the conductivity distribution.

Optimal current: One of a set of a current patterns computed for a particular conductivity distribution that produce data with maximum possible SNR.

Pixel: The conductivity distribution is usually represented as a set of connected piecewise uniform patches. Each of these patches is a pixel. The pixel may take any shape, but square or triangular shapes are most common.

Resistivity: The specific electrical resistance of an electrical conducting material. The inverse of conductivity.

Static imaging: The same as absolute imaging.

References

Avill RF, Mangnall RF, Bird NC, et al. 1987. Applied potential tomography: A new non-invasive technique for measuring gastric emptying. Gastroenterology 92:1019.

Barber DC, Brown BH. 1990. Progress in electrical impedance tomography. In D Colton, R Ewing, W Rundell (eds), Inverse Problems in Partial Differential Equations, pp 149–162. New York, SIAM.

Barber DC, Seagar AD. 1987. Fast reconstruction of resistive images. Clin Phys Physiol Meas 8(A):47.

Bayford R. 1994. Ph.D. thesis. Middlesex University, U.K.

Boone K, Barber D, Brown B. 1992. Imaging with electricity: Report of the European Concerted Action on Impedance Tomography. J Med Eng Tech 21:6 pp 201–232.

Breckon WR. 1990. Image Reconstruction in Electrical Impedance Tomography. Ph.D. thesis, School of Computing and Mathematical Sciences, Oxford Polytechnic, Oxford, U.K.

Brown BH, Barber DC, Seagar AD. 1985. Applied potential tomography: Possible clinical applications. Clin Phys Physiol Meas 6:109.

Brown BH, Barber DC, Wang W, et al. 1994. Multifrequency imaging and modelling of respiratory related electrical impedance changes. Physiol Meas 15:A1.

Brown DC, Seagar AD. 1987. The Sheffield data collection system. Clin Phys Physiol Meas 8(suppl A):91–98.

Cheney MD, Isaacson D, Newell J, et al. 1990. Noser: An algorithm for solving the inverse conductivity problem. Int J Imag Syst Tech 2:60.

Cole KS, Cole RH. 1941. Dispersion and absorption in dielectrics: I. Alternating current characteristics. J Chem Phys 9:431.

Cook RD, Saulnier GJ, Gisser DG, Goble J, Newell JC, Isaacson D. 1994. ACT3: A high-speed high-precision electrical impedance tomograph. IEEE Trans Biomed Eng 41:713–722.

Cusick G, Holder DS, Birkett A, Boone KG. 1994. A system for impedance imaging of epilepsy in ambulatory human subjects. Innovation Technol Biol Med 15(suppl 1):34–39.

Dawids SG. 1987. Evaluation of applied potential tomography: A clinician's view. Clin Phys Physiol Meas 8(A):175.

Erol RA, Smallwood RH, Brown BH, Cherian P, Bardham KD. 1995. Detecting oesophageal-related changes using electrical impedance tomography. Physiol Meas 16(suppl 3A):143–152.

Gisser DG, Newell JC, Salunier G, Hochgraf C, Cook RD, Goble JC. 1991. Analog electronics for a high-speed high-precision electrical impedance tomograph. Proc IEEE EMBS 13:23–24.

Goble J, Isaacson D. 1990. Fast reconstruction algorithms for three-dimensional electrical tomography. In IEEE EMBS Proceedings of the 12th Annual International Conference, Philadelphia, pp 285–286.

Hampshire AR, Smallwood RH, Brown BH, Primhak RA. 1995. Multifrequency and parametric EIT images of neonatal lungs. Physiol Meas 16(suppl 3A):175–189.

Harris ND, Sugget AJ, Barber DC, Brown BH. 1988. Applied potential tomography: A new technique for monitoring pulmonary function. Clin Phys Physiol Meas 9(A):79.

Holder DS, Brown BH. 1990. Biomedical applications of EIT: A critical review. In D Holder (ed), Clinical and Physiological Applications of Electrical Impedance Tomography, pp 6–41. London, UCL Press.

Hua P, Webster JG, Tompkins WJ. 1988. A regularized electrical impedance tomography reconstruction algorithm. Clin Phys Physiol Meas 9(suppl A):137–141.

Isaacson D. 1986. Distinguishability of conductivities by electric current computed tomography. IEEE Trans Med Imaging 5:91.

Jossinet J, Trillaud C. 1992. Imaging the complex impedance in electrical impedance tomography. Clin Phys Physiol Meas 13(A):47.

Kim H, Woo HW. 1987. A prototype system and reconstruction algorithms for electrical impedance technique in medical imaging. Clin Phys Physiol Meas 8(A):63.

Kohn RV, Vogelius M. 1984a. Determining the conductivity by boundary measurement. Commun Pure Appl Math 37:289.

Kohn RV, Vogelius M. 1984b. Identification of an unknown conductivity by means of the boundary. SIAM-AMS Proc 14:113.

Koire CJ. 1992. EIT image reconstruction using sensitivity coefficient weighted backprojection. Physiol Meas 15(suppl 2A):125–136.

Leathard AD, Brown BH, Campbell J, et al. 1994. A comparison of ventilatory and cardiac related changes in EIT images of normal human lungs and of lungs with pulmonary embolism. Physiol Meas 15:A137.

Lidgey FJ, Zhu QS, McLeod CN, Breckon W. 1992. Electrode current determination from programmable current sources. Clin Phys Physiol Meas 13(suppl A):43–46.

McAdams ET, McLaughlin JA, Anderson JMcC. 1994. Multielectrode systems for electrical impedance tomography. Physiol Meas 15:A101.

Metherall P, Barber DC, Smallwood RH, Brown BH. 1996. Three-dimensional electrical impedance tomography. Physiol Meas 15:A101.

Morucci JP, Marsili PM, Granie M, Dai WW, Shi Y. 1994. Direct sensitivity matrix approach for fast reconstruction in electrical impedance tomography. Physiol Meas 15(suppl 2A):107–114.

Riu PJ, Rosell J, Lozano A, Pallas-Areny RA. 1992. Broadband system for multi-frequency static imaging in electrical impedance tomography. Clin Phys Physiol Meas 13(A):61.

Smith RWM. 1990. Design of a Real-Time Impedance Imaging System for Medical Applications. Ph.D. thesis, University of Sheffield, U.K.

Sylvester J, Uhlmann G. 1986. A uniqueness theorem for an inverse boundary value problem in electrical prospection. Commun Pure Appl Math 39:91.

Wexler A, Fry B, Neuman MR. 1985. Impedance-computed tomography: Algorithm and system. Appl Opt 24:3985.

Yorkey TJ. 1986. Comparing Reconstruction Algorithms for Electrical Impedance Imaging. Ph.D. thesis, University of Wisconsin, Madison.

Zadehkoochak M, Blott BH, Hames TK, George RE. 1991. Special expansion in electrical impedance tomography. J Phys D: Appl Phys 24:1911–1916.

Zhu QS, McLeod CN, Denyer CW, Lidgey FL, Lionheart WRB. 1994. Development of a real-time adaptive current tomograph. Clin Phys Physiol Meas 15(suppl 2A):37–43.

Further Information

All the following conferences were funded by the European commission under the biomedical engineering program. The first two were directly funded as exploratory workshops, the remainder as part of a Concerted Action on Electrical Impedance Tomography. Electrical Impedance Tomography—Applied Potential Tomography. 1987. Proceedings of a conference held in Sheffield, U.K., 1986. Published in Clin Phys Physiol Meas 8:Suppl.A. Electrical Impedance Tomography—Applied Potential Tomography. 1988. Proceedings of a conference held in Lyon, France, November 1987. Published in Clin Phys Physiol Meas 9:Suppl.A. Electrical Impedance Tomography. 1991. Proceedings of a conference held in Copenhagen, Denmark, July 1990. Published by Medical Physics, University of Sheffield, U.K. Electrical Impedance Tomography. 1992. Proceedings of a conference held in York, U.K., July 1991. Published in Clin Phys Physiol Meas 13:Suppl.A. Clinical and Physiologic Applications of Electrical Impedance Tomography. 1993. Proceedings of a conference held at the Royal Society, London, U.K. April 1992. Ed. D.S. Holder, UCL Press, London. Electrical Impedance Tomography. 1994. Proceedings of a conference held in Barcelona, Spain, 1993. Published in Clin Phys Physiol Meas 15:Suppl.A.

16

Medical Applications of Virtual Reality Technology

Walter Greenleaf
Greenleaf Medical

Tom Piantanida
Greenleaf Medical

Virtual Reality (VR) is the term commonly used to describe a novel human-computer interface that enables users to interact with computers in a radically different way. VR consists of a computer-generated, *multidimensional* environment and interface tools that allow users to:

1. *immerse* themselves in the environment,
2. *navigate* within the environment, and
3. *interact* with objects and other inhabitants in the environment.

The experience of entering this environment—this computer-generated virtual world—is compelling. To enter, the user usually dons a helmet containing a head-mounted display (HMD) that incorporates a sensor to track the wearer's movement and location. The user may also wear sensor-clad clothing that likewise tracks movement and location. The sensors communicate position and location data to a computer, which updates the image of the virtual world accordingly. By employing this garb, the user "breaks through" the computer screen and becomes completely immersed in this multidimensional world. Thus immersed, one can walk through a virtual house, drive a virtual car, or run a marathon in a park still under design. Recent advances in computer processor speed and graphics make it possible for even desktop computers to create highly realistic environments. The practical applications are far reaching. Today, using VR, architects design office buildings, NASA controls robots at remote locations, and physicians plan and practice difficult operations.

0-8493-1810-6/03/$0.00+$1.50

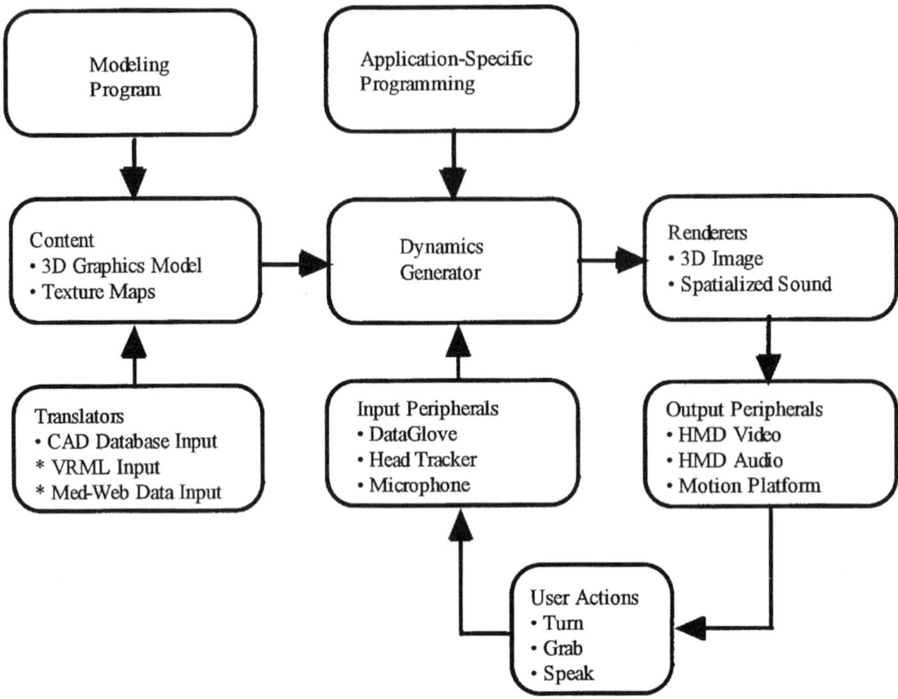

FIGURE 16.1 A complete VR system.

Virtual reality is quickly finding wide acceptance in the medical community as researchers and clinicians alike become aware of its potential benefits. Several pioneer research groups have already demonstrated improved clinical performance using VR imaging, planning, and control techniques.

16.1 Overview of Virtual Reality Technology

The term "virtual reality" describes the experience of interacting with data from within the computer-generated data set. The computer-generated data set may be completely synthetic or remotely sensed, such as x-ray, MRI, PET, etc. images. Interaction with the data is natural and intuitive and occurs from a first-person perspective. From a system perspective, VR technology can be segmented as shown in Fig. 16.1.

The computer-generated environment, or virtual world *content* consists of a *3D graphic model,* typically implemented as a spatially organized, object-oriented database; each object in the database represents an object in the virtual world.

A separate *modeling program* is used to create the individual objects for the virtual world. For greater realism, *texture maps* are used to create visual surface detail.

The data set is manipulated using a real-time *dynamics generator* that allows objects to be moved within the world according to natural laws such as gravity and inertia, or according to other variables such as spring-rate and flexibility that are specified for each particular experience by *application-specific programming.*

The dynamics generator also tracks the position and orientation of the user's head and hand using *input peripherals* such as a *head tracker* and *DataGlove.*

Powerful *renderers* are applied to present 3D images and 3D spatialized sound in real time to the observer.

The common method of working with a computer (the mouse/keyboard/monitor paradigm), based as it is on a two-dimensional desktop metaphor, is inappropriate for the multidimensional virtual

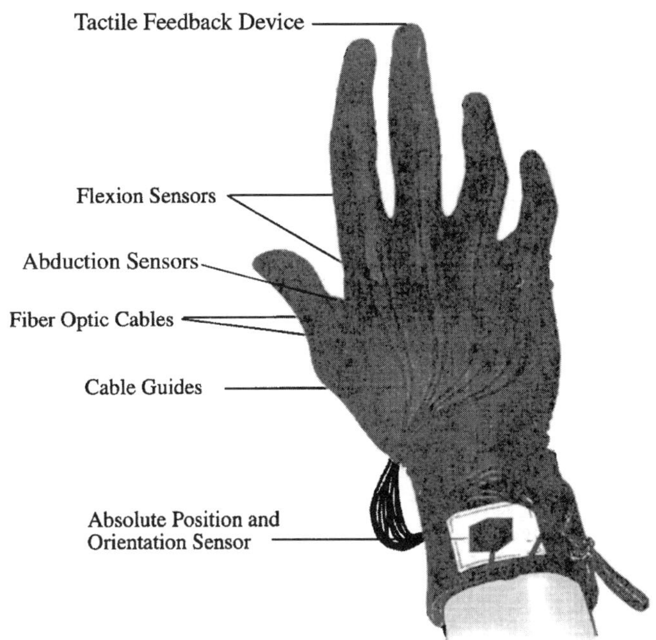

FIGURE 16.2 The DataGlove™, a VR control device.

world. Therefore, one long-term challenge for VR developers has been to replace the conventional computer interface with one that is more natural, intuitive, and allows the computer—not the user—to carry a greater proportion of the interface burden. Not surprisingly, this search for a more practical multidimensional metaphor for interacting with computers and computer-generated artificial environments has spawned the development of a new generation of computer interface hardware. Ideally, the interface hardware should consist of two components: (1) sensors for controlling the virtual world and (2) effectors for providing feedback to the user. To date, three new computer-interface mechanisms, not all of which manifest the ideal sensor/effector duality, have evolved: Instrumented Clothing, the Head Mounted Display (HMD), and 3D Sound Systems.

Instrumented Clothing

The DataGlove™ and DataSuit™ use dramatic new methods to measure human motion dynamically in real time. The clothing is instrumented with sensors that track the full range of motion of specific activities of the person wearing the glove or suit, for example, as the wearer bends, moves, grasps, or waves.

The DataGlove is a thin lycra glove with bend-sensors running along its dorsal surface. When the joints of the hand bend, the sensors bend and the angular movement is recorded by the sensors. These recordings are digitized and forwarded to the computer, which calculates the angle at which each joint is bent. On screen, an image of the hand moves in real time, reflecting the movements of the hand in the DataGlove and immediately replicating even the most subtle actions.

The DataGlove is often used in conjunction with an absolute position and orientation sensor that allows the computer to determine the three space coordinates, as well as the orientation of the hand and fingers. A similar sensor can be used with the DataSuit and is nearly always used with an HMD.

The DataSuit is a customized body suit fitted with the same sophisticated bend-sensors found in the DataGlove. While the DataGlove is currently in production as both a VR interface and as a data-collection instrument, the DataSuit is available only as a custom device. As noted, DataGlove and DataSuit are utilized as general-purpose computer interface devices for VR. There are several potential applications of this new technology for clinical and therapeutic medicine.

Head-Mounted Display (HMD)

The best-known sensor/effector system in VR is a *head-mounted display* (HMD). It supports first-person immersion by generating an image for each eye, which, in some HMDs, may provide stereoscopic vision. Most lower cost HMDs ($6000 range) use LCD displays; others use small CRTs. The more expensive HMDs ($60,000 and up) use optical fibers to pipe the images from remotely mounted CRTs. An HMD requires a position/orientation sensor in addition to the visual display. Some displays, for example, the BOOM System [Bolas, 1994], may be head-mounted or may be used as a remote window into a virtual world.

3D Spatialized Sound

The impression of immersion within a virtual environment is greatly enhanced by inclusion of 3D spatialized sound [Durlach, 1994; Hendrix and Barfield, 1996]. Stereo-pan effects alone are inadequate since they tend to sound as if they are originating inside the head. Research into 3D audio has shown the importance of modeling the head and pinea and using this model as part of the 3D sound generation. A Head Related Transfer Function (HRTF) can be used to a generate the proper acoustics [Begault and Wenzel, 1992; Wenzel, 1994]. A number of problems remain, such as the "cone of confusion" wherein sounds behind the head are perceived to be in front of the head [Wenzel, 1992].

Other VR Interface Technology

A sense of motion can be generated in a VR system by a motion platform. These have been used in flight simulators to provide cues that the mind integrates with visual and spatialized sound cues to generate perception of velocity and acceleration.

Haptics is the science of touch. Haptic interfaces generate perception of touch and resistance in VR. Most systems to date have focused on providing force feedback to enable users to sense the inertial qualities of virtual objects, and/or kinesthetic feedback to specify the location of a virtual object in the world [Salisbury and Srinivasan, 1996, 1997]. A few prototype systems exist that generate tactile stimulation, which allows users to feel the surface qualities of virtual objects [Minsky and Lederman, 1996]. Many of the haptic systems developed thus far consist of exoskeletons that provide position sensing as well as active force application [Burdea et al., 1992].

Some preliminary work has been conducted on generating the sense of temperature in VR. Small electrical heat pumps have been developed that produce sensations of heat and cold as part of the simulated environment. (See, for example, Caldwell and Gosney [1993]; Ino et al. [1993].)

Olfaction is another sense that provides important cues in the real world. Consider, for example, a surgeon or dentist examining a patient for a potential bacterial infection. Inflammation and swelling may be present, but a major deciding factor is the odor of the lesion. Very early in the history of virtual reality, Mort Heilig patented his Sensorama Simulator, which incorporated olfactory, as well as visual, auditory, and motion cues (U.S. patent 3850870, 1961). Recently, another pioneer of virtual reality, Myron Kreuger [Kreuger, 1994, 1995a, 1995b], has been developing virtual olfaction systems for use in medical training applications. The addition of virtual olfactory cues to medical training systems should greatly enhance both the realism and effectiveness of training.

16.2 VR Application Examples

Virtual reality had been researched for years in government laboratories and universities, but because of the enormous computing power demands and associated high costs, applications have been slow to migrate from the research world to other areas. Continual improvements in the price/performance ratio of graphic computer systems, however, have made VR technology more affordable and, thus, used more commonly in a wider range of application areas. In fact, there is even a strong "Garage VR" movement—groups of interested parties sharing information on how to build extremely low-cost VR systems using inexpensive off-the-shelf components [Jacobs, 1994]. These home-made systems are often inefficient, uncomfortable to use (sometimes painful), and slow, but they exist as a strong testament to a fervent interest in VR technology.

VR Applications

Applications today are diverse and represent dramatic improvements over conventional visualization and planning techniques:

Public Entertainment: VR made its first major inroads in the area of public entertainment, with ventures ranging from shopping mall game simulators to low-cost VR games for the home. Major growth continues in home VR systems, partially as a result of 3D games on the Internet.

Computer-Aided Design: Using VR to create "virtual prototypes" in software allows engineers to test potential products in the design phase, even collaboratively over computer networks, without investing time or money for conventional hard models. All of the major automobile manufacturers and many aircraft manufacturers rely heavily on virtual prototyping.

Military: With VR, the military's solitary cab-based systems have evolved to extensive networked simulations involving a variety of equipment and situations. There is an apocryphal story that General Norman Schwartzkopf was selected to lead the Desert Storm operation on the basis of his extensive experience with simulations of the Middle East battle arena.

Architecture/Construction: VR allows architects and engineers and their clients to "walk through" structural blueprints. Designs may be understood more clearly by clients who often have difficulty comprehending them even with conventional cardboard models. Atlanta, Georgia credits its VR model for winning it the site of the 1996 Olympics, while San Diego is using a VR model of a planned convention center addition to compete for the next convention of the Republican Party.

Data Visualization: By allowing navigation through an abstract "world" of data, VR helps users rapidly visualize relationships within complex, multidimensional data structures. This is particularly important in financial-market data, where VR supports faster decision making.

VR is commonly associated with exotic "fully immersive applications" because of the over-dramatized media coverage on helmets, body suits, entertainment simulators, and the like. Equally important are the "Window into World" applications where the user or operator is allowed to interact effectively with "virtual" data, either locally or remotely.

16.3 Current Status of Virtual Reality Technology

The commercial market for VR, while taking advantage of advances in VR technology at large, is nonetheless contending with the lack of integrated systems and the frequent turnover of equipment suppliers. Over the last few years, VR users in academia and industry have developed different strategies for circumventing these problems. In academic settings, researchers buy peripherals and software from separate companies and configure their own systems to maintain the greatest application versatility. In industry, however, expensive, state-of-the-art VR systems are vertically integrated to address problems peculiar to the industry.

Each solution is either too costly or too risky for most medical organizations. What is required is a VR system tailored to the needs of the medical community. Unfortunately, few companies offer integrated systems that are applicable to the VR medical market. This situation is likely to change in the next few years as VR-integration companies develop to fill this void.

At the same time, the nature of the commercial VR medical market is changing as the price of high-performance graphics systems continues to decline. High-resolution graphics monitors are becoming more cost-effective even for markets that rely solely on desktop computers. Technical advances are also occurring in networking, visual photo-realism, tracker latency through predictive algorithms, and variable-resolution image generators. Improved database access methods are under way. Hardware advances, such as eye gear that provides an increased field of view with high-resolution, untethered VR systems and inexpensive intuitive input devices, e.g., DataGloves, have lagged behind advances in computational, communications, and display capabilities.

16.4 Overview of Medical Applications of Virtual Reality Technology

Within the medical community, the first wave of VR development efforts have evolved into six key categories:

1. Surgical Training and Surgical Planning
2. Medical Education, Modeling, and Non-Surgical Training
3. Anatomical Imaging and Medical Image Fusion
4. Ergonomics, Rehabilitation, and Disabilities
5. Telesurgery and Telemedicine
6. Behavioral Evaluation and Intervention

The potential of VR through education and information dissemination indicates there will be few areas of medicine not taking advantage of this improved computer interface. However, the latent potential of VR lies in its capacity to be used to manipulate and combine heterogeneous multidimensional data sets from many sources, for example, MRI, PET, and x-ray images. This feature is most significant and continues to transform the traditional applications environment.

Surgical Training and Surgical Planning

Various projects are under way to utilize VR and imaging technology to plan, simulate, and customize invasive (as well as minimally invasive) surgical procedures. One example of a VR surgical-planning and training system is the computer-based workstation developed by Ciné-Med of Woodbury, Connecticut [McGovern, 1994]. The goal was to develop a realistic, interactive training workstation that helps surgeons make a more seamless transition from surgical simulation to the actual surgical event.

Ciné-Med focused on television-controlled endosurgical procedures because of the intensive training required for endosurgery and the adaptability of endosurgery to high-quality imaging. Surgeons can gain clinical expertise by training on this highly realistic and functional surgical simulator. Ciné-Med's computer environment includes life-like virtual organs that react much like their real counterparts, and sophisticated details such as the actual surgical instruments that provide system input/output (I/O). To further enhance training, the simulator allows the instructor to adapt clinical instruction to advance the technical expertise of learners. Surgical anomalies and emergency situations can be replicated to allow practicing surgeons to experiment and gain technical expertise on a wide range of surgical problems using the computer model before using an animal model. Since the steps of the procedure can be repeated and replayed at a later time, the learning environment surpasses other skills-training modalities.

The current prototype simulates the environment of laparoscopic cholecystectomy for use as a surgical training device. Development began with the creation of an accurate anatomic landscape, including the liver, the gallbladder, and related structures. Appropriate surgical instruments are used for the system I/O and inserted into a fiberglass replica of a human torso. Four surgical incisional ports are assigned for three scissors grip instruments and camera zoom control. The instruments, retrofitted with switching devices, read and relay the opening and closing of the tips, with position trackers located within the simulator. The virtual surgical instruments are graphically generated on a display monitor where they interact with fully textural, anatomically correct, three-dimensional virtual organs. The organs are created as independent objects and conform to object-oriented programming.

To replicate physical properties, each virtual organ must be assigned appropriate values to dictate its reaction when contacted by a virtual surgical instrument. Collision algorithms are established to define when the virtual organ is touched by a virtual surgical instrument. Additionally, with the creation of spontaneous objects resulting from the dissection of a virtual organ, each new object is calculated to have independent physical properties using artificial intelligence (AI) subroutines. Collision algorithms drive the programmed creation of spontaneous objects.

To reproduce the patient's physiologic reactions during the surgical procedure, the simulation employs an expert system. This software subsystem generates patient reactions and probable outcomes derived from surgical stimuli, for example, bleeding control, heart rate failure, and, in the extreme, a death outcome. The acceptable value ranges of these factors are programmed to be constantly updated by the expert system while important data are displayed on the monitor.

Three-dimensional graphical representation of a patient's anatomy is a challenge for accurate surgical planning. Technological progress has been seen in the visualization of bone, brain, and soft tissue. Heretofore, three-dimensional modeling of soft tissue has been difficult and often inaccurate owing to the intricacies of the internal organ, its vasculature, ducts, volume, and connective tissues.

As an extension of this surgical simulator, a functional surgical planning device using VR technology is under development that will enable surgeons to operate on an actual patient, in virtual reality, prior to the actual operation. With the advent of technological advances in anatomic imaging, the parallel development of a surgical planning device incorporating real-time interaction with computer graphics that mimic a patient's anatomy is possible. Identification of anatomic structures to be modeled constitutes the initial phase for development of the surgical planning device. A spiral CAT scanning device records multiple slices of the anatomy during a single breath inhalation by the patient. Pin-registered layers of the anatomy are thus provided for the computer to read.

Individual anatomic structures are defined at the scan level according to gray scale. Once the anatomic structures are identified and labeled, the scans are stacked and connected. The result is a volumetric polygonal model of the patient's actual anatomy. A polygon-reduction program is initiated to create a wire frame that can be successfully texture-mapped and interacted with in real time. As each slice of the CAT scan is stacked and linked together, the result is a fully volumetric, graphic representation of the human anatomy. Since the model, at this point, is unmanageable by the graphics workstation because of the volume polygons, a polygon-reduction program is initiated to eliminate excessive polygons.

Key to the planning device is development of a user-friendly software program that will allow the radiologist to define anatomic structures, incorporate them into graphical representations, and assign physiologic parameters to the anatomy. Surgeons will then be able to diagnose, plan, and prescribe appropriate therapy to their patients using a trial run of a computerized simulation.

Several VR-based systems currently under development allow real-time tracking of surgical instrumentation and simultaneous display and manipulation of three-dimensional anatomy corresponding to the simulated procedure [Hon, 1994; McGovern, 1994; Edmond et al., 1997]. With this design surgeons can practice procedures and experience the possible complications and variations in anatomy encountered during surgery. Ranging from advanced imaging technologies for endoscopic surgery to routine hip replacements, these new developments will have a tremendous impact on improving surgical morbidity and mortality. According to Merril [1993, 1994], studies show that doctors are more likely to make errors performing their first few to several dozen diagnostic and therapeutic surgical procedures. Merril claims that operative risk could be substantially reduced by the development of a simulator that allows transference of skills from the simulation to the actual point of patient contact.

A preliminary test of Merril's claim was achieved by Taffinder and colleagues [1998]. Following the observations by McDougall et al. [1996] that 2D representations of anatomic imagery are insufficient to develop the eye-hand coordination of surgeons, Taffinder et al. conducted randomized, controlled studies of psychomotor skills developed either through the use of the MIST VR Laparoscopic Simulator or through a standard laparoscopic-surgery training course. They used the MIST VR Laparoscopic Simulator to compare the psychomotor skills of experienced surgeons, surgeon trainees, and non-surgeons. When task speed and the number of correctional movements were compared across subjects, experienced surgeons surpassed trainees and non-surgeons. Taffinder and colleagues also noted that among trainees, training on the VR system improved efficiency and reduced errors, but did not increase the speed of the laparoscopic procedures.

To increase the realism of medical simulators, software tools have been developed to create "virtual tissues" that reflect the physical characteristics of physiologic tissues. This technology operates in real time using three-dimensional graphics, on a high-speed computer platform. Recent advances in creating virtual tissues have occurred as force feedback is incorporated into more VR systems and the computational overhead of finite-element analysis is reduced (see, for example, Grabowski [1998]; McInerny and Terzopoulos [1996]). Bro-Nielsen and Cotin [1996] have been developing tissue models that incorporate appropriate real-time volumetric deformation in response to applied forces. Their goal was to provide surgeons with the same "hands-on" feel in VR that they experience in actual surgery. They used mass-spring systems [Bro-Nielsen, 1997] to simplify finite-element analysis, significantly reduced computational overhead, and thereby achieving near-real-time performance. While advancing the state of the art considerably toward the real-time, hands-on objective, much more work remains to be done.

In another study of the effectiveness of force-feedback in surgical simulations, Baur et al. [1998] reported on the use of VIRGY, a VR endoscopic surgery simulator. VIRGY provides both visual and force feedback to the user, through the use of the Pantoscope [Baumann, 1996]. Because the Pantoscope is a remote-center-of-motion force-reflecting system, Baur et al. were able to hide the system beneath the skin of the endoscope mannequin. Force reflection of tissue interactions, including probing and cutting, was controlled by nearest neighbor propagation of lookup table values to circumvent the computational overhead inherent in finite-element analysis. Surgeons were asked to assess the tissue feel achieved through this simulation.

Evaluation of another surgical simulator system was carried out by Weghorst et al. [1998]. This evaluation involved the use of the Madigan Endoscopic Sinus Surgery (ESS) Simulator (see Edmond et al. [1997] for a full description), developed jointly by the U.S. Army, Lockheed-Martin, and the Human Interface Technology Laboratory at the University of Washington. The ESS Simulator, which was designed to train otolaryngologists to perform paranasal endoscopic procedures, incorporates 3D models of the nasopharyngeal anatomy derived from the National Library of Medicine's Virtual Human Data Base. It employs two 6-DOF force-reflecting instruments developed by the Immersion Corporation to simulate the endoscope and 11 surgical instruments used in paranasal surgery.

Weghorst and colleagues pitted three groups of subjects against each other in a test of the effectiveness of the ESS Simulator: non-MDs, non-ENT MDs, and ENTs with various levels of experience. Training aids, in the form of circular hoops projected onto the simulated nasal anatomy, identified the desired endoscope trajectory; targets identified anatomic injection sites; and text labels identified anatomic landmarks. Successive approximations to the actual task involved training first on an abstract, geometric model of the nasal anatomy with superimposed training aids (Level 1); next on real nasal anatomy with superimposed training aids (Level 2); and, finally, on real nasal anatomy without training aids (Level 3).

Results of the evaluation indicated that, in general, ENTs performed better than non-ENTs on Level 1 and 2 tasks, and that among the ENTs, those with more ESS experience scored higher than those who had performed fewer ESS procedures. The researchers also found that deviations from the optimum endoscope path differentiated ENT and non-ENT subjects. In post-training questionnaires, ENTs rated the realism of the simulation as high and confirmed the validity and usefulness of training on the ESS Simulator.

While the ESS Simulator described above requires a 200 MHz Pentium PC and a 4-CPU SGI Oxyx with Reality Engine 2 graphics to synthesize the virtual nasal cavity, a current trend in surgical simulation is toward lower-end simulation platforms. As computational power of PCs continues to escalate, simulations are increasingly being ported to or developed on relatively inexpensive computers. Tseng et al. [1998] used an Intel-based PC as the basis of their laparoscopic surgery simulator. This device incorporates a 5-DOF force-reflecting effector, a monitor for viewing the end-effector, and a speech-recognition system for changing viewpoint. The system detects collisions between the end effector and virtual tissues, and is capable of producing tissue deformation through one of several models including a finite-element model, a displacement model, or a transmission line model. Computational power is provided by dual Pentium Pro 200 MHz CPUs and a Realizm Graphics Accelerator Board.

Medical Education, Modeling, and Non-Surgical Training

Researchers at the University of California–San Diego are exploring the value of hybridizing elements of VR, multimedia (MM), and communications technologies into a unified educational paradigm [Hoffman, 1994; Hoffman et al., 1995, 1997]. The goal is to develop powerful tools that extend the flexibility and effectiveness of medical teaching and promote lifelong learning. To this end, they have undertaken a multiyear initiative, named the "VR-MM Synthesis Project." Based on instructional design and user need (rather than technology per se), they have planned a linked three-computer array representing the Data Communications Gateway, the Electronic Medical Record System, and the Simulation Environment. This system supports medical students, surgical residents, and clinical faculty running applications ranging from full surgical simulation to basic anatomic exploration and review, all via a common interface. The plan also supports integration of learning and telecommunications resources (such as interactive MM libraries, online textbooks, databases of medical literature, decision support systems, electronic mail, and access to electronic medical records).

The first application brought to fruition in the VR-MM Synthesis Project is an anatomic instructional-aid system called Anatomic VisualizeR [Hoffman et al., 1997] that uses anatomic models derived from the Visible Human Project of the National Library of Medicine. Using the "Guided Lessons" paradigm of Anatomic VisualizeR, the student enters a 3D workspace that contains a "Study Guide." The student uses the study guide to navigate through the 3D workspace, downloading anatomic models of interest, as well as supporting resources like diagrammatic representations, photographic material, and text. Manipulation of the anatomic models is encouraged to provide the student with an intuitive understanding of anatomic relationships. The study guide also incorporates other instructional material necessary for the completion of a given lesson.

Another advanced medical training system based on VR technology is VMET—the Virtual Medical Trainer—jointly developed by the Research Triangle Institute and Advanced Simulation Corp. [Kizakevich et al., 1998]. VMET was developed to provide training in trauma care. The VMET Trauma Patient Simulator (VMET-TPS), which was designed to comply with civilian guidelines for both Basic Trauma Life Support and Advanced Trauma Life Support, incorporates models of (1) physiologic systems and functions, (2) dynamic consequences of trauma to these physiologic systems, and (3) medical intervention effects on these physiologic systems.

VMET provides a multisensory simulation of a trauma patient, including visible, audible, and behavioral aspects of the trauma patient. To maintain cost-effectiveness, VMET is constrained to providing "virtual spaces" at the site of several injuries, including a penetrating chest wound, a penetrating arm wound, laceration to the arm, and a thigh contusion. Within the virtual spaces, the trainee can experience the physiologic effects of the injury and of his intervention in real time, as the physiologic engine updates the condition of the wound.

VMET-TPS was designed to train military personnel in trauma care, so it places emphasis on the medical technology currently and foreseeably available to the military. However, VMET-TPS will find applications in civilian teaching hospitals, as well. Partially because of the cost-constraint requirements of the project, the price of VMET should be within reach of many trauma centers.

In another task-specific program at the Fraunhofer Institute, researchers have been developing an ultrasonic probe training system based on VR components called the UltraTrainer [Stallkamp and Walper, 1998]. UltraTrainer uses a Silicon Graphics workstation and monitor to present images drawn from a database of real ultrasonograms, a Polhemus tracker to determine the position of the user's hand, a joystick representation of the ultrasound probe, and an ultrasound phantom to provide probe position/orientation feedback to the trainee. In using the UltraTrainer, the trainee moves the ultrasound probe against the phantom, which is used in this system as a representation of the virtual patient's body. On the monitor, the trainee sees an image of the probe in relation to the phantom, showing the trainee the position and orientation of the probe with respect to the virtual patient.

The Polhemus tracker determines and records the real-space position of the virtual ultrasound probe, and this tracker information is then used to extract stored ultrasonograms from a database of images.

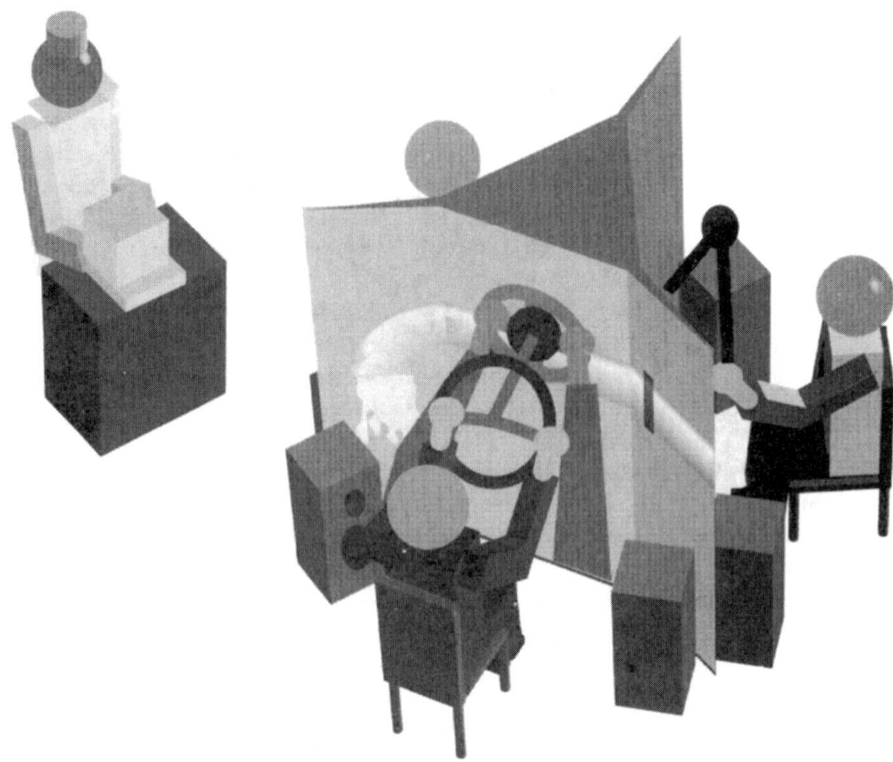

FIGURE 16.3 VR-based rehabilitation workstation.

An ultrasonic image of the appropriate virtual scanfield is presented on the monitor in accordance with the position of the virtual probe on the phantom. As the probe is moved on the phantom, new virtual scanfields are extracted from the database and presented on the monitor. The UltraTrainer is able to present sequential virtual scanfields rapidly enough for the trainee to perceive the virtual ultrasonography as occurring in real time.

Planned improvements to the UltraTrainer include a larger database of stored sonograms that can be customized for different medical specialties, and a reduction in cost by porting the system to a PC and by using a less expensive tracking system. These improvements should allow the UltraTrainer to be accessed by a broader range of users and to move from the laboratory to the classroom, or even to the home.

Three groups of researchers have taken different approaches to developing VR-based training systems for needle insertion, each based on feedback to a different sensory system. At Georgetown University, Lathan and associates [1998] have produced a spine biopsy simulator based on visual feedback; a team from Ohio State University and the Ohio Supercomputer Center have demonstrated an epidural needle insertion simulator based on force feedback [Heimenz et al., 1998]; and Computer Aided Surgery in New York has developed a blind needle biopsy placement simulator that uses 3D auditory feedback [Wenger and Karron, 1998]. Each of these innovative systems draws on technological advances in virtual reality. In the aggregate, they disclose that, given appropriate cognitive constructs, humans are capable of using diverse sensory input to learn very demanding tasks. Imagine how effective virtual reality could be in training complex tasks if all of the sensory information could be integrated in a single system. That is currently one of the goals of the virtual reality community.

Anatomic Imaging and Medical Image Fusion

An anatomically keyed display with real-time data fusion is currently in use at NYU Medical Center's Department of Neurosurgery. The system allows both preoperative planning and real-time tumor

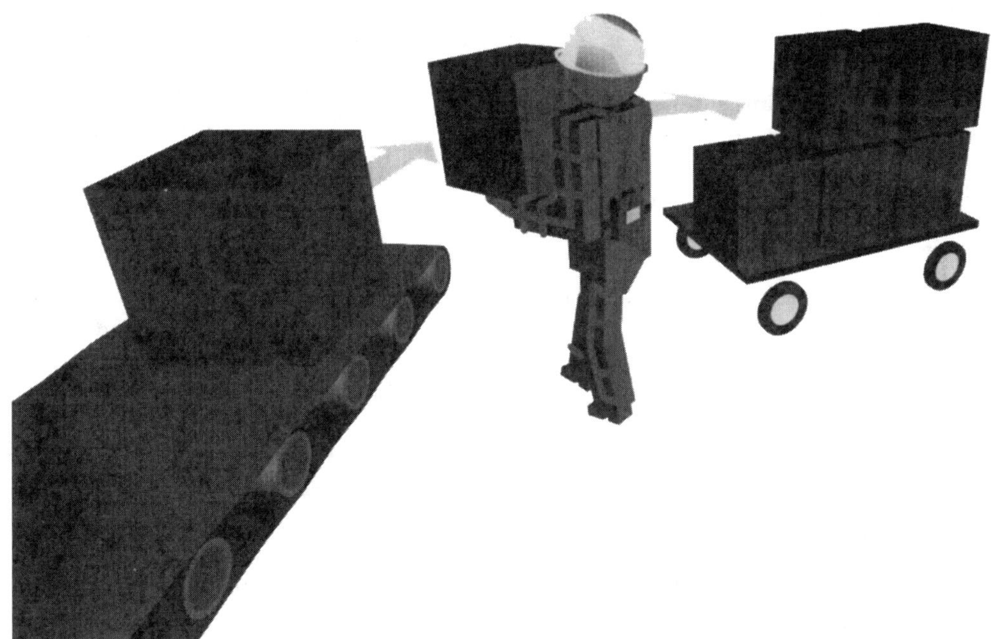

FIGURE 16.4 DataSuit for ergonomic and sports medicine applications.

visualization [Kelly, 1994; Kall, 1994]. The technology offers a technique for surgeons to plan and simulate the surgical procedure beforehand in order to reach deep-seated or centrally located brain tumors. The imaging method (volumetric stereotaxis) gathers, stores, and reformats imaging-derived, three-dimensional volumetric information that defines an intracranial lesion (tumor) with respect to the surgical field.

Computer-generated information is displayed intraoperatively on computer monitors in the operating room and on a "heads up" display mounted on the operating microscope. These images provide surgeons with a CT (computed tomography) and MRI defined map of the surgical field area scaled to actual size and location. This guides the surgeon in finding and defining the boundaries of brain tumors. The computer-generated images are indexed to the surgical field by means of a robotics-controlled stereotactic frame which positions the patient's tumor within a defined targeting area. Simulated systems using VR models are being advocated for high-risk techniques, such as the alignment of radiation sources to treat cancerous tumors. Where registration of virtual and real anatomic features is not an issue, other display technologies can be employed. Two recent examples, based on totally different display modalities, are described below.

Parsons and Rolland [1998] developed a non-intrusive display technique that projects images of virtual inclusions such as tumors, cysts, or abscesses, or other medical image data into the surgeon's field of view on demand. The system relies on retroreflective material, perhaps used as a backing for the surgeon's glove or on a surgical instrument, to provide an imaging surface upon which can be presented images extracted from 2D data sources, for example, MRI scans. The surgeon can access the data by placing the retroreflective screen, e.g., his gloved hand, in the path of an imaging beam. The image of the virtual MRI scan, for example, will appear superimposed along the surgeon's line of sight. Although image registration is not currently possible with this real-time display system, the system does provide a means for the clinician to access critical information without turning to view a monitor or other screen.

For displaying volumetric data, Senger [1998] devised a system based on the FakeSpace Immersive Workbench™ and position-tracked StereoGraphics CrystalEyes™ that presents stereoscopic images derived from CT, MRI, and the Visible Human data sets. The viewer can interact with the immersive data structure through the use of a position/orientation sensed probe. The probe can be used first to identify a region of interest within the anatomic data set and then to segment the data so that particular anatomic features are highlighted. The probe can also be used to "inject" digital stain into the data set and to direct the propagation of the stain into structures that meet predetermined parameters, such as voxel density, opacity, etc. Through the use of the probe, the vasculature, fascia, bone, etc. may be selectively stained. This imaging system takes advantage of the recent advances in VR hardware and software, the advent of programs such as the National Library of Medicine's Visible Human Project, and significant cost reductions in computational power to make it feasible for medical researchers to create accurate, interactive 3D human anatomic atlases.

Suzuki and colleagues [1998] have pushed virtual anatomic imaging a step further by including the temporal domain. In 1987, Suzuki, Itou, and Okamura developed a 3D human atlas based on serial MRI scans. Originally designed to be resident on a PC, the 3D Human Atlas has been upgraded during the last decade to take advantage of major advances in computer graphics. The latest atlas is based on composite super-conducting MRI scans at 4-mm intervals at 4-mm pitch of young male and female humans. In addition to volume and surface rendering, this atlas is also capable of dynamic cardiac imaging.

Rendered on a Silicon Graphics Onyx Reality Engine, this atlas presents volumetric images at approximately 10 frames per second. The user interface allows sectioning of the anatomic data along any plane, as well as extracting organ surface information. Organs can be manipulated individually and rendered transparent to enable the user to view hidden structures. By rendering the surface of the heart transparent, it is possible to view the chambers of the heart in 4D at approximately 8 frames per second. Suzuki and colleagues plan to distribute the atlas over the Internet so that users throughout the world will be able to access it.

Distribution of volumetric medical imagery over the Internet through the World Wide Web (WWW) has already been examined by Hendin and colleagues [1998]. These authors relied on the Virtual Reality Modeling Language (VRML) and VRMLscript to display and interact with the medial data sets, and they used a Java graphical user interface (GUI) to preserve platform independence. They conclude that it is currently feasible to share and interact with medical image data over the WWW.

Similarly, Silverstein et al. [1998] have demonstrated a system for interacting with 3D radiologic image data over the Internet. While they conclude that the Web-based system is effective for transmitting useful imagery to remote colleagues for diagnosis and pretreatment planning, it does not supplant the requirement that a knowledgeable radiologist examine the 2D tomographic images. This raises the question of the effectiveness of the display and interaction with virtual medical images.

The perceived effectiveness of VR-based anatomic imaging systems similar to those described above has been assessed by Oyama and colleagues [1998]. They created virtual environments consisting of 3D images of cancerous lesions and surrounding tissue, derived from CT or MRI scans, and presented these environments to clinicians in one of three modes. The cancers were from the brain, breast, lung, stomach, liver, and colon, and the presentation modes were as surface-rendered images, real-time volume-rendered images, or editable real-time volume-rendered images. Clinicians had to rate the effectiveness of the three modes in providing them with information about (1) the location of the cancer, (2) the shape of the cancer, (3) the shape of fine vessels, (4) the degree of infiltration of surrounding organs, and (5) the relationship between the cancer and normal organs. In each of the five categories, the clinicians rated the editable real-time volume-rendered images as superior to the other modes of presentation. From the study, the authors conclude that real-time surface rendering, while applicable to many areas of medicine, is not suitable for use in cancer diagnosis.

Ergonomics, Rehabilitation, and Disabilities

VR offers the possibility to better shape a rehabilitative program to an individual patient. Greenleaf et al. [1994] have theorized that the rehabilitation process can be enhanced through the use of VR technology. The group is currently developing a VR-based rehabilitation workstation that will be used to (1) decompose rehabilitation into small, incremental functional steps to facilitate the rehabilitation process; and (2) make the rehabilitation process more realistic and less boring, thus enhancing motivation and recovery of function.

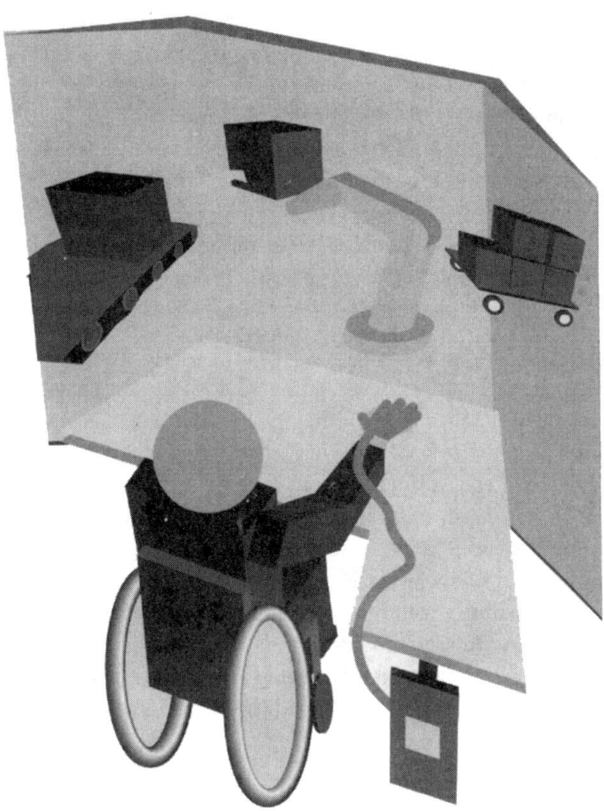

FIGURE 16.5 VR system used as a disability solution.

DataGlove and DataSuit technologies were originally developed as control devices for VR, but through improvements they are now being applied to the field of functional evaluation of movement and to rehabilitation in a variety of ways. One system, for example, uses a glove device coupled with a force feedback system—The Rutgers Master (RM-I)—to rehabilitate a damaged hand or to diagnose a range of hand problems [Burdea et al., 1995, 1997]. The rehabilitation system developed by Burdea and colleagues uses programmable force feedback to control the level of effort required to accomplish rehabilitative tasks. This system measures finger-specific forces while the patient performs one of several rehabilitative tasks, including ball squeezing, DigiKey exercises, and peg insertion.

Another system under development—RM II—incorporates tactile feedback to a glove system to produce feeling in the fingers when virtual objects are "touched" [Burdea, 1994]. In order to facilitate accurate goniometric assessment, improvements to the resolution of the standard DataGlove have been developed [Greenleaf, 1992]. The improved DataGlove allows highly accurate measurement of dynamic range of motion of the fingers and wrist and is in use at research centers such as Johns Hopkins and Loma Linda University to measure and analyze functional movements.

Adjacent to rehabilitation evaluation systems are systems utilizing the same measurement technology to provide ergonomic evaluation and injury prevention. Workplace ergonomics has already received a boost from new VR technologies that enable customized workstations tailored to individual requirements [Greenleaf, 1994]. In another area, surgical room ergonomics for medical personnel and patients is projected to reduce the hostile and complicated interface among patients, health care providers, and surgical spaces [Kaplan, 1994].

Motion Analysis Software (MAS) can assess and analyze upper extremity function from dynamic measurement data acquired by the improved DataGlove. This technology not only provides highly objective measurement, but also ensures more accurate methods for collecting data and performing quantitative analyses for physicians, therapists, and ergonomics specialists involved in job site evaluation and design. The DataGlove/MAS technology is contributing to a greater understanding of upper extremity biomechanics and kinesiology. Basic DataGlove technology coupled with VR media will offer numerous opportunities for the rehabilitation sector of the medical market, not the least of which is the positive implication for enhancing patient recovery by making the process more realistic and participatory.

One exciting aspect of VR technology is the inherent ability to enable individuals with physical disabilities to accomplish tasks and have experiences otherwise denied them. The strategies currently employed for disability-related VR research include head-mounted displays, position/orientation sensing, tactile feedback, eye tracking, 3D sound systems, data input devices, image generation, and optics. For physically disabled persons, VR will provide a new link to capabilities and experiences heretofore unattainable, such as:

- An individual with cerebral palsy who is confined to a wheelchair can operate a telephone switchboard, play hand ball, and dance [Greenleaf, 1994] within a virtual environment.
- Patients with spinal cord injury or CNS dysfunction can relearn limb movements through adaptive visual feedback in virtual environments [Steffin, 1997].
- Disabled individuals can be in one location while their "virtual being" is in a totally different location. This opens all manner of possibilities for participating in work, study, or leisure activities anywhere in the world without leaving home.
- Physically disabled individuals could interact with real-world activities through robotic devices they control from within the virtual world.
- Blind persons could practice and plan in advance navigating through or among buildings if the accesses represented in a virtual world were made up of 3D sound images and tactile stimuli [Max and Gonzalez, 1997].

One novel application of VR technology to disabilities has been demonstrated by Inman [1994a,b; 1996] who trained handicapped children to operate wheelchairs without the inherent dangers of such training. Inman trained children with cerebral palsy or orthopedic impairments to navigate virtual worlds that contained simulated physical conditions that they would encounter in the real world. By training in a virtual environment, the children acquired an appreciation of the dynamics of their wheelchairs and of the dangers that they might encounter in the real world, but in a safe setting. The safety aspect of VR training is impossible to achieve with other training technologies.

VR will also enable persons with disabilities to experience situations and sensations not accessible in a physical world. Learning and working environments can be tailored to specific needs with VR. For example, since the virtual world can be superimposed over the real world, a learner could move progressively from a highly supported mode of performing a task in the virtual world, through to performing it unassisted in the real world. One project, "Wheelchair VR" [Trimble, 1992], is a highly specialized architectural software being developed to aid in the design of barrier-free buildings for persons with disabilities.

VR also presents unique opportunities for retraining persons who have incurred neuropsychological deficits. The cognitive deficits associated with neurophysiologic insults are often difficult to assess and for this and other reasons, not readily amenable to treatment. Several groups have begun to investigate the use of VR in the assessment and retraining of persons with neuropsychological cognitive impairments. Pugnetti and colleagues [1995a,b; 1996] have begun to develop VR-based scenarios based on standardized tests of cognitive function, for example, card-sorting tasks. Because the tester has essentially absolute control over the cognitive environment in which the test is administered, the effects of environmental distractors can be both assessed and controlled. Initial tests by the Italian group suggests that VR-based cognitive tests offer great promise for both evaluation and retraining of brain-injury-associated cognitive deficits.

Other groups have been developing cognitive tests based on mental rotation of virtual objects [Buchwalter and Rizzo, 1997; Rizzo and Buchwalter, 1997] or spatial memory of virtual buildings [Attree et al., 1996]. Although VR technology shows promise in both the assessment and treatment of persons with acquired cognitive deficits, Buchwalter and Rizzo find that the technology is currently too cumbersome, too unfamiliar, and has too many side effects to allow many patients to benefit from its use.

Attree and associates, however, have begun to develop a taxonomy of virtual reality applications in cognitive rehabilitation. Their study examined the differences between active and passive navigation of virtual environments. They report that active navigation improves spatial memory of the route through the virtual environment, while passive navigation improves object recognition for landmarks within the virtual environment. This report sends a clear message that VR is capable of improving cognitive function, but that much more work is required to understand how the technology interacts with the human psyche.

One researcher who is actively pursuing this understanding is Dorothy Strickland [1995, 1996], who has developed a virtual environment for working with autistic children. Strickland's premise is that VR technology allows precise control of visual and auditory stimuli within virtual environments. Frequently, autistic children find the magnitude of environmental stimuli overwhelming, so it is difficult for them to focus. Strickland has developed a sparse virtual environment into which stimuli can be introduced as the autistic child becomes capable of handling more environmental stimulation. Essentially, she produces successive approximations to a real environment at a rate that the autistic child can tolerate. Her work has shown that autistic children can benefit greatly by exposure to successively richer environments and that the advances that they make in virtual environments transfer to the real world.

Max and Burke [1998], also using VR with autistic children, report that contrary to expectations, their patients were able to focus on the virtual environment, rather than "fidgeting" as they are prone to do in other environments. These researchers also found that in the absence of competing acoustic stimuli, autistic children were drawn to loud music and shunned soft choral music. These findings may provide important insights into the etiology of autism that could not be observed in the "real-world" setting.

Telesurgery and Telemedicine

Telepresence is the "sister field" of VR. Classically defined as the ability to act and interact in an off-site environment by making use of VR technology, telepresence is emerging as an area of development in its own right. Telemedicine (the telepresence of medical experts) is being explored as a way to reduce the cost of medical practice and to bring expertise into remote areas [Burrow, 1994; Rosen, 1994; Rovetta et al., 1997; Rissam et al., 1998].

Telesurgery is a fertile area for development. On the verge of realization, telesurgery (remote surgery) will help resolve issues that can complicate or compromise surgery, among them:

- The patient is too ill or injured to be moved for surgery.
- A specialist surgeon is located at some distance from the patient requiring specialized attention.
- Accident victims may have a better chance of survival if immediate, on-the-scene surgery can be performed remotely by an emergency room surgeon at a local hospital.
- Soldiers wounded in battle could undergo surgery on the battlefield by a surgeon located elsewhere.

The surgeon really does operate—on flesh, not a computer animation. And while the distance aspect of remote surgery is a provocative one, telepresence is proving an aid in non-remote surgery as well. It can help surgeons gain dexterity over conventional methods of manipulation. This is expected to be particularly important in laparoscopic surgery. For example, suturing and knot-tying will be as easy to see in laparoscopic surgery as it is in open surgery because telepresence enables the surgery to look and feel like open surgery.

As developed at SRI International [Satava, 1992; Hill et al., 1995, 1998], telepresence not only offers a compelling sense of reality for the surgeon, but also allows the surgeon to perform the surgery according to the usual methods and procedures. There is nothing new to learn. Hand motions are quick and precise. The visual field, instrument motion, and force feedback can all be scaled to make microsurgery easier than it would be if the surgeon were at the patient's side. While the current technology has been implemented in prototype, SRI and Telesurgical Corporation, based in Redwood City, California, are collaborating to develop a full system based on this novel concept.

The system uses color video cameras to image the surgical field in stereo, which the remote surgeon views with stereo shutter glasses. The remote surgeon grasps a pair of force-reflecting 6-DOF remote manipulators linked to a slaved pair of end effectors in the surgical field. Coordinated visual, auditory, and haptic feedback from the end effectors provides the remote surgeon with a compelling sense of presence at the surgical site.

Because the remote manipulators and end effectors are only linked electronically, the gain between them can be adjusted to provide the remote surgeon with microsurgically precise movement of the slaved instruments with relatively gross movement of the master manipulators. Researchers at SRI have demonstrated the microsurgery capabilities of this system by performing microvascular surgery on rats.

Again, because only an electronic link exists between manipulator and end effector, separation of the remote surgeon and the surgical field can be on a global scale. To demonstrate this global remote surgery capability, Rovetta and colleagues [1998] established Internet and ISDN networks between Monterey, California, and Milan, Italy, and used these networks to remotely control a surgical robot. By manipulating controls in Monterey, Professor Rovetta was able to perform simulated biopsies on liver, prostate, and breasts in his laboratory in Milan, Italy. Using both an Internet and ISDN network facilitated the transmission of large amounts of image data and robotic control signals in a timely manner.

Prior to the telesurgery demonstration between Monterey and Milan, Rovetta and colleagues [1997] established a link between European hospitals and hospitals in Africa as part of the Telehealth in Africa Program of the European Collaboration Group for Telemedicine. Among the objectives of this program was a demonstration of the feasibility of transmitting large amounts of medical data including x-ray and other diagnostic images, case histories, and diagnostic analyses. Once established, the data link could be used for teleconsulting and teletraining.

Teleconsulting is becoming commonplace. Within the last year, the U.S. Department of Veteran Affairs has established a network to link rural and urban Vet Centers. This network, which will initially link 20 Vet Centers, will provide teleconsultation for chronic disease screening, trauma outreach, and psychosocial care. In Europe, where telemedicine is making great strides, the Telemedical Information Society has been established. (See Marsh [1998], for additional information.) At the International Telemedical Information Society '98 Conference held in Amsterdam in April 1998, a number of important issues pertaining to teleconsultation were addressed. Among these were discussions about the appropriate network for telemedicine, e.g., the World Wide Web, ATM, and privacy and liability issues.

Privacy, that is, security of transmitted medical information, will be a continuing problem as hackers hone their ability to circumvent Internet security [Radesovich, 1997]. Aslan and colleagues [1998] have examined the practicality of using 128-bit encryption for securing the transmission of medical images. Using software called Photomailer™, Aslan at Duke Medical Center and his colleagues at Boston University Medical Center and Johns Hopkins encrypted 60 medical images and transmitted them over the Internet. They then attempted to access the encrypted images without Photomailer™ installed on the receiving computer. They reported complete success and insignificant increases in processing time with the encrypting software installed.

Behavioral Evaluation and Intervention

VR technology has been successfully applied to a number of behavioral conditions over the last few years. Among the greatest breakthoughs attained through the use of this technology is the relief of akinesia, a symptom of parkinsonism wherein a patient has progressively greater difficulty initiating and sustaining walking. The condition can be mitigated by treatment with drugs such as L-dopa, a precursor of the natural neural transmitters dopamine, but usually not without unwanted side effects. Now, collaborators at the Human Interface Technology Laboratory at the University of Washington, along with the University's Department of Rehabilitation Medicine and the San Francisco Parkinson's Institute, are using virtual imagery to simulate an effect called kinesia paradoxa, or the triggering of normal walking behavior in akinetic Parkinson's patients [Weghorst, 1994].

Using a commercial, field-multiplexed, "heads-up" video display, the research team has developed an approach that elicits near-normal walking by presenting collimated virtual images of objects and abstract visual cues moving through the patient's visual field at speeds that emulate normal walking. The combination of image collimation and animation speed reinforces the illusion of space-stabilized visual cues at the patient's feet. This novel, VR-assisted technology may also prove to be therapeutically useful for other movement disorders.

In the area of phobia intervention, Lamson [Lamson, 1994, 1997; Lamson and Meisner, 1994] has investigated the diagnostic and treatment possibilities of VR immersion on anxiety, panic, and phobia of heights. By immersing both patients and controls in computer-generated situations, the researchers were able to expose the subjects to anxiety-provoking situations (such as jumping from a height) in a controlled manner. Experimental results indicated a significant subject habituation and desensitization through this approach, and the approach appears clinically useful.

The effectiveness of VR as a treatment for acrophobia has been critically examined by Rothbaum and associates [1995a,b]. They used a procedure in which phobic patients were immersed in virtual environments that could be altered to present graded fear-inducing situations. Patient responses were monitored and used to modify the virtual threats accordingly. Rothbaum et al. report that the ability to present graded exposure to aversive environments through the use of VR technology provides a very effective means of overcoming acrophobia. Transfer to the real world was quite good.

The use of VR technology in the treatment of phobias has expanded in recent years to include fear of flying [Rothbaum et al., 1996; North et al., 1997], arachnophobia [Carlin et al., 1997], and sexual dysfunction [Optale et al., 1998]. In each of these areas, patients attained a significant reduction in their phobias through graded exposure to fear-provoking virtual environments. In the treatment of arachnophobia, Carlin and associates devised a clever synthesis of real and virtual environments to desensitize patients to spiders. Patients viewed virtual spiders while at the same time touching the simulated fuzziness of a spider. The tactile aspect of the exposure was produced by having the patient touch a toupé.

Before leaving the subject of VR treatment of phobias, a word of caution is necessary. Bloom [1997] has examined the application of VR technology to the treatment of psychiatric disorders and sounds a note of warning. Bloom notes the advances made in the treatment of anxiety disorders, but also points out that there are examples of physiologic and psychological side effects from immersion in VR. While the major side effects tend to be physiologic, mainly simulator sickness and Sopite Syndrome (malaise, lethargy), psychological maladaptations, such as "unpredictable modifications in perceptions of social context" and "fragmentation of self" [Bloom, 1997, p 12] reportedly occur.

16.5 Summary

VR tools and techniques are being developed rapidly in the scientific, engineering, and medical areas. This technology will directly affect medical practice. Computer simulation will allow physicians to practice surgical procedures in a virtual environment in which there is no risk to patients, and where mistakes can be recognized and rectified immediately by the computer. Procedures can be reviewed from new, insightful perspectives that are not possible in the real world.

The innovators in medical VR will be called upon to refine technical efficiency and increase physical and psychological comfort and capability, while keeping an eye on reducing costs for health care. The mandate is complex, but like VR technology itself, the possibilities are very exciting. While the possibilities—and the need—for medical VR are immense, approaches and solutions using new VR-based applications require diligent, cooperative efforts among technology developers, medical practitioners, and medical consumers to establish where future requirements and demand will lie.

Defining Terms

For an excellent treatment of the state of the art of VR and its taxonomy, see the ACM SIGGRAPH publication *Computer Graphics*, Vol. 26, #3, August 1992. It covers the U.S. Government's National Science Foundation invitational workshop on Interactive Systems Program, March 23–24, 1992, which served to identify and recommend future research directions in the area of virtual environments. A more in-depth exposition of VR taxonomy can be found in the MIT Journal *Presence*, Vol. 1, #2.

References

Aslan, P., Lee, B., Kuo, R., Babayan, R.K., Kavoussi, L.R., Pavlin, K.A., and Preminger, G.M. (1998). Secured Medical Imaging over the Internet. *Medicine Meets Virtual Reality: Art, Science, Technology: Healthcare (R)Evolution* (pp. 74-78). IOS Press, San Diego, CA.

Attree, E.A., Brooks, B.M., Rose, F.D., Andrews, T.K., Leadbetter, A.G., and Clifford, B.R. (1996). Memory Processes and Virtual Environments: I Can't Remember What Was There, But I Can Remember How I Got There. Implications for Persons with Disabilities. *Proceedings of the European Conference on Disability, Virtual Reality, and Associated Technology* (pp. 117-121).

Begault, D.R. and Wenzel, E.M. 1992. Techniques and Applications for Binaural Sound Manipulation in Human-Machine Interfaces. *International Journal of Aviation Psychology,* 2, 1-22.

Bloom, R.W. (1997). Psychiatric Therapeutic Applications of Virtual Reality Technology (VRT): Research Prospectus and Phenomenological Critique. *Medicine Meets Virtual Reality: Global Healthcare Grid* (pp. 11-16). IOS Press, San Diego, CA.

Bolas, M.T. (1994, January). Human Factors in the Design of an Immersive Display. *IEEE Computer Graphics and Applications,* 14(1), 55-59.

Buchwalter, J.G. and Rizzo, A.A. (1997). Virtual Reality and the Neuropsychological Assessment of Persons with Neurologically Based Cognitive Impairments. *Medicine Meets Virtual Reality: Global Healthcare Grid* (pp. 17-21). IOS Press, San Diego, CA.

Burdea, G., Zhuang, J., Roskos, E., Silver, D., and Langrana, N. (1992). A Portable Dextrous Master with Force Feedback. *Presence,* 1(1), 18-28.

Burdea, G., Goratowski, R., and Langrana, N. (1995). Tactile Sensing Glove for Computerized Hand Diagnosis. *Journal of Medicine and Virtual Reality,* 1, 40-44.

Burdea, G., Deshpande, S., Popescu, V., Langrana, N., Gomez, D., DiPaolo, D., and Kanter, M. (1997). Computerized Hand Diagnostic/Rehabilitation System Using a Force Feedback Glove. *Medicine Meets Virtual Reality: Global Healthcare Grid* (pp. 141-150). IOS Press, San Diego, CA.

Burrow, M. (1994). A Telemedicine Testbed for Developing and Evaluating Telerobotic Tools for Rural Health Care. *Medicine Meets Virtual Reality II: Interactive Technology & Healthcare: Visionary Applications for Simulation Visualization Robotics* (pp. 15-18). Aligned Management Associates, San Diego, CA.

Caldwell, G. and Gosney, C. (1993). Enhanced Tactile Feedback (Tele-taction) Using a Multi-Functional Sensory System. *Proceedings of the IEEE International Conference on Robotics and Automation,* 955-960.

Carlin, A.S., Hoffman, H.G., and Weghorst, S. (1997). Virtual Reality and Tactile Augmentation in the Treatment of Spider Phobia: A Case Study. *Behavior Research and Therapy,* 35(2), 153-158.

Durlach, N.I., Shinn-Cunningham, B.G., and Held, R.M. (1993, Spring). Supernormal Auditory Localization. I. General Background. *Presence: Teleoperators and Virtual Environments,* 2(2), 89-103.

Edmond, C.V., Heskamp, D., Sluis, D., Stredney, D., Sessanna, D., Weit, G., Yagel, R., Weghorst, S., Openheimer, P., Miller, J. Levin, M., and Rosenberg, L. (1997). ENT Endoscopic Surgical Training Simulator. *Medicine Meets Virtual Reality: Global Healthcare Grid* (pp. 518-528). IOS Press, San Diego, CA.

Grabowski, H.A. (1998). Generating Finite Element Models from Volumetric Medical Images. *Medicine Meets Virtual Reality: Art, Science, Technology: Healthcare (R)Evolution* (pp. 355-356). IOS Press, San Diego, CA.

Greenleaf, W. (1992). DataGlove, DataSuit and Virtual Reality. *Virtual Reality and Persons with Disabilities: Proceedings of the 7th Annual Conference* (pp 21-24). March 18-21, 1992. Los Angeles, CA. Northridge, CA. California State University. 1992. Available from: Office of Disabled Student Services, California State University, Northridge. 18111 Nordhoff Street—DVSS. Northridge, CA 91330.

Greenleaf, W.J. (1994). DataGlove and DataSuit: Virtual Reality Technology Applied to the Measurement of Human Movement. *Medicine Meets Virtual Reality II: Interactive Technology & Healthcare: Visionary Applications for Simulation Visualization Robotics* (pp. 63-69). Aligned Management Associates, San Diego, CA.

Hendin, O., John, N.W., and Shochet, O. (1998). Medical Volume Rendering over the WWW Using VRML and JAVA. *Medicine Meets Virtual Reality: Art, Science, Technology: Healthcare (R)Evolution* (pp. 34-40). IOS Press, San Diego, CA.

Hendrix, C. and Barfield, W. (1996). The Sense of Presence within Audio Virtual Environments. *Presence,* 5, 295-301.

Hiemenz, L., Stredney, D., and Schmalbrock, P. (1998). Development of a Force-Feedback Model for an Epidural Needle Insertion Simulator. Surgical Simulation. *Medicine Meets Virtual Reality: Art, Science, Technology: Healthcare (R)Evolution* (pp. 272-277). IOS Press, San Diego, CA.

Hill, J.W., Jensen, J.F, Green, P.S., and Shah, A.S. (1995). Two-Handed Tele-Presence Surgery Demonstration System. *Proc ANS Sixth Annual Topical Meeting on Robotics and Remote Systems,* 2, 713-720. Monterey, CA.

Hill, J.W., Holst, P.A., Jensen, J.F., Goldman, J., Gorfu, Y., and Ploeger, D.W. (1998). Telepresence Interface with Applications to Microsurgery and Surgical Simulation. *Medicine Meets Virtual Reality: Art, Science, Technology: Healthcare (R)Evolution* (pp. 96-102). IOS Press, San Diego, CA.

Hoffman, H.M. (1994). Virtual Reality and the Medical Curriculum: Integrating Extant and Emerging Technologies. *Medicine Meets Virtual Reality II: Interactive Technology & Healthcare: Visionary Applications for Simulation Visualization Robotics* (pp. 73-76). Aligned Management Associates, San Diego, CA.

Hoffman, H.M., Irwin, A.E., Ligon, R., Murray, M., and Tohsaku, C. (1995). Virtual Reality-Multimedia Synthesis: Next Generation Learning Environments for Medical Education. *J. Biocomm.*, 22 (3), 2-7.

Hoffman, H.M., Murray, M., Danks, M., Prayaga, R., Irwin, A., and Vu, D. (1997). A Flexible and Extensible Object-Oriented 3D Architecture: Application in the Development of Virtual Anatomy Lessons. *Medicine Meets Virtual Reality: Global Healthcare Grid* (pp. 461-466). IOS Press, San Diego, CA.

Holler, E. and Breitwieser, H. (1994). Telepresence Systems for Application in Minimally Invasive Surgery. *Medicine Meets Virtual Reality II: Interactive Technology & Healthcare: Visionary Applications for Simulation Visualization Robotics* (pp. 77-80). Aligned Management Associates, San Diego, CA.

Hon, D. (1994). Ixion's Laparoscopic Surgical Skills Simulator. *Medicine Meets Virtual Reality II: Interactive Technology & Healthcare:: Visionary Applications for Simulation Visualization Robotics* (pp. 81-83). Aligned Management Associates, San Diego, CA.

Inman, D.P. (1994a). Use of Virtual Reality to Teach Students with Orthopedic Impairments to Drive Motorized Wheelchairs. Paper presented at the Fourth Annual Fall Conference of the Oregon Department of Education, Office of Special Education, Portland.

Inman, D.P. (1994b). Virtual Reality Wheelchair Drivers' Training for Children with Cerebral Palsy. Paper presented to the New York Virtual Reality Expo '94, New York.

Inman, D.P. (1996). Use of Virtual Reality and Computerization in Wheelchair Training. Paper presented to Shriner's Hospital for Crippled Children, Portland, OR.

Ino, S., Shimizu, S., Odagawa, T., Sato, M., Takahashi, M., Izumi, T., and Ifukube, T. (1993). A Tactile Display for Presenting Quality of Materials by Changing the Temperature of Skin Surface. *Proceedings of the Second IEEE International Workshop on Robot and Human Communication* (pp. 220-224).

Jacobs, L. (1994). Garage Virtual Reality, Sams Publications, Indianapolis, IN.

Johnson, A.D. (1994). Tactile Feedback Enhancement to Laparoscopic Tools [abstract]. *Medicine Meets Virtual Reality II: Interactive Technology & Healthcare: Visionary Applications for Simulation Visualization Robotics* (p. 92). Aligned Management Associates, San Diego, CA.

Kall, B.A., Kelly, P.J., Stiving, S.O., and Goerss, S.J. (1994). Integrated Multimodality Visualization in Stereotactic Neurologic Surgery. *Medicine Meets Virtual Reality II: Interactive Technology & Healthcare: Visionary Applications for Simulation Visualization Robotics* (pp. 93-94). Aligned Management Associates, San Diego, CA.

Kaplan, K.L. (1994). Project Description: Surgical Room of the Future. *Medicine Meets Virtual Reality II: Interactive Technology & Healthcare: Visionary Applications for Simulation Visualization Robotics* (pp. 95-98). Aligned Management Associates, San Diego, CA.

Kelly, P.J. (1994). Quantitative Virtual Reality Surgical Simulation, Minimally Invasive Stereotactic Neurosurgery and Frameless Stereotactic Technologies. *Medicine Meets Virtual Reality II: Interactive Technology & Healthcare: Visionary Applications for Simulation Visualization Robotics* (pp. 103-108). Aligned Management Associates, San Diego, CA.

Kizakevich, P.N., McCartney, M.L., Nissman, D.B., Starko, K., and Smith, N.T. (1998). Virtual Medical Trainer. *Medicine Meets Virtual Reality: Art, Science, Technology: Healthcare (R)Evolution* (pp. 309-315). IOS Press, San Diego, CA.

Kreuger, M. (1994). Olfactory Stimuli in Medical Virtual Reality Applications. *Proceedings: Virtual Reality in Medicine—The Cutting Edge* (pp. 32-33). Sig-Advanced Applications, Inc., New York.

Kreuger, M. (1995a). Olfactory Stimuli in Virtual Reality for Medical Applications. *Interactive Technology and the New Paradigm for Healthcare* (pp. 180-181). IOS Press, Washington, D.C.

Kreuger, M. (1995b). Olfactory Stimuli in Virtual Reality Medical Training. *Proceedings: Virtual Reality in Medicine and Developers' Expo.*

Kuhnapfel, U.G. (1994). Realtime Graphical Computer Simulation for Endoscopic Surgery. *Medicine Meets Virtual Reality II: Interactive Technology & Healthcare: Visionary Applications for Simulation Visualization Robotics* (pp. 114-116). Aligned Management Associates, San Diego, CA.

Lamson, R. (1994) Virtual Therapy of Anxiety Disorders. *CyberEdge Journal,* 4 (2), 1-28.

Lamson, R. (1995). Clinical Application of Virtual Therapy to Psychiatric Disorders. *Medicine Meets Virtual Reality III.* IOS Press, San Diego, CA.

Lamson, R. (1997). *Virtual Therapy.* Polytechnic International Press, Montreal.

Lamson, R. and Meisner, M. (1994). The Effects of Virtual Reality Immersion in the Treatment of Anxiety, Panic, & Phobia of Heights. *Virtual Reality and Persons with Disabilities: Proceedings of the 2nd Annual International Conference*; 1994 June 8-10. San Francisco, CA. Sponsored by the Center on Disabilities, California State University, Northridge. 18111 Nordhoff Street—DVSS. Northridge, CA.

Lathan, C., Cleary, K., and Greco, R. (1998). Development and Evaluation of a Spine Biopsy Simulator. Surgical Simulation. *Medicine Meets Virtual Reality: Art, Science, Technology: Healthcare (R)Evolution* (pp. 375-376). IOS Press, San Diego, CA.

Loftin, R.B., Ota, D., Saito, T., and Voss, M. (1994). A Virtual Environment for Laparoscopic Surgical Training. *Medicine Meets Virtual Reality II: Interactive Technology & Healthcare: Visionary Applications for Simulation Visualization Robotics* (pp. 121-123). Aligned Management Associates, San Diego, CA.

Marsh, A. (1998). Special Double Issue: The Telemedical Information Society. *Future Generation Computer Systems,* 14 (1-2). Elsevier, Amsterdam.

Max, M.L. and Burke, J.C. (1997). Virtual Reality for Autism Communication and Education, with Lessons for Medical Training Simulators. *Medicine Meets Virtual Reality: Global Healthcare Grid* (pp. 46-53). IOS Press, San Diego, CA.

Max, M.L. and Gonzalez, J.R. (1997). Blind Persons Navigating in Virtual Reality (VR): Hearing and Feeling Communicates "Reality." *Medicine Meets Virtual Reality: Global Healthcare Grid* (pp. 54-59). IOS Press, San Diego, CA.

McGovern, K.T. and McGovern, L.T. (1994, March). Virtual Clinic: A Virtual Reality Surgical Simulator. *Virtual Reality World,* 2(2), 41-44.

McInerney, T. and Terzopoulos, D. (1996). Deformable Models in Medical Image Analysis. *Medical Image Analysis,* 1(2).

Merril, J.R. (1993, November). Surgery on the Cutting Edge. *Virtual Reality World,* 1(3-4), 34-38.

Merril, J.R. (1994). Presentation Material: Medicine Meets Virtual Reality II. [abstract] *Medicine Meets Virtual Reality II: Interactive Technology & Healthcare: Visionary Applications for Simulation Visualization Robotics* (pp. 158-159). Aligned Management Associates, San Diego, CA.

Minsky, M. and Lederman, S.J. (1996). Simulated Haptic Textures: Roughness. Symposium on Haptic Interfaces for Virtual Environment and Teleoperator Systems. ASME International Mechanical Engineering Congress and Exposition. *Proceedings of the ASME Dynamic Systems and Control Division, DSC-Vol. 58,* 451-458.

North, M.M., North, S.M., and Coble, J.R. (1997). Virtual Reality Therapy for Fear of Flying. *American Journal of Psychiatry,* 154 (1), 130.

Optale, G., Munari, A., Nasta, A., Pianon, C., Verde, J.B., and Viggiano, G. (1998).Virtual Reality Techniques in the Treatment of Impotence and Premature Ejaculation. *Medicine Meets Virtual Reality: Art, Science, Technology: Healthcare (R)Evolution* (pp. 186-192). IOS Press, San Diego, CA.

Oyama, H., Wakao, F., and Takahira, Y. (1998). The Clinical Advantages of Editable Real-Time Volume Rendering in a Medical Virtual Environment: VolMed. *Medicine Meets Virtual Reality: Art, Science, Technology: Healthcare (R)Evolution* (pp. 341-345). IOS Press, San Diego, CA.

Parsons, J. and Rolland, J.P. (1998). A Non-Intrusive Display Technique for Providing Real-Time Data within a Surgeon's Critical Area of Interest. *Medicine Meets Virtual Reality: Art, Science, Technology: Healthcare (R)Evolution* (pp. 246-251). IOS Press, San Diego, CA.

Peifer, J. (1994). Virtual Environment for Eye Surgery Simulation. *Medicine Meets Virtual Reality II: Interactive Technology & Healthcare: Visionary Applications for Simulation Visualization Robotics* (pp. 166-173). Aligned Management Associates, San Diego, CA.

Preminger, G.M. (1994). Advanced Imaging Technologies for Endoscopic Surgery. *Medicine Meets Virtual Reality II: Interactive Technology & Healthcare: Visionary Applications for Simulation Visualization Robotics* (pp. 177-178). Aligned Management Associates, San Diego, CA.

Pugnetti, L. (1994). Recovery Diagnostics and Monitoring in Virtual Environments. *Virtual Reality in Rehabilitation, Research, Experience and Perspectives. Proceedings of the 1st International Congress on Virtual Reality in Rehabilitation.* 1994 June 13-18. Gubbio, Italy.

Pugnetti, L., Mendozzi, L., Motta, A., Cattaneo, A., Barbieri, E., and Brancotti, S. (1995a). Evaluation and Retraining of Adults' Cognitive Impairments: Which Role for Virtual Reality Technology? *Computers in Biology and Medicine,* 25 (2), 213-227.

Pugnetti, L., Mendozzi, L. , Motta, A., Cattaneo, A., Barbieri, E., Brancotti, S., and Cazzullo, C.L. (1995b). Immersive Virtual Reality to Assist Retraining of Acquired Cognitive Deficits: First Results with a Dedicated System. *Interactive Technology and the New Paradigm for Healthcare.* IOS Press, Washington, D.C. (pp. 455-456).

Pugnetti, L., Mendozzi, L., Barbieri, E., Rose, F.D., and Attree, E.A. (1996). Nervous System Correlates of Virtual Reality Experience. *Proceedings of the European Conference on Disability, Virtual Reality and Associated Technology* (pp. 239-246).

Rabinowitz, W.M., Maxwell, J., Shao, Y., and Wei, M. (1993, Spring). Sound Localization Cues for a Magnified Head: Implications from Sound Diffraction about a Rigid Sphere. *Presence: Teleoperators and Virtual Environments,* 2(2), 125-129.

Radesovich, L. (1997). Hackers prove 56-bit DES is not enough. *InfoWorld,* 18 (26), 27.

Rissam, H.S., Kishore, S., Bhatia, M.L., and Trehan, N. (1998). Trans-Telephonic Electro-Cardiographic Monitoring (TTEM)-First Indian Experience. *Medicine Meets Virtual Reality: Art, Science, Technology: Healthcare (R)Evolution* (pp. 361-363). IOS Press, San Diego, CA.

Rizzo, A.A. and Buckwalter, J.G. (1997). The Status of Virtual Reality for the Cognitive Rehabilitation of Persons with Neurological Disorders and Acquired Brain Injury. *Medicine Meets Virtual Reality: Global Healthcare Grid* (pp. 22-33). IOS Press, San Diego, CA.

Rosen, J. (1994). The Role of Telemedicine and Telepresence in Reducing Health Care Costs. *Medicine Meets Virtual Reality II: Interactive Technology & Healthcare: Visionary Applications for Simulation Visualization Robotics* (pp. 187-194). Aligned Management Associates, San Diego, CA.

Rothbaum, B.O., Hodges, L.F., Kooper, I.R., Opdyke, D., Williford, J.S., and North, M. (1995a). Virtual Reality Graded Exposure in the Treatment of Acrophobia: A Case Report. *Behavior Therapy,* 26 (3), 547-554.

Rothbaum, B.O., Hodges, L.F., Kooper, I.R., Opdyke, D., Williford, J.S., and North, M. (1995b). Effectiveness of Computer Generated Graded Exposure in the Treatment of Achrophobia. *American Journal of Psychiatry,* 152(4), 626-628.

Rothbaum, B.O., Hodges, B.F., Watson, B.A., Kessler, G.D., and Opdyke, D. (1996). Virtual Reality Exposure Therapy in the Treatment of Fear of Flying: A Case Report. *Behavior Research and Therapy,* 34 (5/6), 477-481.

Rovetta, A., Falcone, F., Sala, R., and Garavaldi, M.E. (1997). Telehealth in Africa. *Medicine Meets Virtual Reality: Global Healthcare Grid* (pp. 277-285). IOS Press, San Diego, CA.

Rovetta, A., Sala, R., Bressanelli, M., Garavaldi, M.E., Lorini, F., Pegoraro, R., and Canina, M. (1998). Demonstration of Surgical Telerobotics and Virtual Telepresence by Internet + ISDN from Monterey (USA) to Milan (Italy). *Medicine Meets Virtual Reality: Art, Science, Technology: Healthcare (R)Evolution* (pp. 79-83). IOS Press, San Diego, CA.

Salisbury, J.K. and Srinivasan, M. (1996). *Proceedings of the First PHANToM User's Group Workshop*. MIT Press, Cambridge, MA.

Salisbury, J.K. and Srinivasan, M. (1997). *Proceedings of the Second PHANToM User's Group Workshop*. MIT Press, Cambridge, MA.

Satava, R.M. (1992). Robotics, Telepresence and Virtual Reality: A Critical Analysis of the Future of Surgery. *Minimally Invasive Therapy*, 1, 357-363.

Schraft, R.D., Neugebauer, J.G., and Wapler, M. (1994). Virtual Reality for Improved Control in Endoscopic Surgery. *Medicine Meets Virtual Reality II: Interactive Technology & Healthcare: Visionary Applications for Simulation Visualization Robotics* (pp. 233-236). Aligned Management Associates, San Diego, CA.

Senger, S. (1998). An Immersive Environment for the Direct Visualization and Segmentation of Volumetric Data Sets. *Medicine Meets Virtual Reality: Art, Science, Technology: Healthcare (R)Evolution* (pp. 7-12). IOS Press, San Diego, CA.

Shimoga, K.B., Khosla, P.K., and Sclabassi, R.J. (1994). Teleneurosurgery: An Approach to Enhance the Dexterity of Neurosurgeons. *Medicine Meets Virtual Reality II: Interactive Technology & Healthcare: Visionary Applications for Simulation Visualization Robotics* (p. 203). Aligned Management Associates, San Diego, CA.

Stallkamp, J. and Walper, M. (1998). UltraTrainer—A Training System for Medical Ultrasound Examination. *Medicine Meets Virtual Reality: Art, Science, Technology: Healthcare (R)Evolution* (pp. 298-301). IOS Press, San Diego, CA.

Steffin, M. (1997). Computer Assisted Therapy for Multiple Sclerosis and Spinal Cord Injury Patients Application of Virtual Reality. *Medicine Meets Virtual Reality: Global Healthcare Grid* (pp. 64-72). IOS Press, San Diego, CA.

Strickland, D.C. (1995). Virtual Reality Training for Autism. *North Carolina State University, College of Engineering Updates*, May 1995.

Strickland, D.C. (1996). Virtual Reality Helps Children with Autism. *Presence*, 5(3), 319-329.

Suzuki, N., Ito, M., and Okamura, T. (1987). Morphological Reference System of Human Structure Using Computer Graphics. *World Congress on Medical Physics and Biomedical Engineering*, San Antonio, TX.

Suzuki, N., Takatsu, A., Hattori, A., Ezumi, T., Oda, S., Yanai, T., and Tominaga, H. (1998). 3D and 4D Atlas System of Living Human Body Structure. *Medicine Meets Virtual Reality: Art, Science, Technology: Healthcare (R)Evolution* (pp. 131-136). IOS Press, San Diego, CA.

Szabo, Z., Hunter, J.G., Berci, G. et al. (1994). Choreographed Instrument Movements during Laparoscopic Surgery: Needle Driving, Knot Tying and Anastomosis Techniques. *Medicine Meets Virtual Reality II: Interactive Technology & Healthcare: Visionary Applications for Simulation Visualization Robotics* (pp. 216-217). Aligned Management Associates, San Diego, CA.

Tendick, F., Jennings, R.W., Tharp, G., and Stark, L. (1993). Sensing and Manipulation Problems in Endoscopic Surgery: Experiment, Analysis, and Observation. *Presence: Teleoperators and Virtual Environments*, 2(1), 66-81.

Trimble, J., Morris, T., and Crandall, R. (1992). Virtual Reality. *TeamRehab Report*, 3(8), 33-37.

Wang, Y. and Sackier, J. (1994). Robotically Enhanced Surgery. *Medicine Meets Virtual Reality II: Interactive Technology & Healthcare: Visionary Applications for Simulation Visualization Robotics* (pp. 218- 220). Aligned Management Associates, San Diego, CA.

Weghorst, S., Airola, C., Openheimer, P., Edmond, C.V., Patience, T., Heskamp, D., and Miller, J. (1998). Validation of the Madigan ESS Simulator. *Medicine Meets Virtual Reality: Art, Science, Technology: Healthcare (R)Evolution* (pp. 399-405). IOS Press, San Diego, CA.

Weghorst, S., Prothero, J., and Furness, T. (1994). Virtual Images in the Treatment of Parkinson's Disease Akinesia. *Medicine Meets Virtual Reality II: Interactive Technology & Healthcare: Visionary Applications for Simulation Visualization Robotics* (pp. 242-243). Aligned Management Associates, San Diego, CA.

Wenger, K. and Karron, D.B. (1998). Audio-Guided Blind Biopsy Needle Placement. *Medicine Meets Virtual Reality: Art, Science, Technology: Healthcare (R)Evolution* (pp. 90-95). IOS Press, San Diego, CA.

Wenzel, E.M. (1992). Localization in Virtual Acoustic Displays. *Presence,* 1, 80-107.

Wenzel. E.M. (1994). Spatial Sound and Sonification. In G. Kramer (Ed.) *Auditory Display: Sonification, Audification, and Auditory Interfaces.* Addison-Wesley, Reading, MA (pp. 127-150).

Further Information

Burdea, G. and Coiffet, P. *Virtual Reality Technology.* John Wiley & Sons, New York.

HITL (Human Interface Technology Laboratory), University of Washington, FJ-15, Seattle, WA 98195.

UNC Laboratory, University of North Carolina, Chapel Hill, Computer Science Department, Chapel Hill, NC 27599-3175.

Presence: Teleoperators & Virtual Environments. Professional Tech Papers and Journal, MIT Press Journals, 55 Hayward St., Cambridge MA 02142.

Index

A

B

C

D

Q

R

S

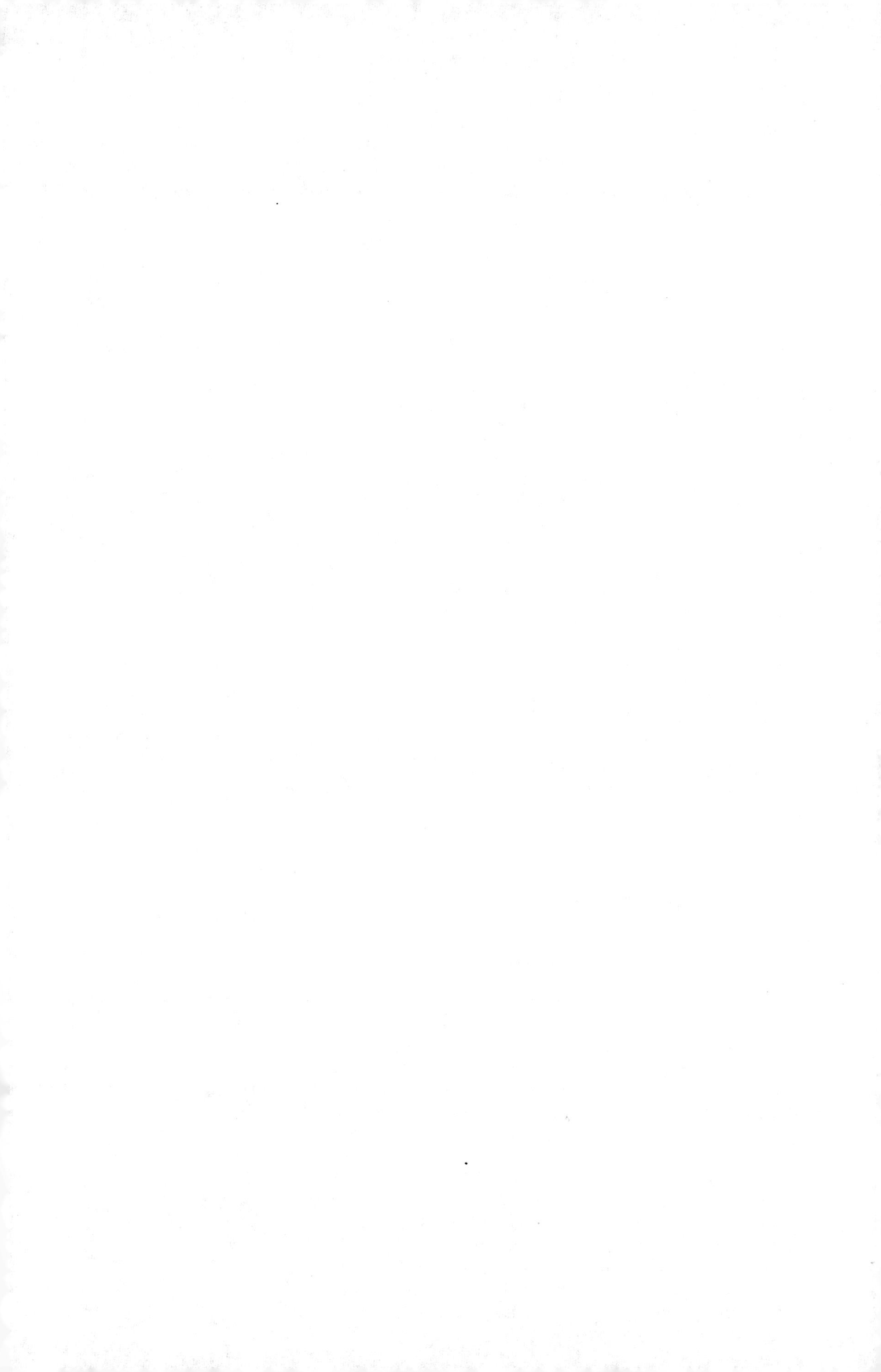